Textbook of Paediatric Anaesthetic Practice

Textbook of Paediatric Anaesthetic Practice

Edited by
EDWARD SUMNER
and
DAVID J. HATCH

The Hospital for Sick Children
Great Ormond Street
London

1989

Baillière Tindall
London Philadelphia Toronto Sydney Tokyo

Baillière Tindall 24–28 Oval Road
W.B. Saunders London NW1 7DX, UK

The Curtis Center,
Independence Square West,
Philadelphia, PA 19106–3399, USA

1 Goldthorne Avenue
Toronto, Ontario M8Z 5T9, Canada

Pty Limited,
32–52 Smidmore Street,
Marrickvillle, NSW 2204, Australia

Harcourt Brace Jovanovich Group Japan Inc.
Ichibancho Central Building, 22–1 Ichibancho
Chiyoda-ku, Tokyo 102, Japan

© 1989 Baillière Tindall

British Library Cataloguing in Publication Data

Textbook of anaesthetic practice
 1. Children. Anaesthesis
 I. Sumner, Edward   II. Hatch, David J.
 617′.96798

 ISBN 0–7020–1336–6

Typeset by Phoenix Photosetting, Chatham, Kent
Printed in bound in Great Britain by
Mackays of Chatham PLC, Chatham, Kent

Contributors

Edward N. Armitage   Royal Alexandra Hospital for Sick Children, Dyke Road, Brighton, UK

Edward F. Battersby   The Hospital for Sick Children, Great Ormond Street, London, UK

Edward J. Bennett   Seton Medical Center, Austin, Texas, USA

John C. Berridge   Addenbrookes Hospital, Cambridge, UK

Frederic A. Berry   Professor of Anaesthesiology and Pediatrics, University of Virginia Medical Center, Charlottesville, Virginia, USA

Denis E. Bowyer   Seton Medical Center, Austin, Texas, USA

Peter Booker   Alder Hey Children's Hospital, Eaton Road, Liverpool, UK

Patricia Coyle   (Uganda) c/o Order of the Sacred Heart, 212 Hammersmith Road, London, UK

Alan Duncan   Princess Margaret Hospital for Children, Box D184, G.P.O. Perth, WA, Australia

Elspeth Facer   The Hospital for Sick Children, Great Ormond Street, London, UK

Hans Feychting   Anestersklinaken, St Goran's Hospital, Stockholm, 5–112 81 Sweden

Robert H. Friesen   Denver Children's Hospital, 1056 East 19th Avenue, Colorado, USA

Nishan D. Goudsouzian   Assistant Professor of Anesthesiology, Massachusetts General Hospital, Boston, Massachusetts, USA

David J. Hatch   The Hospital for Sick Children, Great Ormond Street, London, UK

Ian G. James   The Hospital for Sick Children, Great Ormond Street, London, UK

G. G. Johnson   Children's Hospital of Eastern Ontario, 401 Smyth Road, Ottowa, Ontario, Canada

John P. Keneally   The Royal Alexandra Hospital for Children, Pyrmont Bridge Road, Camperdown, Sydney, NSW, Australia

John R. Klinck   Addenbrookes Hospital, Cambridge, UK

R. D. Latimer   Papworth Hospital, Cambridge, UK

Sten G. E. Lindahl   c/o Mayo Clinic, Rochester, Minnesota, USA

Anne M. Lynn   Assistant Professor, Anesthesiology and Pediatrics, Department of Medicine, University of Washington School of Medicine, Children's Orthopedic Hospital and Medical Center, Seattle, Washington, USA

Angela Mackersie   The Hospital for Sick Children, Great Ormond Street, London, UK

William B. McIlvaine   Denver Children's Hopsital, 1056 East 19th Avenue, Colorado, USA

A. Odura-Dominah   Papworth Hospital, Cambridge, UK

E. J. Rhine   Children's Hospital of Eastern Ontario, 401 Smyth Road, Ottowa, Ontario, Canada

A. P. Triscott   Harefield Hospital, Middlesex, UK

Edward Sumner   The Hospital for Sick Children, Great Ormond Street, London, UK

David A. Zideman   Royal Postgraduate Medical School, Hammersmith Hospital, DuCane Road, London, UK

Contents

Preface

With advances in paediatric surgery and child care, today's anaesthetist is expected to be able to deal with an increasingly complex and wide range of clinical problems in children. In addition the applicability and limitations of new drugs and techniques for paediatric use must be fully understood. The aim of this book is to provide a readily accessible source of information on all aspects of modern paediatric anaesthesia to help anaesthetists understand the problems they are likely to face, together with suggested methods of management. Though primarily designed for the general anaesthetist who deals with children as well as adults, and the trainee studying for higher examinations, it is hoped that the specialist paediatric anaesthetist will also find it a useful reference book.

Six of the chapter authors have been chosen from The Hospital for Sick Children, Great Ormond Street, London, where over 10 000 anaesthetics are administered each year. The remainder have been carefully selected from around the world, not only because they are acknowledged experts in their fields, but also because of their ability to express themselves clearly and to give sound, safe advice.

Special attention has been given to the problems of the third world countries, where high percentages of the population are children, and also to recent developments such as heart–lung transplantation.

E.S.
D.J.H.

Acknowledgements

The editors would like to thank all the chapter authors for their excellent contributions, our colleagues at The Hospital for Sick Children, Great Ormond Street, London, for their constructive criticism, Mrs Diana Newlands for her advice, Mrs Dorothy Duranti for her secretarial assistance, and Mr Peter Lewis and Nicola Sumner for their help with the index.

1   *Sten G. E. Lindahl*

Preoperative physical assessment and preparation for surgery

Within the category of 'paediatric patients' a very wide variety of conditions occurs, including congenital malformation, inherited metabolic diseases, renal and cardiac failure, pulmonary insufficiency, diseases of the brain, and so on. In addition, the age of the patient and stage of growth will both affect the total picture. For this reason it is impossible to lay down set guidelines for general use in patient evaluation and the design of programmes for preparation before anaesthesia and surgery. As always, the key factor will be individual judgement, based on careful clinical investigation and adequate family and previous medical histories.

Various opinions on the assessment and relevant preparation of patients are discussed under two headings: firstly, *the normal child* admitted for minor, intermediate and major elective surgical procedures; then *the complicated child*, with all kinds of disturbances ranging from prematurity to an emergency disease disturbing the body homeostasis of an otherwise normal 12- to 14-year-old.

THE NORMAL CHILD

This category includes children older than 1 month of age, not prematurely born, who are normal apart from the one specific surgical disease that is going to be repaired. *Minor surgical procedures* such as circumcisions, repair of inguinal hernias, adenoidectomies and other similar operations can all be performed on a day-stay basis and without laboratory tests and urinalysis, provided the physical examination and previous medical and family histories are normal. In ethnic groups of patients with higher incidences of sickle cell anaemia a determination of the haemoglobin level and a sickle screening test should always be carried out before any anaesthesia or surgical procedure.

The child with a runny nose could be suffering from an allergic disease, and if no exacerbation of the allergy is present the routine surgical procedure can probably be done, in which case symptomatic treatment should be instituted. But, if the runny nose is caused by an infection, anaesthesia and surgery ought to be postponed, since airway problems during induction of anaesthesia occur more frequently in these cases and tracheal intubation may infect the lower respiratory tract as well. A period of 1 month should elapse after the last symptoms of an upper respiratory tract infection, croup or one of the acute exanthems have subsided.

In *intermediate* and *major* paediatric surgical cases such as correction of undescended testicles, implantation of ureters, oesophago-gastrointestinal surgery and orthopaedic operations, laboratory tests for haemoglobin concentration, blood grouping and cross-matching of blood, plasma electrolyte concentrations, plasma–urea determinations and urinalysis are frequently indicated. The guidelines for appropriate preoperative analysis as presented in Table 1.1 are, however, valid only if the physical examination and the previous family and medical histories are negative for other diseases than the one for which the patient is undergoing elective surgery.

Table 1.1. Preoperative preparation routines in the normal child scheduled for an elective surgical procedure

	Physical examination Fam. and med. histories	Haemo-globin	BG CM	Chemical plasma analysis Electro-lytes	Urea	Liver tests	Coagulation system	Blood gases
Minor procedures	+	–	–	–	–	–	–	–
Intermediate to major procedure	+	+	+	(+)	(+)	(–)	(–)	(–)

BG = blood grouping; CM = cross-matching.
(+) = in cases where disturbances might be anticipated or where postoperative total parenteral nutrition will be needed; (–) = only in special cases.

For preoperative evaluation of normal children subjected to elective minor, intermediate and major surgical procedures:

1. these children could be prepared for anaesthesia and surgery according to the scheme presented in Table 1.1;
2. age-dependent variations of normal values for haemoglobin, haematocrit, blood volume, blood pressure and heart rate have to be taken into account (Table 1.2).

Table 1.2. Some normal values in infancy and childhood

Age	0–1 week	3 months	6–12 months	Preschool
Haemoglobin (g/l)	170–220	105–120	110–120	115–125
Haematocrit (%)	55–70	35–40	34–41	37–41
Blood volume (ml/kg)	80 (preterm 90)	80	75	70
Systolic/diastolic blood pressure (mmHg)	75/45	80/55	85/60	90/60
Heart rate (beats/min)	105–175	120–180	110–175	70–125

THE COMPLICATED CHILD

This category includes children with additional disease along with the surgical illness; patients who have been born preterm, have immature reactions and are younger than 6 months of age and those born at term but younger than 4 weeks of age and still in the adaptive phase from an intra- to an extrauterine life. The child may have a craniofacial malformation, upper airway obstruction, lung disease, decreased lung function after a period of neonatal intensive care, heart failure, renal or liver failure, neurological or musculoskeletal disease and many more aberrations and conditions which in one way or other may influence the behaviour before and during anaesthesia and surgery and which may require special attention pre-operatively.

These children have often been in and out of hospital and may also have been anaesthetized and operated upon many times. The case notes from these patients may therefore often not be so easy to survey. Nevertheless, it is important to do so since there is often most valuable information from previous behaviour during induction and maintenance of anaesthesia as well as from previous postoperative periods. These earlier reactions need to be accounted for so that treatment is optimized. It is also of great importance to have the patient as well investigated as possible and no effort should be spared to get the patient's actual medical status carefully delineated. *Anticipated* anaesthetic problems are frequently solved by a good preoperative examination and preparation. *Unforeseen* difficulties become, on the other hand, too often hazardous for the child.

Anaemia and sickle cell disease

In red blood cells of neonates, fetal haemoglobin dominates over adult, which means that haemoglobin in the neonatal period has a greater affinity for oxygen. Hence, oxygen content and oxygen-carrying capacity are higher. These conditions are most prominent during the first months of life. At 6–8 months of age, most of the fetal haemoglobin is exchanged for the adult type.

A haemoglobin level below 100 g/l is generally considered to be abnormal and may need further preoperative investigation. This figure is not a definitive level above which an anaesthetic can be safely given, although the haemoglobin level is an important factor to evaluate. The attitude should be to consider the overall situation and whether oxygen transport is great enough to supply the amount of oxygen needed for the kind of surgery planned. Surgery should, therefore, not be delayed for a haemoglobin level just below 100 g/l, but it may be an indication for an earlier intraoperative blood transfusion. If anaemia is to be corrected by transfusion preoperatively, this should be done at least 48 hours before surgery to allow levels of 2,3-diphosphoglycerate (DPG) to return to normal.

A sickle cell screening test should be performed on all patients of African origin after the age of 3 months. If this is positive, quantitative electrophoresis should follow to determine exactly the haemoglobinopathy. Patients with sickle cell disease (HbSS) for planned surgery may be given two transfusions with fresh blood, the first one 3 weeks and a second 3 days preoperatively, to raise the Hb to not more than 120 g/l. Repeat electrophoresis should show a pattern more like that of the heterozygous form (HbSA) which carries a very low risk with general anaesthesia.

Prematurity

Due to a shortened intrauterine time preterm babies have a thin subcutaneous layer of fat, poor glycogen storage and a relatively large body surface area which predisposes to heat loss and hypoglycaemia. Precautions should be taken to keep the body temperature normal by covering the skin, by the use of heating pads and the frequent use of incubators, and preoperative starvation periods ought to be limited to 4 hours for milk products and 2 hours for clear (glucose) fluids. In preterm babies who have had a few weeks of parenteral nutrition the plasma concentrations of both calcium and phosphorus are often lowered and may need to be supplemented preoperatively. These babies also have a lower iron storage than at term and since fetal haemoglobin (HbF) is less bound to 2,3–DPG the affinity for oxygen is increased and the dissociation curve of HbF is shifted to the left of the curve for adult haemoglobin (HbA). This may compromise oxygen delivery, which may be even more limited when blood pressure is lowered. The maintenance of a normal blood pressure depends, in these preterm babies, to a large extent on the ability to keep the extracellular volume (ECV) high, since ECV sometimes exceeds 50% of the total body water in the premature baby (Figure 1.1) (Cheek, 1961; Friis-Hansen, 1971). Furthermore, a lowered systemic blood pressure, for instance due to a decreased ECV, may turn the circulation into a fetal pattern again since there is a physiological pulmonary hypertension and the ductus arteriosus is still anatomically open. It is also important to remember that the myocardium is immature from an anatomical and histological point of view, which means that it is virtually impossible for the preterm and neonatal heart to increase its stroke volume, i.e. the cardiac output depends on the heart rate and increased cardiac output occurs up to heart rates of about 200 beats/minute.

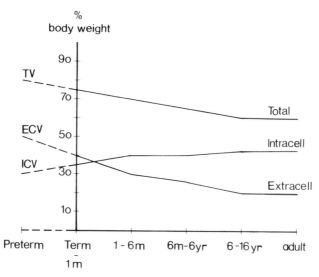

Figure 1.1. Changes in the total body fluid volume (TV), extracellular volume (ECV) and intracellular volume (ICV) in percentage of body weight at various ages. Modified from Friis-Hansen (1971).

Other organ immaturities that may be most important for the anaesthetist are probably those of the airways and lungs and of the central nervous system. In the prematurely born baby the interrupted development of terminal airways and unfinished alveolization, the decreased production of surfactant and the weaker function of the diaphragm and chest wall all contribute to increased work of breathing for gas exchange at this age.

Myelination of the central nervous system proceeds during the first years of life. The maturation is most rapid for the first 6 months of life in those prematurely born. Central nervous depressant drugs at this age must be used with extreme caution. The postoperative observation period also has to be extended to a time when potent analgesics used peroperatively and muscle relaxants are no longer likely to have residual effects. On this basis, day-stay treatment of even minor procedures is not to be advised during the first 6 months of life of a prematurely born child.

To sum up, the prematurely born infant should be delivered to anaesthesia and surgery:

1. in an incubator to prevent heat loss;
2. without having starved for milk products more than 4 hours and for clear fluids more than 2 hours to prevent hypoglycaemia;
3. with a normal Hb value for its age;
4. with an adequate ECV;
5. with an evaluation of respiratory pattern, lung function and gas exchange;
6. from a specialized nursing ward that will keep the patient at least till the day after anaesthesia and surgery.

Neonates

Much of what has been stated for the prematurely born child is also valid for the term newborn during its first 4 weeks of life. The ECV is high, Hb values need to be kept within normal limits (Table 1.1) and possibilities for the development of a persistent fetal circulation are present during this first month of life. Neonates need to be kept warm in an incubator before coming to theatre and should not be starved more than 4 hours for milk products and 2 hours for clear fluids.

Most surgical diseases in this period of life are congenital malformations. Some, like diaphragmatic hernias, neonatal ileus due to malrotation with volvulus and threatening strangulation as well as gastroschisis need to be taken care of immediately while many other congenital malformations (cardiac malformations will be discussed later) do not need such urgent treatment and surgery may be delayed for up to 24 hours.

The recent development of ultrasonographic techniques now enables a well trained obstetrician to make a likely antenatal diagnosis of conditions like diaphragmatic hernias, gastroschisis and huge hydroureter and hydronephrosis caused by urethral valves (Gauderer et al, 1984). It is perhaps better to transport the mother before delivery of the baby in these cases so that the newborn may be treated surgically before vital homeostatic functions have deteriorated too far.

In addition to what was stated for the preterm baby it should also be noted that:

1. in cases where an antenatal diagnosis has revealed urgent neonatal surgical disease the delivery must, where possible, take place close to a well trained team for neonatal anaesthesia and surgery;
2. acute operations in non-life-threatening neonatal states should never be performed before corrections of fluid, electrolyte and acid–base balance have been done;
3. rehydration should start after an estimated dehydration of 5–10% of the body weight;
4. 10 ml of fluid per kg should be added to maintenance fluid requirements over a 3-hour period for each percentage of body weight estimated dehydration. Detailed discussion of fluid and electrolyte therapy is presented in Chapter 8.

After neonatal intensive care

Most neonates subjected to non-surgical intensive care suffer from immaturity and pulmonary diseases with or without concomitant disturbances such as cerebral haemorrhages, septicaemia, renal insufficiency and nutritional disorders. In a few cases minor surgical diseases are diagnosed while the neonate is in the intensive care unit; these ought to be treated before the baby moves home from hospital. In these rare cases it is helpful to obtain as much information as possible about lung function prior to anaesthesia and surgery. Measurements of pulmonary function can now be obtained even in sick neonates.

Measurements of minute ventilation ($\dot{V}_E$), tidal volume (V_T), respiratory rate (f), dynamic compliance (C_{dyn}) and total pulmonary resistance (TPR), inspiratory (T_I) and expiratory (T_E) times, occlusion pressure (P_{occl}) and end tidal CO_2 concentration can be done at the bedside with pneumotachography and in-line capnography. The equipment for this is shown in Figure 1.2 and the results from these kinds of measurements can give information on important functional variables not only of pulmonary ventilation but also of inspiratory drive as reflected by P_{occl} and mean inspiratory flow (V_T/T_I). Furthermore, in-line CO_2 meters have nowadays sufficiently short response time to enable a functional analysis of the expired CO_2 curve.

More sophisticated tests, including the plethysmographic measurement of thoracic gas volume and airway resistance (Ahlström and Jonson, 1974; Stocks et al, 1978; Helms, 1982) are available for the detailed assessment of complex lung problems, but are at present only performed in specialized centres.

After a long period of time on a ventilator it is known that dynamic compliance is reduced (Lindroth et al, 1980), and periodic breathing sometimes with apnoeic episodes exists together with immature central nervous reactions. In some fortunately very rare cases bronchopulmonary dysplasia has developed; this is characterized by a low dynamic compliance, oxygen dependence, pulmonary hypertension and development of cor pulmonale

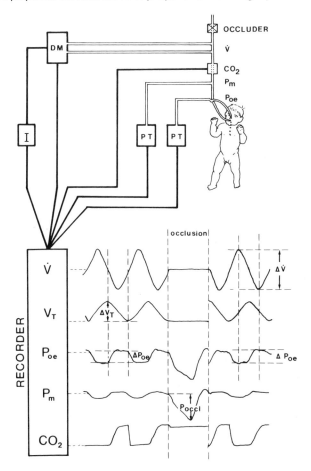

Figure 1.2. Schematic presentation of apparatus for bedside lung function tests. P_{oe} = oesophageal pressure; P_m = airway pressure; CO_2 = the position of the in-line CO_2 meter; $\dot{V}$ = the position of the pneumotachograph. The airway occluder is also indicated. PT = pressure transducers; DM = differential pressure manometer; I = integrator. Occlusion pressure is given, the CO_2 curve is recorded and calculations of dynamic compliance, $\Delta V_T/\Delta P_{oe} - \Delta P_m$, and total pulmonary resistance, $\Delta P_{oe} - \Delta P_m/\Delta \dot{V}$, are shown.

with backward cardiac failure. All these conditions mean an increased risk for anaesthesia and surgery which obviously should be postponed as long as possible until clinical improvements have occurred. If this is not possible the clinical state should be brought into an optimal condition. Lung function may be improved by an adrenergic selective β_2-agonist (i.e. terbutaline) and by the use of corticosteroids. Whether these drugs should be used preoperatively or not should be objectively evaluated by a series of lung mechanics measurements with documented improvements in lung function. Anticongestive treatment with diuretics may also be useful in these cases, although digitalization may not help patients with cor pulmonale.

Newborns recovering from a longer period of artificial ventilation have:

1. decreased lung function;
2. apnoeic attacks and immature central nervous reactions;
3. sometimes developed bronchopulmonary dysplasia with cor pulmonale;
4. an increased risk during anaesthesia and surgery;
5. sometimes an improved lung function by treatment with β_2-agonists, corticosteroids and diuretics.

Congenital cardiac malformations (see Chapter 13)

As with other congenital malformations, some cardiac malformations require immediate treatment while others can be conservatively treated and followed. In the neonatal period transposition of the great vessels needs to be palliated by a balloon-atrioseptostomy for the mixing of blood; pulmonary atresia or a very tight pulmonary stenosis needs a systemic pulmonary shunt of some kind or, if possible, in the case of a stenosis a commissurotomy to improve pulmonary perfusion. A patient with a preductal coarctation or an interrupted aortic arch will also need an urgent operation to widen the aorta and improve the circulation in the lower part of the body. Patients with pulmonary atresia with intact septum, tight pulmonary stenosis and preductal coarctation are in a fairly good condition as long as the ductus arteriosus is still open. When it closes, however, perfusion of the lung and of the lower part of the body decreases critically and the patient will rapidly deteriorate. Previously, these patients died at this stage of their disease or were brought to the operating theatre in such a bad clinical condition that they did not survive the operation. Today, the ductus arteriosus can be kept open pharmacologically by the use of prostaglandin E_1 or E_2 (Freed et al, 1981), which has a relaxing effect on the ductus. The ordinary starting dose is 0.05–0.1 µg/kg/min which is then, after a positive effect has been reached, reduced to the lowest possible maintenance dose. This treatment *must* continue until the operative correction has been performed and can then gradually be decreased and terminated postoperatively. This is, however, a potent treatment with serious side-effects of which apnoea, fever and skin rash are the most frequently reported (Lewis et al, 1981). The risk of apnoea means that this kind of treatment should not be routinely used by hospitals which do not have facilities for artificial ventilation of newborns. However, if the treatment is started on correct indications it should be commenced at the local hospital and continued during transportation provided adequate monitoring and supervision are organized during the transport. With a rapid institution of this treatment for these kinds of malformation the outcome of surgical treatment has been very much improved and prostaglandin E_1 or E_2 is a valuable tool for the preoperative preparation of these patients.

Whenever a congenital cardiac malformation is present a paediatric cardiologist should be consulted preoperatively. For a clinically nonsignificant patent ductus arteriosus, atrial or small ventricular septal defect there would probably not be any increased anaesthetic risk with these

patients when subjected to minor or intermediate non-cardiac surgical procedures. It must, however, be emphasized that even tiny air bubbles
injected intravenously may pass into the left heart and systemic arteries and
techniques for avoiding this by, for instance, three-way stopcocks or air
filters, are advisable. Pre- and postoperatively all patients with congenital
malformations should be prophylactically treated with antibiotics in order to
decrease the risk of bacterial endocarditis.

The patient with a large left-to-right shunt caused by a ventricular septal
defect may require digitalization preoperatively and perhaps also an intensified anticongestive treatment with diuretics. This is a case that will probably
need open heart surgery generally at the age of 8 to 12 months, so it might be
better for minor non-cardiac surgical procedures to be postponed till after
the closure of such a large ventricular septal defect. If, however, urgent
non-cardiac surgery is needed, good preoperative preparation will lower the
risks involved. But intensified diuretic treatment often results in intracellular hypopotassaemia which is best revealed by an acid–base balance
showing metabolic alkalosis.

Cyanotic congenital cardiac malformations with a right-to-left shunt, such
as the tetralogy of Fallot, are likely to be more critical since clinical fitness
depends to such a large extent on lung perfusion. Again, it is stressed that
injection of air bubbles must be avoided and if the non-cardiac surgery can
be postponed a total correction of the cardiac malformation should be done
first. Otherwise, the anaesthesia should be given at a hospital where anaesthetists are trained to give anaesthetics to children with cardiac malformations and have a close co-operation with a paediatric cardiologist.
Digitalization is not indicated in these patients as digitalis increases the risk
of infundibular spasm which is also known to occur with other positive
inotropic drugs. The anaesthetist should be prepared to give morphine as
well as β-blockers if signs of decreasing pulmonary perfusion suddenly
occur.

A high risk of anaesthesia and surgery is also involved in patients with
tight aortic stenosis which is a malformation that in stressful situations could
give rise to cardiac standstill and death. Therefore, all non-cardiac surgical
procedures should be postponed until the cardiac failure is controlled. If this
is not possible a calm and stress-free preoperative period and good premedication are mandatory. Drugs with a positive chronotropic effect like
atropine, isoprenaline or ketamine should be avoided.

All other more complicated cardiac malformations increase the risk of
anaesthesia and surgery and should not be undertaken unless the paediatric
cardiologist has had time to prepare the patient. The anaesthesia should be
given at a hospital accustomed to anaesthetizing children with complicated
congenital cardiac malformations.

For children with congenital cardiac malformations it can be stated that:

1. these patients should be evaluated by a paediatric cardiologist preoperatively;
2. preoperative treatment with prostaglandin E_1 or E_2 is valuable to keep the
   ductus arteriosus open in patients with pulmonary stenosis and atresia
   with intact septum, as well as in patients with preductal coarctation of the
   aorta;

3. the anaesthetic risk for patients with clinically non-significant patent ductus arteriosus, atrial and ventricular septal defects is not increased during minor or intermediate non-cardiac surgery;
4. patients with more complicated cardiac malformations should be dealt with at hospitals used to these problems;
5. injection of air bubbles intravenously must be avoided;
6. antibiotic protection should always be used to prevent bacterial endocarditis.

Craniofacial malformations and upper airway obstruction
(see Chapter 2)

These malformations are often connected with congenital malformations within other organ systems. The most common deformities are uni- or bilateral cleft lip and palate but syndromes such as the Pierre Robin syndrome with micrognathia, macroglossia and a cleft palate and the Treacher Collins syndrome with micrognathia, microstomia, aplastic zygomatic arches, choanal atresia as well as congenital lymph- and haemangiomata in the neck and face are also relatively common. For these cases preoperative information of breathing pattern and the child's ability to maintain a clear airway are most important. Indirect investigations of the mouth and upper airways and X-ray investigations of the face, larynx, trachea and of the lungs for possible aspiration should be made and reviewed by the anaesthetist to get as much information as possible about prevailing anatomic conditions such as laryngeal webs, cleft larynx, laryngomalacia or various tumours. In the neonatal period an awake intubation of the trachea could sometimes be planned for the most difficult cases. Otherwise, intubation is generally performed under inhalation anaesthesia with spontaneous breathing being maintained. In older children where a difficult intubation is anticipated it might be wise to make preparations for a fibre-optic intubation technique.

Acquired conditions such as haematomas in mouth and throat, bleeding tonsils, peritonsillar abscesses, acute epiglottitis and foreign bodies are all emergency cases where the time for preanaesthetic evaluations is limited and time-consuming preoperative investigations should therefore be avoided. In these situations as well as for craniofacial malformations it is wise for the experienced anaesthetist to arrange for the co-operation of an experienced ear, nose and throat (ENT) specialist during induction of inhalation anaesthesia and intubation of the trachea and to have easy access to equipment for a possible emergency tracheostomy.

For children with craniofacial malformations:

1. additional congenital malformations should be sought;
2. assessment of preoperative respiratory pattern and breathing capability is important;
3. investigation of the upper airway condition and anatomy is vital for the treatment;
4. surprising, unknown airway aberrations may occur;

5. awake intubation of the neonate is sometimes justified;
6. inhalation anaesthesia with spontaneous breathing should be used;
7. co-operation with an experienced ENT specialist is advised.

For the child with an acquired upper airway obstruction:

1. these cases are generally acute;
2. there will be no time for extensive preoperative investigations;
3. inhalation anaesthesia with spontaneous breathing should be used;
4. co-operation with an experienced ENT specialist is also advised.

Pulmonary disorders

Disturbances in lung function have previously been discussed for the neonatal period. An acute respiratory tract infection is a contraindication to elective surgery because of the high risk of postoperative pulmonary complications and of generalized pulmonary infection which may sometimes require prolonged postoperative ventilator treatment.

Bronchiolitis and croups, 40% of which are caused by respiratory syncytial virus, cause distal air-trapping because of blockage of bronchioles, leading to increased resistance to airflow and $\dot{V}/\dot{Q}$ (ventilation/perfusion) changes with oxygen dependence. These functional changes may reverse in a few days, but at least 70% of patients may have lung abnormalities of increased resistance and reduced compliance for up to 1 year after acute bronchiolitis.

Occasionally, paediatric patients come to surgery for treatment of mediastinal masses. They may be in a fairly good clinical condition without cardiorespiratory symptoms. Some of these masses may affect the pericardium as well as the heart; this justifies preoperative echocardiography. Others affect airways, causing problems with the induction of anaesthesia, especially after muscle relaxation, and may cause life-threatening respiratory obstruction. Nowadays not only a chest X-ray, but also a computerized tomography scan and flow volume loops should be done preoperatively so that patients who are at risk can be identified prior to anaesthesia. Flow volume loops will, for instance, make it possible to differentiate between extra- and intrathoracic airway obstructions (Figure 1.3). Using these extensive preoperative investigations, the anaesthetist is able to choose a safe induction technique and to organize for rigid bronchoscopy if necessary and perhaps, in extreme cases, even for standby femoral vein-to-artery bypass oxygenation.

Pulmonary complications are more frequent in patients with asthma or cystic fibrosis, and it is important for these patients to be anaesthetized and operated upon during optimal conditions. This means that the treatment of the asthmatic patient and the child with cystic fibrosis should be intensified for at least a 2-week period before anaesthesia. For the asthmatic child, repeated lung function tests should be used to assess the effect of inhalation therapy, selective β_2-agonists and perhaps also corticosteroids. For the child with cystic fibrosis, the drainage treatment and physiotherapy need to be intensified.

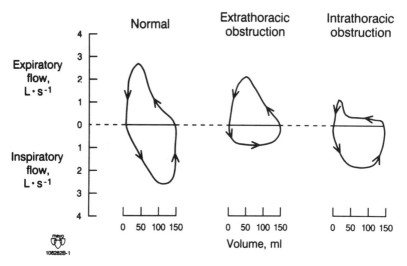

Figure 1.3. Three schematic examples of flow volume loops in the normal situation; with extrathoracic obstruction, and with intrathoracic obstruction. The intrathoracic obstruction pattern is typical for the patient with a severe obstruction, for instance caused by a mediastinal mass. (Modified from Miller and Hyatt, 1969.)

It can be stated in summary that:

1. elective cases with pulmonary infections must be postponed;
2. children who have had severe bronchiolitis may have lung abnormalities almost up to 1 year after their acute disease;
3. children who have mediastinal masses are challenging cases, requiring extensive preoperative investigations.

It is important for the asthmatic child and the child with cystic fibrosis that:

1. preoperative intensive respiratory therapy is given;
2. symptomatic treatment with β_2-agonists and perhaps steroids may be of help to optimize pulmonary function preoperatively in the *asthmatic* child;
3. symptomatic antibiotic treatment and physiotherapy should be started early to improve lung function in the child with *cystic fibrosis.*

Neurosurgical disease (see Chapter 16)

Before anaesthesia and surgery for patients with intracranial diseases it is important to evaluate the intracranial pressure level. Will the intracranial compliance be low with an increased risk for tentorial or foramen magnum herniation? If this is the case, often suspected because of a variable state of consciousness and papilloedema, preparations for active treatment of suddenly raised intracranial pressure should be organized. The choice is corticosteroid injections or mannitol infusions which, together with barbiturates and hyperventilation, will contribute to the decrease of suddenly raised intracranial pressure in the preoperative period. If premedication is to be used, potent respiratory depressants like opioids should be avoided and the doses of sedatives and anxiolytics should be reduced compared with patients in whom no risk of increased intracranial pressure exists. The technique for induction of anaesthesia in neurosurgical patients with a risk of increased intracranial pressure should be planned so that CO_2 retention is avoided and so that stress-free laryngoscopy and tracheal intubation can be performed.

In a child with a neurosurgical disease it is of great importance to:

1. evaluate the intracranial pressure;
2. be prepared to treat suddenly increased intracranial pressure;
3. avoid opioids and reduce doses of sedatives/anxiolytics for premedication;
4. avoid raised intracranial pressure during induction of anaesthesia and tracheal intubation.

Cerebral palsy and muscle diseases

For the paediatric anaesthetist the most common problems with cerebral palsy are connected with the patients who suffer from the most complicated cerebral palsy syndromes. The dominating sign is increased salivation and these children may also have cerebral convulsions requiring a variety of anticonvulsant drugs. The anticonvulsant treatment should not be terminated before anaesthesia. It may, in fact, be given on the morning of operation with a sip of water.

The child with a muscle disease affecting only peripheral muscle groups does not usually have impaired gas exchange. But when muscles of the chest wall and sometimes even of the diaphragm are weaker than normal, lung function and gas exchange are affected. These functions are further reduced by conventional doses of anaesthetic agents which predispose to postoperative pulmonary complications. Physiotherapy should be used preoperatively to improve the condition of these children and to decrease the risk of postoperative pulmonary complications. Sedative premedication should be used with care. Peripheral muscle disorders are also known to affect the myocardium, particularly in children over 8–10 years of age with an increased incidence of cardiac arrhythmias. ECG and a chest X-ray are needed in these children before anaesthesia and surgery. It has also been noted recently that patients with muscle disorders have a greater tendency to malignant hyperpyrexia in connection with the use of suxamethonium, halothane or other triggering agents.

In children with advanced cerebral palsy syndromes:

1. most have increased salivation;
2. most have complex convulsions for which treatment is necessary.

In children with muscle diseases:

1. respiration may be impaired if breathing muscles are affected;
2. sedative premedication should be used with care;
3. the myocardium may also become affected with a high incidence of cardiac arrhythmias;
4. patients with muscle disorders are more inclined to develop malignant hyperpyrexia.

Rheumatoid arthritis

The child with a rheumatoid disease may have suffered from the illness for many years, although still young. Joints are progressively destroyed and may require surgery, which most frequently is performed under general anaesthesia in childhood. Sometimes laryngeal manifestations and restricted movements of the mandible create intubation difficulties. All rheumatoid children should be investigated with an X-ray of the cervical spine to show possible pathological movements of the atlanto-occipital and atlanto-axial joints. Due to the myocardial involvement in this disease an ECG should also be available preoperatively. Sometimes these patients are treated with large doses of corticosteroids, which necessitates the use of steroid protection for possible iatrogenic adrenal hypofunction. This protective steroid treatment should always be given if the patient has been put on prolonged maintenance corticosteroid treatment that is continued or was terminated within the last 2 months. A dose of hydrocortisone 25 mg intravenously every fourth hour is recommended until the ordinary maintenance treatment can be started again.

Children with rheumatoid arthritis:

1. are more frequently operated upon under general anaesthesia and may create intubation difficulties;
2. often have extremely mobile atlanto-occipital and atlantoaxial joints;
3. are often treated with corticosteroids and need corticosteroid protection during anaesthesia and surgery.

Malignant diseases

These patients are also frequently put on a steroid treatment and should in such cases have corticosteroid protection, as described above. The patients in this group suffer either from solid tumours such as intracranial tumours or neuro- or nephroblastoma requiring a combined treatment with extensive surgery and chemotherapy. Paediatric patients with malignant diseases also suffer from various kinds of leukaemia and from different lymphomas. This latter group receive mainly chemotherapy, although staging laparotomies form part of their routine treatment. Patients with malignancy are treated with extremely potent and toxic drugs that depress the bone marrow. Some drugs, such as doxorubicin, are also known to be cardiotoxic, so a preoperative ECG and a paediatric cardiological consultation are indicated. Other agents such as bleomycin and methotrexate are toxic to the lung with development of an interstitial pneumonitis which may be aggravated by high oxygen tensions (Bennet and Reich, 1979). Hence, care must be taken with oxygen administration in these patients.

Neuroblastoma, which is the commonest solid tumour of childhood, may secrete catecholamines and although vanillylmandelic acid is raised in 85% of patients, only 12–15% have symptoms of high catecholamine levels such as hypertension. These symptomatic patients need preoperative α- and β-adrenergic blockade.

Paediatric patients with malignant diseases may have:

1. solid tumours located intracranially or presenting as neuro- or nephro-blastoma;
2. various forms of leukaemia and lymphoma;
3. a treatment that depresses the bone marrow and is cardiotoxic;
4. a treatment that may give an interstitial pneumonitis that could be aggravated by high inspired oxygen concentrations.

Renal disease and hypertension

In the term neonate renal function is adequate for its needs but has a greater capability of excreting sodium ions than preserving them. Therefore, sodium-free solutions should not be used in this age group.

Known renal insufficiency requires special treatment. Preoperatively analysis of plasma protein, electrolytes, creatinine and urea as well as an acid–base balance and urinalysis for protein, osmolality, pH, blood and electrolytes are desirable. Renal function tests such as glomerular filtration rate and concentration capability of the kidneys are also of great importance. Deviations from normal values are corrected and if the child is being dialysed, preoperative dialysis should always be performed.

Frequently, renal disease causes hypertension that needs to be treated. Treatment with the antihypertensive drugs should continue till the day before anaesthesia and surgery. On the operating day the ordinary morning dose of β-blocking agents and of clonidine should be taken to eliminate the rebound phenomenon and if needed injected intravenously during the operation. Antihypertensive treatment with other agents can be terminated until normal function returns and the hypertensive disease should in the meantime be controlled intravenously as required on an individual basis.

For infants and children with renal disease and hypertension:

1. sodium-free solutions should not be used in the neonate;
2. acid–base balance, plasma electrolytes and renal function tests should be analysed preoperatively;
3. preoperative dialysis should be done in children on a regular chronic dialysis schedule;
4. antihypertensive drugs should be continued until the evening before surgery;
5. β-blockers and clonidine should be given on the morning of the operation to prevent a rebound phenomenon.

Endocrine disease

The most common endocrine disorder is diabetes mellitus which is nearly always insulin-dependent in childhood. The diabetic patient in perfect control does not need to be admitted to hospital several days before surgery. Plasma analysis of acid–base balance, glucose and ketone bodies as well as a test for glycosuria should, however, be performed preoperatively.

A straightforward diabetic patient undergoing minor surgery may be managed by omitting the morning insulin and breakfast, but for more complex surgery, an infusion of insulin is more satisfactory. 0.1 µg/kg/h of soluble insulin is infused with the hourly fluid requirements as 5% dextrose (+10 mmol K^+ in 500 ml). Insulin is absorbed by plastic so the infusion should be from a hard plastic syringe. Frequent blood sugar estimations are mandatory.

Diabetic children with acute infections or with other acute medical conditions may develop diabetic ketoacidosis. This is a serious medical condition which rapidly results in severe dehydration, metabolic acidosis and derangements of electrolyte balance. For emergency surgery, these children require specialist consultation, preoperative rehydration, and careful observations of potassium levels and acidosis. If possible, these cases should be postponed and surgery delayed until blood glucose, electrolytes, and acid–base status are normal. Autonomic neuropathy may be present even in young diabetics and this group may also have cardiomyopathy as a further complicating factor.

Adrenocortical hypofunction may be caused by adrenal haemorrhage, hypoplasia, adrenocorticotrophic hormone (ACTH) insufficiency, congenital unresponsiveness to ACTH, fulminating infection, Addison's disease or an iatrogenic adrenal insufficiency. One of the most common adrenocortical hypofunctions is the 21-hydroxylase deficiency which gives rise to the adrenogenital syndrome. These patients are nowadays treated with subcutaneous implantation of desoxycortisone acetate (DOCA) pellets. When DOCA pellets are not used or when the child is unable to take medication orally, DOCA may be administered intramuscularly. It is of the utmost importance to control the plasma levels of electrolytes preoperatively in patients with adrenocortical hypofunction, and hydrocortisone 25 mg should be given on the evening before operation, 25 mg on the morning of surgery and then 25 mg prior to induction of anaesthesia.

Sometimes patients with craniopharyngioma develop diabetes insipidus owing to deficiency of antidiuretic hormone (ADH). Rarely this tumour compresses the pituitary and hypothalamus, resulting in multiple endocrine abnormalities. When symptoms of low ADH secretion exist it is necessary to treat the patient with aqueous vasopressin subcutaneously or vasopressin nasal spray to control polyuria. Fluid and electrolyte balance must be closely controlled preoperatively. Furthermore, additional hydrocortisone should be prepared for immediate use in case of an acute adrenal insufficiency.

Hyperthyroidism needs treatment with antithyroid drugs to render the patient euthyroid prior to anaesthesia and surgery. β-blockers may also be used to control an unnecessarily high heart rate.

Hypothyroidism is almost always detected before anaesthesia and surgery so that the patients will have been put on substitution therapy. If anaesthesia and surgery have to be performed in a hypothyroid patient it is advisable to use small doses of sedatives preoperatively. Furthermore, a preoperative ECG and X-ray of heart and lungs are necessary since heart failure so frequently occurs in a myxoedematous state.

Approximately 90% of children suffering from phaeochromocytoma are hypertensive. Multiple tumours occur more frequently (30%) than in adults (5%; Heikkinen and Akerblom, 1977). These children often have a decreased blood volume. Preoperatively they should be treated for at least 2 weeks with some kind of adrenergic-blocking agent. Currently, the most frequently used drug is phenoxybenzamine (Dibenyline) with a starting dose of 5–10 mg which is then gradually increased up to 1–2 mg/kg twice daily over 2–3 days until orthostatic hypotension occurs. β-blockade with propranolol may also be necessary.

In children with endocrine diseases it is most valuable to:

1. postpone, if possible, an operation in a diabetic patient with ketoacidosis;
2. substitute with hydrocortisone (25 mg intravenously every fourth hour) in patients with adrenocortical hypofunction until the ordinary substitution therapy can be continued;
3. treat a patient suffering from adrenogenital syndrome with DOCA and hydrocortisone injections if maintenance treatment is insufficient;
4. be aware of ADH deficiency in patients with craniopharyngioma;
5. be sure that patients with hypo- or hyperthyroidism are euthyroid in connection with anaesthesia and surgery;
6. use an adrenergic-blocking treatment 2 or 3 weeks prior to operation for a phaeochromocytoma.

Liver disease and coagulopathies

Liver disease may, in advanced cases, decrease glycogen storage and predispose to hypoglycaemia. Furthermore, albumin plasma concentration and coagulation factors may be low. Liver enzymes, bilirubin conjugated and unconjugated and serum proteins should be estimated and clotting studies performed preoperatively.

A coagulopathy frequently occurs in the neonatal period; this is partly due to vitamin K deficiency in the neonatal liver and is consequently treated by injections of vitamin K_1. But coagulation disorders are also inherited with specific deficiencies in the production of coagulation factors. Preoperatively, a complete laboratory coagulation profile has to be measured and fibrinolysis as well as thrombocytopenia should be looked for. Preoperatively, specific agents like factor VIII and fresh frozen plasma (containing coagulation factors) or even fresh blood should be present in the operating theatre; when signs of fibrinolysis exist inhibitors such as epsilonaminocaproic acid should be given. Platelets should be available for thrombocytopenic patients and may be given preoperatively or kept in reserve for intraoperative bleeding.

In children with advanced liver disease one ought to be prepared for:

1. hypoglycaemia;
2. low albumin and coagulation factors.

In children with coagulation disorders it is important that:

1. the coagulopathy is investigated prior to anaesthesia and surgery;
2. fibrinolysis and thrombocytopenia are looked for;
3. factor VIII, fresh frozen plasma and platelets are available when necessary;
4. epsilonaminocaproic acid is given in the case of fibrinolysis.

REFERENCES

Ahlström H & Jonson B (1974) Pulmonary mechanics in infants. Methodological aspects. *Scandinavian Journal of Respiratory Diseases* **55**: 129–134.

Bennet JM & Reich JD (1979) Bleomycin. *Annals of Internal Medicine* **90**: 945–948.

Cheek DB (1961) Extracellular volume: its structure and measurement and the influence of age and disease. *Journal of Pediatrics* **58**: 103–107.

Freed MD, Heyman MA, Lewis AB, Roehl SL & Kensey RC (1981) Prostaglandin E_1 in infants with ductus arteriosus-dependent congenital heart disease. *Circulation* **64**: 899–905.

Friis-Hansen B (1971) Body composition during growth. In vivo measurements and biochemical data correlated to differential anatomical growth. *Pediatrics* **47**: 264–274.

Gauderer MWL, Jassani MN & Izant RJ Jr (1984) Ultrasonographic antenatal diagnosis: Will it change the spectrum of neonatal surgery? *Journal of Pediatric Surgery* **19**: 404–407.

Heikkinen ES & Akerblom HK (1977) Diagnostic and operative problems in multiple pheochromocytomas. *Journal of Pediatric Surgery* **12**: 157–163.

Helms P (1982) Problems with plethysmographic estimation of lung volume in infants and young children. *Journal of Applied Physiology* **53**: 698–702.

Lewis AB, Freed MD & Heyman MA (1981) Side effects of therapy with prostaglandin E_1 in infants with critical congenital heart disease. *Circulation* **64**: 893–898.

Lindroth M, Svenningsen NW, Ahlström H & Jonson B (1980) Evaluation of mechanical ventilation in newborn infants. Pulmonary and neurodevelopmental sequelae in relation to original diagnosis. *Acta Paediatrica Scandinavica* **69**: 151–158.

Miller RD & Hyatt RE (1969) Obstructing lesions of the larynx and trachea: clinical and physiological characteristics. *Mayo Clinic Proceedings* **44**: 145–161.

Stocks J, Godfrey S & Reynolds EOR (1978) Airway resistance following various treatments for hyaline membrane disease, including prolonged high levels of inspired oxygen. *Pediatrics* **60**: 178–183.

Psychological preparation for surgery and premedication

INTRODUCTION

It is probably quite true, as many have suggested, that a personal visit is more important than medication in the alleviation of a patient's anxiety before anaesthesia and surgery. That this is generally recognized in the profession is reflected in the fact that although there are many enthusiastic reports on the excellent effects of a large number of drugs, only a standard few continue to be used. It is reasonable to assume that in many cases the excellent effects are attributable not solely to the drug, but to the fact that the anaesthetist's own heightened concern in using a new drug will inevitably be conveyed to the patient and parents in the form of greater than normal interest. This raised level of care, whether explained or not, will be much appreciated, and will itself create a considerable placebo effect and lead to many of the reported favourable results. Why else have so many 'wonder' drugs been so quickly discarded? Why do they work for some users and not for others? The preoperative visit is, then, the most important element in good psychological preparation.

Nevertheless, an appropriate drug will sometimes be very helpful, especially in situations where preoperative visiting must be minimal or omitted altogether, in day-stay surgery for example, or in countries where the shortage of anaesthetists precludes regular visiting.

Obviously children suffering from preoperative pain should always be given pain relief.

At any age, anaesthesia and surgery represent a major event in the life of a child, and of its family even when the surgical procedure is a minor one. We cannot expect the child to have any knowledge of anaesthetic technicalities. Parents too often have very limited knowledge and may be anxious about the anaesthesia, while they accept surgery in a more matter-of-fact way. To enable them to give their child proper moral support, their own anxieties must be dealt with.

PSYCHOLOGICAL FACTORS RELATED TO AGE

Infants (up to 2 years)

Infants may not show definite symptoms of separation. However, in a hospital ward, sensory stimulation is bound to be much less than at home and comfort, when needed, may not be given as readily. Therefore, parents should be given every opportunity to involve themselves in the care of their infant during the stay in the ward. Preoperatively, the anaesthetist should explain the anaesthetic procedure to them, while realizing that many adults may have exaggerated fears because of the small size of the patient.

Toddlers (2–3 years)

Toddlers are likely to be very upset by hospitalization and separation from their parents. Toddlers are at a stage when they find that they can master their surroundings most of the time and get instant attention by crying. Being in a hospital will mean considerable restraints on the child's freedom to move and on the capacity to command the attention he or she is used to. The toddler will react by showing anger and by crying. At a later stage of separation, these reactions may give way to quietness and docility. These are very serious signs indeed and must never be confused with good behaviour or being brave. Liberal visiting hours may go a long way towards minimizing separation syndromes.

A British paediatrician, Damon, once tried to convey what a 2-year-old child feels like in hospital by asking an adult to imagine himself deported to some foreign country without knowing why, for what possible offence or for how long. His fears would be numerous: what might these foreigners do to him? How often would the person he most loved be able to visit him? Would the visits stop? Would he ever return home?

Preschool children

Preschool children are at a very vulnerable stage of development, being more aware of reality than the toddler but not yet having the defence mechanisms, experience and knowledge of a later age. They fear mutilation and death and may have the strangest notions of what is going to happen to them, not infrequently interpreting surgery as punishment for having been naughty.

Schoolchildren

Schoolchildren have an increasing sense of reality and have gained greater ability to communicate with adults. Yet some still suffer from strange misconceptions of what is to be done to them. A Danish child who was interviewed by Jacoby (1981, personal communication) appeared to be exceptionally afraid of needles. It transpired that he believed his skin was a large sack keeping his blood contained and he was convinced that, when his skin was punctured, his blood would leak out and he would die.

It is important to give straight answers to a child's questions and to avoid the analogies adults love to use to disguise unpleasant realities. If you try 'pulling his leg' he or she may literally be afraid it could come off.

Adolescents

Adolescents are at a stage of development where they are trying to enter the world of adults. Their self-esteem is fragile yet they want to present a tough appearance. This conflict may present itself in a rebellious attitude requiring a lot of patience to overcome. As anaesthetists of the adult world well know, quite a few patients never pass beyond this stage.

FAMILY PROBLEMS

Social problems

Children from families with social difficulties of some kind are likely to be more uncertain and vulnerable at each developmental stage and should be given special consideration and more flexibility than children from normal families.

Religious problems

Children of Jehovah's Witnesses parents present special problems: there is a legal as well as a psychological aspect to the issue of whether or not blood transfusions are acceptable.

Most countries do not accept that the religious convictions of the parents should be allowed to put a child's life in any danger. There may exist a well established social network to deal rapidly with these matters, in extreme situations even temporarily revoking the parents' legal rights regarding their children. Sometimes, however, the legal procedures involved may be time-consuming, creating awkward problems in the acute case outside office hours. There is considerable divergence of opinion on how best to handle this sensitive situation, though all agree that direct conflict with the parents is far better avoided where possible.

Before any legal procedures are considered, the anaesthetist could engage himself in a serious discussion with the parents offering to go to great lengths to respect their belief yet being unwaveringly clear that in any situation involving great blood loss, blood transfusion will have to be given in order to save the child's life.

Haemodilution techniques have been used successfully to minimize the need for blood transfusion not only in these situations but also as a general method in major surgery (Singler, 1983). In order reasonably to guarantee that blood transfusion can be avoided, the haematocrit must be brought down to 20% or even lower while meticulously maintaining normovolaemia. At these haematocrit levels, the oxygen-carrying capacity becomes very small. Accordingly, haemodilution techniques require a detailed protocol as well as collaboration with the hospital blood bank and will certainly not be suitable for the occasional case.

Working in a country where the social network allows almost instantaneous decisions, I find that parents, once forced to comply, most often experience a readily observed relief, perhaps feeling that they have done their utmost to meet the requirements of their religion. It may be useful to bear this in mind in a situation when parents seem utterly obstinate. Perhaps then, a firm approach may win the argument in the end. It must not be forgotten, however, that refusing to discuss the problem and only using legal means may create great problems afterwards, since it is in the nature of this particular religion to consider anyone having received a blood transfusion as unclean. Having had to give a blood transfusion, the anaesthetist may wish to engage in further discussions with the parents to ensure that the risk for the child to be excluded from proper parental care is minimized.

ORGANIZED PREOPERATIVE CARE

Recognizing the importance of psychological preparation, some anaesthetic departments go to great lengths to convey information and to create trust in the patient. Hain (1983, personal communication), visiting five European and Canadian children's hospitals outside Britain, found arrangements ranging from regular educational programmes with considerable involvement of staff, most often on a voluntary spare-time basis, to no organized preparation at all.

Organization can take the form of school education with lectures given by an anaesthetist or open days at the hospital where children may familiarize themselves with the hospital surroundings and some of the equipment. Alternatively, for a child coming into hospital, films or videotapes covering the preoperative procedures may be run in the presence of the family. Hain (1983, personal communication) himself, besides running a videotape, also gives a guided tour of the wards when the children are given an opportunity to meet the ward staff, to see what kind of bed they will be sleeping in, what nightdress they will be wearing, what the lavatory looks like and other equally important matters.

Anaesthetic departments, with insufficient time or resources to engage in such extensive schemes or which find themselves opposed by trade unions taking an unfavourable attitude towards engaging members on a non-monetary basis, may have to rely on simpler solutions. One is to make a photographic album or booklet with a series of pictures covering the stay in hospital, such as the child's arrival on the ward, being in bed, being visited by parents, being prepared for going to theatre, being transported in the big elevator, being wheeled along vast corridors and meeting the anaesthetic staff, ending with happily meeting mother on awakening in the recovery room. Such an album with a short, accurate text can be made at very low cost and distributed to all wards to be readily available at the preoperative visit. It should be used as a complement to the preoperative visit, not as a substitute.

Information

Information should be given in simple terms. Anxious families cannot cope with too many details. They will want straight answers to essential questions, such as: Will the induction be very unpleasant? Will the child be likely to wake up in the middle of the operation and feel pain? Will it hurt very much afterwards? Will the child be given any pain relief?

It is wise to start the visit by asking what information the family feel they have received from the surgeon. It will sometimes seem that the family have very confused ideas of what is going to happen. This is particularly true in cases where major procedures are considered and when the underlying disease has a sudden onset. Parents may state that they have received very scanty information when, in fact, the surgeon has described his intentions at length. This phenomenon of 'blocking' information should be recognized and medical staff must be prepared to repeat information several times without appearing impatient.

Most people are sensitive to body language. Standing up and looking down at people implies that you are in a hurry. Leaning against a doorpost or supporting your head in your hands will give a supercilious or disinterested impression. In order to create a relaxed and unhurried impression when talking to a family, *always sit down* and adopt an interested attitude. The act of bringing forward a chair and seating yourself on it will convey the impression that you are really ready to listen to their problems.

If old enough, the child should be addressed directly, in the presence of his or her mother. This will make the child feel that you really care about him or her and make it possible for the mother to expand on certain topics afterwards.

Many parents raise the question of whether they will be allowed to be present during the induction of anaesthesia. Indeed, parental presence seems to be becoming more widely accepted. In some countries, parents' associations are even bringing pressure to bear on anaesthetic departments to adopt this practice. In the author's view, parents can help their child, not only by being present at the induction but also by being able to give assurance beforehand that they will not be deserting their child as long as he or she is awake.

Some anaesthetists disapprove of parental presence because it may upset very rapid induction techniques, which require co-operation between a skilled anaesthetist and an experienced technician. In high-risk inductions the presence of a parent may increase the risks by distracting the anaesthetist. Other anaesthetists fear that parental anxiety may be transferred to the child and that some parents may be upset and even faint during the induction. Indeed, some parents do not want to come with their child and may resent pressure put on them to do so.

If you feel able to give consent to parents being present during the induction this consent should not be given grudgingly. It will be of no comfort to a mother to feel from the attitudes of the staff that she is a nuisance. She will then be likely to take a defensive or rebellious attitude, and this sentiment will convey itself to the child. The child will then feel surrounded by a crowd of enemies.

If you do not want parents to be present tell them in plain language that you find you manage better on your own and that their presence will inhibit you. Most parents will respect that. Subterfuge, however, such as telling them that their presence will increase the risk of spreading infection, is likely to create resentment.

Another frequent parental request is to be allowed to be present during the recovery from anaesthesia. All paediatric anaesthetic departments should allow parents to be with their child as soon as possible after surgery. Adult recovery rooms which receive the occasional child may have difficulties in making room for a mother as well, although in a spacious recovery room ways to cope with this problem can always be found. Where children are sent back almost immediately to the general ward, parents should be allowed to be present in the ward on their return. Surprisingly, some staff seem to feel that mothers cannot cope with seeing their child vomit or thrash about in the bed when awakening. This is of course untrue: the close bonding between mothers and children is invaluable in this period. Therefore, it should always be possible during a preoperative visit to promise the child that his or her mother will be present when he or she wakes up. Furthermore, any child thrashing about in bed postoperatively is likely to need some pain relief.

Bothe and Galdston (1972), Korsch (1975), Melamed (1977) and Pinkerton (1981) have published more comprehensive studies on the subject of psychological preparation of children and allied subjects.

REPEATED ANAESTHESIA

Children requiring repeated anaesthesia present different problems of preanaesthetic handling.

Children with *leukaemia* and *other malignant diseases* must have bone marrow biopsies taken from time to time and particularly frequently when on cytostatic drug treatment. In addition to worrying about the anaesthesia, they suffer from all the side-effects of the drug treatment. Most of these children come to hospital for the occasion and expect to return home later in the day.

These children want to meet the same anaesthetist on every occasion and some have a tendency to ritualize the induction down to the smallest detail in order to feel secure. Within reason, this should be granted. Once this ritual is established the main concern of the anaesthetist will be to keep his calendar in order and never fail an appointment.

There are some children, however, who will always be extremely unhappy, not only because of the anaesthesia but because of the many blood tests being taken or injections being given. These children are greatly helped by implantation of a central venous line with a subcutaneous access port. The part of the skin covering the access port may be pretreated with an ointment containing a eutectic mixture of lignocaine and prilocaine (EMLA) 1 hour before puncture.

Whenever possible, simple procedures should be carried out in well known surroundings, preferably in the ward. It should not be too difficult to keep the necessary anaesthetic equipment there permanently. It will also seem more natural to have parents present during the induction when it takes place away from the operating area.

Children with *extensive burns, recurring malignant tumours, Crohn's disease* or *congenital megacolon* may have to undergo repeated major surgery. The immediate main worry of these children is usually the postoperative pain which they may have experienced previously and the discomfort of bowel paralysis after laparotomy.

During recent years the techniques of regional blocks have become increasingly widespread and continuous infusion of morphine has proved to be a safe technique. It should therefore be possible when preparing these children for anaesthesia to promise them a minimum of postoperative pain.

Clearly, preparing children for repeated anaesthesia is very different from the single preoperative visit. A more long-term relationship has to be established, founded on mutual trust. More time has to be spent, at least initially, on how things are going to be handled and how pain can be mastered in different ways. These children often show considerable interest in technical details as if a thorough knowledge helps to keep evil forces at a distance. Some children aged over 12 may even handle a self-administration pump for analgesia with confidence.

PHARMACOLOGICAL PREPARATION

The aim of pharmacological preparation is:

1. to abolish unwanted effects of anaesthetic agents;
2. to abolish preoperative pain;
3. to supplement anaesthesia;
4. to allay anxiety and facilitate a smooth induction.

Since children dislike needles intensely, a non-painful route should be used if possible. Children of different nationalities may have different views on whether the rectal route is really preferable to needles. A Scandinavian child will think nothing of having a catheter put into his rectum while children from other countries consider their rectum a most private part not to be readily manipulated by strangers.

The oral route is widely used and is quite satisfactory for the average child having minor surgery. Intestinal absorption, however, may be unreliable, especially in the anxious patient, and attempts to administer oral drugs to an uncooperative patient may be more traumatic than an intramuscular injection. The intramuscular route is preferred by many when reliable pharmacological preparation is required as, for instance, in mentally handicapped children or where the narcotic effect of the premedication is meant to supplement the anaesthesia. In very sick children or children undergoing cardiac surgery, for example, efficient premedication allows the use of reduced doses of anaesthetic drugs, with fewer harmful side-effects than doses of equivalent drugs given intravenously during anaesthesia.

Anticholinergic drugs

These drugs are given to counteract side-effects of anaesthetic agents, most of which are cholinergic, and to reduce excessive secretions from the airways. Small children may show very rapid vagal responses to manipulation of the airways and even such an apparently innocent manoeuvre as passing a nasogastric tube may cause disturbing bradycardia. Therefore, it is generally agreed that an anticholinergic drug should be included in the premedication of children or be given at induction.

Atropine is the most common drug for these purposes. It is a powerful vagolytic drug and has moderate but satisfactory antisialagogue properties. In most cases it produces a moderate degree of tachycardia which is normally of no untoward consequence. For children with a tendency to paroxysmal tachycardia and with certain types of congenital heart disease, tachycardia may become excessive or cause impaired cardiac output.

Atropine inhibits sweat gland activity. Since evaporation of sweat is the main means of removing heat in individuals after the neonatal period, children who have been given atropine may appear in the operating theatre with a slightly flushed face and running a slight fever. Once they are anaesthetized these phenomena usually disappear and are of no consequence.

The onset of action will be complete within 30 minutes whether the drug is given intravenously or intramuscularly. The usual dose is 0.02 mg/kg by either route with a minimum of 0.1 mg. The dose may also be given orally or rectally. Olsson et al (1983) found by measuring plasma levels of atropine that an intramuscular dose of 0.02 mg/kg gave a mean peak plasma level of 2.40 ng/ml after 5–10 minutes, while the same dose given rectally reached a mean peak plasma level of 0.76 ng/ml after 15 minutes. Vagolytic as well as antisialagogue effects were reported to be satisfactory at both plasma levels. In a recent double-blind study of the clinical effects of rectal atropine on three groups of children, the first of which was given no atropine, the second 0.02 mg/kg and the third 0.04 mg/kg, Olsson (1987, personal communication) found that 0.04 mg/kg administered rectally gave the most satisfactory clinical result.

Most children seem to suffer from excessive dryness of the mouth after atropine. Therefore, some anaesthetists prefer to give atropine intravenously immediately after the induction. This works particularly well with intravenous induction when atropine may be given as soon as a needle is inserted.

Scopolamine (hyoscine) has never gained the same popularity as atropine in young children, although it is commercially available combined with papaveretum for premedication of older children. It is a less potent vagolytic agent compared with atropine but a more powerful antisialagogue. Indeed, the drying effect is in excess of what is really desirable. The greater drying effect also extends to the sweat glands which may sometimes cause problems with heat removal. Unlike atropine, scopolamine has a central nervous effect producing amnesia and sedation – in small children even confusion. It should therefore be avoided in children under 2 years of age. The dose is the same as for atropine. Hyoscine is poorly absorbed after oral administration so should be given in increased dosage (Gupta et al, 1972).

Glycopyrrolate (glycopyrronium) is a quaternary ammonium anticholinergic compound. It is used as premedication because of its reported lesser tendency to increase the heart rate. Mirakhur et al (1982) found that both atropine and glycopyrrolate increased the heart rate, although the latter less so. Oduro (1975), giving the drugs intravenously, found that after 2 minutes atropine produced the greater increase, while after 5 minutes, glycopyrrolate did. Hunsley et al (1982) found that neither drug fully protected children against oculocardiac reflexes; both drugs had the same effect.

Studies available until now do not convincingly demonstrate any advantage of glycopyrrolate in children compared to atropine.

The recommended dose of glycopyrrolate is half that of atropine.

Pain-relieving drugs

Derivates of opiates, especially morphine, are widely favoured by paediatric anaesthetists, not only for pain relief but also for sedation. Opiates are respiratory depressants. A moderate overdose will lower the respiratory rate while a still larger dose will cause slow, uneven respiration and signs of upper airway obstruction. When given for pain relief, the stronger the pain, the less will be the respiratory depression. The reverse will also hold true, which is especially important to remember when a regional block is considered for postoperative pain relief (Hatch et al, 1984). A sudden disappearance of pain by a successful block may cause respiratory depression in the presence of an opiate.

Morphine seems to be the most widely used opiate. As well as relief of pain, in most cases morphine will produce a mild euphoria. Occasionally, however, some degree of dysphoria or nausea may be seen. Its respiratory depressant action is particularly evident in children under 1 year of age, and it should not be given as a sedative below this age unless the child is receiving ventilatory support.

Children under 1 year of age, and especially newborn babies, less frequently show signs of suffering from pain than do older children. Those signs are restlessness, crying that will not stop when the child is comforted and tachycardia without hypovolaemia. Occasionally, however, infants and even newborn babies, may benefit from morphine preoperatively when they are on a ventilator or suffering from decompensated heart failure due to congenital heart disease.

Morphine for pain relief may be given in doses of 0.1 mg/kg for children 1–4 years of age and 0.2 mg/kg for those 5 years of age or older. The limit for a single dose should be 10 mg. Since preoperative pain will usually appear in connection with an illness serious enough to warrant intravenous fluids or plasma expanders, morphine may preferably be given *slowly* intravenously. A too rapid injection is likely to cause nausea and vomiting. It can also be given intramuscularly, but the onset is much slower.

When using *morphine for sedation* and hoping that some of its pain-relieving effect may be present postoperatively, careful consideration should be given to the anaesthetic technique to be used and especially to whether spontaneous or controlled ventilation is intended. Vivori (1981), when describing the Liverpool regimen of premedication for elective surgery, recommends trimeprazine tartrate 1.5 mg/kg orally 3 hours preoperatively and morphine 0.25 mg/kg intramuscularly 1 hour before the operation. With this premedication, in addition to being a sedative, morphine will also act as a supplement to the anaesthetic. A combination of morphine 0.15–0.2 mg/kg and diazepam 0.2 mg/kg has been used successfully in some centres.

If it is intended to give some of the modern, potent anaesthetic agents with spontaneous ventilation it will be best to postpone morphine until it may be needed for postoperative pain relief.

Morphine may also be given by the rectal route. Lindahl et al (1981) gave a series of children rectally a mixture of diazepam 0.5 mg/kg, morphine 0.15 mg/kg and scopolamine 0.01 mg/kg dissolved in propylene glycol. Morphine plasma levels of 10–20 ng/kg were reached; the mixture was administered 1 hour preoperatively. The mixture proved satisfactory as sedation but gave insufficient pain relief. The lowest plasma level of morphine to give adequate pain relief was found by Dahlström et al (1979) to be 65 ng/kg.

Papaveretum (0.4 mg/kg), a semisynthetic mixture of opium alkaloids, is probably the opiate premedication which is most widely used in Britain in adults. Conventionally given with scopolamine (0.008 mg/kg), it is satisfactory for use in children weighing over 15–20 kg, in a dose of 0.4 mg/kg intramuscularly.

Pethidine (meperidine, Demerol) is a potent analgesic drug. It will give much less sedation than morphine and is said to cause less respiratory depression. There is, however, no recent support for this claim. Until proved with modern techniques, it would be wise to assume that the depressant action of pethidine on respiration is of the same magnitude as morphine. The equipotent dose is 10-fold that of morphine.

Pethidine has been widely used in some countries in combination with promethazine and chlorpromazine in the mixture known as pethidine compound or Toronto mixture (Smith et al, 1958). Each 1 ml of the mixture contains pethidine 25 mg, promethazine 6.25 mg and chlorpromazine 6.25 mg. The intramuscular dose is 0.06–0.08 ml/kg up to 14 kg. It should be kept in mind, however, that this dose will be in excess of the equipotent dose of morphine stated above.

The Toronto mixture was originally suggested as a superior alternative during heart catheterization and is still favoured by some paediatric cardiologists. Increasingly, modern radiological techniques, such as computerized tomography scan, place considerable demands on the resources of anaesthetic departments. The problem often has to be solved by giving a suitable sedative such as the Toronto mixture in the absence of an anaesthetist. Radiologists, who are less aware than cardiologists of the potential dangers of potent analgesic mixtures, should be thoroughly advised about the hazards and discouraged from increasing the dose.

Pentazocine is a benzomorphane-derivate. Acting as a morphine antagonist, it was once believed not to cause addiction. This has, however, subsequently been proved untrue. The side-effects are the same as for morphine. In addition, quite a few children may suffer from extremely unpleasant hallucinations. This property, once seen, is enough to warn against its use in children.

Sedative drugs (Table 2.1)

In this group are classified barbiturates, benzodiazepines and phenothia-

Table 2.1. Recommended oral and rectal doses of sedative drugs

Drug	Oral dose (mg/kg)	Rectal dose (mg/kg)
Pentobarbital	2–3	2–4
Diazepam	0.3–0.5	0.5*
Trimeprazine	1.5–4	

*Commercially available solutions of diazepam in propylene glycol have very rapid and predictable onset. Suppositories are slow and unpredictable.

zines. Among the first, pentobarbital is widely favoured because of its relatively short action. In the second group, diazepam has become quite common while some others, such as midazolam, have been tested but not gained widespread popularity (Taylor et al, 1986). In the third group, trimeprazine is the most common while promethazine, once quite popular, seems to have been abandoned.

There also seem to exist certain national preferences. Pentobarbital is used widely in the USA and to a lesser degrèe in European countries. Diazepam is used in many countries and is quite popular in Scandinavia. Trimeprazine is favoured by some British anaesthetists.

Ketamine, although mostly used as an anaesthetic, in reduced doses has been used for premedication. However, it seems to have lost favour in most centres because of its hallucinatory properties.

Fasting before anaesthesia (for day-stay requirements see p. 466)

Fasting for 4–6 hours before anaesthesia is generally recommended to minimize the risk of aspiration of gastric contents. Is there any risk of hypoglycaemia during the fasting period?

Jensen et al (1982), in a study of 134 children ranging from 6 months to 9 years of age and fasting from bedtime the previous day, found only one instance of moderate hypoglycaemia. Nilsson et al (1984) in a study of 70 children aged from 2 weeks to 22 months and after 5.8 hours mean fasting time, found no hypoglycaemia. A fuller discussion of glucose requirements may be found in Chapter 8.

It may be concluded that 4 hours' fasting is a safe precaution for infants. It is now recommended that a drink of 5% dextrose is given 4 hours preoperatively, though no solid food is given for 6 hours. Newborn babies who are having frequent feeds may have their last feed omitted; this may be 2–3 hours before the anaesthetic.

REFERENCES

Bothe A & Galdston R (1972) The child's loss of consciousness: a psychiatric view of pediatric anesthesia. *Pediatrics* 50: 252–263.

Dahlström B, Bolme P, Feychting et al (1979) Morphine kinetics in children. *Clinical Pharmacology and Therapeutics* **26:** 354–365.

Gupta RK, Blades HR & Hatch DJ (1972) Oral premedication in children. Atropine or hyoscine with triclofos. *Anaesthesia* **27:** 32–36.

Hatch DJ, Hulse MG & Lindahl SGE (1984) Caudal analgesia in children. *Anaesthesia* **39:** 873–878.

Hunsley JE, Bush GH & Jones CJ (1982) A study of glycopyrrolate and atropine in the suppression of the oculocardiac reflex during strabismus surgery in children. *British Journal of Anaesthesia* **54:** 459–464.

Jensen BH, Wernberg M & Andersen M (1982) Preoperative starvation and blood glucose concentrations in children undergoing inpatient and outpatient anaesthesia. *British Journal of Anaesthesia* **54:** 1071–1074.

Korsch B (1975) The child and the operating room. *Anesthesiology* **43:** 251–257.

Lindahl S, Olsson AK & Thomson D (1981) Rectal premedication in children. *Anaesthesia* **36:** 376–379.

Melamed BG (1977) Psychological preparation for hospitalization. In Rachman S (ed) *Contributions to Medical Psychology*, vol. 1. London: Pergamon Press.

Mirakhur RK, Jones CJ, Dundee JW et al (1982) I.m. or i.v. atropine or glycopyrrolate for the prevention of oculocardiac reflex in children undergoing squint surgery. *British Journal of Anaesthesia* **54:** 1059–1063.

Nilsson K, Larsson LE, Andreasson S et al (1984) Blood glucose concentrations during anaesthesia in children. Effects of starvation and peroperative fluid therapy. *British Journal of Anaesthesia* **56:** 375–381.

Oduro KA (1975) Glycopyrrolate methobromide. 2. Comparison with atropine sulphate in anaesthesia. *Canadian Anaesthetists' Society Journal* **22:** 466–473.

Olsson GL, Bejersten A, Feychting H et al (1983) Plasma concentrations of atropine after rectal administration. *Anaesthesia* **38:** 1179–1182.

Pinkerton P (1981) Preventing psychotrauma in childhood anaesthesia. In Jackson Rees G & Gray TC (eds) *Paediatric Anaesthesia. Trends in Current Practice*, pp 1–18. London: Butterworths.

Singler RC (1983) Acute normovolemic hemodilution. In Gregory GA (ed) *Pediatric Anesthesia*, pp 564–575. New York: Churchill Livingstone.

Smith C, Rowe RD & Vlad P (1958) Sedation of children for cardiac catheterization with an ataractic mixture. *Canadian Anaesthetists' Society Journal* **5:** 35–40.

Taylor MB, Vine PR & Hatch DJ (1986) Intramuscular midazolam premedication in small children: a comparison with papaveretum and hyoscine. *Anaesthesia* **41:** 21–26.

Vivori E (1981) Preparation for surgery and premedication. In Jackson Rees G & Gray TC (eds) *Paediatric Anaesthesia. Trends in Current Practice*, pp 93–100. London: Butterworths.

Inhalation agents in paediatric anaesthesia

INTRODUCTION

The concept of what constitutes the anaesthetized state has undergone
major rethinking in the past several years. This has resulted from firstly, the
introduction of potent narcotics that blunt or eliminate the stress response
and secondly, recent studies that suggest a better outcome in patients who
have a blunted stress response. The stress response refers to the hormonal
response of the body to the stress of anaesthesia and surgery. The complete
nature of the stress response has not been fully characterized, but at the
present time there have been identified increases in plasma adrenaline, noradrenaline, glucagon, aldosterone, corticosterone, antidiuretic
hormone, and β-endorphin immunoreactivity. These increases result in a
mobilization of energy stores and a redistribution of blood flow from unes-
sential organs (such as the kidney and liver) to the heart, brain, and lungs,
resulting in an increased demand upon the circulatory system. In the
healthy patient, these changes have little apparent impact. In contrast, in
the patient undergoing major surgery who may already have respiratory or
circulatory limitations, these changes may have greater significance. In
Roizen et al's (1987a) study of patients undergoing aortic reconstruction
comparing isoflurane and sufentanil, the patients receiving isoflurane had
higher plasma levels of adrenaline and a higher incidence of postoperative
complications (renal insufficiency and congestive heart failure). Anand and
colleagues' studies (Anand and Hickey, 1987; Anand et al, 1988) in the
neonate demonstrate that light anaesthesia results in a stress response that
is even greater than the adult's and that neonates who have the stress
response may have increased postoperative morbidity and mortality compared with infants who were randomly treated with high-potency narcotics.
These infants had a minimal stress response with fewer metabolic and
circulatory perturbations.

The classic triad of general anaesthesia is usually thought to consist of:

1. hypnosis or loss of consciousness;
2. analgesia;
3. muscle relaxation.

Now it appears that there may be another factor of importance—blunting
the stress response. Conventional inhalational anaesthesia with moderate

concentrations of nitrous oxide and volatile agents supplemented with pentothal and morphine will partially block the stress response but not apparently to the same degree as the more potent narcotics.

It appears that we are in the early stages of determining what comprises the ideal anaesthetic state and what concentrations of the various anaesthetic agents are required to accomplish this condition. One approach that has been used to assess anaesthetic depth of inhalational anaesthetics is the concept of MAC (Merkel and Eger, 1963). MAC is usually defined as the minimal anaesthetic concentration in the alveolus (i.e. end-tidal) at which 50% of patients move in response to a surgical incision (Saidman and Eger, 1964). Of course, it also means that 50% of the patients do not move. This definition of MAC does not address the issue of awareness, but at these depths of inhalational anaesthetics, there was no awareness. Varying concentrations of the inhalational agents and narcotics were used to arrive at this anaesthetic depth. As an example, in an adult, 70% nitrous oxide decreases the halothane MAC by 61% (Saidman and Eger, 1964) and enflurane decreases MAC by 60% (Torri et al, 1974). This concept of anaesthetic depth was extended to the narcotics, and it was determined that 5 mg/kg morphine in the dog reduces the halothane MAC by 63% (Murphy and Hug, 1982) and that high-dose sufentanil reduces the halothane MAC by 90% (Hecker et al, 1983). Narcotics have a ceiling effect as far as their ability to reduce the MAC of volatile agents is concerned. The ceiling effect means, for example, that regardless of the dose of morphine (i.e. 20 mg/kg) the maximum reduction of MAC is 90% (Lake et al, 1985). This has resulted in something of a paradox as far as determining the anaesthetic depth and the ideal anaesthetic state. MAC concentrations of halothane and other inhalational agents eliminate awareness but are not able to blunt the stress response completely. However, moderate doses of the potent narcotics are able to blunt the stress response but awareness may still be present. The concept of 'MAC awareness' will become more important as the anaesthetist attempts to induce the ideal anaesthetic state. Recently fentanyl was studied in newborns undergoing surgery, and it was found that a dose of 10–12 µg/kg was sufficient to blunt the cardiovascular response to anaesthesia and surgery (Yaster, 1987). In another study of preterm infants undergoing patent ductus arteriosus (PDA) ligation, the addition of 10 µg/kg of fentanyl to 50% nitrous oxide prevented the stress response (Anand et al, 1987). However, in the older child and adult, these concentrations of anaesthetics would result in an unacceptably high level of awareness. Therefore, in the rush to create the ideal anaesthetic state, the concept of creating an anaesthetized state where there is no awareness must be kept in mind, in addition to blunting the stress response.

There is a price to be paid for the administration of any anaesthetic. The use of high doses of potent narcotics, particularly in the neonate, has resulted in varying degrees of depression of ventilation and the need for prolonged intubation and ventilation (Koehntop et al, 1986), not because of the nature of the surgery but because of the altered pharmacokinetics of the fentanyl. It is obvious that the anaesthetist must learn to balance the risks and benefits of the various anaesthetic techniques. The inhalational agents have great advantages because they are relatively painless to administer and their action can be terminated by ventilation without the need for reversal agents. The judicious use of narcotics in addition to the inhalation agents may achieve the hoped-for ideal anaesthetic state.

There is some confusion about terminology in deciding what concentration of volatile agent the patient is receiving or the concentration of anaesthetic in the brain, i.e. end-tidal concentration. The mass spectrometer has greatly clarified the issue since accurate determinations of inspired and expired (end-tidal) concentrations are displayed. The confusion about what concentration the patient is receiving is due to anaesthetic circuit differences and the uptake and distribution of anaesthetics. With a non-rebreathing or almost completely non-rebreathing circuit the concentration of halothane from the vaporizer (i.e. dialled concentration) is the same as the inspired concentration. With a circle system the inspired concentration is determined by the ratio of the fresh gas flow (the dialled concentration) to the rebreathing volume where the anaesthetic concentration is the end-tidal. Therefore, the inspired concentration will be lower than the vaporizer concentration and higher than end-tidal. In an infant or child for the first 5–10 minutes, the inspired concentration of a circle system is about 60–70% of the concentration of the vaporizer and increases up to about 80% of the dialled concentration after 20–30 minutes. For relatively minor surgical procedures the anaesthetic concentrations needed (end-tidal) are 1 MAC whereas with bronchoscopy 2–3 MAC anaesthetic concentrations may be required and concentrations can be administered for long periods. The pulse and blood pressure are followed and the concentrations regulated accordingly.

INHALATIONAL ANAESTHETICS

Nitrous oxide

Nitrous oxide is a weak inhalation agent. In normal healthy patients, nitrous oxide by itself cannot predictably produce surgical anaesthesia since the MAC is 105%. Nitrous oxide is a very safe anaesthetic when used in concentrations that maintain normal oxygenation. Its safety is related to its lack of potency and for this reason, other drugs need to be added to accomplish the anaesthetized state. Nitrous oxide is frequently used in paediatric anaesthesia. Several different techniques for its use will be discussed. Nitrous oxide is used as an induction agent, to reduce the MAC of volatile anaesthetics, and in balanced anaesthesia.

Nitrous oxide is an insoluble anaesthetic agent and will rapidly equilibrate in the bloodstream. Figure 3.1 shows the relationships between end-tidal and inspired concentrations of nitrous oxide and other inhalation agents. In 5 minutes the end-tidal concentration of nitrous oxide will be approximately 90% of inspired concentration. This also has clinical significance at the end of anaesthesia since the nitrous oxide will offload in the same manner. This rapid clearing of nitrous oxide at the end of surgery is responsible for a condition referred to as diffusion hypoxia. This rapid efflux of nitrous oxide from the lungs will dilute the oxygen in the inspired gas. If the inspired gas is room air then the concentration of inspired oxygen may be reduced

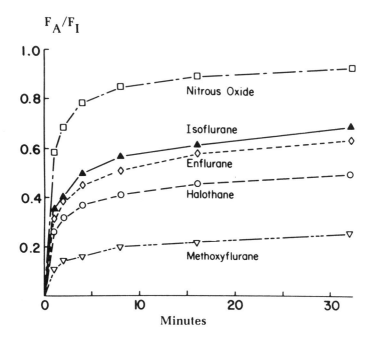

Figure 3.1. Volunteers breathed trace to subanaesthetic concentrations of isoflu-rane (Cromwell et al, 1971a,b) or nitrous oxide, enflurane, halothane and meth-oxyflurane (Munson et al, 1978). Alveolar (F_A) and inspired (F_I) concentrations were measured by gas chromatography. The plot of the ratio of F_A/F_I expressed the rapidity with which the alveolar concentration approaches the concentration being inspired. It is most rapid with the least soluble anaesthetic, nitrous oxide, and least rapid with the most soluble anaesthetic, methoxyflurane. From Eger (1981), with permission.

significantly, resulting in diffusion hypoxia. For this reason, increased con-centrations of inspired oxygen should be given at the end of surgery for several minutes.

Nitrous oxide undergoes very little, if any, biotransformation. It is rapidly eliminated through the respiratory system and expired gas, with a very small amount being excreted through the skin. Nitrous oxide is contra-indicated in certain conditions. It may be contraindicated if there are gas pockets within the body. These gas pockets will expand with the addition and equilibration of nitrous oxide. The blood gas partition coefficient for nitrous oxide is 34 times that for nitrogen. Therefore, the nitrous oxide will rapidly equilibrate in any pocket of trapped gas, causing an expansion of the volume of the gas-containing compartment. Nitrous oxide will increase the size of the gas pocket in direct proportion to its concentration, so that 50% nitrous oxide will double and 66% nitrous oxide will triple the size of the gas compartment. Situations in which this may occur include pneumothorax, lung cysts, pneumoencephalogram, trapped gas within obstructed loops of bowel, and the middle ear.

The other situation when nitrous oxide may be relatively contraindicated is in severely ill children who are hypoxic secondary to a disease process such as pneumonia or congenital heart disease, where a high inspired oxygen concentration is required to maintain oxygenation. The haemodynamic responses of 50% nitrous oxide have been studied in infants (Hickey et al, 1986). There is a statistically significant depression of systemic haemodynamics but these changes are felt to be clinically insignificant, except perhaps in severely compromised infants. The changes in pulmonary haemodynamics are minimal. The contraindication for nitrous oxide is relative and depends upon the inspired oxygen concentration the child requires to maintain normal oxygenation.

Nitrous oxide as an induction agent and in reducing the MAC of volatile anaesthetics

Nitrous oxide is frequently used as the initial anaesthetic in inhalation inductions where a volatile agent is also to be added. In this technique, high-flow (6–10 l/min) nitrous oxide in a concentration of 70–80% is used to begin the induction of anaesthesia. Nitrous oxide is almost odourless but does have a slightly sweet smell. When rubber delivery hoses are used, they often have more odour than the nitrous oxide. The mask can be held away from the child's face and slowly advanced until tolerated. Various scents have been used on anaesthetic masks to camouflage the odour of the anaesthetics. When the child has tolerated the nitrous oxide for a minute or so the volatile agent is added slowly in 0.5% concentrations. As he or she tolerates the volatile agent for 15–20 seconds, the concentration is increased by another 0.5%. At times the child will hold the breath, cough, and so on. At that point the concentration needs to be held constant until the reaction to the volatile agent ceases. The concentration of the volatile agent can then be increased again until induction is accomplished.

Nitrous oxide is used to reduce the MAC requirements of the various volatile agents. In this situation, nitrous oxide is used in a 50–70% concentration. Since the MAC value for nitrous oxide is 105%, whatever the concentration of nitrous oxide used will reduce the MAC requirement of the volatile agent by approximately the same percentage. As an example, nitrous oxide in a 50% concentration will reduce the MAC requirement of halothane by 50% in a 6-year-old child from an end-tidal concentration of 1% to one of 0.5%. Nitrous oxide by itself has little clinical effect upon circulation or respiration (Wren et al, 1986) but when added to the volatile agents it will produce some degree of effect if the concentration of volatile agent is not reduced accordingly (second gas effect). A recent report by Roizen et al (1987b) describes 10 patients with atrioventricular junctional rhythm thought to be associated with nitrous–narcotic and nitrous–volatile anaesthesia. The aetiology of the observation has not been delineated.

Nitrous oxide in balanced anaesthesia

Balanced anaesthesia means different things to different anaesthetists. The definition used in this discussion is a narrow one, referring to a combination of nitrous oxide, narcotics, sedative hypnotics and muscle relaxants. When nitrous oxide is used in the balanced technique usually the induction of anaesthesia is accomplished with the intravenous administration of barbiturates or similar drugs; muscle relaxation is accomplished with curare or other muscle relaxants; narcotics are given for additional analgesia and nitrous oxide is administered in the concentration of approximately 70%. The advantages of this technique are that the patient undergoes a rapid induction; operating conditions as far as muscle relaxation is concerned are excellent and the patient recovers very rapidly from the anaesthetic as the muscle relaxants are reversed and the nitrous oxide discontinued. The disadvantages of the balanced technique are the limited possibilities of changing inspired oxygen concentration or depth of anaesthesia and a level of anaesthesia just below the awareness level where slight breaches in technique may allow awareness to surface.

Balanced anaesthesia for spinal fusion will be discussed as one application of the balanced technique. This discussion will include some of the potential problems that occur with this technique and the use of the various anaesthetic adjuvants to accomplish the desired surgical and anaesthetic effects. Many orthopaedic surgeons have requested the 'wake-up test' for spinal fusion operations, although the use of evoked potentials makes this less common (see p. 400). This technique requires patients to be awakened at mid-surgery after instrumentation in order to determine if the spinal cord is intact. The anaesthetics are discontinued and the patient is asked to move the extremities. The use of volatile agents makes this wake-up test very difficult or prolonged. Therefore, in this situation, the use of a balanced technique which can rapidly be reversed so that the spinal cord can be rapidly evaluated has gained a great deal of popularity. Some of the problems reported with this technique which will be discussed are firstly, unless hypotensive techniques are used the patient may become relatively hypertensive, resulting in increased blood loss and longer surgery, and secondly, the stress response associated with this type of anaesthesia may result in dilutional hyponatremia in the postoperative period if hypotonic intravenous fluids are administered.

Balanced anaesthesia and deliberate hypotension (for specific situations see p. 400 and p. 407).   Various techniques can be used to accomplish hypotensive anaesthesia. Nitrous oxide is administered in a concentration of 70%. Intravenous morphine in a dose of 0.2–0.3 mg/kg or fentanyl in a dose of 5–10 µg/kg are administered in the induction period as an analgesic. The choice of muscle relaxants is quite important. Pancuronium is known to cause varying degrees of stimulation of the adrenergic nervous system, leading to an increase in heart rate and blood pressure. It is a poor choice of muscle relaxant when normotensive or hypotensive anaesthesia is desired. The muscle relaxants of choice are curare (d-tubocurarine), metocurine, atracurium or vecuronium. Curare and, to a lesser extent, atracurium will produce a dose-related release of histamine. Histamine is a vasodilator and reduces the blood pressure. There is minimal histamine release in children under 6 years of age. In older children, dividing the curare dose into several increments will modulate the histamine release and the hypotension. Sodium nitroprusside can be used as a hypotensive agent in a dose of 2–3 µg/kg/min. It should be administered by an infusion pump so that the dosage may be more accurately controlled. The renin angiotensin aldosterone system will respond to the hypotension caused by the sodium nitroprusside. This may lead to a reactive tachycardia which will increase the blood pressure. Therefore, a β-blocker such as propranolol can be titrated in doses of 0.01 mg/kg in order to control the heart rate (Marshall et al, 1981). Another very useful agent is labetalol (up to 1 mg/kg) which is both an α- and β-blocker.

In summary, depending upon the technique that is used to create hypotensive anaesthesia, the pharmacological approach is usually a two-phase process. The initial phase is the administration of the hypotensive agent, i.e. sodium nitroprusside, hydralazine, and so on. The body attempts to overcome the hypotensive state by a series of compensatory steps, such as the activation of the renin angiotensin aldosterone response or the baroreceptor response, causing tachycardia and an increase in arterial blood pressure. Phase two is the administration of pharmacological agents to block these compensatory mechanisms. A knowledge of the compensatory responses greatly enhances the ability of the anaesthetist to manipulate the pharmacological agents appropriately in order to create the desired control of blood pressure. Isoflurane has become a popular hypotensive agent because the hypotensive effect is related to a decrease in peripheral vascular resistance and not a decrease in cardiac output. However, it is difficult to use in spinal fusions when the wake-up test is requested because of the delay in recovery.

Balanced anaesthesia and the stress response.   Light levels of anaesthesia are associated with the stress response, which results in the release of antidiuretic hormone. Therefore, in the postoperative period, if hypotonic intravenous fluids are administered, the increased levels of antidiuretic hormone will cause an increased reabsorption of free water through the distal tubule and collecting duct, resulting in a dilutional hyponatremia (Burrows et al, 1983). The fluid of choice in the perioperative period is a balanced salt solution (isotonic).

VOLATILE INHALATION ANAESTHETICS

The volatile anaesthetics are the most frequently used primary anaesthetic agents in paediatric anaesthesia. The two major potential complications of the volatile agents are hepatotoxicity and triggering an episode of malignant hyperthermia. These will be discussed later. The three volatile agents in current use are: halothane, enflurane, and isoflurane. Halothane is by far the most popular of the three because of the low cost, ease of administration, and operator familiarity. The other two have both practical and theoretical advantages as well as disadvantages but until their cost decreases, they will not replace halothane. One theoretical advantage of isoflurane is that it is more insoluble than halothane (blood gas partition coefficient 1.4 vs. 2.3), which means that the alveolar concentration will rise rapidly towards the inspired concentration and hence the child should be induced more rapidly.

The theoretical advantage has never been realized in practice when isoflurane is used as an induction agent since it is <u>more pungent</u> than halothane and the pungency provokes coughing and breath-holding, thereby prolonging induction. There have also been episodes of <u>laryngospasm</u> which have the potential for disaster. The use of nitrous oxide to facilitate induction reduces the pungency but halothane still remains the gentlest of the volatile inhalation agents. One study compared halothane, enflurane, and isoflurane for outpatient anaesthesia (Fisher et al, 1984). The children in the study were not premedicated, and all three agents were administered with nitrous oxide. The results of the study demonstrated that halothane had the fastest induction time with the lowest incidence of excitement. Enflurane was similar to halothane except that the excitement period was longer. Isoflurane had the highest incidence of coughing, and laryngospasm on induction, and the highest incidence of coughing on emergence and in the recovery room. The conclusion of the study was that in a busy outpatient practice, the rapid and smooth induction makes halothane the agent of choice.

Metabolism of volatile anaesthetics

Another theoretical advantage of isoflurane and enflurane is the low degree of metabolism these drugs undergo, compared with halothane (Table 3.1). This potential advantage has not been a dominant factor in paediatric patients but it does have advantages in adult patients, particularly obese ones.

Table 3.1. Metabolism of inhaled anaesthetics

Anaesthetic	Absorbed anaesthetic recovered as metabolites (%)
Nitrous oxide	0.004
Isoflurane	0.17
Enflurane	2.4
Halothane	20

Theoretically, it should also be important in obese paediatric patients but to date there have been no reports to substantiate this advantage. Even without documented advantage, some anaesthetists prefer to use the less soluble anaesthetic agents in obese paediatric patients because of the reduced requirement for muscle relaxants and the theoretical advantage that the patients will wake more quickly from their anaesthetic because there will be less agent dissolved in the fat tissue and less agent biotransformed to potentially harmful metabolites. Halothane is often used initially because of the smoother induction and then changed over to isoflurane.

Further comparisons of inhalation agents

The next section will compare the effects of the volatile agents on the circulation, respiration, muscle relaxation, and intracranial pressure. The majority of the reported studies were done on healthy, unpremedicated adult volunteers in the absence of disease, drugs, and surgical stimulation. This fact needs to be kept in mind when transferring the data to patients who have concurrent disease and are on various medications. There is controversy about coronary and cerebral 'steal' with isoflurane. At the present time there is considerable heat but not much light in this debate. The effects on the vast majority of paediatric patients are minimal.

The circulatory system

The effects of the volatile agents will be discussed with special emphasis on blood pressure, cardiac output and peripheral resistance. What the anaesthetist really would like to know, as anaesthetics are administered, is what is happening to myocardial performance, i.e. cardiac output. Cardiac output can be measured but it requires invasive monitoring. The ECG is non-invasive and has been used to assess ventricular function in children during both isoflurane and halothane anaesthesia, but it is primarily a research tool in the operating room at the present time. Perhaps in the future intraoperative ECG measurements of cardiac performance will become practicable.

Arterial blood pressure

The volatile agents cause a dose-related decrease in arterial blood pressure. Nitrous oxide alone usually does not alter blood pressure in the fit patient. When nitrous oxide is used with a volatile agent and the volatile agent is reduced by the MAC equivalent of nitrous oxide then there is less of a blood pressure depression at the same anaesthetic dose. The effects of nitrous oxide, halothane, enflurane, and isoflurane on blood pressure are depicted in Figure 3.2.

Cardiac output

There is a dose-dependent reduction in cardiac output with enflurane and halothane. However, isoflurane at 1–2 MAC does not cause a reduction in cardiac output (Neal et al, 1984). In adult patients nitrous oxide is associated with an increase in cardiac output. This is thought to be due to a weak sympathomimetic effect of this drug. Figure 3.3 depicts these findings. The decrease in cardiac output demonstrated with halothane closely parallels the changes in blood pressure. The same is true for enflurane. This factor magnifies the importance of monitoring blood pressure as a method of determining the effect of these agents upon the cardiovascular system. The

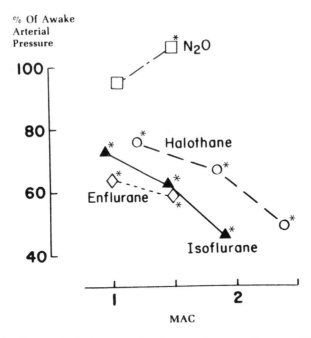

Figure 3.2. Isoflurane, halothane and enflurane, but not nitrous oxide, decrease arterial blood pressure from preanaesthetic values in a dose-related fashion (asterisks indicate a significant change). Data from Stevens et al (1971) and Winter et al (1972), with permission.

values for the anaesthetic agents are given in end-tidal MAC concentrations. Barash et al (1978) studied ventricular function in children during halothane anaesthesia and reported a dose-dependent depression of ventricular function. The changes found in their study were felt to be both rate-dependent and due to myocardial depression. Figure 3.4 shows these effects; the values of halothane in the figure are inspired concentrations of halothane, not end-tidal. The administration of atropine (0.2 mg) resulted in a rapid improvement in cardiac output and in all the rate-dependent variables. However, the other indices of myocardial performance, such as the ejection fraction and the left ventricular end diastolic volume, still showed depression. Studies in children using ECG assessment of ventricular function during isoflurane and halothane anaesthesia suggest that there is little if any reduction in ventricular function at 1.3 MAC concentrations (end-tidal concentrations) of isoflurane, whereas there is significant depression of ventricular function with halothane at these concentrations (McNeil et al, 1984). There was little change in heart rate but there was a progressively significant fall in mean blood pressure with both agents.

Peripheral vascular resistance

The volatile anaesthetics have different effects on systemic vascular

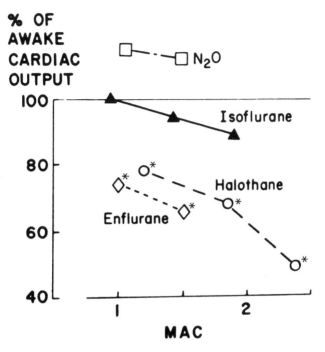

Figure 3.3. Neither isoflurane nor nitrous oxide depressed cardiac output below awake levels in volunteers. In contrast, both halothane and enflurane decreased output significantly (asterisks) and did so to a greater extent at deeper levels of anaesthesia. Data from Stevens et al (1971) and Winter et al (1972), with permission.

resistance. Halothane has little effect, whereas isoflurane and to a lesser extent enflurane produce a dose-dependent reduction in calculated systemic vascular resistance (Fig. 3.5). There is a common clinical misconception that halothane reduces peripheral resistance because of the cutaneous vasodilatation which occurs.

In neonates, where the balance between pulmonary and systemic vascular resistance is easily disturbed, and in children with congenital heart disease, particularly those with balanced shunts, fall in systemic resistance can lead to serious right-to-left shunting and hypoxia.

Baroreceptors

There is a dose-dependent depression of baroreceptors with volatile inhalation anaesthesia. This has been demonstrated in the preterm infant (Gregory, 1982) as well as the more mature infant and adult (Cameron et al, 1984). One of the compensatory responses of the infant for hypotension is activation of the baroresponse, which increases the heart rate. It is evident that the depression of the baroresponse would limit the ability of the infant to increase heart rate to compensate for hypotension. In the study of isoflu-

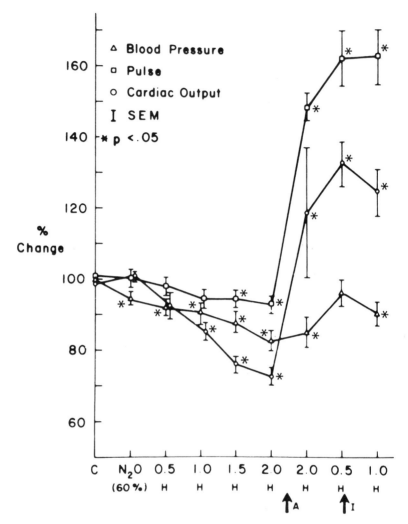

Figure 3.4. Changes in blood pressure, pulse and cardiac output with increasing concentrations of halothane (H). A = atropine; I = intubation. From Barash et al (1978), with permission.

rane in preterm infants, 1 MAC of isoflurane significantly depressed the baroresponse so that there was no response of heart rate in spite of significant decreases in systolic blood pressure (LeDez and Lerman, 1987).

Summary of cardiovascular effects of volatile anaesthetics

The inhalational agents have specific effects upon the circulation. All of the volatile agents are myocardial depressants and will depress isolated heart

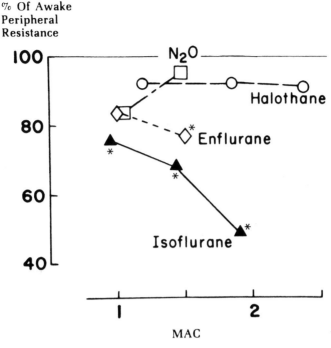

Figure 3.5. Isoflurane and to a lesser extent enflurane cause peripheral vasodilatation while halothane and nitrous oxide do not (asterisks indicate significant changes from awake values). Data from Eger et al (1970), Stevens et al (1971), Winter et al (1972) and Calverley et al (1978a,b), with permission.

muscle in a physiological solution. However in the intact system the effects on peripheral vascular resistance also determine the effect on cardiac output. The studies shown are in normal patients. Patients who have decompensation of the various organ systems may respond to volatile anaesthetics by varying degrees of decompensation. Careful attention to dose–response relationships will allow the safe administration of the volatile anaesthetics to most sick patients. All of the volatile agents will cause a dose-dependent reduction in arterial blood pressure. In the case of isoflurane, the reduction in blood pressure is due to a decrease in peripheral resistance while the cardiac output remains normal. On the other hand, both halothane and enflurane have dose-dependent reductions in cardiac output to account for the reduction in arterial blood pressure. There is little effect of halothane on peripheral vascular resistance.

Ventilation

The volatile anaesthetic agents produce a dose-dependent effect on ventilation. The respiratory pattern changes to a regular rhythm, the rate increases and the tidal volume decreases in the anaesthetized state. Exhalation becomes an active process which results in an increase in abdominal muscle tone during exhalation. This is the reason why when ventilation is controlled and the P_aCO_2 is below the apnoeic threshold the abdominal muscles are more relaxed. At times the relaxation produced by controlled ventilation and moderate levels of volatile anaesthetics (1 MAC) may produce sufficient relaxation for surgery. If not, titrated doses of muscle relaxants can be added. The effects of anaesthetics on the carbon dioxide response curve are well known as there is a dose-dependent depression (Fig. 3.6), with enflurane having the greatest respiratory depressant effect (O'Neill et al, 1982; Murat et al, 1987). There is a greater effect of anaesthetics on the hypoxic ventilatory drive than on the response to hypercarbia. A report by Knill and Clement (1984) examined the effects of halothane on the peripheral chemoreflex pathway. Although this study was done in healthy adult volunteers, there is no reason to believe that there would be differences in infants and children. The authors examined the effect of subanaesthetic concentrations of halothane (0.15–0.30% inspired) and found a profound depression of the peripheral chemoreflex pathway via the depression of the carotid bodies. The subjects of the study were somewhat drowsy, but coherent and had full recall of the experiment.

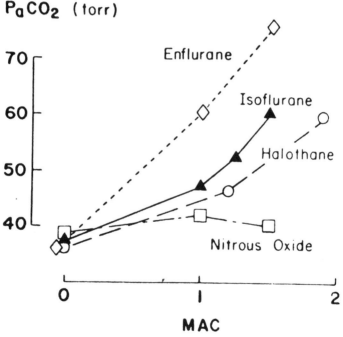

Figure 3.6. Healthy male volunteers were given one of four anaesthetics in oxygen. Increasing levels of enflurane, isoflurane and halothane but not nitrous oxide increased P_aCO_2. The order of their ability to depress respiratory function (from highest to lowest) was as follows: enflurane (Calverley et al, 1978a), isoflurane (Cromwell et al, 1971a,b), halothane (Bahlman et al, 1972) and nitrous oxide (Winter et al, 1972). Nitrous oxide was given in a pressure chamber at 1.1 and 1.55 atmospheres (total pressure in both cases was 1.9 atmospheres). Reprinted with permission.

One of the actions of the peripheral chemoreflex pathway is to protect the body from hypoxia. When the carotid bodies are stimulated by hypoxia, a cascade of protective physiological defences is activated. These defences are tachypnoea with an increase in minute ventilation, hypertension, and a favourable redistribution of cardiac output. In the unanaesthetized state, there is also central nervous system arousal. The clinical implications are clear—not only for small infants but for all patients. The post-anaesthetized patient is at great risk. This, along with the other handicaps of the infant, is why most anaesthetists intubate almost all young infants and leave them intubated until they are awake and have recovered their protective airway reflexes. The drowsy patient may have sufficient residual anaesthesia to depress the peripheral chemoreflex pathway, resulting in a risk of obstruction, since their hypoxic respiratory protective reflexes are depressed. The period of recovery in the post-anaesthesia room is critical as the child eliminates the anaesthetics from his or her system and attempts to return to the unanaesthetized state. For this reason, any child who is still unconscious or semi-conscious from anaesthesia needs to be monitored as if anaesthetized, not as if he or she is in the almost awakened state.

Cerebral blood flow

For patients in whom intracranial pressure (ICP) is an issue, there are two factors to consider with inhalation anaesthetics—cerebral blood flow (CBF) and cerebrospinal fluid (CSF) volume. The effects of inhalation anaesthetics on CBF (Fig. 3.7) and ICP have been thoroughly studied in adult volunteers and patients. At light levels of volatile anaesthetics, defined as 0.6% MAC end-tidal concentrations, there is no effect on CBF by any of the agents. At 1.2% MAC end-tidal concentration, halothane and enflurane increase CBF. Increases in CBF are associated with an increase in ICP. The increases in both CBF and ICP can be partially reversed by inducing hypocapnia. Isoflurane has minimal effect on CBF compared to enflurane and halothane at 1.2% MAC. In addition, isoflurane and fentanyl will increase the reabsorption of spinal fluid and decrease ICP (Artru, 1984). Enflurane, halothane and ketamine result in a decreased rate of absorption of CSF, resulting in increased CSF flow and ICP (Artru, 1983). The message for use of these agents in neurosurgical anaesthesia is: if there is a question about ICP, use lower concentrations of isoflurane and control P_aCO_2 to levels of 25–30 mmHg (see Chapter 16).

FACTORS INFLUENCING THE TECHNIQUES OF INHALATION ANAESTHESIA IN INFANTS

Since the uptake of inhalation anaesthetics primarily depends upon the ventilatory system, a brief description of the similarities and differences between the infant and adult respiratory systems will be given.

Table 3.2 lists the normal respiratory values for the newborn compared with those of the adult. Perusal of the values reveals that there are many similarities and differences.

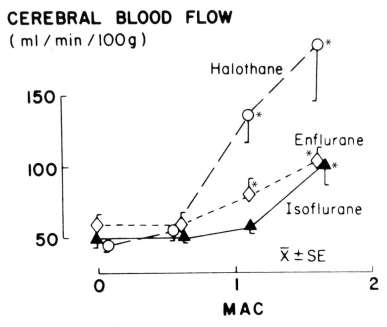

CEREBRAL BLOOD FLOW
(ml / min / 100 g)

Figure 3.7. Cerebral blood flow was measured in volunteers at various levels of MAC for three anaesthetic agents. The volunteers were paralysed with d-tubocurarine and their P_aCO_2 and systemic blood pressure were kept at normal levels. Flow increased at light levels of enflurane and halothane anaesthesia, but did not increase at the same levels of isoflurane. All three agents increased flow at 1.6 MAC. From Murphy et al (1974), with permission.

Table 3.2. Comparison between normal respiratory values of infant and adult

	Infant	Adult
Respiratory frequency (breaths/min)	30–50	12–16
Tidal volume (ml/kg)	6–8	7
Dead space (ml/kg)	2–2.5	2.2
Alveolar ventilation (ml/kg/min)	100–150	60
Function residual capacity (ml/kg)	27–30	30
Oxygen consumption (ml/kg/min)	6–8	3

The dead space:tidal ventilation (VD:VT) ratio and functional residual capacity (FRC) are essentially the same. The major difference in respiratory values is the very large oxygen consumption of the infant compared with the adult. Since tidal ventilation is the same and oxygen consumption is 2–3 times greater it becomes evident that the respiratory frequency must be 2–3 times greater in order to deliver the oxygen requirement of the infant. This, in turn, results in an increase of the same magnitude in the resting alveolar ventilation. The ratio of alveolar ventilation to FRC is 5:1 in the infant and 1.5:1 in the adult. The ratio of minute ventilation to FRC in the pregnant woman at term is similar to the infant because of the reduced FRC due to the elevation of the diaphragm by the large uterus. The results and implications are exactly the same for infants and pregnant women.

There are advantages and disadvantages in a large ratio of minute ventilation to FRC. The major advantage is that there will be a much more rapid induction of inhalation anaesthesia and a more rapid awakening at the end of surgery when the inhalation anaesthetics are discontinued. The FRC acts as the oxygen reservoir for the body. When airway obstruction occurs, the oxygen remaining in the lungs must sustain life until the airway can be re-established. The elevated oxygen requirement in the infant is not matched by an elevated oxygen reserve in the FRC. Therefore, the infant will use up the oxygen reserve much more quickly than the older child or adult. The pregnant woman has a decreased FRC and hence reduced oxygen reserve.

The question of preferred anaesthetic technique for infants depends upon the experience and training of the anaesthetist as well as the condition of the infant. The two major inhalational techniques are balanced techniques and volatile agent, nitrous oxide and relaxant. The proponents of both techniques are well aware of the advantages and disadvantages of both. In infants who are moribund or quite ill, a third technique is oxygen, relaxant, and narcotics or ketamine. Ketamine supports the circulation better than any of the other anaesthetics (Friesen and Henry, 1986). At times this type of anaesthetic falls into the category of a resuscitation. As the infant is successfully resuscitated and begins to respond to the surgical stimulus as evidenced by an increase in blood pressure, anaesthetic techniques should be modified in accordance with the response of the patient.

The advantages of using a volatile anaesthetic are that it allows for a reduced dosage of muscle relaxant, reduces tracheobronchial reactivity, allows for control of blood pressure, and allows a higher inspired oxygen concentration to be administered. The disadvantage of volatile agents is that they require a slightly greater degree of skill to manage myocardial depression as well as to awaken the infant at the termination of surgery. At times, in spite of efforts to the contrary, significant myocardial depression still occurs. Careful attention to ensure adequate fluid volume and frequent monitoring will minimize these problems. The advantage of the balanced technique is that there is less cardiovascular depression, but at the same time there is less upward control of the blood pressure and a potential for increased bleeding with surgery. The risks of hepatitis and acquired immune deficiency syndrome (AIDS) have greatly raised interest in anaesthetic techniques that control blood pressure and reduce the need for transfusions. Nitrous oxide techniques cannot be used when there is the problem of gas pockets within the body.

In infants, hypotension is certainly one of the concerns when volatile agents are used. The incidence of hypotension is well documented (Diaz and Lockhart; 1979; Friesen and Lichtor, 1982, 1983). The reasons for the hypotension are several. There is a more rapid uptake of halothane and other inhalational anaesthetics in infants compared with adults. This has been well documented in the studies by Brandom et al (1983). Figure 3.8 compares a computer simulation and in vivo measurements of the uptake and distribution of halothane in infants. It is evident that the infant equilibrates halothane approximately 30% faster than the adult. The reasons for more rapid uptake of anaesthetic by the infant are the ratio of alveolar minute ventilation to FRC, and the reduced muscle mass of the infant which results in centralizing the cardiac output towards the vessel-rich group, including the heart and the brain. The clinical implication is that after 10 minutes of inhalation the ratio of end-tidal halothane to inspired halothane in an adult will be approximately 50%, whereas in an infant, it may well be 80%. Many of the studies that report hypotension with halothane use 3% inspired halothane concentration for the induction. This means that after 10 minutes the end-tidal halothane would approach 2.4%. For the neonate this represents a relatively high concentration of halothane and requires frequent circulatory monitoring. The other possible reason for the hypotension is the maturational state of the infant's myocardium, i.e. a lower amount of contractile mass per gram of cardiac tissue, as well as the increased parasympathetic tone of infants.

The maturational state of the myocardium was described by Friedman (1972). His studies revealed that in the fetus 30% of the cardiac muscle is contractile mass, whereas it is 60% in the adult. The clinical implication of this finding is that the infant will have relatively less myocardial contractile ability for the same amount of cardiac muscle compared with the adult and that there will be a reduced compliance or stretchability of the ventricle. The infant is less able to increase stroke volume to increase cardiac output and must depend, to a great degree, upon an increase in heart rate. In addition,

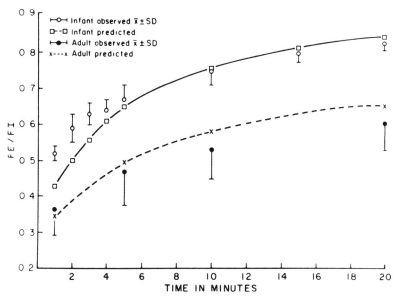

Figure 3.8. Predicted versus observed F_E/F_I (expired/inspired fraction) for halothane in infants and adults. Predicted F_E/F_I values are those generated by a computer program of anaesthetic uptake and distribution. In infants minute ventilation averaged 1.9 l; in adults minute ventilation was 6.9 l. The inspired fraction of halothane was 0.5% in both cases. From Brandom et al (1983), with permission.

it has been found that the infant has incomplete sympathetic innervation of the myocardial muscle. These factors result in less myocardial reserve in the infant; this reserve increases with maturation. Infants appear to have a higher degree of vagal tone than older children and adults. They are quite prone to develop varying degrees of bradycardia with what would appear to be minimal vagal stimulation.

The anaesthetic requirements of infants

The initial studies demonstrating age-dependent MAC requirements (Gregory et al, 1969) have been supplemented at the younger ages for halothane (Lerman et al, 1983) and have been determined for isoflurane (Fig. 3.9). The anaesthetic concentrations for the volatile anaesthetics isoflurane and halothane as determined in these studies of MAC demonstrated that the 1–6-month-old infant had the highest requirement. For isoflurane, the MAC of preterm infants <32 weeks' gestational age is 1.28; 32–37 weeks' is 1.41; full term at 1 month 1.6%; 1–6 months 1.87%; 6–12 months 1.8%; 1–5 years 1.6%, and for young adults 1.28% (LeDez and Lerman, 1987). All concentrations for MAC determinations of isoflurane and halothane are end-tidal

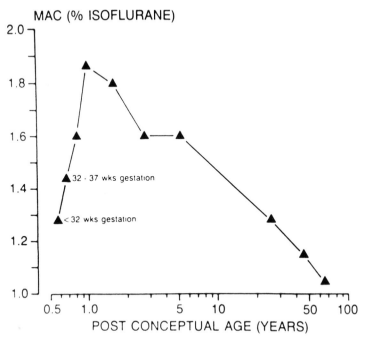

Figure 3.9. The MAC of isoflurane and postconceptual age. Values for postconceptual age were obtained by adding 40 weeks to the mean postnatal age for each age group. The MAC of isoflurane in preterm neonates is significantly less than in full-term neonates and older infants 1–6 months of age (p <0.005). From LeDez and Lerman (1987), with permission.

determinations. For halothane, the MAC of preterm infants <32 weeks' gestational age is 0.55; 0–1 month 0.87%; 1–6 months 1.2%; 1–5 years 1%, and for young adults 0.87%.

Three possible reasons are postulated for the low MAC in the neonate: elevated progesterone levels; immature central nervous system, and a combination of high circulating β-endorphins and an immature central nervous system. The pregnant woman has a decrease in MAC at term of approximately 30% and this is thought to be related to the circulating levels of progesterone. The progesterone from the mother undergoes transplacental passage into the fetus and the levels are measurable for the first 10 days of life. This is postulated as one of the possible reasons for the lower anaesthetic requirement of the neonate. The second reason is that the immature central nervous system of the neonate may result in a lower appreciation of pain or conversely a higher threshold to elicit the pain response. The third factor is that it has been shown that neonates have higher circulating levels of β-endorphins than do adults (Moss et al, 1982). Normally the β-endorphins do not cross the blood–brain barrier and therefore have little effect upon the central nervous system. However, it has been postulated that in neonates the immature central nervous system and immature blood–brain barrier may allow passage of the β-endorphins and therefore result in a lower MAC value.

Cyclopropane

This agent, introduced into clinical practice in the 1930s, continues to be used for induction of anaesthesia in children in many centres around the world. Its manufacture and use will continue in the foreseeable future in spite of its explosive properties. It is the simplest of hydrocarbons and the most potent of gases used for anaesthesia. Its solubility coefficient in blood is 0.415, which accounts for the rapid induction achieved with cyclopropane. It is eliminated from the circulation within 5 minutes of cessation of administration and it does not undergo biotransformation to any degree. The mixture 50:50 with oxygen is heavier than air so it will gravitate towards the floor.

Because it is a pleasant, sweet-smelling gas when mixed 50% with oxygen it is usually very well accepted even by a fractious child if drifted over the mouth and nose. The average time from starting the induction to loss of eyelash reflex is approximately 35 seconds, after which the cyclopropane is turned off and another agent substituted or the patient is paralysed, intubated and ventilated. No other induction agent offers the advantages of high inspired oxygen concentration, speed and smoothness of induction and yet with these doses leaves both the cardiovascular and respiratory systems completely unaffected. An infant, for example, with severe congenital heart disease maintains a normal blood pressure, pulse rate and cardiac output. The drug is also ideal for the induction of preterm babies in whom awake intubation carries the risk of intraventricular cerebral haemorrhage with subsequent neurodevelopmental handicap.

It should never be forgotten that the 50:50 cyclopropane:oxygen mixture is very explosive. Its use is confined solely to induction rooms in operating departments. It is never used in investigation suites in the close presence of electrical equipment. All the induction room equipment and floors must be antistatic and must undergo regular checks. All the clothing of patients and staff should be made of cotton; a high level of ambient humidity must be maintained, and monitoring equipment for induction such as ECG and pulse oximeter must be kept at least 2 metres away from the gas source.

Some interactions of drugs with volatile anaesthetics

Two major interactions of volatile anaesthetics with agents used in surgery will be discussed. These are the use of adrenaline solutions, and the use of non-depolarizing muscle relaxants.

Volatile anaesthetics and adrenaline solutions

Shortly after the introduction of halothane, it was noted that adrenaline under certain circumstances caused ventricular dysrhythmia. Johnston et al (1976) reported on the comparative interaction of adrenaline with enflurane, isoflurane, and halothane. The patients studied were all adults in ASA (American Society of Anesthesiology) status 1 or 2. Ventilation was controlled to maintain a P_aCO_2 between 30 and 40 mmHg. The adrenaline solutions used were 1:100 000, 1:150 000, and 1:200 000 adrenaline in saline (10, 6.7 or 5 µg/ml). One group of the halothane patients received adrenaline 1:200 000 in 0.5% lignocaine solution. The patients were anaesthetized with the various volatile agents and the anaesthetic gas tensions were adjusted to 1.25 times MAC. The median effective dose (ED_{50}) of adrenaline was determined. This was defined as the appearance of 3 premature ventricular contractions (PVC) at any time during or immediately following adrenaline injection. The results are given in Figure 3.10. The ED_{50} for adrenaline and halothane in adults is 2.1 µg/kg; the ED_{50} for halothane, lignocaine–adrenaline is 3.7 µg/kg. The ED_{50} for enflurane is 10.9 µg/kg and 6.7 µg/kg for isoflurane.

There have been several reports of the adrenaline–halothane interaction in children. The report by Ueda et al (1983) in spontaneously breathing children concluded that a mean dose of adrenaline of 7.8 µg/kg given together with lignocaine could be used safely. In the study of Karl et al (1983), the authors felt that at least 10 µg/kg adrenalin could safely be used in normocarbic and hypocarbic paediatric patients who did not have congenital heart disease. Some of the patients in their series had lignocaine administered with the adrenaline while others did not.

It is evident from comparing the studies done in adults and children that there is a different interaction between adrenaline and halothane in children compared with that seen in adults. The reasons for this difference are not clear. It is felt by most authors that the addition of lignocaine to the adrenaline solution increases the margin of safety since the lignocaine will treat the ventricular dysrhythmias caused by the interaction. As a practical matter, it

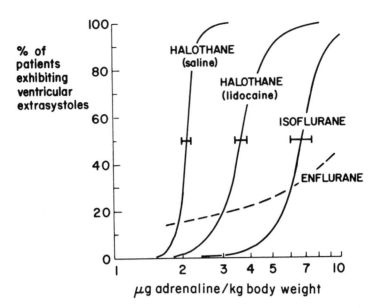

Figure 3.10. Patients were given 1.25 MAC enflurane, halothane, or isoflurane in oxygen. For halothane the ED_{50} was 2.1 μg/kg when the medium for adrenaline injection was saline, and 3.7 μg/kg when the medium was 0.5% lignocaine. For isoflurane, the ED_{50} was 6.7 μg/kg (adrenaline in saline). The curve for enflurane is flatter than that for halothane or isoflurane: a few patients given enflurane developed extrasystoles at relatively low doses of adrenaline. From Johnston et al (1976), with permission.

would appear that the dosage recommendation for children should be at least 10 μg/kg adrenaline; if dysrhythmias develop they should be treated with intravenous lignocaine 1 mg/kg. If the dysrhythmias continue then the patient must be evaluated for hypoxia and hypercarbia. If the dysrhythmias continue for no obvious reason then switching to either enflurane or isoflurane would be appropriate since, at least in adults, there is a much higher threshold for the development of dysrhythmias due to the interaction with adrenaline.

Dosage requirements for non-depolarizing muscle relaxants used with volatile anaesthetics

Figure 3.11 demonstrates the dose-dependent reduction in the dose of non-depolarizing muscle relaxant needed when volatile anaesthetic agents are being used. In adults, isoflurane and enflurane potentiate the effects of d-tubocurarine more than halothane, and the same may be true in children. The dose of non-depolarizing muscle relaxants should be guided with the use of a nerve stimulator (see Chapter 5). This results not only in a more satisfactory dose–response of muscle relaxant during the surgical procedures, but the use of the nerve stimulator also serves as a diagnostic tool at the termination of surgery to determine the reversal of the muscle relaxants.

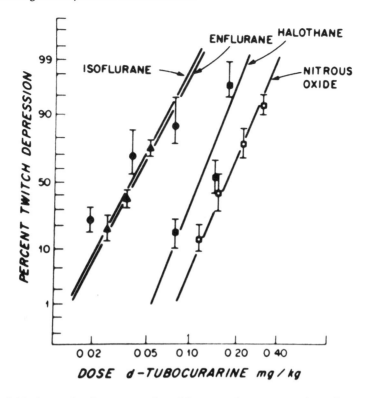

Figure 3.11. Anaesthesia was produced in normal normocapnic patients with a balanced technique or with 1.25 MAC enflurane, halothane, or isoflurane. Halothane potentiated the effect of d-tubocurarine more than the balanced technique with nitrous oxide. Isoflurane and enflurane, in turn, produced a greater potentiation (by a factor of 2 or 3) than did halothane. From Ali and Savarese (1976), with permission.

Complications

There are potential complications from the use of volatile anaesthetic agents related to technique as well as to the fact that the drug was used. Technique complications include laryngospasm, bronchospasm etc. and will not be discussed here.

Malignant hyperthermia

There is an association between the volatile anaesthetics and the triggering of malignant hyperthermia (Brown and Gandolfi, 1987). This condition will be discussed in Chapter 21.

Renal toxicity

Inorganic fluoride in high concentrations has been associated with renal damage (50 μmol/l). The infamous example of this is methoxyflurane. One of the metabolic products of enflurane is inorganic fluoride. However, as a practical matter the inorganic fluoride levels with enflurane do not usually achieve the levels associated with renal damage. Obese patients do have higher levels of inorganic fluoride than non-obese patients (Strube et al, 1987). This is thought to be secondary to the large amount of fat tissue which traps more of the anaesthetic gas and allows for more metabolism of the enflurane. It would appear to have no clinical consequences, however.

Analgesia

None of the three commonly used inhalational agents have significant analgesic properties.

Hepatitis

The patient who develops jaundice in the postoperative period represents an enormous dilemma for the anaesthetist. There are many causes of post-operative jaundice but the one that the anaesthetist is most concerned about is whether or not the patient has drug-induced hepatitis from the volatile anaesthetic. There is good evidence that halothane hepatitis is a multifac-torial disease. Possibilities to explain the hepatotoxicity of halothane include: metabolite-mediated hepatotoxicity, genetic predisposition, immu-nologically mediated hepatotoxicity and hypoxic liver injury.

Metabolite-mediated hepatotoxicity.   When one considers the degree of biotransformation that the various inhalation anaesthetics undergo, halothane is by far the leader (Cousins et al, 1987). Approximately 20% of the inhaled halothane will be metabolized. Approximately 2.4% of enflurane and 0.17% of isoflurane will undergo biotransformation and metabolism within the body. In general, the metabolism of halothane is predominantly oxidative but it is felt that under conditions where halothane undergoes reductive metabolism there may be the formation of free radicals which are capable of covalent binding, and that this may lead to direct liver cell membrane injury. The other possibility is that the damaged cell mem-brane may result in the formation of a hapten and an immunological response. In addition the whole process may be accentuated by hypoxia secondary to a reduction in liver blood flow. Seyde et al (1986) have shown a reduction in liver blood flow with the administration of halothane and nitrous oxide.

Genetic factors.   There appears to be a very small number of patients with a genetic predisposition to the development of halothane hepatitis

(Cousins et al, 1981). Hoft et al (1980) reported the development of halothane hepatitis in three pairs of closely related women. Farrell et al (1985) demonstrated a nucleophilic attack using a phenytoin preparation and the white cells of patients who developed hepatic necrosis after halothane. Some 50% of the family members showed a similar nucleophilic attack even though no one else in the family had ever had a problem of halothane hepatitis. Studies in three strains of guinea-pigs who underwent multiple exposures to halothane demonstrated the generation of an antibody response to a reactive intermediate of halothane (Siadat-Pajouh et al, 1987). A genetic predisposition to developing halothane hepatitis is poorly expressed in children and this may be one reason why children have such a low incidence of halothane hepatitis compared with adults. The incidence in adults ranges from 1/10 000 to 1/35 000 whereas in children the incidence in one study was 1/82 000 patients (Wark, 1983).

Immunologically mediated hepatotoxicity. The diagnosis of halothane hepatitis is usually made by an exclusionary process after checking for viral antibodies as well as the history of transfusions etc. It is most helpful if the diagnosis of halothane hepatitis can be made in a positive fashion. There has been strong suggestion in recent years that halothane can cause a specific immunological injury (Neuberger et al, 1983). Vergani (1986) studied a group of patients with halothane hepatitis, a control group, a group of patients exposed to halothane who did not develop hepatitis, and a group of patients who developed hepatitis without exposure. He took hepatocytes from rabbits who had been exposed to halothane and incubated them with the serum from the various patient groups. The hypothesis was that if there was an immunological injury, the circulating antibodies in the patients would then be directed against the hepatocytes which had been altered by halothane and this would be detected by immunofluorescent techniques. Nine of 13 patients with presumed severe halothane hepatitis demonstrated the antibodies, whereas sera from normal controls, patients exposed to halothane without hepatitis and patients with non-halothane hepatitis were negative when tested for antibodies. There is some disagreement about the reliability of this test but it is a step in the appropriate direction of being able to make a positive diagnosis of halothane hepatitis.

Enflurane and isoflurane hepatitis. Alteration in liver enzyme can be demonstrated not only in halothane anaesthesia but also with enflurane and isoflurane. However, several reviews of cases of reported enflurane alterations of liver enzymes (Eger et al, 1986) and isoflurane hepatitis strongly suggest that the incidence of hepatitis with these two agents is extremely low.

Clinical considerations in halothane hepatitis. Inhalation anaesthetics provide the basis for most paediatric anaesthetics. The objective of the anaesthetist is to provide the surgeon with ideal operating conditions and to provide the child with a safe anaesthetic. This can be done by understanding the advantages and limitations of the various inhalation anaesthetics (Table 3.3) and their alternatives. This provides conditions as near as possible to the ideal anaesthetic state and, in addition, gives the anaesthetist enormous satisfaction.

Table 3.3. Relative properties of commonly used inhalational agents

	Halothane	Enflurane	Isoflurane
Acceptability	+++	++	+
Rapid uptake	+++	++	+
Rapid elimination	+	++	+++
CVS stability			
Cardiac output	++	++	+++
SVR	+++	++	+
Adrenaline	+	+++	++
RS stability	+++	+	++
Muscle relaxation	+	+++	+++
ICP	++	+	+++
Nephrotoxicity	+++	+	+++
Analgesia	—	—	—
Metabolism	+	++	+++

+++ Most satisfactory; ++ less satisfactory; + least satisfactory.
CVS, cardiovascular system; SVR, systemic vascular resistance; RS, respiratory system; ICP, intracranial pressure.

All drugs have a risk:benefit ratio. There is no question but that the risk: benefit ratio for halothane hepatitis in adults is greater than for either enflurane or isoflurane. There are certain patients who have a higher predisposition to develop halothane hepatitis. These categories include repeated anaesthetics, obesity and females. Halothane hepatitis has been reported in children, although it appears to be much rarer than in adults. Only one death from halothane hepatitis has so far been reported in a child in the UK. Many paediatric anaesthetists still feel that the benefits of halothane in children outweigh the risks (Battersby et al, 1987; Black et al, 1987).

A high percentage of adult patients who have developed fatal or severe halothane hepatitis have a history that the previous halothane anaesthetic resulted in a mild degree of hepatitis characterized by pyrexia and/or malaise. The same history may be found in children (Whitburn and Sumner, 1986). Therefore, it appears that careful history and attention to previous records would help to reduce the incidence of halothane hepatitis. If there is any questionable history after a halothane anaesthetic alternate techniques should be considered.

REFERENCES

Ali HH & Savarese JJ (1976) Monitoring of neuromuscular function. *Anesthesiology* **45:** 216–249.
Anand KJS & Hickey PR (1987) Randomised trial of high-dose sufentanil anesthesia in neonates undergoing cardiac surgery: effects on the metabolic stress response. *Anesthesiology* **67:** A502.

Anand KJS, Sippell WG & Aynsley-Green A (1987) Randomised trial of fentanyl anaesthesia in preterm babies undergoing surgery: effects on the stress response. *Lancet* **i:** 243–248.

Anand KJS, Sippell WG, Schofield NM & Aynsley-Green A (1988) Does halothane anaesthesia decrease the metabolic and endocrine stress responses of newborn infants undergoing operation? *British Medical Journal* **296:** 668–671.

Artru AA (1983) Relationship between cerebral blood volume and CSF pressure during anesthesia with halothane or enflurane in dogs. *Anesthesiology* **58:** 533–539.

Artru AA (1984) Relationship between cerebral blood volume and CSF pressure during anesthesia with isoflurane or fentanyl in dogs. *Anesthesiology* **60:** 575–579.

Bahlman SH, Eger EI II, Halsey MJ et al (1972) The cardiovascular effects of halothane in man during spontaneous ventilation. *Anesthesiology* **36:** 494–502.

Barash PG, Glanz S, Katz JD, Taunt K & Talner NS (1978) Ventricular function in children during halothane anesthesia: an echocardiographic evaluation. *Anesthesiology* **49:** 79–85.

Battersby EF, Bingham R, Facer E et al (1987) Halothane hepatitis in children. *British Medical Journal* **295:** 117.

Black GW, Hatch DJ & Morris P (1987) Halothane hepatitis in children. *British Medical Journal* **295:** 117.

Brandom BW, Brandom RB & Cook DR (1983) Uptake and distribution of halothane in infants: in vivo measurements and computer simulations. *Anesthesia and Analgesia* **62:** 404–410.

Brown BR & Gandolfi AJ (1987) Adverse effects of volatile anaesthetics. *British Journal of Anaesthesia* **59:** 14–23.

Burrows FA, Shutack JG & Crone RK (1983) Inappropriate secretion of antidiuretic hormone in a postsurgical pediatric population. *Critical Care Medicine* **11:** 527.

Calverley RK, Smith NT, Jones CW, Prys-Roberts C & Eger EI II (1978a) Ventilatory and cardiovascular effects of enflurane anesthesia during spontaneous ventilation in man. *Anesthesia and Analgesia* **57:** 610–618.

Calverley RK, Smith NT, Prys-Roberts C, Eger EI II & Jones CW (1978b) Cardiovascular effects of enflurane anesthesia during controlled ventilation in man. *Anesthesia and Analgesia* **57:** 619–628.

Cameron CB, Robinson S & Gregory GA (1984) The minimum alveolar concentration of isoflurane in children. *Anesthesia and Analgesia* **63:** 418–420.

Cousins MJ, Gourlay GK, Hall P de la M & Adams J (1981) Genetics and halothane hepatitis. *British Medical Journal* **283:** 1334.

Cousins MJ, Gourlay GK, Knights KM, Hall P de la M, Lunam CA & O'Brien P (1987) A randomized prospective controlled study of the metabolism and hepatotoxicity of halothane in humans. *Anesthesia and Analgesia* **66:** 299–308.

Cromwell TH, Eger EI II, Stevens WC & Dolan WM (1971a) Forane uptake, excretion, and blood solubility in man. *Anesthesiology* **35:** 401–408.

Cromwell TH, Stevens WC, Eger EI II et al (1971b) The cardiovascular effects of compound 469 (Forane) during spontaneous ventilation and CO_2 challenge in man. *Anesthesiology* **35:** 17–25.

Diaz JH & Lockhart CH (1979) Is halothane really safe in infancy? *Anesthesiology* **51:** S313.

Eger EI II (1981) *Isoflurane (Forane): A Compendium and Reference.* Madison, Wisconsin: Ohio Medical Products.

Eger EI II, Smith NT, Stoelting RK et al (1970) Cardiovascular effects of halothane in man. *Anesthesiology* **32:** 396–409.

Eger EI II, Smuckler EA, Ferrell LD, Goldsmith CH & Johnson BH (1986) Is enflurane hepatotoxic? *Anesthesia and Analgesia* **65:** 21–30.

Farrell G, Prendergast D & Murray M (1985) Halothane hepatitis. Detection of a constitutional susceptibility factor. *New England Journal of Medicine* **313:** 1310.

Fisher DM, Robinson S, Brett C, Gregory GA & Perin G (1984) Comparison of enflurane, halothane, and isoflurane for outpatient pediatric anesthesia. *Anesthesiology* **61**: A427.

Friedman WF (1972) The intrinsic physiologic properties of the developing heart. *Progress in Cardiovascular Diseases* **15**: 87–111.

Friesen RH & Henry DB (1986) Cardiovascular changes in preterm neonates receiving isoflurane, halothane, fentanyl and ketamine. *Anesthesiology* **64**: 238–242.

Friesen RH & Lichtor JL (1982) Cardiovascular depression during halothane anesthesia in infants: a study of three induction techniques. *Anesthesia and Analgesia* **61**: 42.

Friesen RH & Lichtor JL (1983) Cardiovascular effects of inhalation induction with isoflurane in infants. *Anesthesia and Analgesia* **62**: 411–414.

Gregory GA (1982) The baroresponses of preterm infants during halothane anaesthesia. *Canadian Anaesthetists Society Journal* **29**: 105–107.

Gregory GA, Eger EI II & Munson ES (1969) The relationship between age and halothane requirement in man. *Anesthesiology* **30**: 488–491.

Hecker BR, Lake CL, DiFazio CA, Moscicki JC & Engle JS (1983) The decrease of the minimum alveolar anesthetic concentration produced by sufentanil in rats. *Anesthesia and Analgesia* **62**: 987–990.

Hickey PR, Hansen DD, Strafford M, Thompson JE, Jonas RE & Mayer JE (1986) Pulmonary and systemic hemodynamic effects of nitrous oxide in infants with normal and elevated pulmonary vascular resistance. *Anesthesiology* **65**: 374–378.

Hoft RH, Bunker JP, Goodman HI & Gregory PB (1980) Halothane hepatitis in three pairs of closely related women. *New England Journal of Medicine* **304**: 1023.

Johnston RR, Eger EI II & Wilson C (1976) A comparative interaction of epinephrine with enflurane, isoflurane, and halothane in man. *Anesthesia and Analgesia* **55**: 709–712.

Karl HW, Swedlow MD, Lee KW & Downes JJ (1983) Epinephrine–halothane interactions in children. *Anesthesiology* **58**: 142–145.

Knill RL & Clement JL (1984) Site of selective action of halothane on the peripheral chemoreflex pathway in humans. *Anesthesiology* **61**: 121–126.

Koehntop DE, Rodman JH, Brundage DM, Hegland MG & Buckley JJ (1986) Pharmacokinetics of fentanyl in neonates. *Anesthesia and Analgesia* **65**: 227–232.

Lake CL, DiFazio CA, Moscicki JC & Engle JS (1985) Reduction in halothane MAC: comparison of morphine and alfentanil. *Anesthesia and Analgesia* **64**: 807–810.

LeDez KM & Lerman J (1987) The minimum alveolar concentration (MAC) of isoflurane in preterm neonates. *Anesthesiology* **67**: 301–307.

Lerman J, Robinson S, Willis MM & Gregory GA (1983) Anesthetic requirements for halothane in young children 0–1 month and 1–6 months of age. *Anesthesiology* **59**: 421–424.

Marshall WK, Bedford RF, Arnold WP et al (1981) Effects of propranolol on the cardiovascular and renin–angiotensin systems during hypotension produced by sodium nitroprusside in man. *Anesthesiology* **55**: 277–280.

McNeil AM, Lerman J & Gregory GA (1984) Echocardiographic assessment of ventricular function in children during isoflurane anesthesia. *Anesthesiology* **61**: A426.

Merkel G & Eger EI II (1963) A comparative study of halothane and halopropane anesthesia. *Anesthesiology* **24**: 346.

Moss IR, Conner H, Yee WFH, Iorio P & Scarpelli EM (1982) Human β-endorphin-like immunoreactivity in the perinatal/neonatal period. *Journal of Pediatrics* **101**: 443–446.

Murat I, Chaussain M, Hamja J et al (1987) The respiratory effects of isoflurane, enflurane and halothane in spontaneously breathing children. *Anaesthesia* **42**: 711–718.

Munson ES, Eger EI II, Tham MK & Embro WJ (1978) Increase in anesthetic uptake, excretion and blood solubility in man after eating. *Anesthesia and Analgesia* **57**: 224–231.

Murphy FL Jr, Kennell EM, Johnstone RE et al (1974) The effects of enflurane, isoflurane, and halothane on cerebral blood flow and metabolism in man. *Abstracts of Scientific Papers, Annual Meeting of the American Society of Anesthesiologists*, pp 61–62.

Murphy MR & Hug CC (1982) The enflurane sparing effect of morphine, butorphanol and nalbuphine. *Anesthesiology* **57**: 489–492.

Neal MB, Peterson MD, Gloyna D et al (1984) Hemodynamic and cardiovascular effects of halothane and isoflurane anesthesia in children. *Anesthesiology* **61**: A437.

Neuberger J, Gimson AES, Davis M & Williams R (1983) Specific serological markers in the diagnosis of fulminant hepatic failure associated with halothane anaesthesia. *British Journal of Anaesthesia* **55**: 15–19.

O'Neill MP, Sharkey AJ, Fee JPH & Black GW (1982) A comparative study of enflurane and halothane in children. *Anaesthesia* **37**: 634–639.

Roizen MF, Lampe GH, Benefiel DJ & Sohn YJ (1987a) Is increased operative stress associated with worse outcome? *Anesthesiology* **67**: A1.

Roizen MF, Plummer GO & Lichtor JL (1987b) Nitrous oxide and dysrhythmias. *Anesthesiology* **66**: 427–431.

Saidman LJ & Eger EI II (1964) Effect of nitrous oxide and of narcotic premedication on the alveolar concentration of halothane required for anesthesia. *Anesthesiology* **25**: 302.

Seyde WC, Ellis JE & Longnecker DE (1986) The addition of nitrous oxide to halothane decreases renal and splanchnic flow and increases cerebral blood flow in rats. *British Journal of Anaesthesia* **58**: 63–68.

Siadat-Pajouh M, Hubbard AK, Roth TP & Gandolfi AJ (1987) Generation of halothane-induced immune response in a guinea pig model of halothane hepatitis. *Anesthesia and Analgesia* **66**: 1209–1214.

Stevens WC, Cromwell TH, Halsey MJ et al (1971) The cardiovascular effects of a new inhalation anesthetic, Forane, in human volunteers at constant arterial carbon dioxide tension. *Anesthesiology* **35**: 8–16.

Strube PJ, Hulands GH & Halsey MJ (1987) Serum fluoride levels in morbidly obese patients: enflurane compared with isoflurane anaesthesia. *Anaesthesia* **42**: 685–689.

Torri G, Damia G & Fabiani ML (1974) Effect of nitrous oxide on the anesthetic requirement of enflurane. *British Journal of Anaesthesia* **46**: 468.

Ueda W, Hirakawa M & Mae O (1983) Appraisal of epinephrine administration to patients under halothane anesthesia for closure of cleft palate. *Anesthesiology* **58**: 574–576.

Vergani D (1986) Immunological aspects of liver function and halothane hepatotoxicity. Halothane and the liver: The problem revisited. Proceedings of a symposium at Bristol University Medical School, April.

Wark HJ (1983) Postoperative jaundice in children. *Anaesthesia* **38**: 237–242.

Whitburn RH & Sumner E (1986) Halothane hepatitis in an 11-month-old child. *Anaesthesia* **41**: 611–613.

Winter PM, Hornbein TF, Smith G, Sullivan D & Smith KH (1972) Hyperbaric nitrous oxide anesthesia in man: determination of anesthetic potency (MAC) and cardiorespiratory effects. *Abstracts of Scientific Papers, Annual Meeting of the American Society of Anesthesiologists*, pp 103–104.

Wren WS, Allen P, Synnott A & O'Griofa P (1986) Effects of nitrous oxide on the respiratory pattern of spontaneously breathing children—a reappraisal. *British Journal of Anaesthesia* **58**: 274–279.

Yaster M (1987) The dose response of fentanyl in neonatal anesthesia. *Anesthesiology* **66**: 433–435.

Intravenous agents in paediatric anaesthesia

INTRODUCTION

It is now well recognized that infants and children cannot merely be thought of as 'little adults' with respect to either drug effects or disposition. Paediatric pharmacology and therapeutics deal with an immature individual in a continuous state of development of anatomical and physiological function. There is no simple or reliable means of extrapolating to children drug dosage guidelines determined in adults. Dosage schedules based on body weight may be insufficient to achieve a given plasma concentration, or conversely, may result in toxic effects. Dosage based on surface area usually has more validity because this parameter correlates with some of the physiological changes that are important in determining differences in pharmacokinetics in patients of different ages, but has to be predicted rather than measured. Doses of intravenous sedative and analgesic agents must be modified in patients who have received sedative premedication and in those receiving inhalational agents.

This chapter does not aim to provide a comprehensive review of all drugs that may be administered intravenously by anaesthetists to paediatric patients. Examination of the pharmacokinetic data and clinical studies that relate to some commonly used intravenous anaesthetic agents may enable the reader better to comprehend the basic principles involved in the selection and administration of any drug to young patients.

Before discussing pharmacokinetic data and dosage schedules for individual drugs, it may be helpful to explain firstly some of the concepts embodied in the terminology of pharmacokinetic data, and secondly, to examine the changes in pharmacokinetic functions that occur in the developing infant and child.

PHARMACOKINETICS

The study of drugs is conventionally considered under two main headings—pharmacokinetics and pharmacodynamics. Pharmacokinetics involves the quantitative study of drug absorption, distribution, metabolism and excretion, while pharmacodynamics is the study of the effects of a drug.

The principles of pharmacokinetics are based on models. In the simplest model, the body is considered to be a single compartment within which the drug is uniformly and rapidly distributed. The apparent volume of distribution (Vd) of the drug is the total amount of drug in the body divided by its concentration in plasma. Thus if a drug is concentrated in extravascular tissues, the Vd can be very large. The removal of drug from this compartment is usually exponential or first order, which means that the same fraction of drug is eliminated in any given time period. The rate of this exponential process may be expressed as its half-life, which is the time necessary for a 50% reduction in drug plasma concentration. It follows that the half-life of a drug is independent of dosage unless the elimination process becomes saturated. If this occurs, then zero order kinetics are followed; in this case a constant amount of drug is eliminated in a given time. The total body clearance (CI) of a drug is the volume of plasma from which all available drug is completely removed per unit of time, and is a product of Vd and the elimination rate constant. It can be measured by dividing the total dose of a drug by the area under the concentration–time curve following a single intravenous injection.

A more useful pharmacokinetic representation is the two-compartment model in which redistribution of a drug from plasma into tissues is taken into account. In this model, the change in plasma drug concentration with time can be represented by two exponential decay curves, as shown in Figure 4.1. The first and faster decay represents redistribution from a central to a peripheral compartment, and the second represents elimination. Although each phase has its own half-life (the distribution half-life, t½α and the elimination half-life, t½β), it should be appreciated that the process of distribution of drugs between compartments continues throughout the elimination phase, as long as the drug is present in the body. Similarly, the processes of metabolism and excretion begin as soon as the drug reaches the appropriate tissues.

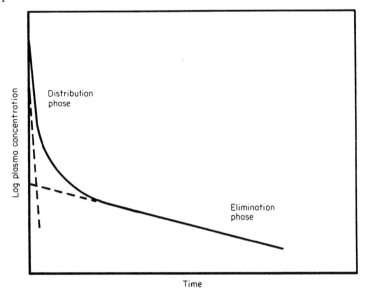

Figure 4.1. Diagrammatic representation of a plasma decay curve for drug disposition in a two-compartment model after a single injection.

The pharmacological effect of a drug bears no inherent relationship to its half-life. The correlation of concentration with response varies depending on the drug; often it is very tenuous. However, from some drugs, such as morphine or fentanyl, knowledge of the elimination half-life may help to predict the rate at which drug response decays following cessation of therapy. For many drugs the relation between elimination half-life and effect is non-existent; drugs which are enzyme inhibitors or which bind covalently to receptors are examples. For drugs whose effect can be related to plasma drug concentration, it may be possible to give guidelines for dosage regimes by using pharmacokinetic data and desired blood levels, e.g.:

Loading dose (mg/kg) = Vd (ml/kg) × plasma concentration required (mg/ml)
Infusion rate (mg/kg/min) = CL (ml/min/kg) × plasma concentration required (mg/ml)

However, it must be remembered that there is often great interpatient variability both in pharmacokinetic and pharmacodynamic processes. Thus the above equations must be used only as guidelines and dosages should be reviewed in the light of clinical experience.

Developmental factors affecting pharmacokinetics

Changes in apparent volume of distribution (Vd)

There is of course a continuous change in body weight and relative body composition throughout childhood. The limited data that are available on distribution volumes in the paediatric patient suggest that the Vd is often relatively greater (in terms of l/kg body weight) in the newborn period and throughout childhood as compared to the adult. These changes in body composition affecting Vd can be broadly divided into three—changes in lipid content, changes in water content and distribution, and protein binding.

Changes in lipid content. The relative body lipid content is lower in the newborn, especially in the preterm infant, but the central nervous system (CNS) constitutes a greater proportion of lipid mass in infancy. In addition, the blood–brain barrier of the newborn may allow for increased passage of some drugs across it. The relative amount of subcutaneous fatty tissue increases to its greatest value at 9 months of age, decreases until 6 years, then begins to rise again as adolescence approaches. These changes will affect the distribution of lipid-soluble drugs.

Changes in water content (see Figure 4.2). There is a gradual decrease in the water content of the fetus during development such that water constitutes 95% by weight of the small embryo, compared with 75% in the term neonate. By 1 year of age, total body water (TBW) has fallen to adult proportions (55% of body weight). From this point there is a linear relationship between TBW and lean body mass until old age. These changes in TBW

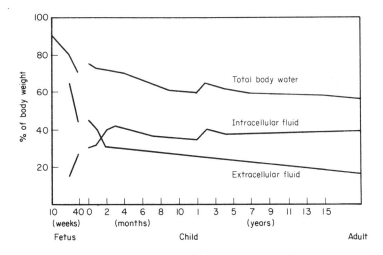

Figure 4.2. Age-related differences in body water distribution.

are of particular relevance for predominantly water-soluble drugs, such as midazolam, rather than for lipophilic drugs such as opioids. At equilibrium, non-ionized water-soluble drugs will be uniformly distributed throughout the TBW and these changes in TBW will have a significant effect on the distribution volume of drugs that have small or moderate values for Vd.

Conventionally, body water is divided into discrete compartments: intracellular (ICF) and extracellular fluid (ECF). The latter accounts for approximately 45% of the full-term newborn weight, but this proportion falls steeply during the first weeks of life to reach 30% at 6 months. The fall in the ECF fraction continues for much longer than does the change in TBW, and it is still well above the adult value of 16% at 10 years. This fall in the percentage of ECF is greater than the fall in TBW because there is a simultaneous rise in ICF. The proportion of ICF shows an increase from 30% of body weight at birth to the adult value of 40% at 7 years. Ionized drugs tend to be confined to the extracellular compartment, so that changes in the relative sizes of the two compartments during growth will influence the effective concentration of these drugs.

Protein binding.   Many drugs bind to proteins or other macro-molecules and this drug–protein complex differs from the free drug in that it may lack pharmacological activity, cannot penetrate cell membranes and is often not directly available for biotransformation and elimination. Changes in protein binding will therefore cause changes in both the apparent volume of distribution and the elimination half-life of a drug. In preterm infants the serum albumin concentration may be low, as levels tend to rise with increasing gestational age (Hyvarinen et al, 1973). During the neonatal period variable amounts of fetal albumin, which has a lower affinity for drugs than adult albumin, may also persist. The concentrations of γ-globulins and lipoproteins (which have a major contribution to fentanyl binding, for instance) are also lower.

When all plasma protein-binding sites are occupied, the addition of more drug increases the unbound fraction by a disproportionate amount, thus making more drug available to the tissues. This can be a particular problem in the neonatal period when high levels of unconjugated bilirubin or free fatty acids are not uncommon, as these substances compete with acidic drugs at albumin-binding sites. Thus, compared with the adult, protein binding of many drugs is much reduced in the neonate, leading to increased concentration of the free drug. In fact, protein binding of acidic drugs does not reach adult values for 2–3 years and adult levels of γ-globulin may only be reached by 7–12 years (Morselli et al, 1983). The relationship between the degree of drug–protein binding, changes that occur in the amount of free drug, and the resultant concentration is not a straightforward one. Increased amounts of free drug will increase availability to receptors, but also to some metabolic and excretory functions. In addition, some hepatic and renal tubular functions can act on both bound and free drug. The Vd of the drug, therefore, may be altered without a change in the elimination half-life, and it becomes difficult to predict the resultant net effect on the pharmacokinetics of a particular drug.

Changes in elimination of drugs with age

Metabolism and excretion together constitute the body's mechanisms for eliminating drugs. There are marked variations in rates of drug elimination in infants and children compared to adults.

Hepatic function. The liver is quantitatively the most important organ for drug metabolism in all age groups. There is a change in the relative hepatic size with increasing age: the fetal liver is 4% of TBW compared to 2% in the adult. This provides the child with a theoretical relative increase in hepatic surface area available for drug metabolism.

The second important variable for drug metabolism is the quantitative change in the hepatic drug-metabolizing enzyme systems with increasing postconceptional age. In vitro studies have shown that at term cytochrome P-450 and NADPH-cytochrome-C-reductase activity is only about one-half of adult values (Aranda et al, 1974). Although human fetal liver can catalyse the glucuronidation of morphine (Pacifici et al, 1982), conjugation with glucuronic acid reaches adult values only after 3 years of age. Tserng et al (1983), studying theophylline metabolism in preterm infants 28–42 weeks post conception, demonstrated a gradual change from methylation to oxidation and demethylation pathways, suggesting differential development of different forms of hepatic cytochrome P-450. For theophylline at least, it seems that drug metabolism increases with postconceptual age, and reaches adult levels by 7 months of age. Other drugs studied in the neonatal period include paracetamol and aspirin, where elimination half-lives are close to those of the adult. This is due to the use of different metabolic pathways for these drugs in the neonate. Paracetamol, for instance, is excreted predominantly as a sulphate conjugate in neonates and only to a minor degree as the glucuronide, whereas the opposite occurs in adults.

Conventionally, drugs which are cleared by the liver are often divided into those whose clearance is mainly dependent on hepatic blood flow and those whose clearance depends largely on metabolism by the liver cells. For drugs with a high hepatic extraction ratio, such as morphine, the $t\frac{1}{2}\beta$ should tend to reflect hepatic blood flow and be relatively unaffected by microsomal activity. In fact, this generalization is only valid once hepatic metabolism has achieved a critical value, and does not always remain true throughout the neonatal period. For drugs with a low hepatic extraction ratio, the $t\frac{1}{2}\beta$ will tend to reflect differences in hepatic enzyme activity. These differences can change dramatically during the first few years of life.

The neonatal period, a time of reduced metabolic degradation, is usually followed by a dramatic increase in the metabolic rate of mainly phase one reactions such as oxidation or demethylation; the drug disposition rate may pass from that of one-fifth of the adult to one five times faster than in adults (Morselli et al, 1983). This increased drug-metabolizing activity is usually evident from 2–3 months up to 3 years of age, when values gradually decline to reach those of adults at puberty.

Renal function (see also p. 194).   Excretion is the ultimate route for drug elimination from the body, either as unchanged drug or as metabolites produced by the liver or other tissues. Excretion may occur through bile, faeces, urine or lungs, with the kidney being the primary drug-excretory organ for drugs administered intravenously. As with the liver, there are developmental changes that occur in the renal drug-eliminating processes. Although the ratio of the neonatal kidney mass to body weight is twice that of adults, the organ is anatomically and physiologically immature, with all aspects of renal function being reduced.

A progressive rise in glomerular filtration rate (GFR) in the neonatal period is related to increasing renal perfusion and to a marked decrease in renal arteriolar vascular resistance. However, although GFR is about one-quarter of that expected when related to size, glomerular function is still relatively more mature than tubular function in the newborn. Postnatal growth of the kidney is largely accounted for by an increase in tubular mass which is accompanied by an improvement in function. The immature kidney is relatively poor at concentrating urine, but this is due, at least in part, to the lower level of production and excretion of urea, resulting in low osmotic gradients in the renal papillae. Nevertheless, there is some residual deficiency in renal concentrating capacity which improves with age and which reflects the fewer and shorter loops of Henle in the developing kidney; adult renal function is achieved by about 2 years of age.

The importance of immature renal function with respect to the metabolism and elimination of various drugs is not always clear, but may sometimes be more important than was previously thought (see morphine elimination, p. 79). Certainly there are drugs, such as antibiotics, that depend primarily on renal excretion for elimination from the body. Caution must be exercised when repeated administration of any drug to patients with poor renal function is being considered, and if possible, drug plasma concentrations should be monitored to avoid drug accumulation and possible toxic effects.

General factors affecting pharmacokinetics

Hypovolaemia and hypotension

Hypovolaemia and/or hypotension will result in reduced tissue perfusion which can have profound effects on drug pharmacokinetics. The distribution of drugs between the blood and poorly perfused tissues will be restricted, which may result in greater distribution to those tissues whose perfusion is maintained, such as the brain. In addition, drug may become sequestered in fat or muscle, only to return to the vascular compartment and thus to other tissues when perfusion is restored to normal. If renal or hepatic blood flow is reduced by hypovolaemia or hypotension, drug elimination may also be markedly affected. In the neonate, because of poor autoregulation mechanisms, a reduction of cerebral blood flow with a preferential perfusion of brainstem structures may occur secondary to systemic hypotension. This in turn may lead not only to modified brain distribution of lipophilic drugs (which are flow-dependent), but also to alterations in their absorption and excretion rates.

Hypothermia

The effects of hypothermia are similar to those following hypotension and hypovolaemia, though in addition the metabolic rate may be decreased, if there is no shivering. In profound hypothermia, as produced commonly for open heart surgery, drug metabolism and elimination will be severely restricted. However, these effects will be overshadowed in most cases by the dilution with bypass prime blood.

Ventilation/pH changes

Drug ionization is affected by the pH of the tissues, and the degree of ionization will influence the distribution of drugs between the body compartments. This is potentially important in relation to drug distribution to the brain which may also be affected directly by changes in blood flow induced by hyper- or hypocarbia.

INDIVIDUAL INTRAVENOUS DRUGS

Induction agents

The perfect intravenous induction agent has yet to be discovered. Although there are many drugs that have been used to produce unconsciousness, at the present time there is no one drug that can reliably induce anaesthesia within one arm–brain circulation time, allow complete recovery within a few minutes, and yet be totally free from unwanted effects.

The drugs that are considered under this section are quite diverse in their chemical formulation. However they share one characteristic: they all reliably produce loss of consciousness in one arm–brain circulation time. Other drugs that can induce anaesthesia, albeit more slowly and/or less reliably, are considered under separate sections.

Thiopentone

Thiopentone is the most commonly used intravenous induction agent in both adult and paediatric anaesthetic practice. It remains the standard against which all other induction agents are compared.

Pharmacokinetics.   Thiopentone has a rapid onset of action: peak concentrations are reached in the heart and brain usually within one circulation time and diffusion into the CNS is facilitated by its high lipid solubility. As thiopentone has a pK of 7.6, changes in blood pH can lead to significant changes in the degree of ionization of the drug. An alkalosis, for example, will cause an increase in ionization of thiopentone with a decrease in both potency and the apparent volume of distribution.

Approximately 87% of thiopentone is reversibly bound to plasma albumin (Sorbo et al, 1984). This value is apparently the same for infants, children and young adults, though it decreases with age thereafter. The plasma decay of thiopentone can usually be fitted to a bi- or tri-exponential curve, representing a two- or three-compartment model. The initial decline in plasma concentration is over 2–4 min, representing the extensive redistribution of drug to other tissues including muscle and fat. This is followed by a slower distribution phase lasting 40–50 min. These values are apparently unaffected by age.

Metabolism and excretion.   Thiopentone is almost completely metabolized in the liver; its high lipid solubility precludes significant renal excretion. The main metabolic pathway is by oxidation which produces a pharmacologically inactive metabolite. There is very little metabolism of thiopentone in the first 15 min following administration and hepatic function does not contribute significantly to the recovery time.

Elimination of the drug is limited by the metabolic capacity of the liver and is unaffected by hepatic blood flow. In infants and children the elimination half-life following a single dose has been calculated at 6.1($\pm$3.3) h (Sorbo et al, 1984). This compares with values of 6–12 h obtained in healthy adults (Table 4.1). Pharmacokinetic data on similar drugs studied in the newborn infant suggest that a prolongation of elimination half-life for thiopentone should be expected for this age group (Morselli et al, 1983).

Clinical effects.   All short-acting barbiturates cause direct myocardial depression. The degree of depression is related both to the dose and rate of administration, as these are the prime determinants of the peak blood level obtained. Experimental work on dogs and healthy adult volunteers has suggested that decreases in myocardial contractility are usually compen-

Table 4.1. Age-related differences in pharmacokinetic parameters for induction agents (pooled data)

Drug		Apparent volume of distribution (l/kg)	Elimination half-life (min)	Clearance (ml/kg/min)
Thiopentone	Infant	—	—	—
	Child	2.1	360	6.6
	Adult	2.2	540	3.2
Methohexitone	Infant	—	—	—
	Child	2.1	193	18.0
	Adult	2.2	230	11.5
Propofol	Infant	—	—	—
	Child	—	—	—
	Adult	4.6	78	29.0
Ketamine	Infant	—	—	—
	Child	1.9	100	16.8
	Adult	2.6	185	16.0

sated for by increases in heart rate. This in turn increases myocardial oxygen utilization which may be important in patients with compromised myocardial perfusion. Short-acting barbituates, when given in single doses, seem to have little effect on systemic vascular resistance (SVR) and alterations in arterial blood pressure are secondary to changes in cardiac output. The transient mild to moderate hypotension often seen following thiopentone administration is of no clinical significance to the healthy patient. However, patients who are hypovolaemic or who are being supported by high levels of endogenous sympathetic activity may be acutely decompensated by normally safe doses of thiopentone. This is because thiopentone administration not only decreases myocardial contractility but also results in increased distensibility of the peripheral venous system and thus an increase in the volume of blood occupying the venous capacitance vessels. It also reduces sympathetic outflow from the CNS. Todd and co-workers (1985) have demonstrated some of the haemodynamic consequences of thiopentone given by infusion in high dosage (75 mg/kg/h) to 10 neurosurgical patients aged 12 to 42 years. Significant increases in heart rate (116% of control), and decreases in arterial pressure (87% of control), stroke volume index (87% of control), SVR (84%) and both left and right ventricular stroke work indices (66 and 69% of control, respectively), were observed. There were no changes in pulmonary arterial pressure or vascular resistance (PVR).

The only other important side-effect of thiopentone is respiratory depression, the extent depending on the dose and speed of injection or previous opioid administration. Transient apnoeas are common, but do not normally require intervention unless the dose has been unusually large. True allergic reactions are extremely rare, but can be life-threatening when they do occur.

Dosage and administration.   Thiopentone should never be given in a concentration greater than 2.5%. Higher concentrations offer no advantages but have a reduced margin of safety and increased local toxicity. The sleep dosage required for healthy premedicated infants and children normally varies between 4 and 5 mg/kg but may be greatly reduced in the very sick infant or child. Whenever practical it is best to titrate the drug against effect by administering in incremental doses. However, in the wriggling infant or the very apprehensive child this may not always be easy or even desirable. The judgement of the smallest dose that will produce the desired effect will often have to be determined in advance and the experience of the anaesthetist then becomes even more important.

In healthy unpremedicated infants and children, dose requirements of thiopentone required to abolish lid and corneal reflexes increase to 5–7 mg/kg and do not seem to vary with age (Brett and Fisher, 1987). However, the dose of thiopentone required to produce loss of laryngeal reflexes is probably larger in paediatric patients than adults, and the dose needed to abolish response to fitting of a facemask is higher in infants than in older children (Jonmarker et el, 1987). Neonates, however, need less thiopentone than older infants to achieve the same loss of reflexes and 2–4 mg/kg should not be exceeded.

Methohexitone

Although methohexitone has been in use since 1957, it is only very recently that pharmacokinetic studies have been carried out in children. No information is available regarding its use in neonates and infants. Adult studies have demonstrated that the recovery from a single intravenous injection of methohexitone produces a faster and more complete recovery than that following an equipotent dose of thiopentone, though in fact this potential advantage has never been confirmed in children.

Pharmacokinetics.   Methohexitone is less lipid-soluble than thiopentone but has an equally rapid onset of action. It has a pK of 7.9 and about 75% is bound to plasma proteins.

A recent study performed on six children aged between 4 and 7 years by Bjorkman et al (1987) has demonstrated that, following a single intravenous injection of methohexitone, the decay in plasma concentration can usually be fitted on to a tri-exponential function. Distribution phases were very rapid ($t\frac{1}{2}\alpha$ 2.4 min; $t\frac{1}{2}\beta$ 23 min), and were much shorter than adult values of 5.6 and 58.3 min respectively (Hudson et al, 1983). The elimination half-life was calculated at 3.2 h, slightly shorter than the 3.9 h previously reported for adults (Hudson et al, 1983; Ghoneim et al, 1985). A clearance value of 18.9 ml/kg/min in children is higher than adult figures of 8.7–11.5 ml/kg/min, though the apparent volume of distribution seems similar in all age groups (1.2–2.2 l/kg).

The difference in the values for elimination half-life of methohexitone and thiopentone (see Table 4.1) would appear to be due to the higher clearance rates for methohexitone. Although redistribution is the major determinant for the duration of unconsciousness after a single dose of either drug, barbiturate metabolism is probably the most important determinant of the time required for complete psychomotor recovery. Thus, based solely upon its pharmacokinetic properties, methohexitone would seem preferable to thiopentone whenever a more rapid and full recovery from anaesthesia is desired, particularly after large or repeated doses.

Metabolism. Methohexitone is cleared predominantly by hepatic oxidative metabolism. This process is more influenced by variations in hepatic blood flow than is thiopentone which has a low hepatic extraction ratio of 0.15 compared to a value of 0.5–0.67 for methohexitone (Richter et al, 1980; Hudson et al, 1983).

Clinical effects. The effects of methohexitone on the cardiovascular system are very similar to those of thiopentone when administered in comparable dosages. Todd and co-workers (1984), in a similar study to that reported for thiopentone (see above), examined the cardiovascular effects of high doses of methohexitone (0.4 mg/kg/min) on eight neurosurgical patients aged from 12 to 58 years. They concluded that doses of methohexitone sufficient to produce profound electroencephalogram suppression were accompanied by both vasodilatation and some depression of myocardial function, even when ventricular filling pressures were maintained.

Dosage and administration. Methohexitone is usually given intravenously as a 1% solution. When given to healthy unpremedicated infants and children for intravenous induction of anaesthesia, the usual sleep dose is 1.5 mg/kg. Injection into small veins commonly causes pain, which can be minimized by adding 1 mg lignocaine to each 1 ml of solution. Compared to thiopentone, induction of anaesthesia with methohexitone is associated with a higher incidence of excitatory phenomena such as twitching, coughing or hiccup. For rectal use see Chapter 6.

Propofol

Propofol (2,6 di-isopropyl phenol) is a relatively new drug (now reformulated in Intralipid) which has been used successfully in both children and adults to induce and maintain anaesthesia. No pharmacokinetic data have as yet been reported for children, but preliminary pharmacokinetic evaluation has been performed in adults (Cockshott et al, 1987; Kay et al, 1986b). These studies have demonstrated a rapid decline in blood propofol concentrations following a single dose, with very short distribution ($t\frac{1}{2}\alpha$ 2–8 min) and elimination phases ($t\frac{1}{2}\beta$ 56–109 min). Although for each patient there is usually a good correlation between concentration and effect, there is wide intersubject variability in the pharmacodynamics of a given mg/kg dose.

Propofol is highly lipophilic and is bound to plasma proteins to an unknown extent. It appears to be rapidly metabolized in the liver to conjugated metabolites, principally propofol glucuronide, which are subsequently eliminated in the urine (Simons et al, 1985).

Clinical effects, dosage and administration.   When comparing the
induction characteristics of propofol with thiopentone in 60 children aged
3–16 years, Purcell-Jones et al (1987) found that a dose of 2–2.5 mg/kg
propofol was necessary to induce anaesthesia in these heavily premedicated
patients. Despite using a large vein in the antecubital fossa, pain on injection
was observed in 24% of children in the propofol group. Subsequent experience has shown that this can be reduced by the addition of lignocaine.
Induction times for both groups of patients were about 30 s, except for two
patients receiving propofol who took 45 and 60 s. Apnoeas of greater than
30 s duration occurred in 13% of patients in each group. The incidence of
spontaneous movement was greater in the propofol group (33%) than in the
thiopentone group (13%), but were all short-lived and not considered
troublesome.

Significantly greater decreases in systolic blood pressure were noted after
induction with propofol (−20%), and the heart rate did not increase in this
group, as it did with thiopentone (+10%).

Overall the authors regarded thiopentone as a better induction agent and
certainly the problems regarding pain on injection and hypotension may
preclude the more general use of propofol in this role. However, the preliminary clinical work and the pharmacokinetic studies in adults suggest that
a more appropriate use for this drug may be as part of an intravenous
anaesthetic technique (see also total intravenous anaesthesia, p. 85). The
relatively large volume of distribution in infants and young children suggests that recovery may be prolonged after an infusion technique.

Etomidate

Etomidate is a water-soluble carboxylated imidazole which has been used
for induction and maintenance of anaesthesia. Despite the demonstration of
adrenocortical suppression produced by this drug when given by infusion
(Ledingham et al, 1983), this does not occur following a single dose (Duthie
et al, 1985), and etomidate has been retained for use as an induction agent.
The main advantage it is claimed to possess in this role is its lack of depressant effects on the cardiovascular system. It is short-acting and its duration of
effect is less dependent on redistribution than is the case with the barbiturates, and recovery is good. However, the high incidence of pain on
injection (30%) and myoclonia (10%) has meant that etomidate is now only
used rarely in paediatric anaesthesia. Although etomidate has been advocated for the induction of anaesthesia in critically ill patients, it is the
author's view that for the high-risk patient, the safest course is to use an
agent with which one is familiar, albeit judiciously, rather than change
technique and use a drug with which one has little experience.

Dosage and administration.   In unpremedicated children the dose
of etomidate needed to produce a clinically acceptable induction of
anaesthesia is 0.3–0.4 mg/kg. Children who have received opioid premedication will usually only require a dose of 0.2 mg/kg (Kay, 1976).

Ketamine

Ketamine hydrochloride is a non-barbiturate cyclohexamine-derivative which produces a state of dissociative anaesthesia, characterized by profound analgesia and light sleep. Its mechanism of action has not been clarified but may involve opioid receptors (Finck and Ngai, 1982) and mono-aminergic systems (Pekoe and Smith, 1982).

Pharmacokinetics. Grant et al (1983) studied nine healthy children aged 4–9 years who were given either 2 mg/kg ketamine i.v. or 6 mg/kg i.m. They found that the apparent volume of distribution (Vd) was 1.9(±0.6) l/kg, compared to (previously studied) adult values of 2.3(±0.4) l/kg. Elimination half-life values were 100(±19) min in the children compared to 153(±27) min in adults. Adult values for ketamine clearance, 12.6(±2.2) ml/min/kg, were compared to values of 16.8(±3.3) ml/min/kg in the children. Absorption of ketamine from the intramuscular injection site appeared to be faster in children than in adults, probably related to the differences in muscle mass and perfusion. In infants less than 3 months of age the Vd is similar to that in older children but the $t\frac{1}{2}\beta$ is prolonged and clearance increased (Cook, 1986). Reduced metabolism and renal excretion are presumed to be the cause.

Metabolism. Ketamine is metabolized in the liver by n-demethylation to norketamine, a metabolite which has anaesthetic activity in the rat, though its action in man is not known. Plasma norketamine concentrations are greater in children than in adults, however, despite their shorter recovery times (Grant et al, 1983).

Clinical effects. One of the advantages claimed for ketamine is that it does not cause respiratory depression or loss of pharyngeal or laryngeal reflexes. In fact, most series report some degree of airway obstruction requiring treatment in 8–20% of patients. Ketamine tends to produce cardiovascular stimulation and a 10% rise in heart rate and blood pressure is usually seen. Pulmonary artery pressures and PVR are not thought to be affected in normal infants or those with pulmonary hypertension (Hickey et al, 1984). Postoperative nausea, vomiting or anorexia appear to be uncommon in young children. As ketamine can cause excessive salivation, the inclusion of an antisialogogue in the premedication is always indicated.

One of the major problems associated with the use of ketamine, especially in older children and adults, is the occurrence of unpleasant dreaming, hallucinations and delirium during recovery. The incidence of emergence phenomena is probably dose-related and tends to increase with age. In children under 5 years of age the incidence of reactions is about 5% when using ketamine as a sole agent, but can be further reduced if sedative premedication is given, nitrous oxide is administered peroperatively and disturbance during recovery is kept to an absolute minimum (Wessels et al, 1973). Other problems of ketamine anaesthesia, which are also probably dose-related, include muscle rigidity and non-purposeful random movements. If these become troublesome, supplementation with other anaesthetic agents, including muscle relaxants, may become necessary.

These side-effects have confined the indications for the use of ketamine in most centres to infants and young children needing multiple anaesthetics for radiotherapy or burns and occasionally for patients in severe shock (when preoperative resuscitation is not possible).

Dosage and administration.   When administered intravenously to healthy premedicated children, a dose of 2 mg/kg will produce a state of surgical anaesthesia within 30 s, lasting for 5–10 min. An intramuscular dose of 10 mg/kg will produce anaesthesia within 2–3 min, with a duration of effect of about 25 min, though interpatient variability can be marked. It has been suggested that dose requirements vary inversely with age, with infants less than 6 months of age requiring up to four times the dose of ketamine needed in children 5–6 years of age (Lockhart and Nelson, 1974).

Repeated intravenous doses may be given without significant cumulative effects, though repeated intramuscular doses can lead to unpredictably long and variable recovery times (Page et al, 1972). An intravenous infusion of ketamine may be a more logical approach (Idvall et al, 1979), as the total dose of ketamine needed using this technique may be significantly less than one using intermittent administration. A loading dose of 2 mg/kg is followed by an infusion of 40 μg/kg/min. For rectal administration see Chapter 6.

Benzodiazepines

This group of compounds with tranquillizing properties are singularly free from toxic effects. Their actions are complex but are probably a result of potentiation of the neural inhibition that is mediated by γ-aminobutyric acid (GABA). The drugs that are of particular interest to anaesthetists also have powerful anxiolytic, hypnotic and amnesic properties. They have been used in a variety of ways, including premedication, sedation, induction of anaesthesia or as part of a total intravenous anaesthetic technique (TIVA).

Diazepam

Current indications for the administration of diazepam in anaesthetic practice are now confined to premedication and sedation. Diazepam has previously been utilized as an induction agent and as an adjuvant in the maintenance of anaesthesia. However, it has been superseded in this respect by midazolam, which has a similar pharmacodynamic profile to diazepam, but does not have the problem of prolonged recovery. Diazepam is insoluble in water; the solution for injection contains several organic solvents which results in a rather viscid solution which cannot be diluted. A newer formulation (Diazemuls) in an oil-in-water emulsion can, however, be diluted with water or dextrose solutions. This new formulation has also greatly reduced the high incidence of local pain on injection and thrombophlebitis that used to follow diazepam injection.

Pharmacokinetics.   Diazepam is highly lipid-soluble and is extensively bound to plasma proteins—nearly 98% in adults and children and 85% in neonates. Following a single intravenous injection, plasma concentrations of diazepam are best described by a three-compartment model. There is rapid uptake of diazepam into highly vascular organs such as the brain and the concentration in the cerebrospinal fluid approximates the concentration of free drug in the plasma. This is followed by a rapid redistribution phase into tissues that are less well perfused, especially muscle and fat.

The apparent volume of distribution in neonates and infants (1.3–2.6 l/kg) is similar to adult values (1.6–3.2 l/kg). Elimination half-lives of 40–400 h have been observed in preterm newborns, while in full term neonates half-life values range from 20–50 h, reducing further to 8–14 h in infants (Morselli et al, 1983). No information is available on the disposition rate of desmethyldiazepam in either neonates or infants. The slower clearance of diazepam in the newborn period is due to reduced hydroxylation and subsequent conjugation, while demethylating activities are less impaired.

Metabolism. Diazepam is metabolized by several different microsomal enzyme systems in the liver generating a number of active metabolities, which in turn are biotransformed more slowly than the parent compound. The duration of action of the drug is thus not necessarily apparent from its elimination half-life, especially when repeated injections have been given. Another complication that is seen with diazepam administration is due to a significant enterohepatic circulation; pharmacologically active diazepam metabolites excreted in the bile and reabsorbed from the gastrointestinal tract can cause a rebound effect hours after the initial injection.

Clinical effects, dosage and administration. Other than when used as an anticonvulsant, diazepam should only be given in single doses, and is probably best avoided before the age of 1 year. As is common with all the benzodiazepines, there is great interpatient variability of dose–response. However, a dose of 0.3 mg/kg will induce unconsciousness in about 1 min in 90% of premedicated healthy children (Cole, 1982).

Effects on the respiratory and cardiovascular systems are not significantly different to those produced by midazolam.

Midazolam

Midazolam is a water-soluble benzodiazepine that has been used successfully in both adults and children as an induction agent, a sedative agent and as part of a total intravenous anaesthetic technique.

Pharmacokinetics. Following a single dose the plasma decay curve of midazolam can usually be fitted to a bi-exponential curve, representing a two-compartment model.

In older children and adults, midazolam is extensively bound to plasma albumin leaving only 2–5% as free drug. No data regarding protein binding in infants and young children are available.

The elimination half-life of midazolam given as a single dose to 21 children was calculated at 1.45($\pm$0.5) h, and the apparent volume of distribution (Vd) as 1.50($\pm$0.5) l/kg (Salonen et al, 1987). The clearance varied from 4.83 to 11.2 ml/min/kg and could be correlated with increasing dose (0.075–0.6 mg/kg). It was suggested that plasma protein-binding sites may have become saturated or that other anaesthetic agents may have affected hepatic metabolism. These results suggest a faster elimination in children compared to adults, but this has not been confirmed by other workers administering midazolam to children by infusion (Lloyd-Thomas and Booker, 1986). However, as clearance values seem to increase with increasing dosage, it is possible that these differing results are not incompatible, but merely reflect dose-dependent elimination in children.

Metabolism. Midazolam is cleared from plasma almost exclusively by liver oxidative processes involving cytochrome P-450, less than 1% appearing unchanged in the urine. Midazolam is converted to 1-hydroxy-methyl- and 4-hydroxy-midazolam, which, although possessing some hypnotic activity, are conjugated quickly and contribute little to the pharmacological effect. Following a single dose the peak concentrations of these metabolites are seen 5–20 min after administration and at 1 h have fallen to 10% of peak values. During an infusion of midazolam, hydroxy-midazolam concentrations are approximately 25% of midazolam concentrations.

The hepatic extraction ratio of midazolam varies from 0.3 to 0.7, so that drug clearance will depend on both the intrinsic hepatic clearance and the hepatic blood flow.

Although no pharmacokinetic data are available for neonates and young infants, the involvement of cytochrome P-450 systems in midazolam metabolism suggests that elimination rates would be prolonged in this age group.

Clinical effects, dosage and administration. When used as an induction agent, midazolam has a relatively slow onset of action (1–2 min) and does not reliably cause loss of consciousness. The average induction dose needed in healthy premedicated children is 0.15–0.25 mg/kg. About 4% of children may need higher doses than this or be almost completely resistant. For these patients, it is probably better to supplement with another agent, e.g. thiopentone 1–2 mg/kg.

Effects on the cardiovascular system in healthy children seem minimal, with falls in blood pressure of about 10% from baseline being observed in about 10% of patients and rises in heart rate of more than 10% occurring in about 33%. These changes in cardiovascular parameters are not a problem in healthy children but, as with most induction agents, may become important in sick or hypovolaemic children.

Transient apnoeas and tachypnoeas are common following fast injection, but do not usually warrant intervention. Excitation phenomena are rarely seen. Recovery times following a single dose of midazolam are significantly longer than those resulting from thiopentone administration, and are similar to those following a single dose of diazepam.

When given by infusion at rates of 2–5 µg/kg/min, midazolam has no clinically significant effects on cardiovascular or respiratory parameters.

This dosage regime will provide useful sedation for most infants and children, but will require supplementation with other agents in about 5% of patients (Booker et al, 1986). In children with normal hepatic function, midazolam does not accumulate when given at these infusion rates, and recovery times on stopping the infusion are not usually related to the duration of the infusion. In patients with abnormal hepatic function, midazolam clearance may be decreased and accumulation will occur unless infusion rates are decreased accordingly. The benzodiazepine antagonist (anexate) may also be useful in patients with abnormal hepatic function to determine whether or not their altered conscious state is due to midazolam overdosage (Sage et al, 1987).

In addition to having sedative, anxiolytic and hypnotic properties, midazolam is a powerful amnesic agent. This can make it a particularly useful drug in the intensive care unit or as part of a total intravenous anaesthetic technique (see total intravenous anaesthesia, p. 85).

Opioids

The term opioid is used to designate both drugs with morphine-like actions, and drugs which antagonize those actions. They interact with several closely related receptors and share some of the properties of certain naturally occurring peptides, the enkephalins, endorphins and dynorphins. Studies of the binding of opioids to specific sites in the CNS and other organs have suggested the existence of up to eight types of receptors. Further discussion of this constantly expanding field is beyond the scope of this chapter.

No attempt has been made to be comprehensive and only opioids which are commonly used in paediatric practice will be discussed. The section is divided into three—opioid agonists, opioid antagonists and partial agonists.

Opioid agonists

These are morphine-like substances which act as agonists primarily at μ, $\varkappa$ and perhaps λ receptors.

Morphine

Morphine is still probably the most widely used opioid administered to children for postoperative analgesia. It has certainly been the most investigated analgesic drug in paediatric practice and remains the standard with which all other strong analgesics should be compared. It is still commonly used for premedication and intraoperative anaesthesia and analgesia.

Pharmacokinetics. Morphine has a pK of 7.9 and is only poorly lipid-soluble. Although the primary site of action is in the CNS, only small quantities pass the blood–brain barrier. About 40% is bound to plasma albumin in adults and older children, though in neonates this value falls to about 30%. There is also some evidence to suggest that morphine crosses the blood–brain barrier more easily in neonates (Kupferberg and Way, 1963; Koren et al, 1985).

One of the first studies to examine morphine kinetics in children was performed by Dahlstrom and co-workers in 1979. They measured plasma morphine concentrations in 53 children aged between 1 month and 15 years, following a single intravenous dose of morphine (0.15 mg/kg), and found that the kinetics of morphine for all age groups could usually be adequately described by a tri-exponential function. The rapid initial distribution phase had a half-life of about 2.5 min and the secondary and tertiary phases had half-lives of 13.3 and 133 min respectively. The clearance in children older than 1 year was calculated at 6.45 ml/min/kg, which was similar to previously published adult values (Stanski et al, 1976). Pharmacokinetic investigations on both children and adults carried out since then, however, have demonstrated significantly higher clearance values (Stanski et al, 1978; Vandenberghe et al, 1983; Aitkenhead et al, 1984). Nevertheless, the general conclusions reached by all workers, that there are no significant age-related differences in kinetic parameters in the age groups studied apparently remains valid (Table 4.2). The discrepancies are at least partially due to the shorter sampling times in the earlier studies and changes in the analytical methods employed.

Table 4.2. Age-related differences in pharmacokinetic parameters for opioids and benzodiazepines (pooled data)

Drug		Apparent volume of distribution (l/kg)	Elimination half-life (min)	Clearance (ml/kg/min)
Diazepam	Infant	1.9	840	—
	Child	—	—	—
	Adult	1.6	2400	0.38
Midazolam	Infant	—	—	—
	Child	1.5	105–240	8.0
	Adult	1.4	180	6.0
Morphine	Neonate	3.4	629	7.0
	Infant	5.1	235	23.8
	Child	1.3	120	6.5–20.5
	Adult	3.3	180	15.0
Fentanyl	Neonate	4.7	293	18.0
	Infant	3.4	233	18.0
	Child	2.8	184	12.0
	Adult	4.0	222	13.0
Alfentanil	Infant	—	—	—
	Child	1.0	63	11.0
	Adult	1.0	96	7.6
Sufentanil	Infant	1.6	53	27.5
	Child	3.0	55	18.1
	Adult	2.9	164	12.7
Naloxone	Neonate	2.0	185	9.5
	Child	—	—	—
	Adult	2.0	72	25.0

Kinetic studies involving neonates have demonstrated a different picture. Koren and co-workers in Toronto (1985) studied 12 neonates of 35–41 weeks' gestation at 1–49 days after birth. The patients were administered morphine infusions for postoperative analgesia for 3.5–105 h (mean 59.5 ± 10.2 h). The infusion rates varied between 6.2 and 40 µg/kg/h (mean 21 µg/kg/h). They calculated an elimination half-life of 13.9(±6.4) h in eight babies, the value being even higher in the other four (24.8 ± 4.6 h). Clearance rates were 7.8 ± 1.9 ml/kg/min, with large variability in values.

Lynn and Slattery (1987) administered infusions of morphine at 20–100 µg/kg/h to seven newborn babies less than 5 days old and three infants 17–65 days old. They calculated an elimination half-life of 6.81 ± 1.63 h for the neonates and 3.91(±1.0) h for the infants. Clearance rates were 6.3 ml/kg/min in the newborns compared to 23.8 ml/kg/min in the infants. They suggested that the 'adult' values for $t\frac{1}{2}\beta$ and clearance obtained in the infant group may be related to their capability to form a sulphate conjugate of morphine, analogous to the alternate metabolic pathway available for paracetamol.

Metabolism and elimination. Morphine is mainly metabolized in the liver but has a number of active metabolites, including morphine-6-glucuronide and normorphine. Extrahepatic metabolism of morphine in the gastrointestinal tract and kidney has also been postulated (McQuay and Moore, 1984; Park, 1985): certainly patients in severe hepatic failure are capable of metabolism and elimination of morphine without any prolongation of clinical effect (Shelly et al, 1986). An adequate urinary output is probably important for the elimination of active (and inactive) metabolites and termination of clinical effect.

Clinical effects. Morphine and related opioids produce their major effects on the CNS and the gastrointestinal tract. Their effects are diverse and include analgesia, sedation, changes in mood, respiratory depression, decreased gastrointestinal motility, nausea, vomiting and alterations of the endocrine and autonomic nervous systems.

Of particular interest to the anaesthetist using morphine intraoperatively is its relative lack of effect on the cardiovascular system. Even very large doses (1 mg/kg) given intravenously to patients with compromised myocardial function may have little effect on cardiac index though small infants with severe lesions may become hypotensive. Myocardial oxygen consumption, left ventricular end diastolic pressure and cardiac work may all be reduced (Sethna et al, 1982). However, morphine does cause variable histamine release, which may be involved in the aetiology of the peripheral arteriolar and venous dilatation that also occurs.

There have been many attempts to correlate effect with plasma concentrations of morphine. Dahlstrom and co-workers (1979) found that a concentration of 64.5(±18) µg/l was necessary to prevent sweating, increases of blood pressure or heart rate during anaesthesia with 70% nitrous oxide. This compares with minimum analgesic concentrations of 12–25 µg/l apparently required in the postoperative period (Lynn et al, 1984). These figures must be interpreted with some caution however, as there is great interpatient variability in the pharmacokinetic and pharmacodynamic effects of morphine.

Administration and dosage.　　The use of large doses of morphine in paediatric anaesthesia is usually limited to those infants and children undergoing major abdominal, scoliosis or cardiothoracic surgery. Elective postoperative ventilation for these patients may be indicated and makes the administration of large doses of morphine peroperatively safe and relatively complication-free. For those children whom the anaesthetist expects to extubate at the end of surgery, the dosage of morphine needs to be more critically determined, so that postoperative respiratory depression can be avoided. In a comparison of three balanced anaesthesia techniques, 60 children below the age of 5 years were given halothane, isoflurane or morphine to supplement a nitrous oxide/relaxant anaesthetic (Chinyanga et al, 1984). Morphine was administered in a loading dose of 60 µg/kg, followed by an infusion at 2 µg/kg/min, resulting in a mean concentration of 55.9(±2.4) µg/l. Intraoperative anaesthetic conditions, as assessed by heart rate and blood pressure changes, were similar in all three groups, though the morphine group tended to exhibit consistently higher blood pressure measurements. Recovery times were not prolonged in the morphine group and most patients were pain-free for the first 2 h postoperatively, in comparison to those children in the other groups who needed immediate postoperative analgesia.

The determination of an appropriate dose of morphine for patients having operations not expected to last more than 1 h can be difficult. For patients over 1 year of age a dose of 100 µg/kg is usually sufficient and will not prolong recovery in most children. Infants under 6 months of age are probably best given morphine postoperatively, when the effects can be more easily determined, and then in increments of 25 µg/kg. Infants of 6–12 months of age will usually tolerate a single dose of 25–50 µg/kg without prolonging recovery too severely. Alternatively, a shorter-acting opioid such as fentanyl or alfentanil may be a more appropriate choice of drug peroperatively, with administration of the longer-acting morphine being deferred until the postoperative period. For postoperative infusion rates see Chapter 10.

Administration of morphine to neonates or infants under the age of 6 months should only be undertaken peroperatively when postoperative intensive monitoring and a one-to-one nurse:patient ratio can be guaranteed. In addition to the problem of a prolonged elimination half-life in this age group, there are also great variations in serum concentrations, following any given µg/kg dose. Serum morphine concentrations can also increase despite cessation of an infusion, which may be due to enterohepatic circulation (Koren et al, 1985). Sensitivity to the effects of morphine is also probably greater in this age group. For these reasons, infusion rates above 10–15 µg/kg/h are undesirable, and almost always unnecessary.

Fentanyl

Fentanyl is still commonly used as a peroperative analgesic, though a greater understanding of its pharmacokinetic profile has made anaesthetists realize the potential problems that may occur from repeated dosage, particularly in the very young. It also retains a role as an anaesthetic agent, when given in large doses, for children undergoing cardiac surgery, due to its lack of cardiovascular depression.

Fentanyl has a pK of 8.4 and changes in tissue pH from 7.4 to 7.0 will increase the unbound fraction of fentanyl by 52% (Meuldermans et al, 1982). It is the most lipid-soluble of all the opioids discussed in this chapter and is extensively distributed to all tissues. Fentanyl binds to red cells (40%) to a similar extent to its binding to plasma albumin and lipoproteins (44%; Meuldermans et al, 1982).

Pharmacokinetics.   A number of studies have been performed that demonstrate age-related differences in fentanyl pharmacokinetics (Baskoff and Stevenson, 1981; Johnson et al, 1984; Koren et al, 1984; Singleton et al, 1984; Koehntop et al, 1986). Following single-dose administration of 20–50 µg/kg, plasma concentrations are usually best described by a two-compartment model. Apparent volumes of distribution vary from 4.7 l/kg in the neonate, to 3.4 l/kg in infants, and 2.8 l/kg in young children, compared to values of 4.0 l/kg in adults. Values for elimination half-life are prolonged in neonates (294 min), but are similar in all age groups thereafter (see Table 4.1). Total body clearances for fentanyl are higher in the neonate and infant (18.0 ml/kg/min) than in children and adults (12–13.0 ml/kg/min). The surprisingly high value for Vd in neonates does not correlate with their low volume/kg of fat and muscle, and may relate to tissue sequestration and/or perfusion. The increased clearance in the very young may be related to the higher hepatic blood flow/kg body weight in this age group.

Metabolism.   Elimination of fentanyl is almost entirely due to hepatic metabolism by 'mixed function' oxidase enzymes and, due to its high hepatic extraction ratio, is perfusion-dependent.

Transient rebounds in plasma fentanyl levels (and resultant clinical effects) have been observed in all age groups and probably reflect sequestering and subsequent release.

Clinical effects, dosage and administration.   Hickey and co-workers (1985), in their study of the response to 25 µg/kg of fentanyl administered to 12 infants recovering from open heart surgery, found no significant changes in heart rate, cardiac index, pulmonary artery pressure or PVR 5 min after administration. There were clinically insignificant (<5%) decreases in mean arterial pressure and SVR.

In common with all opioids, fentanyl can cause severe respiratory depression, especially in the very young. In children and adults, a strong correlation exists between fentanyl concentrations in plasma and cerebrospinal fluid and respiratory depression. However, Koehntop et al (1986), who administered 10–50 µg/kg fentanyl to 14 neonates undergoing thoracoabdominal procedures, observed profound respiratory depression requiring prolonged postoperative ventilation in four patients, despite plasma levels of only 0.05–0.77 ng/ml at time of extubation. These compare with plasma levels of 2.0–4.6 ng/ml which were necessary to produce 50% depression of the carbon dioxide response curve in healthy adults (Fung and Eisele, 1980; Cartwright et al, 1983). They concluded that, in addition to the pharmacokinetic differences already discussed, neonates are also particularly sensitive to the respiratory depressant effects of fentanyl, though the particular mechanism is not known. They also emphasized the highly variable disposition of fentanyl in neonates, which compounds the difficulty in predicting full and permanent ventilatory recovery after fentanyl anaethesia in this age group. In spontaneously breathing children an appropriate dose range is 1–3 µg/kg, for ventilated premedicated patients 5 µg/kg, for unpremedicated patients up to 10 µg/kg. Higher doses may be administered to patients who require postoperative ventilation. For postoperative infusion rate see p. 329.

Alfentanil

Alfentanil, a fentanyl analogue, is a relatively new synthetic opioid with a pK of 6.5; 'free' alfentanil levels are much less affected by pH changes than morphine or fentanyl (Hull, 1983). Despite being only moderately lipid-soluble, there is rapid transfer across the blood–brain barrier (Stanski and Hug, 1982). Binding to plasma proteins (mostly glycoproteins) is similar in both adults and children—about 88–92%.

Pharmacokinetics.   Following a single intravenous dose of 20 µg/kg given to 20 children (aged 10 months to 6 years) and 10 adults, plasma alfentanil concentrations decreased in a curve best described by a bi-exponential function (Roure et al, 1987). In the children the distribution phase had a half-life of about 5 min and the elimination phase a mean half-life of 63(±24) min, significantly shorter than comparative adult values of 95(±20) min. This decrease in $t\frac{1}{2}\beta$ in children is due to increased clearance, 11.1(±3.9) ml/kg/min as opposed to 5.9(±1.6) ml/kg/min in adults. The apparent volume of distribution has been calculated at 1.03(±0.71) l/kg, very similar to adult values of 0.82(±0.3) l/kg. Similar studies in 3–11-month-old infants have not shown any significant differences in pharmacokinetic parameters obtained between infants and children (Den Hollander et al, 1986).

This increase in biotransformation of alfentanil in children may be partially due to the general increase in hepatic microsomal activity in children under 3 years of age. The increase in hepatic blood flow in young children, related to the increased hepatic mass:body weight ratio and cardiac index, may also be significant, as the hepatic extraction ratio is 0.4–0.7.

Clinical effects, dosage and administration.   The cardiovascular responses to a single very large dose (120 µg/kg) of alfentanil may include decreases in heart rate, blood pressure and cardiac index, though the myocardial oxygen supply:demand ratio may improve (Rucquoi and Camu, 1983). Loading doses of 50 µg/kg or less do not usually produce any clinically significant effects on the cardiovascular system, particularly if atropine has been previously administered.

Alfentanil has potent respiratory depressant effects but can be administered to spontaneously breathing patients if the dosage is carefully controlled (Kay, 1986a). However, the dosage regime that may be necessary to provide adequate operating conditions and ablate cardiovascular responses to surgical stimuli often precludes spontaneous respiration. Most published studies in children have used controlled ventilation and this is undoubtedly a much easier and safer technique.

Because the action of a single dose of alfentanil has a duration of action of only a few minutes, nearly all operations will require either repeated doses or an infusion. A typical regime would include a loading dose of 10–20 µg/kg followed by an infusion rate of about 1 µg/kg/min. Infusion rates can be altered in anticipation of different surgical stimuli or when blood pressure changes are observed, as different rates (and thus different plasma concentrations), will be required to block varying intensities of stimuli. The infusion should be stopped about 5–10 min before the anticipated end of surgery if the patient is to be extubated.

Usually recovery is excellent within 10–15 min of stopping an infusion, though the duration of the infusion and total dose administered will become more relevant as these latter figures increase. Cessation of the alfentanil infusion also means that analgesia will wear off rapidly and may require subsequent recommencement of the infusion at a lower dose.

Sufentanil

Sufentanil is a new fentanyl derivative that is highly lipophilic and extensively bound to plasma proteins (90%), mostly glycoproteins and albumin. It is 5–10 times more potent than fentanyl and in high doses has been used as a primary anaesthetic agent for infants and children undergoing cardiac surgery.

Pharmacokinetics. Following a single intravenous injection, the decay curve for sufentanil concentrations is best described by a biexponential equation. The values that have been obtained for elimination half-life in infants (53 ± 15 min) are not significantly different to those obtained for children (55 ± 10 min; Davis et al, 1987), though both are significantly smaller than adult values (164 min); Bovill et al, 1984). Clearance values for both infants and children are 18.1–27.5 ml/kg/min, significantly higher than adult figures of 12.7 ml/kg/min. The apparent volume of distribution in infants is significantly smaller (1.6 ± 0.46 l/kg) than values obtained in children (3.0 l/kg) or adults (2.9 l/kg).

Metabolism. Animal studies indicate that sufentanil is metabolized by O-demethylation and N-dealkylation (Meuldermans et al, 1980). The increased clearance in infants and young children may be explained by the larger hepatic:body weight ratio and increased microsomal P-450 enzyme activity.

Clinical effects, dosage and administration. Following a single dose of 15 µg/kg, administered to 20 infants and children undergoing open heart surgery, Davis et al (1987) observed a 25% decrease in systolic and diastolic blood pressures and a 15% decrease in heart rate, which returned to baseline values following surgical stimulus. Thereafter, they found sufentanil reliably suppressed major changes in blood pressure and heart rate. In another study (Moore et al, 1985), bolus doses of 5, 10 or 20 µg/kg given to children 4–12 years of age undergoing cardiac surgery provided a haemodynamically stable state during induction of anaesthesia. The use of pancuronium as a muscle relaxant and the older age of the children may explain this difference from the above-mentioned study. In common with Hickey and Hansen (1984), the authors found a 1–4 min interval between initiation of anaesthetic induction and loss of eyelash reflex.

In conclusion, these studies have shown that sufentanil, when given to infants and children undergoing open heart surgery, is safe in doses that will effectively block systemic haemodynamic responses to noxious stimuli. However, it is not yet clear whether this drug offers any advantage over fentanyl or alfentanil, for example, or whether high-dose opioid administration as a concept is a particularly valuable one for the paediatric cardiac patient.

Opioid antagonists

Naloxone

Naloxone, a derivative of oxymorphine, is now the only drug commonly used in anaesthesia for the purpose of antagonizing opioid-induced respiratory depression and sedation. It binds competitively to all types of opioid receptor, albeit with widely differing affinities. Although naloxone has been regarded traditionally as a pure opioid antagonist without agonist activity, there is some evidence to suggest that this may not be entirely true. For example, it has been shown that naloxone can increase blood pressure in patients with endotoxic shock (Peters et al, 1981). The mechanism for this action is not fully understood as yet, though antagonism of endogenous opioids, a centrally mediated increase in sympathetic tone, and an increase in catecholamine levels may all be involved. Naloxone may also cause an increase in cerebral and spinal cord blood flow, probably mediated through opioid receptors found in CNS vessels. In addition, anecdotal reports and experimental data have suggested that naloxone may have many other neurophysiological effects, most of which can be explained on the basis of antagonism of the endogenous opioid peptide system (Smith and Pinnock, 1985).

Metabolism and pharmacokinetics.   Naloxone is metabolized in the liver, principally by conjugation with glucuronic acid. There are no pharmacokinetic data relating to children, though neonates have prolonged elimination, probably due to their reduced conjugating capacity (Moreland et al, 1980).

Dosage and administration.   When used for opioid antagonism, naloxone can be administered to all age groups, by intravenous or intramuscular injection, in a dose of 5–10 μg/kg. When given intravenously, the drug should be administered slowly in order to titrate the minimum dose possible against the desired effect. In less urgent situations, the intramuscular route may be superior and will decrease the risk of acute arousal. In view of the disparities in duration of action between naloxone and many opioid drugs, prevention of a rebound opioid agonist effect may require repeated doses or an intravenous infusion of naloxone, starting at 10–20 μg/kg/h (Tenenbein, 1984).

Partial agonists

Buprenorphine

Little work has been published regarding the administration of buprenorphine to children, and this probably reflects the lack of advantages for this drug compared to other opioids in the younger age groups. Buprenorphine is a highly lipid-soluble drug and also has a very high receptor affinity which is associated with a long duration of action and resistance to reversal by naloxone. No evidence has yet been forthcoming of any advantage over morphine, and this expensive drug can certainly cause respiratory depression and has addiction potential, despite initial reports in adults which suggested otherwise. A dose of 50 μg/kg does not usually result in any clinically significant respiratory depression in older children and provides useful analgesia for up to 8 h.

Total intravenous anaesthesia

Although drugs administered for the intravenous induction of anaesthesia have often been tried as sole anaesthetic agents, early experiences were frequently disastrous, as the pharmacokinetics and toxicity of these drugs were not fully understood. Since the development of drugs with more suitable pharmacokinetic and pharmacodynamic profiles, however, the concept of total intravenous anaesthesia is again being examined with interest. In addition, the increasing realization that long-term exposure to anaesthetic gases may harm operating room personnel, and the difficulties of safely and effectively scavenging paediatric anaesthetic circuits, have increased the potential advantages of a totally intravenous technique.

At present no single intravenous anaesthetic drug possesses all the attributes of an ideal agent. The concept of balanced anaesthesia, using a combination of drugs to achieve a desired effect, with suppression of harmful stress response without cardiovascular depression seems a logical approach. Accordingly, separate drugs can be used to provide hypnosis, muscle relaxation and suppression of reflex responses to noxious stimuli.

The concept of minimum infusion rate (MIR) was introduced by Sear and Prys-Roberts (1979) as an equivalent to MAC for inhalational agents. MIR defines the ED_{50} of an i.v. anaesthetic agent which suppresses movement in response to the surgical incision in 50% of patients, although this rate does not necessarily correlate with the concentration of the anaesthetic in the blood.

The hypnotic agent needs to be free from undesirable side-effects, easy to administer and guaranteed to prevent awareness. In addition it should be rapidly distributed and eliminated so that significant cumulation does not occur. The recovery time after the end of surgery should compare with other conventional techniques. The only drug which at the present time appears to fulfil most of these desirable qualities is propofol, which has been used successfully in this role in adults (de Grood et al, 1985; Hilton et al, 1986; Kay, 1986b), but may not be so suitable in young children. Other drugs which have been used in a similar fashion (in adults), with varying success, include midazolam (Person et al, 1987) and methohexitone (Kay, 1986b).

An opioid is usually required to suppress reflex responses to noxious stimulation, as most hypnotic agents are relatively poor in this respect, unless their dose is increased to a degree such that cardiovascular depression occurs. Although opioids, if given in sufficiently large doses, can virtually eliminate all these reflex responses, for spontaneously breathing patients ventilatory depression will limit the dose that can be given. However, if muscle relaxants and controlled ventilation are employed, then the dose of opioid is not under the same constraints, although large dosage regimes may still result in postoperative respiratory depression.

On the currently available drugs, the opioid with the smallest distribution volume and fastest elimination rate is alfentanil. It is probably the drug of choice for total intravenous anaesthesia if the patient is being extubated at the end of surgery. An alternative technique that is particularly suitable for paediatric anaesthetic practice is the use of local analgesia to block noxious stimuli. Opioids are not needed, postoperative analgesia is provided and the risk of respiratory depression in the recovery period minimal.

The third modality of this balanced total intravenous anaesthesia technique, muscle relaxation, can be maintained by muscle relaxant drugs, using the same intermittent or infusion dosage regimes and criteria for administration as in conventional anaesthesia. If necessary, neuromuscular blockade can be monitored using a nerve stimulator.

One of the problems highlighted by total intravenous anaesthesia, but encountered with all anaesthetic techniques employing muscle relaxants, is the paucity of clinical signs relating to depth of anaesthesia. As Russell (1986) has demonstrated in adults, the incidence of awareness may be low, but nevertheless exists, mainly because of the interpatient variability in pharmacokinetic and pharmacodynamic responses to any given μg/kg drug dose. Logically, these problems should be minimized by titrating the amount of drug administered according to other easily measured responses such as increases in blood pressure or heart rate. Unfortunately, the suppression of cardiovascular reflex responses does not necessarily mean that the patient is not capable of being aware, or of retaining memory of an intraoperative event: different sensory modalities have different degrees of conscious representation and will not be affected by a given concentration of anaesthetic agent to the same extent. In fact, the difficulties involved in monitoring the depth of anaesthesia remain, to a large extent, unsolved. This is, at least in part, because 'consciousness' as opposed to 'unconsciousness' is not an all-or-none phenomenon but is part of a continuum. In addition, depth of anaesthesia does not necessarily correlate with the brain content of an anaesthetic agent or even with the amount of neuronal activity, but is a measure of efficiency of performance of brain function (Mori, 1987). The attempt to monitor brain performance, as opposed to brain activity, remains one of our major challenges.

REFERENCES

Aitkenhead AR, Vater M, Achola K, Cooper CMS & Smith G (1984) Pharmacokinetics of single dose i.v. morphine in normal and patients with end-stage renal failure. *British Journal of Anaesthesia* **56**: 813–819.

Aranda JV, MacLeod SM, Renton KW & Eade NR (1974) Hepatic microsomal drug oxidation and electron transport in newborn infants. *Journal of Pediatrics* **85**: 534–542.

Baskoff JD & Stevenson RL (1981) Fentanyl pharmacokinetics in children with heart disease. *Anesthesiology* **55**: A194.

Bjorkman S, Gabrielsson J, Quaynor H & Corbey M (1987) Pharmacokinetics of i.v. and rectal methohexitone in children. *British Journal of Anaesthesia* **59**: 1541–1547.

Booker PD, Beechey A & Lloyd-Thomas AR (1986) Sedation of children requiring artificial ventilation using an infusion of midazolam. *British Journal of Anaesthesia* **58**: 1104–1108.

Bovill JG, Sebel P, Blackburn CL, Oei-Lim V & Heykants JJ (1984) The pharmacokinetics of sufentanil in surgical patients. *Anesthesiology* **61**: 502–506.

Brett CM & Fisher DM (1987) Thiopental dose–response relations in unpremedicated infants, children and adults. *Anesthesia and Analgesia* **66**: 1024–1027.

Cartwright P, Prys-Roberts C, Gill K, Dye A, Stafford M & Gray A (1983) Ventilatory depression related to plasma fentanyl concentrations during and after anesthesia in humans. *Anesthesia and Analgesia* **62**: 966–974.

Chinyanga HM, Vandenberghe H, MacLeod S, Soldin S & Endrenyi L (1984) Assessment of immediate post-anesthetic recovery in young children following intravenous morphine infusions, halothane and isoflurane. *Canadian Anesthetists Society Journal* **31**: 28–35.

Cockshott ID, Briggs LP, Douglas EJ & White M (1987) Pharmacokinetics of propofol in female patients. *British Journal of Anaesthesia* **59**: 1103–1110.

Cole WHJ (1982) Midazolam in paediatric anaesthesia. *Anaesthesia and Intensive Care* **10**: 36–39.

Cook DR (1986) Newborn anesthesia: pharmacological considerations. *Canadian Anesthetists Society Journal* **33**(suppl): 38–42.

Dahlstrom B, Bolme P, Feychting H, Noack G & Paalzow L (1979) Morphine kinetics in children. *Clinical Pharmacology and Therapeutics* **26**: 354–365.

Davis PJ, Cook R, Stiller RL & Davin-Robinson KA (1987) Pharmacodynamics and pharmacokinetics of high-dose sufentanil in infants and children undergoing cardiac surgery. *Anesthesia and Analgesia* **66**: 203–208.

de Grood PMRM, Ruys AHC, van Egmond J, Booij LDHJ & Crul JF (1985) Propofol emulsion for total intravenous anaesthesia. *Postgraduate Medical Journal* **61**(suppl 3): 65–69.

Den Hollander JM, Hennis PJ, Quaegebeur JM, Burm AGL & Olofsen S (1986) Pharmacokinetics of alfentanil in infants and children with congenital heart defects. Abstract 815. European Congress on Anaesthesiology. Vienna.

Duthie DJR, Fraser R & Nimmo WS (1985) Effect of induction of anaesthesia with etomidate on corticosteroid synthesis in man. *British Journal of Anaesthesia* **57**: 156–159.

Finck AD & Ngai SH (1982) Opiate receptor mediation of ketamine analgesia. *Anesthesiology* **56:** 291–293.

Fung DL & Eisele JH (1980) Narcotic concentration–respiratory effect curves in man. *Anesthesiology* **53:** A397.

Ghoneim MM, Chiang CK, Shoenwald RD, Lilbum JK & Dhanaraj J (1985) The pharmacokinetics of methohexital in young and elderly subjects. *Acta Anaesthesiologica Scandanavica* **29:** 480–485.

Grant IS, Nimmo WS, McNicol LR & Clements JA (1983) Ketamine disposition in children and adults. *British Journal of Anaesthesia* **55:** 1107–1111.

Hickey PR & Hansen DD (1984) Fentanyl and sufentanil-oxygen-pancuronium for cardiac surgery in infants. *Anesthesia and Analgesia* **63:** 117–124.

Hickey PR, Hansen DD & Cramolini GM (1984) Pulmonary and systemic hemodynamic responses to ketamine in infants with normal and elevated pulmonary vascular resistance. *Anesthesiology* **61:** 3A, A438.

Hickey PR, Hansen DD, Wessel DL, Lang P & Jones RA (1985) Pulmonary and systemic hemodynamic responses to fentanyl in infants. *Anesthesia and Analgesia* **64:** 483–486.

Hilton P, Dev VJ & Major E (1986) Intravenous anaesthesia with propofol and alfentanil. The influence of age and weight. *Anaesthesia* **41:** 640–643.

Hudson RJ, Stanski DR & Burch PG (1983) Pharmacokinetics of methohexital and thiopental in surgical patients. *Anesthesiology* **59:** 215–219.

Hull CJ (1983) The pharmacokinetics of alfentanil in man. *British Journal of Anaesthesia* **55:** 157S–164S.

Hyvarinen M, Zeltzer P, Oh W & Stiehm ER (1973) Influence of gestational age on serum levels of α-1 fetoprotein, IgG globulin, and albumin in newborn infants. *Journal of Pediatrics* **82:** 430–437.

Idvall J, Ahlgren I, Aronsen KF & Stenberg P (1979) Ketamine infusions: pharmacokinetics and clinical effects. *British Journal of Anaesthesia* **51:** 1167–1173.

Johnson KL, Erickson JP, Holley FO & Scott JC (1984) Fentanyl pharmacokinetics in the pediatric population. *Anesthesiology* **61:** A441.

Jonmarker C, Westrin P, Larsson S & Werner O (1987) Thiopental requirements for induction of anesthesia in children. *Anesthesiology* **67:** 104–107.

Kay B (1976) A clinical assessment of the use of etomidate in children. *British Journal of Anaesthesia* **48:** 207–210.

Kay B (1986a) Alfentanil infusion in paediatric dental anaesthesia. Abstract 813, European Congress on Anaesthesiology, Vienna.

Kay B (1986b) Propofol and alfentanil infusion. A comparison with methohexitone and alfentanil for major surgery. *Anaesthesia* **41:** 589–595.

Kay NH, Sear JW, Uppington J, Cockshott ID & Douglas EJ (1986) Disposition of propofol in patients undergoing surgery. *British Journal of Anaesthesia* **58:** 1076–1079.

Koehntop DE, Rodman JH, Brundage DM, Hegland MG & Buckley JJ (1986) Pharmacokinetics of fentanyl in neonates. *Anesthesia and Analgesia* **65:** 227–232.

Koren G, Goresky G, Crean P, Klein J & MacLeod S (1984) Pediatric fentanyl dosing based on pharmacokinetics during cardiac surgery. *Anesthesia and Analgesia* **63:** 577–582.

Koren G, Butt W, Chinyanga H, Soldin S, Tan Y-K & Pape K (1985) Postoperative morphine infusion in newborn infants: assessment of disposition characteristics and safety. *Journal of Pediatrics* **107:** 963–967.

Kupferberg HJ & Way EL (1963) Pharmacologic basis for the sensitivity of the newborn rat to morphine. *Journal of Pharmacological Experimental Therapeutics* **141:** 105–112.

Ledingham I McA, Finlay WEI, Watt I & McKee JI (1983) Etomidate and adrenocortical function. *Lancet* **i:** 1434–1437.

Lloyd-Thomas AR & Booker PD (1986) Infusion of midazolam in paediatric patients after cardiac surgery. *British Journal of Anaesthesia* **58:** 1109–1115.

Lockhart CH & Nelson WL (1974) The relationship of ketamine requirements to age in pediatric patients. *Anesthesiology* **40**: 507–508.

Lynn AM & Slattery JT (1987) Morphine pharmacokinetics in early infancy. *Anesthesiology* **66**: 136–139.

Lynn AM, Opheim KE & Tyler DC (1984) Morphine infusion after pediatric cardiac surgery. *Critical Care Medicine* **12**: 863–867.

McQuay H & Moor A (1984) Metabolism of narcotics. *British Medical Journal* **228**: 237–240.

Meuldermans W, Hurkmans R & Hendricks J (1980) Plasma levels, excretion, and metabolism of tritium-labelled sufentanil following intravenous administration in dogs. *Janssen Preclinical Research Report* **R33**: 800–808.

Meuldermans WEG, Hurkmans RMA & Heykants JJP (1982) Plasma protein binding and distribution of fentanyl, sufentanil, alfentanil and lofentanil in blood. *Archives Internationales de Pharmacodynamie et de Thérapie* **257**: 4.

Moore RA, Yang SS, McNicholas KW, Gallagher JD & Clark DL (1985) Hemodynamic and anesthetic effects of sufentanil as the sole anesthetic for pediatric cardiovascular surgery. *Anesthesiology* **62**: 725–731.

Moreland TA, Brice JEH, Walker CHM & Parija AC (1980) Naloxone pharmacokinetics in the newborn. *British Journal of Clinical Pharmacology* **9**: 609–612.

Mori K (1987) Editorial: The EEG and awareness during anaesthesia. *Anaesthesia* **42**: 1153–1155.

Morselli PL, Franco-Morselli R & Bossi L (1983) Clinical pharmacokinetics in newborns and infants. In Gibaldi M & Prescot L (eds) *Handbook of Clinical Pharmacokinetics*, pp 98–141. New York: Adis Health Science Press.

Pacifici GM, Sawe J, Kager L & Rane A (1982) Morphine glucuronidation in human fetal and adult liver. *European Journal of Clinical Pharmacology* **22**: 553–558.

Page P, Morgan M & Loh L (1972) Ketamine anaesthesia in paediatric procedures. *Acta Anaesthesialogica Scandinavica* **16**: 155–160.

Park GR (1985) Effect of morphine on gastric emptying. *Anaesthesia* **40**: 82.

Pekoe GM & Smith DJ (1982) The involvement of opiate and mono-aminergic systems in the analgesic effects of ketamine. *Pain* **12**: 57–61.

Persson P, Nilsson A, Hartrig P & Tansen A (1987) Pharmacokinetics of midazolam in total i.v. anaesthesia. *British Journal of Anaesthesia* **59**: 548–556.

Peters WP, Johnson MW, Friedman PA & Mitch WE (1981) Pressor effect of naloxone in septic shock. *Lancet* **i**: 529–532.

Purcell-Jones G, Yates A, Baker JR & James IG (1987) Comparison of the induction characteristics of thiopentone and propofol in children. *British Journal of Anaesthesia* **59**: 1431–1436.

Richter E, Epping J, Fuchshofen-Rockel M, Heusler H & Zilly W (1980) Arzneimittelmetabolisms bei Patienten mit Lebererkrankungen. *Leber Magen Darm* **10**: 234–238.

Roure P, Jean N, Leclerc A-C, Cabanel N, Leyron J-C & Duvaldestin P (1987) Pharmacokinetics of alfentanil in children undergoing surgery. *British Journal of Anaesthesia* **59**: 1437–1440.

Rucquoi M & Camu F (1983) Cardiovascular responses to large doses of alfentanil and fentanyl. *British Journal of Anaesthesia* **55**: 223S–230S.

Russell IF (1986) Comparison of wakefulness with two anaesthetic regimens. Total i.v. v. balanced anaesthesia. *British Journal of Anaesthesia* **58**: 965–968.

Sage DJ, Close A & Boas RA (1987) Reversal of midazolam with anexate. *British Journal of Anaesthesia* **59**: 459–464.

Salonen M, Kanto J, Iisalo E & Himberg J-J (1987) Midazolam as an induction agent in children: a pharmacokinetic and clinical study. *Anesthesia and Analgesia* **66**: 625–628.

Sear JW, Prys-Roberts C (1979) Dose related haemodynamic effects of continuous infusions of Althesin in man. *British Journal of Anaesthesia* **51**: 867–873.

Sethna DH, Moffitt EA, Gray RJ et al (1982) Cardiovascular effects of morphine in patients with coronary arterial disease. *Anesthesia and Analgesia* **61:** 109–114.

Shelly MP, Cory EP & Park GR (1986) Pharmacokinetics of morphine in two children before and after liver transplantation. *British Journal of Anaesthesia* **58:** 1218–1223.

Simons PJ, Cockshott ID, Douglas EJ, Gordon EA, Hopkins K & Rowland M (1985) Blood concentrations, metabolism and elimination after a subanaesthesia intravenous dose of ^{14}C-propofol to male volunteers. *Postgraduate Medical Journal* **61**(suppl 3): 64 (abstract).

Singleton MA, Rosen JL & Fisher DM (1984) Pharmacokinetics of fentanyl for infants and adults. *Anesthesiology* **61:** A440.

Smith G & Pinnock C (1985) Editoral: Naloxone-paradox or panacea? *British Journal of Anaesthesia* **57:** 547–549.

Sorbo S, Hudson RJ & Loomis JC (1984) The pharmacokinetics of thiopental in pediatric surgical patients. *Anesthesiology* **61:** 666–670.

Stanski DR & Hug CC (1982) Alfentanil—a kinetically predictable narcotic analgesia. *Anesthesiology* **57:** 435–439.

Stanski DR, Greenblatt DJ, Lappas DG, Koch-Weser J & Lowenstein E (1976) Kinetics of high dose intravenous morphine in cardiac surgery patients. *Clinical Pharmacology and Therapeutics* **19:** 752–756.

Stanski DR, Greenblatt DJ & Lowenstein E (1978) Kinetics of intravenous and intramuscular morphine. *Clinical Pharmacology and Therapeutics* **24:** 52–59.

Tenenbein M (1984) Continuous naloxone infusion for opiate poisoning in infancy. *Journal of Pediatrics* **105:** 645–648.

Todd MM, Drummond JC & Sang UH (1984) The hemodynamic consequences of high-dose methohexital anaesthesia in humans. *Anesthesiology* **61:** 495–501.

Todd MM, Drummond JC & Sang UH (1985) The hemodynamic consequences of high-dose thiopental anesthesia. *Anesthesia and Analgesia* **64:** 678–687.

Tserng K-Y, Takeiddine FN & King KC (1983) Developmental aspects of theophylline metabolism in premature infants. *Clinical Pharmacology and Therapeutics* **33:** 525–528.

Vandenberghe H, MacLeod S, Chinyanga H, Endrenyi L & Soldin S (1983) Pharmacokinetics of i.v. morphine in balanced anaesthesia: studies in children. *Drug Metabolism Review* **14:** 887–903.

Wessels JV, Allen GW & Slogoff S (1973) The effect of nitrous oxide on ketamine anesthesia. *Anesthesiology* **39:** 382–396.

Relaxants in paediatric anaesthesia

Until about 20 years ago, the practice of paediatric anaesthesia depended in part on only two neuromuscular blocking agents, which were usually administered in single bolus doses. By contrast, at least seven such agents are now clinically available, with the promise of a few others currently under evaluation. The various properties of the drugs themselves allow for a more carefully tailored anaesthesia course. As practice has grown more sophisticated, varied modes of administration have also entered routine use, the clinician now having at his or her disposal such methods as priming, drugs in combination, and continuous infusion. To meet the demands for prolonged surgical relaxation, an intermediate-acting agent might be given in sequential doses or via infusion; a long-acting agent might be substituted, there being a predictable rate of recovery even after lengthy procedures. Because the newer agents have no appreciable cumulative properties, the anaesthetist can time recovery to the conclusion of surgery or can quickly and easily reverse residual effects. There are even added extraclinical decisions: since the cost of the newer drugs is two to three times higher than that of the older ones, the anaesthetist can at times choose freely only within the limits of his or her own hospital's fiscal restraints.

This chapter reviews and classifies the neuromuscular blocking agents currently available to the modern paediatric anaesthetist and makes suggestions for their practical use.

SHORT-ACTING RELAXANTS

Succinylcholine

Succinylcholine (SCh) is the only short-acting relaxant presently available for use in children. Though its rapid onset of action is unsurpassed, its unique mode of action (sustained depolarization) causes side-effects which are markedly different from those of other agents. Interestingly, some of these side-effects are dissimilar in children and in adults.

Early in 1955 Stead observed that infants require more SCh than adults according to body weight. Cook and Fischer (1975) later confirmed with twitch recording that 1 mg/kg SCh in small infants produced neuromuscular blockade equal to that produced by 0.5 mg/kg in older children. At these equipotent doses there was no significant difference between the recovery time to 50 and 90% of neuromuscular transmission. It is now postulated that SCh undergoes a first-order pharmacokinetic elimination (Cook, 1981). Since the extracellular volume occupies a larger percentage of body weight in the infant (40 vs. 18% in adults), it may be assumed that the drug is distributed in a larger volume and that the net result is a lower concentration reaching the myoneural junction. In infants, therefore, it would seem reasonable to give a larger dose of SCh (mg/kg) than that given to older children. In fact the usual recommended i.v. dose for neuromuscular blockade is 2 mg/kg in the infant and only 1 mg/kg in the older child (Stead, 1955; Cook, 1981; Goudsouzian and Gionfriddo, 1984). If given intramuscularly 5 mg/kg (Liu et al, 1981) suffices for infants and 4 mg/kg for children (Liu and Goudsouzian, 1982).

When SCh is administered to infants and children via continuous intravenous infusion, tachyphylaxis and phase II block develop as in adults. Clinical evaluations have shown that tachyphylaxis may occur in children after the administration of 3 mg/kg over an interval of 23 min and phase II block after a total of 4 mg/kg has been given (DeCook and Goudsouzian, 1980). A longer infusion period (100 min) may lead to the development of bradyphylaxis because of decreased requirements subsequent to the establishment of phase II block (Bevan et al, 1986). In infants tachyphylaxis is seen after 4 mg/kg with phase II block occurring after 5 mg/kg (Goudsouzian and Liu, 1984). Interestingly, in some very young infants (5 days to 4 months of age) marked resistance to the neuromuscular effects of SCh has been detected; demonstrating a threefold difference in dosage requirement, these infants go on to recover within the short span of 5 min after discontinuation of infusion. As yet there is no definitive explanation for this marked resistance. It was originally suggested that such infants might have a high level of plasma cholinesterase but investigators have found that cholinesterase levels are lower in infants than in adults (Szigmond and Downs, 1971). Differences in distribution volume may be partially responsible, but the threefold difference in requirement remains something of a mystery. Probably there exists an inherent resistance of the myoneural junction to SCh in very young infants but this has yet to be demonstrated with certainty.

Side-effects

Most of the side-effects associated with SCh are benign in nature and resolve spontaneously. The most frequently observed are bradyarrhythmias in the form of premature atrial or nodal contractions lasting for a few beats and then disappearing without any specific treatment. In adults most arrhythmias are seen after a second i.v. dose (Stoelting and Peterson, 1975), but in children they can frequently be spotted after a single dose (Leigh et al, 1957; Craythorne et al, 1960a; Goudsouzian, 1981); they are not seen following i.m. administration of the drug (Hannallah et al, 1986). These arrhythmias are most reliably prevented by i.v. atropine 0.01 mg/kg just prior to SCh administration (Goudsouzian, 1981). Adequate premedicating doses of atropine also prevent arrhythmias.

In healthy children SCh does not cause any significant hyperkalaemia; only a slight potassium increase of 0.23 nmol has been reported (Keneally and Bush, 1974). In the presence of burns, tetanus and paraplegia, however, marked hyperkalaemia can occur (McCaughey, 1982); in children with cerebral palsy it does not (Dierdorf and McNiece, 1984). Though of frequent occurrence in adults following i.v. SCh, fasciculations rarely develop in children less than 4 years of age. Some gross muscle movements are, however, occasionally present (Cozantis et al, 1987). Children do not demonstrate the rise in intragastric pressures seen in their older counterparts (Salem et al, 1972).

Masseter spasm has been frequently associated with the use of SCh, especially in the presence of halothane (Schwartz et al, 1984). Upon investigation, some patients will be found to have a rise in serum phosphokinase levels, and some will prove positive on biopsy for malignant hyperthermia.

Whereas adults are usually free of the risk of myoglobinuria subsequent to SCh administration, children may show a significant increase in serum myoglobin concentrations (although of a small magnitude; Ryan et al, 1971). This increase is even greater during the concomitant administration of halothane (Harrington et al, 1984) but can be easily managed by the prior administration of tubocurarine (Asari et al, 1984) or pancuronium (Blanc et al, 1986). Malignant hyperthermia, when it occurs, is frequently associated with the use of SCh, together with halothane anaesthesia.

Intraocular pressure may rise after SCh whether the patient fasciculates or not. This effect is due mostly to contraction of the extraocular muscles. The rise in pressure begins about 1 min after administration of the drug, reaches its peak in about 3 min and subsides in 7 min (Craythorne et al, 1960b). In the clinical situation it is advisable to wait at least this long before tonometry in children. Although the use of SCh without untoward side-effects has been reported in several cases of open eye injury (Libonati et al, 1985), many anaesthetists feel it is prudent to refrain from its use in situations of penetrating ocular wounds unless the eye is not salvageable (see p. 451).

Because SCh has the fastest onset of the presently available neuromuscular blocking agents, it remains the most suitable, despite its side-effects, if rapid tracheal intubation is needed. Although satisfactory intubating conditions can be achieved with 1 mg/kg in children, the author's inclination is to use 1.5 mg/kg to achieve a faster and more reliable onset (Cunliffe et al, 1986). If the main inhalation anaesthetic is halothane, pretreatment with atropine 0.01 mg/kg i.v. is advisable to decrease the incidence of arrhythmias.

INTERMEDIATE-ACTING RELAXANTS

The recent availability of the non-depolarizers atracurium and vecuronium has made a significant impact on the practice of paediatric anaesthesia. The major advantage of these two agents lies in the fact that at clinical doses they cause virtually no change in the pulse rate or blood pressure. Since they are also free from the side-effects of SCh and have a comparatively short duration of action, they can be satisfactorily used in the many short paediatric procedures.

In assessing the various studies designed to determine the doses of atracurium and vecuronium that effect 50 and 95% depression of the twitch response (ED_{50} and ED_{95}), one needs to be aware that the use of the incremental technique to determine the dose–response sometimes results in higher values than that of the bolus dose technique (Tables 5.1 and 5.2). This is so because with the cumulation method much of the effect of the initial dose is dissipated before the last dose is given (Fisher et al, 1982a), a circumstance not in evidence in the assessment of long-acting non-depolarizing muscle relaxants (Donlon et al, 1980).

Table 5.1. The effective doses of atracurium in infants, children and adolescents

Reference	Anaesthetic agent	Technique	ED_{50} (μg/kg)	ED_{95} (μg/kg)
Infants				
Brandom et al (1984)	Halothane	Bolus	85	150
Goudsouzian et al (1985)	Halothane	Incremental	100	170
Meistelman et al (1988)				
Infants 1–3 months	Halothane	Bolus	86	175
Infants 3–12 months	Halothane	Bolus	131	205
Children				
Brandom et al (1983)	Halothane	Bolus	132	260
Brandom et al (1983)	N_2O:narcotic	Bolus	169	354
Goudsouzian et al (1983a)	Halothane	Incremental	110	170
Goudsouzian et al (1985)	N_2O:narcotic	Incremental	160	240
Adolescents				
Brandom et al (1983)	Halothane	Bolus	101	157
Goudsouzian et al (1983a)	Halothane	Incremental	120	180

Table 5.2. The effective doses of vecuronium in infants, children and adolescents

Reference	Anaesthetic agent	Technique	ED_{50} (μg/kg)	ED_{95} (μg/kg)
Infants				
Fisher and Miller (1983)	Halothane	Bolus	16.5	—
Children				
Fisher and Miller (1983)	Halothane	Bolus	19	—
Goudsouzian et al (1983b)	Halothane	Incremental	33	60
Meistelman et al (1986b)	Halothane	Bolus	31	64
Adolescents				
Goudsouzian et al (1983b)	Halothane	Incremental	23	45

A comparison of data reveals the fact that children generally require more of these two relaxants than do adults to obtain the same degree of neuromuscular blockade. The difference, however, is relatively small and is masked in most statistical analyses by the wide range of individual responses. The effect of potentiation from volatile anaesthetics is also apparent, but it is less marked than that observed with the long-acting neuromuscular blocking agents (Miller et al, 1984).

Some investigators have observed that the atracurium requirement of infants seems to be less than that of older children (Table 5.1). This difference, however, is a small one, and has not appeared in other studies. Most recently this difference has been noticed in very small infants, especially those less than 48 hours postpartum with a temperature less than 36°C (Nightingale, 1986).

Certain differences in atracurium and vecuronium need to be remarked upon. Their respective modes of elimination are of primary importance. Vecuronium is excreted mostly in bile; a small amount (10–25%) is excreted in urine, most of which seems to be in the non-metabolized form. Atracurium by contrast is unique in being metabolized completely through Hofmann elimination and to a lesser extent by ester hydrolysis. As a consequence it is not excreted in bile or urine except in the form of a metabolite, hence, its advantageous use in infants with impaired liver function (Simpson and Green, 1986). Hofmann elimination is a non-biological method of degradation that occurs at normal body temperature and in the alkaline pH of blood. In the blood the quaternary ammonium compound breaks down primarily into laudanosine and a related quaternary acid in the absence of plasma enzymes. These compounds do not have neuromuscular blocking properties (Miller et al, 1984).

In comparing recovery times we find that for both agents the duration of clinical relaxation (recovery of twitch height to 25% of control) is about 25 min in children and the time to complete recovery is about 40–60 min (Table 5.3 and 5.4). Although individual responses vary, there is some indication that vecuronium may be slightly shorter-acting than atracurium. In one study an intubating dose of 80 μg/kg vecuronium provided 25 min of clinical relaxation with full recovery in under 50 min; this period is somewhat shorter than that usually observed with an equipotent dose of atra-

Table 5.3. Recovery times from the action of atracurium

Reference	Dose (μg/kg)	Anaesthetic agent	Recovery from maximum block to 25% (min)	Recovery from maximum block to 95% (min)
Infants				
Brandom et al (1984)	300	Halothane	22	32
Goudsouzian et al (1985)	400	Halothane	37	56
Meretoja and Kalli (1986)	400	N_2O:narcotic	30	53
Children				
Brandom et al (1983)	400	N_2O:narcotic	28	41
Brandom et al (1983)	400	N_2O:narcotic	23	40
Goudsouzian et al (1983a)	400	Halothane	38	59
Goudsouzian et al (1985)	500	N_2O:narcotic	36	51
Meretoja and Kalli (1986)	400	N_2O:narcotic	22	41

Table 5.4. Recovery times from the action of vecuronium

Reference	Dose (μg/kg)	Anaesthetic agent	Recovery from maximum block	
			to 25% (min)	to 95% (min)
Infants				
Fisher and Miller (1983)	70	Halothane		73
Meistelman et al (1986a)	100	Halothane		36(90%)
Children				
Goudsouzian et al (1983a)	80	Halothane	22	43
Ferres et al (1983)	100	Halothane	20	
Friesdorf et al (1986)	80	Thiopental or ketamine	13	27(90%)
Friesdorf et al (1986)	100	Thiopental or ketamine	19	35(90%)
Adolescents				
Goudsouzian et al (1983a)	80	Halothane	26	48

curium (Goudsouzian et al, 1983b). The recovery data from children tend to agree with those from adults for both drugs, but, again, these drugs have on occasion been seen to be somewhat shorter-acting in children (Goudsouzian et al, 1983a,b). In infants vecuronium has a longer duration of action than in children (Fisher and Miller, 1983; Motsch et al, 1985).

Pharmacokinetic data have shown that the distribution volume of atracurium (area) is larger in infants than in children (176 vs. 139 ml/kg) and that the clearance is faster; this explains the shorter duration of action detected in some studies (Brandom et al, 1986). In studies with vecuronium, clearance has been found to be faster in children than in adults, a factor which partly explains the drug's relatively shorter duration of action in the younger patients (Steinbereithner et al, 1984). A comparison of infants with children (Fisher et al, 1985) finds that the plasma concentration causing 50% depression of the twitch (C_{pss50}) is lower in infants. Their requirement, however, tends to be the same as that of older children. This is because the larger volume of distribution in infants dilutes a given dose, counteracting the greater sensitivity of the neuromuscular junction. The mean residence time is, however, longer in infants, a fact which explains the longer duration of action in infants. Further, vecuronium's shorter duration of action relative to pancuronium can be explained by its higher rate of plasma clearance (Meistelman et al, 1986a).

Atracurium and vecuronium are very useful in the paediatric population because of the large number of short surgical procedures (for example, hernia repairs, orchidopexies, tonsillectomies) that are performed in children. Because of their short duration of action, these drugs can be given in one intubating dose (atracurium 0.4–0.6 mg/kg, vecuronium 0.08–0.012 mg/kg), a light anaesthetic level can be maintained throughout the procedure, and the child will be minimally anaesthetized at the conclusion of surgery. Reversal does not seem to be mandatory in all patients. In fact, if more than 45 min has elapsed since the final dose of either drug, one may reasonably assume that the neuromuscular function has nearly recovered. This can, of course, be adequately confirmed by observing four equal twitches during train-of-four stimulation. It is nonetheless essential that an evaluation of *clinical* recovery be made in all cases. Respiratory patterns should be observed and strong movement of all four limbs should be in evidence. Most important, especially in infants, is the return of facial movement and crying.

Because of their desirable properties, atracurium and vecuronium have varied uses. They are particularly useful in children with irritable airways. In paediatric practice we are frequently confronted with children who have repeated airway infection. Ideally one would like to operate when such children are completely free of residual infection, but this becomes a practical impossibility. With atracurium and vecuronium one can maintain the patient at a light level of anaesthesia, provide adequate surgical relaxation, reverse the effect of the relaxant, and have the child's reflexes fully recovered at the end of the surgical procedure. A similar situation pertains to children presenting for bronchoscopy or oesophagoscopy.

Because of the rapidity with which reversal occurs even after extended use, both atracurium and vecuronium can be easily administered via continuous infusion. In children the requirement for atracurium is 9 μg/kg/min during N_2O narcotic anaesthesia, 6–8 μg/kg/min during halothane or isoflurane, and 5 μg/kg/min during enflurane (Figure 5.1) (Brandom et al, 1985; Goudsouzian et al, 1986a; Ridley and Hatch, 1988). Infants seem to require the same infusion rates but show marked individual variation (Goudsouzian, 1988). With vecuronium a rate of about 1.4 μg/kg/min (Mirakhur et al, 1984) is required in adults to maintain 90–99% depression of the twitch during $N_2O:O_2$ narcotic anaesthesia. Children will probably require a slightly higher infusion rate than this.

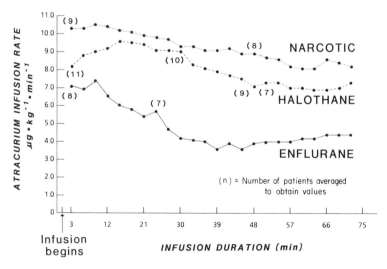

Figure 5.1. Atracurium infusion requirements in children during $N_2O:O_2$ narcotic, halothane and enflurane anaesthesia. From Goudsouzian et al (1986a), with permission.

For all their advantages these agents do have some drawbacks, the main one being a delayed onset of action after an intubating dose. Complete paralysis does not occur until at least 2 min after administration, considerably longer than the 45 s span one is used to with SCh. Several attempts have been made to cut the time to onset of blockade by giving a priming dose of about one-quarter of the original, waiting 5 to 7 min, and then giving a full dose. This has succeeded in reducing the onset time by only one-third (Tsai et al, 1986). It should be realized, however, that complete peripheral neuromuscular relaxation is not an absolute prerequisite for ventilation or tracheal intubation. In an adequately anaesthetized patient who receives a non-depolarizing relaxant, ventilation can be assisted before the occurrence of complete peripheral paralysis, presumably because of early paralysis of the laryngeal and pharyngeal muscles. Furthermore, after relaxants have been given, these patients do not develop laryngospasm if difficulty is experienced during the intubation attempt. Although priming might seem logical in some situations it has very limited use in paediatric practice. One example might serve to illustrate: in the child presenting with 'full stomach', where rapid intubation is desirable, it is wishful thinking to suppose a co-operative subject; to administer a small dose of relaxant and then wait for 5 min while the child is experiencing some muscle weakness is clearly unrealistic. Such a child is liable to be upset, to flail about and retch or vomit, creating a situation much worse than the one the anaesthetist is trying to avoid.

Because these relaxants are virtually free of cardiovascular or vagolytic properties, the clinician should be particularly cautious in those situations in which bothersome bradycardic episodes occur secondary to surgical manipulation (such as when traction is applied to the extraocular muscles or viscera). Such episodes respond satisfactorily to the relaxation of traction or to the administration of vagolytic agents such as atropine. Cases should be monitored closely, assessed individually and treatment given when needed. Interestingly, we have not observed the bradycardic response during tracheal intubation.

One should also realize that atracurium and vecuronium are acidic compounds (pH values between 3 and 4) and as such can be easily deactivated in alkaline media. This fact is especially important for atracurium, since its mode of elimination is alkaline hydrolysis (Hofmann elimination). In a slowly running intravenous system in which thiopentone (ph 10–11) is injected with atracurium, precipitation and loss of the relaxant's potency might conceivably occur. Consequently if these drugs are to be used in tandem the clinician should insure that the thiopentone is washed through the intravenous tubing before the introduction of atracurium. Because dilution may decrease the potency, atracurium is preferably infused undiluted. A further point to be noted is the unsuitability of these agents for intramuscular administration due to their availability only in acidic mixture; in this respect, SCh holds the advantage.

With respect to atracurium, one should be aware of the slight possibility of histamine release. Most of the time this manifests itself as harmless cutaneous reactions in the form of flushing of the neck or the face (Rowlands, 1987). It is in fact commonplace by now to remark that some erythema can frequently be seen with atracurium in children (Lavery and

Mirakhur, 1984). Extremely rare instances of anaphylactoid reactions or bronchospasm have been reported, though it is interesting that these have occurred when atracurium was preceded by thiopentone (Woods et al, 1985; Pollock et al, 1986; Cohen and Frank, 1987). A study designed to assess the possible histaminergic properties of atracurium found histamine release in children to be much less frequent than in adults; even in the presence of high plasma histamine levels, children did not manifest marked cardiovascular effects (Goudsouzian et al, 1986b). Vecuronium seems to be entirely free of such histamine-induced side-effects (Figure 5.2). Laudanosine, one of the degradation products of atracurium, can be detected in the plasma of children who have received the drug. Laudanosine can have convulsant properties, but only at doses far greater than those that may result from the clinical administration of atracurium (Ward et al, 1983). The decay of laudanosine is slower in children with impaired renal function. Lower concentrations (about 2% of plasma levels) can be detected in the cerebrospinal fluid (Harris et al, 1987); however, this low concentration has not been shown to cause any harmful effects.

LONG-ACTING MUSCLE RELAXANTS

Four long-acting neuromuscular blocking agents—pancuronium, tubo-curarine, metocurine and gallamine—have been adequately evaluated in

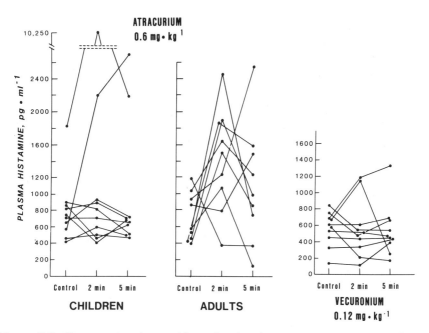

Figure 5.2. Changes in plasma histamine levels upon administration of atracurium 0.6 mg/kg in adults and children, and 0.12 mg/kg vecuronium in children. From Scott et al (1985) and Goudsouzian et al (1986b), with permission.

children. Metocurine and gallamine do not enjoy wide popularity; tubocurarine is still widely used but pancuronium is more popular, largely because of its vagolytic properties (Goudsouzian and Gionfriddo, 1984). Cardiac output in children, and especially in infants, is rate-dependent, the young heart being less compliant than the adult; hence the Frank Starling mechanism is less efficient (Crone, 1984). Consequently, mild tachycardia is a desirable condition in children, and even more so in infants. Because cardiac output can generally be well maintained with pancuronium, this has for many years been the drug of choice in children in whom there is impairment of cardiovascular reserves (Nightingale and Bush, 1973). Its use should probably be avoided in hypertensive patients.

Tubocurarine can usually be used in children without the worry of marked cardiovascular side-effects. A large intubating dose, however, may cause histamine release, especially in adolescents. Such an occurrence manifests as a transient rash and a mild hypotension, but clears spontaneously (Nightingale and Bush, 1973). Metocurine, though carrying the potential for histamine release, does not cause appreciable changes in pulse rate or blood pressure at large intubating doses (0.5 mg/kg; Goudsouzian et al, 1978). Tachycardia does result from the introduction of gallamine and may occasionally last even longer than the drug's neuromuscular effects.

Pancuronium is the most potent of these four drugs, followed by metocurine, tubocurarine and gallamine in a 1:4:7:40 ratio (Figure 5.3) (Goudsouzian

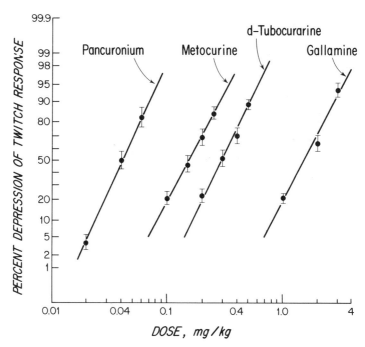

Figure 5.3. The dose–response effects of pancuronium, metocurine, tubocurarine and gallamine in children anaesthetized with $N_2O:O_2$ narcotics, at a frequency of stimulation at 0.1 Hz. From Goudsouzian et al (1984), with permission.

et al, 1984). The latter three have about the same duration of action; an intubating dose gives complete paralysis (no twitch response) for 1 h and satisfactory surgical relaxation (twitch 5–25%) for another 30 min. Pancuronium appears in some studies to have a slightly shorter duration of action (Goudsouzian et al, 1974, 1975, 1984), though it may be masked at times by wide individual variations; this may be particularly so in studies on limited numbers of patients.

The choice between these four relaxants depends on the clinical circumstances and on the habit of the attending anaesthetist. One can, however, make good use of these agents by matching particular side-effects to the given situation. If a mild tachycardia is desirable, pancuronium is preferred; a good indication for its use is in the presence of halothane or fentanyl when the tachycardia will counteract the slowing of the heart rate and help to maintain the blood pressure. If a slow heart rate or mild hypotension is desirable, tubocurarine is a better choice; it can be especially useful if a narcotic $N_2O:O_2$ relaxant technique is to be used. If no particular change in heart rate or blood pressure is desired then metocurine, or perhaps atracurium or vecuronium, would be indicated.

In common paediatric practice, the initial dose of tubocurarine has varied between 0.25 and 0.8 mg/kg. The lower dose is usually used in children already intubated and anaesthetized with a halogenated agent. This dose produces clinical relaxation lasting for about 25 min, whereas the larger dose can be used for tracheal intubation with the clinical effect lasting for about 1 h. Pancuronium similarly has been used in doses of 0.06–0.15 mg/kg. A frequently used dose is 0.1 mg/kg; this will produce satisfactory conditions for intubation in 1.5 min and a clinical effect lasting for 45 min.

Pancuronium is frequently advocated for a variety of cardiac surgical procedures in infants. Infants presenting for ligation of patent ductus arteriosus tolerate the anaesthetic technique of fentanyl–air–oxygen pancuronium satisfactorily (Robinson and Gregory, 1981). The vagolytic effects of pancuronium counteract the bradycardiac effects of fentanyl, and its relaxant properties counteract the muscle stiffness caused by fentanyl. Pancuronium has also been found to be useful for correction of cyanotic and acyanotic congenital cardiac anomalies. In the presence of pancuronium infants tolerate large doses of fentanyl (75 μg/kg) or sufentanil 10 μg/kg (Hickey and Hansen, 1984). Further, in the mechanically ventilated patient, the drug is valuable for decreasing O_2 consumption.

In neonatal intensive care units pancuronium can be employed to achieve easier ventilation, especially for premature infants who actively expire against the positive pressure of the ventilator, increasing the risk of pneumothorax (Henry et al, 1979; Grenough et al, 1984). Since pancuronium increases the heart rate, blood pressure, plasma adrenalin and noradrenaline levels (Cabal et al, 1984), there has been some concern that it might be a contributing factor in cerebral haemorrhage (Reynolds et al, 1985). In patients at risk, it should be noted that nasotracheal intubation or intratracheal suctioning in the presence of pancuronium causes a smaller change in intracranial pressure than such activity in patients not receiving the drug (Finer and Tomney, 1981; Fanconi and Duc, 1987). Adequate sedation is required prior to the introduction of the relaxant. Thus, the best approach to neonatal intubation seems to be the administration of pancuronium with sedation in the intensive care unit or a general anaesthetic in the operating theatre (Friesen et al, 1987). Vecuronium might offer an advantage over pancuronium in that it does not significantly increase the blood pressure, which is directly related to cerebral blood flow (Hamza et al, 1987) and in the intensive care unit is frequently administered by continuous infusion.

In considering the demands of neonatal intensive care, it is further of interest to note that prolonged blockade with pancuronium can be adequately reversed with the usual doses of atropine and neostigmine; this holds true after a period of 10 h subsequent to the last dose of the relaxant and, in fact, as soon as 4 h after the final dose (Goudsouzian et al, 1981).

It has recently been suggested that muscle relaxants should be used in combination to decrease the total amount of medication, in order to minimize side-effects (Lebowitz et al, 1980). The combination of pancuronium with metocurine or tubocurarine has seemed particularly inviting in these respects. Although a case can be made for the use of these combinations in children, one must proceed with great care in the operating theatre due to the risk of miscalculation and dosing error. This technique is perhaps most useful in prolonged surgical procedures (infrequent in children) where adequate neuromuscular monitoring is essential.

Pharmacokinetics

There are two pincipal studies, one by Fisher et al (1982b) and the other by Matteo et al (1984), that have investigated the pharmacokinetics of tubocurarine in infants. Some interesting though conflicting observations have been made. First, since neonates and small infants have twice the extracellular fluid per body weight than do adults, there exists in them a greater distribution volume for tubocurarine. Both studies found further that the elimination half-life was longer in neonates than in older children and adults, suggesting that in neonates the duration of action of multiple doses or a large initial dose might be prolonged. Fisher et al (1982b), however, observed that the plasma concentration causing 50% depression of twitch response was markedly lower in neonates than in adults. By contrast, Matteo et al (1984) did not find significant differences in the effect of plasma concentration response lines between adults, children, infants and neonates. No specific reason can be found for this disagreement. The anaesthetic agent might be a factor; the fact that Fisher's work with general surgical patients who were well hydrated as opposed to Matteo's with neurosurgical patients who were probably fluid-restricted might also be relevant. In reviewing these studies one should also realize that tubocurarine and metocurine bind less to plasma proteins in neonates; hence the free fraction of the muscle relaxant is higher in neonatal than in adult blood due to the lower α_1-acid glycoprotein levels present there (Wood and Wood, 1981). Consequently, these drugs will be more effective in neonates at a lower plasma concentration.

In contrast to those for tubocurarine, the pharmacokinetic data for pancuronium do not differ in children and adults. Pancuronium is mostly excreted by the kidney and renal function does not change after infancy, so changes in pharmacokinetic data are not seen (Meistelman et al, 1986a).

A salient feature of most studies on infants is the wide individual variation; some infants are sensitive to relaxants and some are markedly resistant. This observation is confirmed by the above-referenced pharmacokinetic studies of tubocurarine. One can assume the lower requirement in some infants to be a sign of underdevelopment of the myoneural junction but it is more difficult to explain the resistant individual. A correlation can perhaps be drawn from animal studies in which developing muscle cells are shown to have immature fetal and/or extrajunctional receptors which are resistant to tubocurarine (Goudsouzian and Standaert, 1986).

New muscle relaxants

The recent trend has been to develop new non-depolarizing muscle relaxants with minimal side-effects. Initial evaluations of two long-acting agents, pipecuronium and doxacurium, are promising. These drugs are practically devoid of side effects at doses up to three times the ED_{95}. Doxacurium, which has already been evaluated in children (Goudsouzian et al, 1987, 1988; Sarner et al, 1987), does not have any cardiovascular or histaminergic properties. Its ED_{95}, approximately 30 µg/kg, makes it the most potent neuromuscular blocking agent available. Though it is approximately twice as potent as vecuronium, its duration of action is similar to that of tubocurarine or metocurine. This would be the drug of choice in situations where no changes in cardiovascular parameters are desirable, as in patients with a complicated clinical course.

Mivacurium is an interesting short-acting neuromuscular blocking agent. It is non-depolarizing and at least partially hydrolysed by plasma cholinesterase. Its ED_{95} in children during halothane anaesthesia is about 0.1 mg/kg (Miler et al, 1988). A dose of 0.2 mg/kg provides complete suppression of the twitch response in 1.8 ± 0.2 min. After such a dose children recover to 5, 25 and 95% of control twitch height in 9, 11 and 19 min respectively. In adults who were given large doses of the drug, some evidence of histamine release could be detected. In children the only side-effects yet seen have been an occasional reddening along the tract of the vein or a transient flush.

REVERSAL OF LONG-ACTING RELAXANTS

With the intermediate-acting relaxants not all children need to be reversed if monitored adequately. This rarely holds true, however, for long-acting relaxants, the main reason being the long recovery time—over an hour in most children—from 5 to 95% of control twitch height.

Contrary to previous reports (Cook, 1981) the neostigmine requirement of infants and children is less than that of adults (Fisher et al, 1983). In clinical trials infants have been shown to require only about half as much neostigmine as do adults for reversal of tubocurarine-induced neuromuscular blockade. In contrast to tubocurarine the distribution half-lives and distribution volumes were also similar for infants, children and adults. Based on these data, the recommended dose of neostigmine to reverse tubocurarine blockade in infants and children was set at 20 µg/kg (Fisher et al, 1983). One should, however, realize that in the experimental settings from which these observations were drawn the twitch height before the attempted reversal was at least 10% of control and the return of the twitch was therefore prompt. This desirable situation is not always possible at the end of surgical procedures, so more neostigmine will sometimes be required. It always remains of great importance for the anaesthetist to assess the adequacy of reversal both by clinical signs and by the neuromuscular monitor. The presence of four equal twitches during train-of-four stimulation is a very satisfactory and easily discernible end-point, though the post-tetanic twitch count is more sensitive (Viby-Mogensen et al, 1981). Clinical signs of recovery include adequate airway and respiratory movements, facial expressions, leg-lifting (Mason and Betts, 1980) and, most important in an infant, crying.

In contrast to neostigmine the dose of edrophonium required to antagonize tubocurarine-induced neuromuscular blockade is rather similar or possibly greater in infants and children than in adults. Under controlled circumstances the optimal antagonism has been obtained by administering 1 mg/kg (Meakin et al, 1983; Fisher et al, 1984). Onset and duration of antagonism were observed to be similar in the three age groups while clearance was highest in infants and lowest in adults. Theoretically, this rapid clearance may allow the possibility of recurarization. As with neostigmine, to prevent the vagomimetic effects of edrophonium it is preferable to give atropine 10–20 µg/kg prior to its administration. If atropine is given 30 s prior, heart rate and systolic blood pressure remain constant.

Whether edrophonium offers a specific advantage over neostigmine is a matter of opinion. Edrophonium has a more rapid onset of action, but whether the difference of a few minutes justifies the higher cost of edrophonium is questionable. It is interesting to note that the two agents produce dissimilar patterns of recovery of the train-of-four. The train-of-four ratios (T_4/T_1) at the same twitch height tensions (T_1) are greater with edrophonium than with neostigmine, indicating a greater prejunctional effect of edrophonium (Meakin et al, 1983). It has been further noted that the dose–response relationship for edrophonium varies more in infants and that it may therefore be necessary to administer larger doses of edrophonium (1 mg/kg) to paediatric patients for consistent predictable antagonism of neuromuscular blockade (Fisher et al, 1984).

RELAXANTS IN CERTAIN CLINICAL SITUATIONS

In the presence of certain diseases the response of the patient to a given relaxant may be different from that expected, whereas in some other states an otherwise minor or insignificant side-effect could be catastrophic. The following are some pathological situations in which diversions from the norm are likely to occur.

Progressive muscular dystrophy

The Duchenne form is the most common and severe type of the childhood muscular dystrophies (Smith and Bush, 1985). Caused by an X-linked recessive gene, it usually becomes apparent at 2–6 years with the onset of clumsy, waddling gait and frequent falling. It affects first the proximal muscles of the pelvis and the shoulder; these muscles enlarge from fatty infiltration and become extremely weak (pseudohypertrophy). Eventually the weakness progresses to all the muscles of the body; the young victim loses his or her ability to ambulate and develops contractures. These patients also demonstrate myocardial involvement that manifests itself during anaesthesia as tachycardia or even ventricular fibrillation and cardiac arrest (Delphine et al, 1987).

In these patients SCh causes rhabdomyolysis as evidenced by myoglobinurea, increased creatine phosphokinase, hyperkalaemia and occasionally metabolic acidosis. During anaesthesia a moderate rise of body temperature has been seen in these patients and their biopsied muscles have shown increased sensitivity to halothane and caffeine, suggesting some association between muscular dystrophy and malignant hyperthermia (Rosemberg and Heiman-Patterson, 1983); these two diseases, however, have completely different courses and outcomes.

Because of their prominent cardiac and muscular effects depolarizing muscle relaxants such as SCh should be avoided in these patients, especially in combination with halothane. Non-depolarizing agents can, however, be safely used (Sethna et al, 1988). The fact that these patients have a weakness of the respiratory muscles that may lead to respiratory failure is also important. Consequently, adequacy of reversal should be thoroughly evaluated before any attempt at extubation; if there is any doubt the patient should be ventilated postoperatively.

Myotonia

Myotonic dystrophy (dystrophia myotonica) is an autosomal dominant disease (Aldridge, 1985) which causes facial weakness (expression-less face), wasting of the sternomastoids, ptosis, dysarthria, and a progressive distal muscle weakness with wasting. A characteristic feature of its victims is an inability to relax the hand muscles after stimulation (hence the name myotonia).

In these patients SCh may exacerbate myotonia, causing respiratory and jaw muscle rigidity leading to hypoxia and the inability to relax jaw muscles. Occasionally increased myotonia has been seen following neostigmine, presumably from the stimulating effect of acetylcholine.

Again for these patients safe practice demands the avoidance of SCh and the use of one of the non-depolarizing agents instead. Of those presently available, atracurium seems to be the most favoured because of its predictably rapid recovery rate; this feature obviates the need for reversal agents in most of the clinical situations (Nightingale et al, 1985; Stirt et al, 1985).

Myasthenia gravis

This rare condition may affect an infant of a mother with the disease by passage of antibodies and may last for up to 8 weeks. Other paediatric forms are congenital and juvenile types, and 10% of all cases are under 16 years of age. The disease has an autoimmune background with a reduction in the number of acetylcholine receptor sites at the neuromuscular junction. Thymectomy is a common form of treatment for the young as an adjunct to oral anticholinesterase therapy with, for example, pyridostigmine.

There is no agreement about the best anaesthetic regimen to follow. It should be remembered that respiratory failure with secretion retention may follow surgery and provision should be made for respiratory support post-operatively if necessary. Minimal doses of opioid analgesics should be used if ventilation is not planned. Intubation can be achieved by deep inhalational anaesthesia with halothane, for example, though competitive neuromuscular blocking drugs can be used if treated with great caution. Davies and Steward (1973) recommend a dose one-twentieth of normal and if used, the block should be closely monitored with a peripheral nerve stimulator. At the end of the operation the action of the drug is reversed with the usual dose of atropine and neostigmine. These patients may require respiratory support postoperatively even after simple surgery where no muscle relaxants have been used because of changing requirements of anticholinesterases.

Malignant hyperthermia

The combination of SCh and halothane seems to be the one most likely to trigger malignant hyperthermia (Gronert, 1980). Depolarizing relaxants and halogenated agents should, therefore, be avoided in patients thought to be at risk for this syndrome. The safest general anaesthetic technique is the use of a narcotic–nitrous oxide–oxygen combination with a non-depolarizing relaxant (Michel and Fronefield, 1985). Non-depolarizing agents devoid of side-effects may offer an advantage in not masking tachycardia, which is one of the first signs of malignant hyperthermia (see Chapter 21).

Burns

Since the early reports of cardiac arrest in burned patients receiving SCh (Allan et al, 1961), extensive investigations have sought to define and understand the effects of relaxants in these unfortunate patients (Gronert and Theye, 1975; Martyn et al, 1986). In such patients SCh is known to cause hyperkalaemia, which predisposes to cardiac arrest. It seems to be the case that the more extensive the burn the more likely is the hyperkalaemic response. Although most cases of cardiac arrest have occurred 20–50 days after the burn injury, abnormal elevations of plasma potassium levels can occur within a few days of the burn. The hyperkalaemia probably results from the development of new acetylcholine receptors along the surface of the muscle membrane in the post-burn phase (Kim et al, 1988); such receptors are thought to be supersensitive to the usual doses of agonists such as acetylcholine or SCh, so instead of the discrete potassium movement at the end-plate, there is a more general leakage along the entire muscle membrane.

In burned patients the pharmacodynamic effects of non-depolarizing muscle relaxants are markedly altered. These patients may require two to three times the usual intravenous dose with the resultant increased plasma concentration to produce the desired clinical effect (Martyn et al, 1983). This resistance peaks about 2 weeks after the burn, persists for many months in patients with major burns and decreases gradually with healing; in fact it seems to correlate with both the magnitude of the burn and the period of healing. The resistance can be partially explained by the increased drug binding as a result of increased plasma α_1-acid glycoprotein levels normally found in the presence of a burn.

Although no cases of cardiac arrest have been reported in the first few days following a burn, the use at that time of SCh should be avoided because of the ever-present possibility of hyperkalaemia. The patient can usually tolerate a non-depolarizing relaxant, though in most cases he or she will require up to three times the usual dose. The relaxant effect can, however, be reversed by the usual dose of anticholinesterase.

REFERENCES

Aldridge LM (1985) Anaesthetic problems in myotonic dystrophy. *British Journal of Anaesthesia* **57:** 1119.

Allan CM, Cullen WG & Gillies DM (1961) Ventricular fibrillation in a burned boy. *Canadian Medical Association Journal* **85:** 432.

Asari H, Inoue K, Maruta H et al (1984) The inhibitory effect of intravenous d-tubocurarine and oral dantrolene on halothane induced myoglobinemia in children. *Anesthesiology* **61:** 332.

Bevan JC, Donati F & Bevan DR (1986) Prolonged infusion of suxamethonium in infants and children. *British Journal of Anaesthesia* **58:** 839.

Blanc VF, Vaillancourt G & Brisson G (1986) Succinylcholine fasciculations and myoglobinemia. *Canadian Anaesthetists' Society Journal* **33:** 178.

Brandom BW, Rudd GD & Cook DR (1983) Clinical pharmacology of atracurium in paediatric patients. *British Journal of Anaesthesia* **55:** 117S.

Brandom BW, Woelfel SK, Cook D et al (1984) Clinical pharmacology of atracurium in infants. *Anesthesia and Analgesia* **63:** 309.

Brandom BW, Cook DR, Woelfel SK et al (1985) Atracurium infusion requirements in children during halothane, isoflurane, and narcotic anesthesia. *Anesthesia and Analgesia* **64:** 471.

Brandom BW, Stiller RL, Cook DR et al (1986) Pharmacokinetics of atracurium in anaesthetized infants and children. *British Journal of Anaesthesia* **58:** 1210.

Cabal LA, Siassi B, Artal R et al (1985) Cardiovascular and catecholamine changes after administration of pancuronium in distressed neonates. *Pediatrics* **75:** 284.

Cohen AY & Frank G (1987) Periorbital edema after atracurium administration. *Anesthesiology* **66:** 431.

Cook DR (1981) Muscle relaxants in infants and children. *Anesthesia and Analgesia* **60:** 335.

Cook DR & Fischer CG (1975) Neuromuscular blocking effects of succinylcholine in infants and children. *Anesthesiology* **42:** 662.

Cozantis DA, Erkola O, Klemola UM & Makela V (1987) Precurarisation in infants and children less than three years of age. *Canadian Anaesthetists' Society Journal* **34:** 17.

Craythorne NWB, Turndorf H & Dripps RD (1960a) Changes in pulse rate and rhythm associated with the use of succinylcholine in anesthetized patients. *Anesthesiology* **21:** 465.

Craythorne NWB, Rottenstein HS & Dripps RD (1960b) The effect of succinylcholine on intraocular pressure in adults, infants and children. *Anesthesiology* **21:** 59.

Crone RK (1984) Pediatric critical care: supporting the development of organ system. *State of the Art SCCM V(D):* 1–69.

Cunliffe M, Lucero VM, McLeod ME et al (1986) Neuromuscular blockade for rapid tracheal intubation in children: comparison of succinylcholine and pancuronium. *Canadian Anaesthetists' Society Journal* **33:** 760.

Davies DW & Steward DJ (1973) Myasthenia gravis in children and anaesthetic management for thymectomy. *Canadian Anaesthetists' Society Journal* **20:** 253.

DeCook TH & Goudsouzian NG (1980) Tachyphylaxis and phase II block development during infusion of succinylcholine in children. *Anesthesia and Analgesia* **59:** 639.

Delphine E, Jackson D & Rothstein P (1987) Use of succinylcholine during elective pediatric anesthesia should be reconsidered. *Anesthesia and Analgesia* **66:** 190.

Dierdorf SF & McNiece WL (1984) Effect of succinylcholine on plasma potassium in children with cerebral palsy. *Anesthesiology* **61:** A432.

Donlon JV, Savarese JJ, Ali HH & Teplick RS (1980) Human dose–response curves for neuromuscular blocking drugs. A comparison of two methods of construction and analysis. *Anesthesiology* **53:** 161.

Fanconi S & Duc G (1987) Intratracheal suctioning in sick preterm infants: prevention of intracranial hypertension and cerebral hypoperfusion by muscle paralysis. *Pediatrics* **79:** 538.

Ferres CJ, Crean PM & Mirakhur RK (1983) An evaluation of Org NC 45 (vecuronium) in paediatric anaesthesia. *Anaesthesia* **38:** 943.

Finer NN & Tomney PM (1981) Controlled evaluation of muscle relaxation in the ventilated neonate. *Pediatrics* **67:** 641.

Fisher DM & Miller RD (1983) Neuromuscular effects of vecuronium (Org NC45) in infants and children during N_2O_2 halothane anesthesia. *Anesthesiology* **58:** 519.

Fisher DM, Fahey MR, Cronnelly R et al (1982a) Potency determination for vecuronium (Org NC45): comparison of cumulative and single dose techniques. *Anesthesiology* **57:** 309.

Fisher DM, O'Keeffe C, Stanski DR et al (1982b) Pharmacokinetics and pharmacodynamics of d-tubocurarine in infants, children and adults. *Anesthesiology* **57:** 203.

Fisher DM, Cronnelly R, Miller RD et al (1983) The neuromuscular pharmacology of neostigmine in infants and children. *Anesthesiology* **59:** 220–225.

Fisher DM, Cronnelly R, Sharma M et al (1984) Clinical pharmacology of edrophonium in infants and children. *Anesthesiology* **61:** 428.

Fisher DM, Castagnoli K & Miller RD (1985) Vecuronium kinetics and dynamics in anesthetized infants and children. *Clinical Pharmacology and Therapeutics* **37:** 402.

Friesdorf W, Shultz M, Fosel T et al (1986) Pharmakodynamic von Vecuronium im Kleinkindesalter bei intravenoser Narkoseeinleitung mit Ketamin. *Anaesthetist* **35:** 99.

Friesen RH, Honda AT & Thieme RE (1987) Changes in anterior fontanelle pressure in preterm neonates during tracheal intubation. *Anesthesia and Analgesia* **66:** 874.

Goudsouzian NG (1981) Turbe del ritmo cardiaco durante intubazione tracheale nei bambini. *Acta Anaesthesiologica Italica* **32:** 293.

Goudsouzian NG (1988) Atracurium infusion in infants. *Anesthesiology* **68:** 267.

Goudsouzian NG & Gionfriddo M (1984) Muscle relaxants and children. *Seminars in Anesthesia* **III(1)**: 50.

Goudsouzian NG & Liu LMP (1984). The neuromuscular response of infants to a continuous infusion of succinylcholine. *Anesthesiology* **60**: 97.

Goudsouzian N & Standaert F (1986) The infant and the myoneural junction. *Anesthesia and Analgesia* **65**: 743.

Goudsouzian NG, Ryan JF & Savarese JJ (1974) The neuromuscular effects of pancuronium in infants and children. *Anesthesiology* **41**: 95.

Goudsouzian NG, Donlon JV, Savarese JJ et al (1975) Reevaluation of d-tubocurarine dosage and duration in the pediatric age group. *Anesthesiology* **43**: 416.

Goudsouzian NG, Liu LMP & Savarese JJ (1978) Metocurine in infants and children: neuromuscular and clinical effects. *Anesthesiology* **49**: 266.

Goudsouzian NG, Crone RR & Todres ID (1981) Recovery from pancuronium blockade in the neonatal intensive care unit. *British Journal of Anaesthesia* **53**: 1303.

Goudsouzian NG, Liu LMP, Cote CJ et al (1983a) Safety and efficacy of atracurium in adolescents and children anesthetized with halothane. *Anesthesiology* **59**: 459.

Goudsouzian NG, Martyn JJA, Liu LMP et al (1983b) Safety and efficacy of vecuronium in adolescents and children. *Anesthesia and Analgesia* **62**: 1083.

Goudsouzian NG, Martyn JJA, Liu LMP & Ali HH (1984) The dose response effect of long-acting nondepolarizing neuromuscular blocking agents in children. *Canadian Anaesthetists' Society Journal* **31**: 246.

Goudsouzian NG, Liu LMP, Gionfriddo M & Rudd GD (1985) Neuromuscular effects of atracurium in infants and children. *Anesthesiology* **62**: 75.

Goudsouzian N, Martyn J, Rudd GD et al (1986a) Continuous infusion of atracurium in children. *Anesthesiology* **64**: 171.

Goudsouzian NG, Young ET, Moss J & Liu LMP (1986b) Histamine release during the administration of atracurium or vecuronium in children. *British Journal of Anaesthesia* **58**: 1229.

Goudsouzian NG, Alifimoff JK, Liu LM et al (1987) The dose response of BW A938U in children. *Anesthesiology* **67**: A366.

Goudsouzian NG, Miler V, Foster VJ et al (1988) The efficacy and safety of bolus doses of doxacurium in children. *Anesthesia and Analgesia* **67**: S80.

Grenough A, Wood S, Morley CJ & Davis JA (1984) Pancuronium prevents pneumothorax in ventilated premature babies who actively expire against positive pressure inflation. *Lancet* **i**: 1–3.

Gronert GA (1980) Malignant hyperthermia. *Anesthesiology* **53**: 305.

Gronert GA & Theye RA (1975) Pathophysiology of hyperkalaemia induced by succinylcholine. *Anesthesiology* **43**: 89.

Hamza J, Macquin I, Wood C et al (1987) Cardiovascular effects of vecuronium vs pancuronium in premies with hyaline membrane disease. *Anesthesiology* **67**: A515.

Hannallah RS, Oh T, McGill WA & Epstein BS (1986) Changes in heart rate and rhythm after intramuscular succinylcholine with or without atropine in anesthetized children. *Anesthesia and Analgesia* **65**: 1329.

Harrington JF, Ford DJ & Striker TW (1984) Myoglobinemia after succinylcholine in children undergoing halothane and non-halothane anesthesia. *Anesthesiology* **61**: A431.

Harris MM, Stirt JA, Broaddus WF & Cook DR (1987) Cerebrospinal fluid laudanosine kinetics in children. *Anesthesiology* **67**: A506.

Henry GW, Stevens DC, Schreiner RL et al (1979) Respiratory paralysis to improve oxygenation and mortality in large newborn infants with respiratory distress. *Journal of Pediatric Surgery* **14**: 761.

Hickey P & Hansen DD (1984) Fentanyl- and sufentanyl–oxygen–pancuronium anesthesia for cardiac surgery in infants. *Anesthesia and Analgesia* **63**: 117.

Keneally JP & Bush GH (1974) Changes in serum potassium after suxamethonium in children. *Anaesthesia and Intensive Care* **2**: 147.

Kim C, Fuke N & Martyn JAJ (1988) Burn injury to rat increases nicotinic acetylcholine receptors in the diaphragm. *Anesthesiology* **68:** 401.

Lavery GG & Mirakhur RR (1984) Atracurium besylate in paediatric anaesthesia. *Anaesthesia* **39:** 1243.

Lebowitz PW, Ramsey FM, Savarese JJ et al (1980) Potentiation of neuromuscular blockade in man produced by combinations of pancuronium and metocurine or pancuronium and d-tubocurarine. *Anesthesia and Analgesia* **59:** 604.

Leigh MD, McCoy DD, Belton KM et al (1957) Bradycardia following intravenous administration of succinylcholine chloride to infants and children. *Anesthesiology* **18:** 698.

Libonati MM, Leahy JJ & Ellison N (1985) The use of succinylcholine in open eye injury. *Anesthesiology* **62:** 637.

Liu LMP & Goudsouzian NG (1982) Neuromuscular effect of intramuscular succinylcholine in infants. *Anesthesiology* **57:** A413.

Liu LMP, DeCook T, Goudsouzian NG et al (1981) Dose response to intramuscular succinylcholine in children. *Anesthesiology* **55:** 599.

Martyn JAJ, Goudsouzian NG, Matteo RS et al (1983) Metocurine requirements and plasma concentrations in burned paediatric patients. *British Journal of Anaesthesia* **55:** 263.

Martyn J, Goldhill DR & Goudsouzian N (1986) Clinical pharmacology of muscle relaxants in patients with burns. *Journal of Clinical Pharmacology* **26:** 680.

Mason LJ & Betts EK (1980) Leg lift and maximum inspiratory force: clinical signs of neuromuscular blockade reversal in neonates and infants. *Anesthesiology* **52:** 441.

Matteo RS, Lieberman IG, Salanitre E et al (1984) Distribution, elimination and action of d-tubocurarine in neonates, infants, children and adults. *Anesthesia and Analgesia* **64:** 799.

McCaughey TJ (1962) Hazard of anaesthesia for the burned child. *Canadian Anaesthetists' Society Journal* **9:** 220.

Meakin G, Sweet PP, Bevan JC et al (1983) Neostigmine and edrophonium as antagonists of pancuronium in infants and children. *Anesthesiology* **59:** 316.

Meistelman C, Agoston S, Kersten UW et al (1986a) Pharmacokinetics and pharmacodynamics of vecuronium and pancuronium in anesthetized patients. *Anesthesia and Analgesia* **65:** 1319.

Meistelman C, Loose JP, Saint-Maurice C et al (1986b) Clinical pharmacology of vecuronium in children. *British Journal of Anaesthesia* **58:** 996.

Meistelman C, Debaen B, Saint-Maurice C et al (1988) Potency of atracurium in infants during halothane anesthesia. *Anesthesiology* **65:** A290.

Meretoja OA & Kalli I (1986) Spontaneous recovery of neuromuscular function after atracurium in pediatric patients. *Anesthesia and Analgesia* **65:** 1042.

Michel PA & Fronefield HP (1985) Use of atracurium in a patient with malignant hyperthermia. *Anesthesiology* **62:** 213.

Miler V, Goudsouzian N, Griswold J et al (1988) Dose response of mivacurium in pediatric patients. *Anesthesia and Analgesia* **67:** S149.

Miller RD, Rupp SM, Fisher DM et al (1984) Clinical pharmacology of vecuronium and atracurium. *Anesthesiology* **61:** 444.

Mirakhur RK, Ferres CJ & Pandi SK (1984) Muscular relaxation with an infusion of vecuronium. *Anesthesiology* **61:** A293.

Motsch J, Hutschenreuter K, Ismaily AJ & von Blohn K (1985) Vecuronium bei Saugglingen und Kleinkindern: klinische und neuromuskulare Effekte. *Anaesthetist* **34:** 382.

Nightingale DA (1986) Use of atracurium in neonatal anaesthesia. *British Journal of Anaesthesia* **58:** 32S.

Nightingale DA & Bush GH (1973) A clinical comparison between tubocurarine and pancuronium in children. *British Journal of Anaesthesia* **45:** 63.

Nightingale P, Healy TEJ & McGuinness K (1985) Dystrophia myotonica and atracurium. *British Journal of Anaesthesia* **57**: 1131.

Pollock EM, MacLeod AD & McNicol LR (1986) Anaphylactoid reaction complicating neonatal anaesthesia. *Anaesthesia* **41**: 178.

Reynolds EOR, Hope PL & Whitehead MD (1985) Muscle relaxation and periventricular hemorrhage. *New England Journal of Medicine* **313**: 955.

Ridley SA & Hatch DJ (1988) Post-tetanic count and profonol neuromuscular blockade with atracuronium infusion in paediatric anaesthesia. *British Journal of Anaesthesia* **60**: 31–35.

Robinson S & Gregory GA (1981) Fentanyl-air-oxygen anesthesia for ligation of patent ductus arteriosus in preterm infants. *Anesthesia and Analgesia* **60**: 331.

Rosemberg H & Heiman-Patterson T (1983) Duchennes's muscular dystrophy and malignant hyperthermia: another warning. *Anesthesiology* **59**: 362.

Rowlands DE (1987) Harmless cutaneous reactions associated with the use of atracurium. *British Journal of Anaesthesia* **59**: 693.

Ryan JF, Kagen LJ & Hyman AI (1971) Myoglobinemia after a single dose of succinylcholine. *New England Journal of Medicine* **285**: 824.

Salem MR, Wong AW & Lin YH (1972) The effect of suxamethonium on the intragastric pressure in infants and children. *British Journal of Anaesthesia* **44**: 166.

Sarner JB, Brandom BW, Woelfel SK et al (1987) Neuromuscular effects of BW 938U in anesthetized children. *Anesthesiology* **67**: A365.

Schwartz L, Rockoff M & Koka BV (1984) Masseter spasm with anesthesia: incidence and implications. *Anesthesiology* **61**: 772.

Scott RPF, Savarese JJ, Basta SJ et al (1985) Atracurium: clinical strategies for preventing histamine release and attenuating the haemodynamic response. *British Journal of Anaesthesia* **57**: 550.

Sethna NV, Rockoff MA, Worthen M & Rosnow JM (1988) Anesthesia-related complications in children with Duchenne muscular dystrophy. *Anesthesiology* **68**: 462.

Simpson DA & Green DW (1986) Use of atracurium during major abdominal surgery in infants with hepatic dysfunction from biliary atresia. *British Journal of Anaesthesia* **58**: 1214.

Smith CL & Bush GH (1985) Anaesthesia and progressive muscular dystrophy. *British Journal of Anaesthesia* **57**: 1113.

Stead AL (1955) The response of the newborn infant to muscle relaxants. *British Journal of Anaesthesia* **27**: 124.

Steinbereithner K, Fitzal S, Schwarz S, Gilly H, Semsroth M & Weindlmayr-Goettel (1984) Pharmacocinetique et pharmacodynamique du vecuronium chez l'enfant. *Cahiers d'Anésthesiologie* **32**: 5.

Stirt JA, Stone DJ, Weinberg G et al (1985) Atracurium in a child with myotonic dystrophy. *Anesthesia and Analgesia* **64**: 369.

Stoelting RK & Peterson C (1975) Heart rate slowing and junctional rhythm following intravenous succinylcholine with and without preanesthetic medication. *Anesthesia and Analgesia* **54**: 705.

Szigmond EL & Downs JR (1971) Plasma cholinesterase activity in newborns and infants. *Canadian Anaesthetists' Society Journal* **18**: 278.

Tsai SK, Mok MS, Lee TY et al (1986) The priming effect of vecuronium in children. *Anesthesia and Analgesia* **65**: S160.

Viby-Mogensen J, Howardy-Hansen P & Chraemmer-Jorgensen B (1981) Post tetanic count (PTC); a new method of evaluating an intense non-depolarizing neuromuscular blockade. *Anesthesiology* **55**: 458–461.

Ward S, Neill EAM, Weatherley BC et al (1983) Pharmacokinetics of atracurium besylate in healthy patients (after a single i.v. bolus dose). *British Journal of Anaesthesia* **53**: 113.

Wood M & Wood AJJ (1981) Changes in plasma drug binding and α_1-acid glycoprotein in mother and newborn infant. *Clinical Pharmacology and Therapeutics* **4:** 522.
Woods I, Morris P & Meakin G (1985) Severe bronchospasm following the use of atracurium in children. *Anaesthesia* **40:** 207.

Basic techniques of paediatric anaesthesia

'After all, it is the duty of the anaesthetist to adapt the anaesthetic to the patient, not the patient to the anaesthetic,' Ayre (1937a).

PAEDIATRIC ANAESTHETIC EQUIPMENT

Anaesthetists who work in an environment where infants and children only appear occasionally are often less fortunate than those who work in special paediatric centres. The range of available equipment is usually far less wide, items which have not been used for some time may have fallen into disrepair, vital sizes of tubes or connectors may be missing, and tracheal tubes may not be cut to the correct length. The giving of even a relatively straightforward anaesthetic may become a nightmare in these circumstances, and accepting less than ideal items of equipment may well cause hazards to patient safety. Accepting a tracheal tube which is 0.5 mm too small in a neonate, for example, may cause unacceptably high airway resistance, and one that is too large may lead to severe stridor on extubation and possible subglottic damage. Deficiencies in equipment have been blamed for deaths in young children (Edwards et al, 1956). It is therefore essential that all anaesthetic departments should have a reliable system for ensuring that equipment comes up to the high standard required for paediatric anaesthesia.

Anaesthetic breathing systems

It is fascinating to ponder the great leaps forward made in the development and clinical use of various anaesthetic breathing systems in the 50 years since Philip Ayre described the T-piece technique (Ayre, 1937a,b). To satisfy the anaesthetist's prime directive—*primum non nocere*—the design of a breathing system should meet certain criteria: it should be lightweight, have a minimum number of connections, and be easy to assemble and use without error. It should reliably deliver oxygen, nitrogen, nitrous oxide, and anaesthetic vapours; eliminate carbon dioxide; conserve heat and humidity; be easy to sterilize, and allow scavenging of waste gases. It should minimize dead space and resistance to breathing, and facilitate monitoring of airway pressure and concentrations of inspired and expired gases. It may be influenced by the prior experience and bias of the anaesthetist. In centres where flammable agents are still used non-conductivity is essential.

The most commonly used breathing system for neonates is some version of the Mapleson E or D system (Mapleson, 1954). Ayre's original T-piece was modified by Rees (Rees, 1950) who added an expiratory limb to prevent air dilution and an open-ended 500 ml reservoir bag to allow respiration to be monitored and positive pressure ventilation to be applied (Figure 6.1).

Lightness and ease of use

It is not yet clear whether the recently introduced ADE breathing system (Humphrey, 1983) will gain popularity for paediatric anaesthesia, despite its obvious attractions. At present the T-piece remains the least cumbersome breathing system for infants and young children, with the Magill attachment or Bain system being popular for older patients.

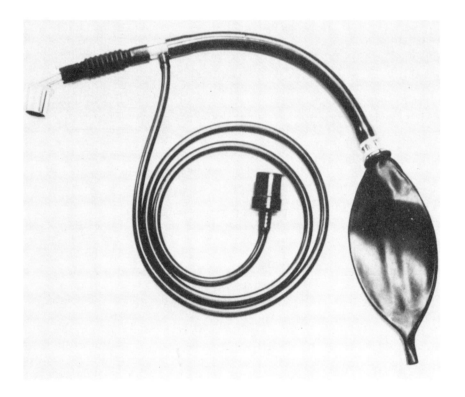

Figure 6.1. The Rees modification of Ayre's T-piece with Levin's facemask adaptor and open-ended reservoir bag. From Hatch and Sumner (1986), with permission.

Carbon dioxide elimination

Elimination of CO_2 from the breathing system is neither a simple problem to discuss nor an easy goal to accomplish in the operating theatre. The concept of variable rebreathing (Nunn, 1977) implies that rebreathing of CO_2 is a dynamic and multifactorial process. The flux of CO_2 in the expiratory limb of a partial rebreathing system depends on the mass of CO_2 produced by the patient and eliminated by alveolar ventilation as well as the distribution of CO_2 in the system. The distribution of CO_2 within the system is determined by the acceleration and deceleration of gas flow with changes in direction during spontaneous or controlled ventilation, and by the dilution of CO_2 caused by the continuous fresh gas flow (Jaeger and Schultetus, 1987). Key factors which determine the anaesthetized patient's arterial CO_2 tension are listed in Table 6.1.

Table 6.1. Variables influencing rebreathing of carbon dioxide in anaesthetic breathing systems

Equipment	Patient
Fresh gas flow rate	Alveolar ventilation
Apparatus dead space	Alveolar perfusion
Compression and distension of system	CO_2 production
Leaks in ventilator, circuit, and around tracheal tube	CO_2 diffusion
Breathing system design	Respiratory drive
Ventilator waveform	Respiratory waveform

Studies done to determine the efficacy of CO_2 elimination by various breathing systems necessarily involve different numbers of patients and a myriad of variables. The key to the reader's application of the studies' results is to determine what is safe for all patients and to apply that standard to meet each patient's unique and variable demands. Fresh gas flow recommendations for specific breathing systems follow.

Classification

The classification of anaesthetic breathing systems permits the user to identify a system's fresh gas flow requirements and CO_2 elimination pattern. This permits the safest and most practical use of any system in a given clinical situation. The classification shown in Table 6.2 is a modification of those proposed by Mapleson (1954), Baraka (1977), and McIntyre (1986). Popular systems are illustrated in Figure 6.2.

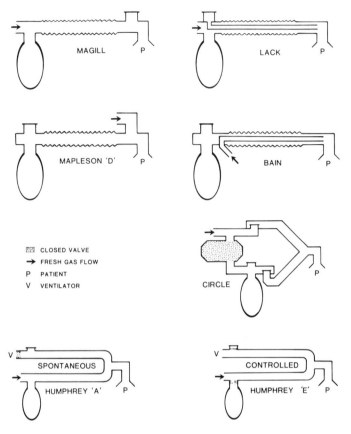

Figure 6.2. Anaesthetic breathing systems for paediatric patients.

Table 6.2. Classification of anaesthetic breathing systems

Carbon dioxide washout systems
Open (no reservoir bag)
  Open mask (drop)
  Insufflation
  Mapleson E (Ayre's T-piece)
Semi-open (with reservoir bag)
  Mapleson A (Magill, Lack)
  Mapleson D (Bain)
  Mapleson F (Rees)
  Universal (Humphrey ADE)
  Non-rebreathing valve systems

Carbon dioxide absorption systems
Closed circle (fresh gas flow = uptake by patient)
Semi-closed circle (fresh gas flow > uptake by patient)

Mapleson A and Humphrey ADE.   Recommendations for fresh gas flow to be used in children during spontaneous ventilation with a Mapleson A system range from a high of two to three times the minute ventilation to a low equal to the alveolar ventilation (Dorsch and Dorsch, 1984). Humphrey and Brock-Utne (1987) compared the A mode of the Humphrey ADE to the T-piece (Mapleson E) for both spontaneous and controlled ventilation in children. The A mode required one-third the fresh gas flow of the T-piece (123 vs. 386 ml/kg/min) to prevent rebreathing during spontaneous ventilation while the E mode functioned identically (139 ml/kg/min) to the T-piece when used during controlled ventilation. Children, having higher oxygen consumption (6–8 ml/kg/min), carbon dioxide production (5–8 ml/kg/min), and minute ventilation (Avery et al, 1981; Crone, 1983), require higher fresh gas flows per kg than adults. For a more detailed analysis of the function of the Humphrey ADE system the reader is referred to the original work (Humphrey, 1983; Humphrey et al, 1986a,b). The Mapleson A should not be used for controlled ventilation because the required fresh gas flow to prevent rebreathing is high and unpredictable (McIntyre, 1986).

Mapleson D, E, F.   These breathing systems, which include the T-piece and coaxial D (Bain) system, are more efficient during controlled than spontaneous ventilation. When fresh gas flow is reduced to a level which permits partial rebreathing, CO_2 containing gas enters the respiratory tract mainly towards the end of inspiration. With minor degrees of rebreathing, this gas only reaches that part of the respiratory tract which is not involved in gas exchange (anatomical dead space) so that alveolar ventilation is not affected. The minimum recommended fresh gas flow required to avoid alveolar rebreathing during controlled ventilation in infants and young children weighing less than 20 kg is 1000 ml + 200 ml/kg (Hatch et al, 1987). Froese and Rose (1982) recommended a slightly lower minimum fresh gas flow in children weighing from 10–30 kg (1000 ml + 100 ml/kg) to give a P_aCO_2 of 4.9 kPa with a minimum fresh gas flow of 3 l/min, combined with a considerably greater degree of mechanical hyperventilation (minute volume = 1.5 × fresh gas flow) than most anaesthetists normally use. The Froese and Rose formula is more appropriate to the upper end of the weight range (20–30 kg). Another recommendation for the fresh gas flow through D and coaxial D systems to maintain normocarbia during controlled ventilation is 2500 ml/m²/min (Rayburn and Watson, 1980). This type of system becomes inefficient during spontaneous ventilation, requiring a much higher fresh gas flow to prevent uncontrolled rebreathing.

Circle.   Because the circle system relies on the soda lime absorber to remove CO_2, a precisely defined fresh gas flow is unnecessary, although it must meet the patient's uptake of oxygen and anaesthetic agents.

To summarize the use of anaesthetic breathing systems in spontaneous and controlled ventilation modes, one might attempt to make a table listing each circuit and the recommended fresh gas flow rates for control of CO_2 in either mode. However, the safe use of a breathing system depends on clinical assessment of the patient and measurement of selected respiratory parameters.

The most important clinical monitor which assists the anaesthetist's visual, tactile and auditory assessment of the patient is arterial oxygen saturation, as measured by pulse oximetry. The second parameter to be measured should be the expired minute ventilation. If a paediatric respirometer is not available, the airway pressure at the breathing system–patient connection should be measured and recorded. The third monitor is the measurement of the composition of the patient's expired and inspired gases. The most important of these is capnometry, which assesses the patient's metabolic status, the breathing system's function, and the anaesthetist's vigilance. Ventilatory monitoring is discussed in Chapter 7.

Humidification

Advantages of humidified gases in the anaesthetized patient include reduced water and heat loss from the patient, protection of the airway mucosa, and potential reduction of pulmonary complications after prolonged surgery (Rayburn and Watson, 1980; Cote et al, 1983; Flynn et al, 1984). When the fresh gas flow is not humidified, the major source of humidification of inspired gases is rebreathing of expired gas. An additional source of water in a circle system is that liberated by the chemical reaction between CO_2 and soda lime. Inspiratory gas in a circle system is primarily dry, fresh gas because the paediatric patient has a low minute ventilation and expiratory flow rate, and the fresh gas inlet is located on the inspiratory side of the circuit.

Using partial rebreathing methods, Mapleson A, D and F systems provide better humidification than do circle systems. Flynn et al (1984) compared the absolute humidity in the inspired gases of Mapleson and circle systems during spontaneous ventilation. At fresh gas flow rates adequate to maintain normocarbia, Mapleson A and F systems provided 16 mg/l absolute humidity, while a 5 l/min flow through a semi-closed circle provided 7 mg/l. Humidification through the circle system improved when a Revell circulator was added. During normocarbic controlled ventilation with a coaxial D system, Rayburn and Watson (1980) measured inspired absolute humidity to be 24 mg/l. The humidity in a closed-circle system increased with time, but did not equal that of the Mapleson D.

Humidification can be improved in breathing systems by adding a servo-controlled heated humidifier (Fonkalsrud et al, 1980), but doing so increases the compression volume of the system and may reduce the efficiency of the system's other functions (Cote et al, 1983).

Virtually any anaesthetic breathing system can be used in any patient with due regard for the patient's needs and the limitations of the system. Clearly some systems will meet the patient's and/or anaesthetist's requirements with greater ease and flexibility, less weight, lower cost and greater adaptability.

Sterilization

Ideally, anaesthetic breathing systems should either be autoclavable or disposable. In practice, because of the damage which repeated autoclaving does to the rubber parts, routine cleansing is often carried out by washing in detergents. Automated washing and drying machines are now available for this purpose. Autoclaving should always be performed after equipment has been used on infected patients.

Scavenging

The T-piece is not easy to scavenge, and the fitting of scavenging devices to the bag-tail seriously detracts from the basic simplicity of the system, increasing the risk of exposing the airway to high pressures and of kinking or disconnection of the system. Exhaust gases can be safely removed by use of a scavenging dish with no direct contact with the T-piece (Hatch et al, 1980).

Dead space

Values for a dead space (V_D), tidal volume (V_T) and $V_T:V_D$ ratio when related to body weight are similar to the adult, so that a 3 kg infant with a tidal volume of 21 ml (7 ml/kg) and a $V_T:V_D$ ratio of 0.3 has a dead space volume of 7 ml. $V_D:V_T$ will rise as V_T decreases during deep anaesthesia with spontaneous ventilation. Dead space can be significantly increased by the apparatus dead space of masks and breathing systems unless steps are taken to minimize it. The Rendell–Baker mask and airway divider help to solve this problem, as does tracheal intubation.

The effective apparatus dead space of the T-piece or Bain systems, whose characteristics are indistinguishable (Rose and Froese, 1979), depends on the fresh gas flow rate as well as the apparatus volume between the patient and fresh gas inlet.

Resistance

During laminar flow through tubes the Hagen–Poiseuille equation applies:

$$Q = \frac{\pi \, p \, r^4}{8 \, l \, n}$$

where Q is flow, p the pressure drop across the tube, r the radius, l the length and n the viscosity of the gas. Pressure across the tube, and hence resistance, at a given flow rate increases according to the fourth power of any reduction in radius, causing a marked increase in the work of breathing during spontaneous ventilation. From the point of view of resistance, therefore, paediatric breathing systems should contain relatively wide-bore tubing, though increase in size may increase dead space and make the system unnecessarily bulky. Resistance is not a significant problem with tubing of 1 cm diameter unless the length of the expired limb is excessive.

Safety checks

The importance of checking the assembly and function of the anaesthetic breathing system immediately before each use cannot be over-emphasized. A visual check of all components to verify correct assembly is the first step. Using the rotameter flow tubes and not the oxygen flush mechanism to fill the circuit and bag while the patient connection is occluded tests the continuity of the system from the wall source to the patient connection and also allows the user to quantitate leaks. When using a coaxial system it is vital to determine visually and functionally the integrity of the inner tube and its attachments. Various tests for the coaxial Mapleson D systems have been devised (Pethick, 1975; Foëx and Crampton Smith, 1977; Robinson and Fisher, 1983; Ghani 1984).

Breathing system connectors

One of the most frustrating experiences in anaesthesia is to be faced with incompatible breathing system connectors, and attempts at standardization are to be encouraged. The subject is not, however, as straightforward for paediatric systems as for adults, since the 15 mm male tracheal tube connector is often too bulky for use in neonates and infants. The sudden change in diameter from a 2.5 mm tracheal tube to a 15 mm connector also causes turbulent flow with increased resistance (Hatch, 1978). Connectors of 8.5 mm are widely used in the UK as an alternative to 15 mm, and disposable 8.5 mm connectors (Figure 6.3) with 15 mm adapters are now available.

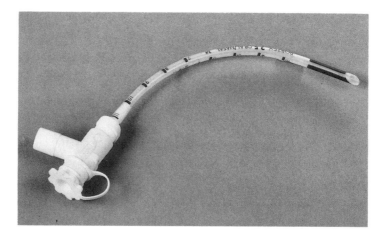

Figure 6.3. Disposable 8.5 mm tracheal tube connector.

Facemasks

The Rendell-Baker–Soucek facemask (Figure 6.4) is designed to provide a contoured fit around the infant's face, with reduction of dead space to about 4 ml for the smallest size (Rendell-Baker and Soucek, 1962). The use of the partitioned facemask adapter described by the same authors ensures that the fresh gas is carried down into the facemask and reduces apparatus dead space still further. The Keats and Hustead elbows act in a similar fashion. Clear plastic facemasks with inflatable rims are widely available but should not be used in the presence of cyclopropane.

With streaming effects of the fresh gas flow within the mask, the subject of mask dead space is less important than it appears at first sight. A little practice is required before the Rendell–Baker Soucek mask can be used for inflating the lungs without leaks occurring between the mask and the face—the lower edge of the mask should fit between the chin and lower lip (Figure 6.5).

Pharyngeal airways

The Guedel airway is now virtually universally used, and is available in five sizes from 2 to 000. Small babies sometimes require a larger airway than expected.

Laryngoscopes

Because of the anterior, highly placed larynx in the neonate, with the large soft epiglottis tending to obscure the laryngeal inlet, a straight-bladed laryngoscope is usually required in the first year or so of life. A variety of

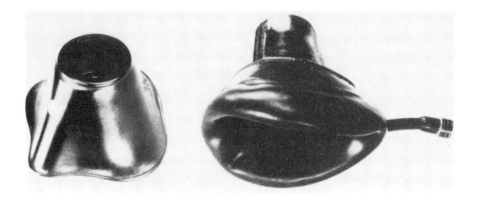

(a)   (b)

Figure 6.4. (a) Rendell-Baker–Soucek facemask; (b) with inflatable rim. From Hatch and Sumner (1986), with permission.

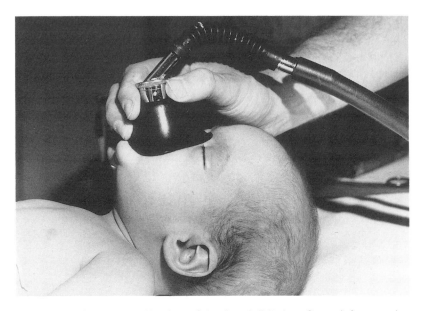

Figure 6.5. Correct application of the Rendell-Baker–Soucek facemask.

shapes of infant blade are available (Figure 6.6) and choice is largely a matter of personal preference. Many of these blades are now becoming available with a fibreoptic light source, which increases reliability as well as improving the intensity of the illumination. The Seward or Robertshaw blades are particularly useful for nasotracheal intubation as they allow Magill forceps to be introduced into the mouth with minimum loss of view. The light-weight handle of the Anderson–Magill laryngoscope with its hook for the index finger is easy to hold but the original light source was unreliable. Most of these blades can be used in the classical Magill fashion, with the tip placed posterior to the epiglottis or like a Mackintosh blade in the vallecula.

Tracheal tubes

A wide range of tracheal tubes, both disposable and reusable, have been used over the years (Figure 6.7; Hatch, 1985). More recently, disposable preformed tubes have become increasingly popular (Figure 6.8; Ring et al, 1975). Rubber tubes are now implantation-tested, which removes one of their main disadvantages, but since they are more difficult to produce accurately than polyvinyl chloride (PVC) tubes, wall thicknesses vary more from tube to tube within the fairly wide tolerances allowed by standards organizations. Internal and external diameters, which are now marked on all tubes, should be checked before use, especially for neonates. Rubber tubes are more rigid than PVC ones, which makes them slightly easier to pass. For prolonged intensive care use, PVC tubes are virtually exclusively used, often by the nasal route.

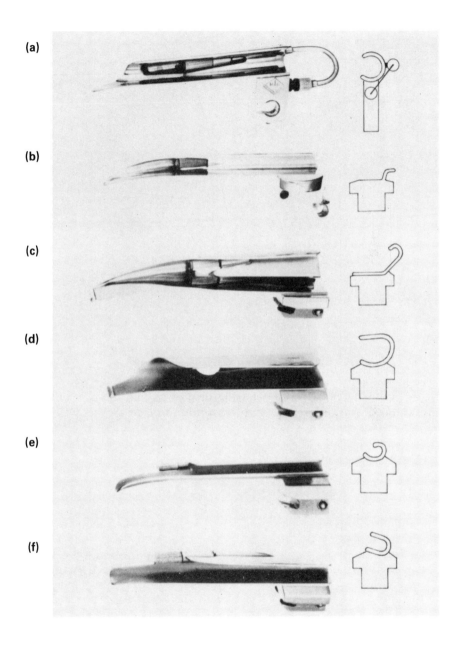

Figure 6.6. Straight laryngoscope blades for use in infancy: **(a)** Anderson–Magill; **(b)** Seward; **(c)** Robertshaw; **(d)** Oxford; **(e)** Miller; **(f)** Wisconsin. From Hatch and Sumner (1986), with permission.

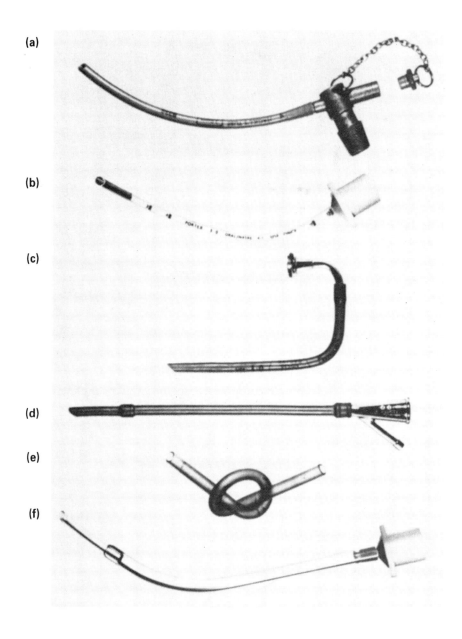

Figure 6.7. Tracheal tubes commonly used in paediatric anaesthesia: **(a)** reusable rubber Magill (with Cardiff connector); **(b)** disposable plain tube; **(c)** Oxford; **(d)** Magill armoured; **(e)** Latex armoured; **(f)** Cole pattern. From Hatch andSumner (1986), with permission.

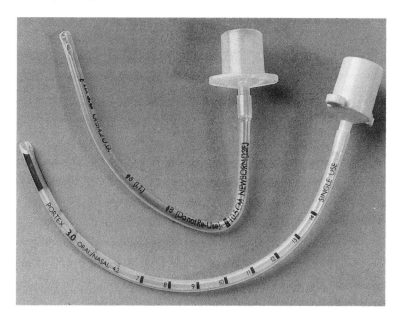

Figure 6.8. Disposable paediatric tracheal tubes: **top** plain and **bottom** Rae pattern with Murphy eye.

The preformed Rae tubes may be useful in operations on the head and neck, though they may become compressed against the lower teeth by the tongue plate of a mouth gag during pharyngeal surgery.

The latex armoured non-kinking tube is particularly popular for neurosurgery, but the wall thickness is too great for neonatal use.

The Cole pattern tube was designed to reduce resistance by limiting the narrow laryngeal section to a short length of the terminal portion of the tube. Unfortunately, however, turbulent flow occurs at the area of sudden change in diameter so that resistance is not significantly different from uniform-born tubes of similar external diameter with appropriate connectors attached. The tube has been popular with neonatologists because of the relative ease with which it can be passed, but long-term use has resulted in laryngeal damage from the pressure of the shoulder on the vocal cords, and its use is decreasing.

Tube size (Table 6.3) is determined by using a formula such as the following (Finholt et al, 1985):

$$\text{Internal diameter} = \frac{16 + \text{age (years)}}{4}$$

After insertion of the tube, proper size is confirmed by testing for an air leak around the tube when positive pressure is applied through the breathing system (Finholt et al, 1985). An air leak at less than 25 cm H_2O pressure indicates appropriate fit (Allen & Steven, 1965; Koka et al, 1977).

Table 6.3. Age and tracheal tube size

Age	Internal diameter (mm)	Type
Neonate < 1500 g	2.5	uncuffed
Neonate > 1500 g	3.0	uncuffed
1–6 months	3.5	uncuffed
7–23 months	4.0	uncuffed
2 years	4.5	uncuffed
3–4 years	5.0	uncuffed
5–6 years	5.5	uncuffed
7–8 years	6.0	uncuffed
9–11 years	6.5 or	uncuffed
	6.0	cuffed
12–13 years	6.5	cuffed
14–18 years	7.0–8.0	cuffed

Uncuffed tracheal tubes are used until the patient is about 10 years of age. Prior to that age, the narrowest portion of the airway is the cricoid cartilage and the larynx has a gradually tapering shape. A cylindrical tracheal tube fits the ring-shaped cricoid well enough to minimize positive pressure air leaks from below and aspiration of pharyngeal contents from above. A cuffed tube effectively reduces the lumen and increases the resistance of the tube. Beyond the age of 9 or 10 years, the vocal cords are the narrowest portion of the airway. The shape of this aperture does not allow a snug fit by a tracheal tube, thus, an inflatable cuff on the distal tube is necessary. Oedema of 1 mm in the infant cricoid ring will reduce the airway by 60%.

For short duration, ortracheal intubation is usually performed, unless the surgical procedure involves the mouth, in which case nasotracheal intubation may be preferred. Long-term intubation in the intensive care unit is best accomplished with a nasotracheal tube because it is less likely to be displaced, is more comfortable and may be associated with less laryngeal damage (Dubick and Wright, 1978). Preterm neonates may be more susceptible to nasopharyngeal damage by long-term nasal tubes, so orotracheal intubation may be preferable in those patients.

The distal end of the tracheal tube should lie in the mid-trachea to decrease the risk of bronchial intubation or accidental extubation. Various formulae are suggested to estimate appropriate tube length:

Length of oral tube at teeth (cm) = internal diameter (mm) × 3

Thus, a 5.0 mm internal diameter tracheal tube would be 15 cm long at the teeth if placed orally and 18 cm long at the nares if placed nasally. Yates et al (1987) suggest that the length of a nasal tube at the nares in cm = internal diameter (mm) × 3 + 2 cm. Distal tube position can change during head and neck movement: neck flexion causes downward movement and neck extension causes upward movement of the tube (Toung et al, 1985). Proper position should be confirmed in all cases by auscultation of the lungs and by chest radiograph for long-term intubation when the tip of the tube is seen to lie between the heads of the clavicles.

SPONTANEOUS VENTILATION

Several factors contribute to significant ventilatory dysfunction in infants during anaesthesia. Contraction of the infant's diaphragm is less efficient than that of the adult because of its horizontal, rather than oblique, angle of insertion (Muller and Bryan, 1979). The infant's rib cage is cartilaginous, rather than bony; its elasticity gives the chest wall a tendency to collapse. Closing capacity approximates—and may exceed—the supine functional residual capacity (FRC) of the lung (Mansell et al, 1972).

In the awake infant, intercostal muscle tone stabilizes the chest wall, preventing collapse and supporting diaphragmatic function. During halo-thane anaesthesia, intercostal muscle function is profoundly impaired (Tusiewicz et al, 1977). A reduction in tidal volume and FRC results, leading to small airways closure, increased work of breathing, loss of oxygen storage capacity in the lung, and decreased P_aO_2. Since diaphragmatic function and ventilatory response to CO_2 are also impaired by halothane, the infant can only compensate by increasing ventilatory rate. While marked increases in spontaneous breathing rates are usually observed in anaesthetized infants, effective minute ventilation remains less than awake levels (Podlesch et al, 1966; Tusiewicz et al, 1977).

The anaesthetist can compensate for the anaesthetized infant's venti-latory dysfunction by assisting ventilation with continuous positive airway pressure, assisted inspiration, or controlled ventilation with or without positive end expiratory pressure. This can be done through the anaesthetic breathing system either manually or by use of a mechanical ventilator.

Controlled ventilation by the T-piece can either be manual compression of the reservoir bag whilst the open limb is simultaneously occluded, or in conjunction with a ventilator. T-piece occluders rely on fresh gas flow to inflate the lungs, and require relatively high flow rates (two to three times the minute volume). When ventilators with a separate source of driving gas are used, fresh gas flow can be separately adjusted to avoid hypocapnia and the low flows described earlier in this chapter can be used.

MECHANICAL VENTILATORS

The descriptive classification of ventilators can be approached from several different perspectives (Pietak, 1983; Smallwood, 1986). Because of inter-national differences in use and availability of specific ventilators, our approach is to take important facts from each classification, the discussion of which may guide the anaesthetist in the selection and use of a ventilator for the individual patient. The following topics will be reviewed: power sources; control systems; pressure and flow generators; gas transmission; cycling, limiting and triggering mechanisms; humidification; scavenging, and monitoring. Important sources of more detailed information are Mushin et al (1980) and Kirby et al (1985).

Power sources

Power can be provided to a ventilator from either the gas source at the wall or cylinder or from electrical mains. The important points are the effect the loss of either source will have on the functioning of the ventilator, the likelihood of such a loss in any given location, the provision of back-up supplies, and alarms to identify the nature of the problem.

Control systems

The individual components of the ventilator require specific, reliable control systems which can be mechanical, electronic, pneumatic or fluidic (Duffin, 1977). Repair by the operator, ease of maintenance and parts availability may be of considerable importance in some locations.

Pressure and flow generators

Many different types of mechanisms have been developed to generate the required flows and pressures necessary for automatic ventilation of the lungs of children. These include piston, solenoid-controlled gate or knife valve, Venturi, compressor, bellows, spring-weighted bellows, and high pressure gas through a flow resistor. From the point of view of function, these mechanisms can be classified as either pressure or flow generators.

The pressure generator generates a constant pressure at the mouth resulting in an exponential increase in volume with respect to time and an exponential decrease in flow over time as alveolar pressure approaches the constant mouth pressure.

The flow generator produces a constant or non-constant flow during the inspiratory cycle with inspired volume increasing linearly with time. The slope of alveolar pressure over time is linear and parallel to the slope of mouth pressure over time.

Gas transmission

Gas may be transferred to the patient by two mechanisms: the first is direct gas transmission from source of pressure or flow to the patient; the second mode uses gas transmission from source to produce subsequent compression of bag or bellows within a bottle. This method separates the driving gas source from the patient's inspired gases. Significance of a leak in the bag or bellows will be determined by the concentration of oxygen in the driving gas and the extent of dilution of the patient's anaesthetic mixture.

Cycling mechanisms

The important phases of the ventilator cycle were described by Mapleson (1962) as inflation; termination of inspiration and change-over to expiration;

expiration, and change-over to inspiration to repeat the cycle. Each component of the phases of the ventilatory cycle is controlled by a cycling mechanism. The key to understanding the cycling mechanism is quite simple. Identify which parameter—pressure, time, flow, volume—is measured. Determine how and where within the system the measurement takes place. Based on this information it is possible to predict how the ventilator will respond to changing clinical parameters of the patient (Figure 6.9).

In order to predict the interaction of the patient's lungs with the ventilator's function, it is important to remember the three vital equations which describe pulmonary function:

$$\text{Compliance} = \text{volume/pressure} \tag{1}$$

Compliance varies with the volume of gas within the lung and also with the tone of the chest wall, the shape of the diaphragm and the pressure exerted by the abdominal contents.

$$\text{Resistance} = \text{pressure/flow} \tag{2}$$

This principle summarizes the Hagen–Poiseuille equation. Remember that resistance varies with gas flow and airway diameter.

$$\text{Compliance} \times \text{resistance} = \text{time constant } (\tau) \tag{3}$$

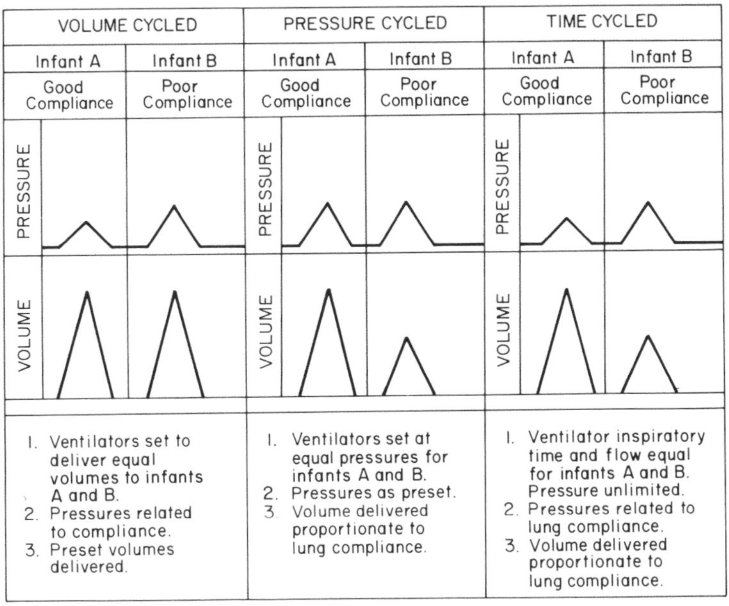

VOLUME CYCLED		PRESSURE CYCLED		TIME CYCLED	
Infant A	Infant B	Infant A	Infant B	Infant A	Infant B
Good Compliance	Poor Compliance	Good Compliance	Poor Compliance	Good Compliance	Poor Compliance
1. Ventilators set to deliver equal volumes to infants A and B. 2. Pressures related to compliance. 3. Preset volumes delivered.		1. Ventilators set at equal pressures for infants A and B. 2. Pressures as preset. 3. Volume delivered proportionate to lung compliance.		1. Ventilator inspiratory time and flow equal for infants A and B. Pressure unlimited. 2. Pressures related to lung compliance. 3. Volume delivered proportionate to lung compliance.	

Figure 6.9. Pressure and volume curves generated by different modes of ventilation. From Goldsmith and Karotkin (1981), with permission.

In one time constant, the process of inflation of the lungs will be 63% complete. After two, three, four and five time constants the process is 87, 95, 98 and 99% complete, respectively (Water and Mapleson, 1964).

Underlying pathological processes or the results of surgical interventions can affect each parameter and thereby disturb the patient–ventilator interaction through either the cycling or limiting mechanisms (Mapleson, 1962). Cycling mechanisms include pressure, time, volume, and flow. In the surgical patient, the use of flow cycling is of limited value.

Pressure cycling terminates inspiration when a preset pressure is reached at the mouth. If a neonate's compliance and time constant are halved by the reduction of a diaphragmatic hernia, the tidal volume delivered by a pressure-cycled pressure generator will also be halved because the preset pressure will be reached twice as quickly. This could present a serious hypoventilation problem if it is not immediately recognized.

Time cycling terminates inspiration when a preset inspiratory duration is reached. If the same neonate was ventilated with a time-cycled pressure generator, the 50% fall in compliance would result in a 50% fall in the tidal volume. Without a change in the length of the total respiratory cycle, the minute ventilation would be similarly reduced and the patient compromised.

Volume cycling terminates inspiration when a preset inspired volume has been achieved. Many ventilators which purport to be volume-cycled are, in fact, time-cycled flow generators. Actual measurement of the inspired volume at the patient connection with termination of inspiration when a preset volume has been delivered is rarely done. Many anaesthetists measure the expired volume with a respirometer and compare it to the preset inspired minute volume. Subsequent adjustment of the preset parameters may be required so that the expired volume meets the anaesthetist's desired goals and the patient's metabolic needs. If a ventilator with such a cycling mechanism was used in the neonate under discussion, the patient's minute ventilation would not be compromised by a change in lung compliance, although a higher peak inspiratory pressure would be generated.

The problems of mechanical ventilation of infants and small children have been a concern since adult ventilators were first modified for use in children (Mushin et al, 1962). The ideal paediatric ventilator must deliver low flows at high rates with precise control over time intervals and pressure limits.

If a 3 kg infant requires a tidal volume of 7 ml/kg at a rate of 40 breaths/min with an inspiration:expiration (I:E) ratio of 1:2, inspiration will deliver 21 ml in 0.5 s at a calculated inspiratory flow rate of 2.5 l/min. With a normal compliance of 6 ml/cm H_2O and resistance of 30 cm $H_2O/l/s$, the infant's time constant would be 0.18 s. After three time constants, or 0.54 s, inflation would be 95% complete.

If the patient's lungs deteriorated, requiring a ventilatory rate of 120 breaths/min with an I:E ratio of 1:2, then inspiration would last 0.166 s and expiration would require 0.332 s. The ventilator, therefore, must have the capacity to measure very short inspiratory intervals with a high degree of accuracy.

Limiting mechanisms

To protect the patient from barotrauma, each ventilator requires devices to terminate the ventilatory cycle immediately in the event that certain predetermined criteria for time, pressure, flow or volume are exceeded. The ventilator's function may appear to continue unabated, but most of the gas may be vented to the outside. The provision of alarms to indicate this condition is vital.

Humidification

Dry, cold gases will be humidified and warmed by the patient with a predictable cost in water and calories. The consequences of this effort during a short surgical procedure may be minimal, but may be important to a tiny patient undergoing a lengthy procedure. The ventilator, therefore, should be designed to accept a humidifier.

Scavenging of waste gases

The evidence is very suggestive that long-term exposure to trace anaesthetic gases may cause significant health problems in operating theatre personnel. The provision of scavenging systems for ventilators, which will safely eliminate exhaled anaesthetic gases, is mandatory in every anaesthetic location.

T-piece occluding ventilators

The range of patients suitable for this type of ventilator is limited by the fresh gas flow for the T-piece. Newton et al (1981) describe a valve with a fixed leak which allows the Nuffield series 200 ventilator (Penlon) to be used even for the smallest neonate. This time-cycled constant-flow generator is compact, reliable and inexpensive. An appropriate fresh gas flow for the size of the patient is delivered from the anaesthetic machine and an appropriate I:E ratio set on the ventilator. The dangers with this type of machine include sticking of the valve because it is on the expiratory limb; this may cause a dangerous rise in pressure in the patient's lungs. The ventilator makes no allowance for changes in pulmonary compliance and the user must be extremely vigilant to ensure adequate ventilation at all times. A disconnection and high-pressure alarm is also necessary. The ventilator will appear to be functioning normally even in the absence of any fresh gas flow.

Monitoring (see Chapter 7)

The importance of constant vigilance with visual, auditory, and tactile assessment of the paediatric patient cannot be over-emphasized because the time constant for physiological change is so short. Significant progress in ventilatory monitoring has been made in recent years with the development of pulse oximetry and capnography. These devices cannot replace a finger on the pulse, a precordial stethoscope, and close inspection of the patient during the anaesthetic, but they can provide valuable information in a timely manner. Ventilators and breathing systems should have ports for access to the respired gas mixture so that appropriate adjustments of ventilatory parameters and fresh gas flow can be made in response to changes in the patient's needs. This important subject is discussed comprehensively in Chapter 7.

VASCULAR ACCESS

Peripheral venous cannulation

A peripheral venous cannula should be inserted in patients undergoing all but the briefest of surgical procedures; the dorsum of the hand is the usual site. The purpose of the peripheral venous cannula is to provide routes, firstly for intravenous fluid therapy to supply basic hydration and caloric requirements and to replace pre- or intraoperative losses of fluid or blood and secondly, for intravenous administration of anaesthetic and other therapeutic or resuscitative drugs. For most elective procedures in healthy children, the cannula can be inserted after induction of anaesthesia. It should be inserted prior to anaesthesia in cases when intravenous anaesthetic induction is planned, when the patient requires preanaesthetic fluid infusion to prepare him or her adequately for the procedure, when an ill patient might require drug injection during induction, and for all newborns.

For the induction of anaesthesia sharp fine needles are required, and these are now available as small as 27 s.w.g. Scalp vein-type needles have wings which can be used to fix the needle down after insertion, and are useful for intermittent injections. They should not, however, be relied upon for fluid replacement during major surgery and care should be taken when injecting irritant drugs, as even in careful hands they can easily cut out of the vein. Fortunately there is now a wide range of intravenous cannulas available in sizes as small as 24 s.w.g., and made of a variety of synthetic plastic materials such as Teflon with its low frictional resistance. These cannulas can be used for peripheral venous, central venous and arterial cannulation at all ages, using percutaneous techniques.

Cannulas should be securely fixed and it is wise to interpose a short length of narrow-bore extension tubing between the cannula and a three-way stopcock to minimize any interference with the cannulation site. Whenever possible Luer lock connections should be made, and this is essential with central venous cannulas if air embolism is to be avoided.

Central venous cannulation (see also Chapter 7)

Insertion of a central venous cannula into the superior vena cava or right atrium is indicated for:

1. monitoring of central venous pressure;
2. infusion of inotropic, vasoactive or other resuscitative drugs;

3. providing a sheath through which other monitoring cannulas, such as those used for cardiac output measurement, pulmonary artery pressure monitoring, or mixed venous oximetry, can be inserted.

The internal jugular vein can be entered by direct percutaneous puncture using 50 mm 20 or 18 g cannulas (16 g 80 mm in older children). One or two cannulas can be used in the same vein. The Seldinger (1953) technique of placing a wire through a needle into the vein and inserting the cannula over the wire can also be used. Cannulation of the right internal jugular vein is the preferred approach. This vein is chosen because it is readily accessible and provides a short, straight route into the right atrium. The patient is placed in the Trendelenberg position with a roll under the shoulders and the head turned about 60° towards the left so there is always positive venous pressure and no danger of air embolism. Firm pressure over the liver will also distend the vein. The neck is cleansed and draped, and sterile technique is observed. The right carotid artery is palpated with the left index finger at a point high in the neck (midway between the mastoid and the suprasternal notch) and medial to the sternocleidomastoid muscle. The vein lies antero-lateral to the artery, so the needle is inserted just lateral to the artery and advanced towards the ipsilateral nipple at a very slight angle from the coronal plane of the body. Continuous slight negative pressure is exerted by a syringe held in the right hand while the needle is advanced. The vein is usually entered after advancement of 1–3 cm, depending on the size of the patient, although blood aspiration may not occur until the needle is slowly withdrawn. A very similar technique is described by Boulanger et al (1976).

After the needle has entered the vein, a flexible angiographic guide wire is inserted through the needle and held in place while the needle is removed. A dilator–sheath combination is placed over the wire, the wire and dilator are removed, and the sheath remains in the superior vena cava. The sheath can be used to monitor central venous pressure by itself or can be used for fluid or drug infusion while other catheters of variable lengths are inserted through it to measure central venous pressure, pulmonary artery pressure, mixed venous oxygen saturation, or cardiac output by thermodilution (Figure 6.10). The equipment should have Luer locking components and suitable sets are made by Cook (Bloomington, IN, USA). It is possible to insert a size 5.5 Fr sheath, through which size 4.0 Fr monitoring catheters may be placed, although a larger sheath is required to accommodate the triple-lumen thermodilution catheter. Simpler double- and triple-lumen catheters are also available for paediatric use (Arrow Ltd.).

For an alternative approach to the internal jugular vein, Prince et al (1976) suggest that the primary landmark should be the apex of the triangle formed by the two heads of the sternocleidomastoid muscle. Other techniques have been described (English et al, 1969; Jernigan et al, 1970; Rao et al, 1977), as has central venous cannulation via the external jugular vein (Blitt et al, 1974). All techniques can also be used on the left side of the neck, though this is usually less satisfactory.

Occasionally central venous cannulation is desired, but use of the neck for insertion is not feasible, such as when craniotomy or craniofacial recon-struction is planned or when neck veins have been cannulated recently. In these cases subclavian vein puncture is used. A needle will enter the sub-

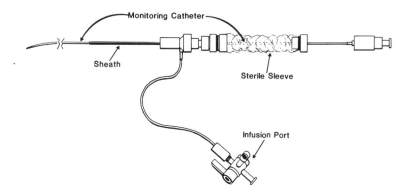

Figure 6.10. Central venous cannulation set: monitoring catheter through a vascular sheath.

clavian vein if passed underneath the clavicle from the junction of its lateral and middle thirds towards the suprasternal notch (Davidson et al, 1963). The femoral vein can also be used in such cases, inserting a long cannula into the right atrium through a sheath (Figure 6.2) placed by Seldinger technique into the femoral vein. The femoral artery is palpated approximately 2 cm below the inguinal ligament. The vein is entered by a needle inserted just medial to the artery and directed cephalad at about a 45° angle from the coronal plane. As with the neck approaches, sterile technique is used.

The most common complication of internal jugular vein cannulation is accidental carotid artery puncture by the needle, occurring in from 2% (Boulanger et al, 1976) to 23% (Prince et al, 1976) of patients. While this can cause haematoma formation, prompt recognition and application of pressure for a few minutes usually prevents this problem. Horner's syndrome can be a transient complication. Pneumothorax and haemothorax are serious complications which are avoided by using the high neck approach.

Late complications of internal jugular vein cannulation in children include infection and thrombosis. Damen (1987) reported a 5.5% incidence of positive bacterial (usually *Staphylococcus epidermidis*) culture of the catheter tip but no positive blood cultures. Duration of catheterization and patient age influenced the incidence. Thrombosis of the superior vena cava occurred in 2 of 235 children (Damen, 1987).

Cannulation of the left internal jugular vein is associated with two further complications. Injury to the thoracic duct can occur during a low neck approach (Rao et al, 1977), and perforation of the superior vena cava is an uncommon late finding (Tocino and Watanabe, 1986).

Peripheral arterial cannulation (see also Chapter 7)

Cannulation of a peripheral artery is indicated when direct arterial pressure monitoring is desired, such as occurs when the planned surgical procedure involves potential for extensive blood loss or rapid changes in cardiovascular status; when a critically ill patient is being cared for in the operating theatre or intensive care unit, or when induced hypotension is planned. Arterial cannulation also provides a port through which blood can be withdrawn for blood gas analysis and other laboratory tests.

The radial artery is the preferred vessel for cannulation because it is readily accessible and is one of two arteries supplying blood to the hand. The cannulation technique is well established and has been previously described (Marshall et al, 1984). The hand is extended about 45° at the wrist and is secured to an arm board. The skin of the wrist is cleansed and sterile technique is observed. The radial artery is palpated or may be visualized by transillumination in an infant. At a point a few millimetres distal to the maximum pulsation, the skin is incised with the tip of an 18 gauge needle to minimize skin resistance to the cannula. While palpating the artery with a finger, the cannula, with its needle stylet, is inserted through the skin incision into the artery. When the artery has been entered, loss of resistance may be felt and blood will flash back into the stylet hub. The stylet and catheter are advanced together 1–2 mm while blood continues to flow into the stylet hub. The stylet is partially removed. If blood flows freely through the stylet, the cannula is advanced up the artery. If blood does not flow through the stylet, transfixion of the artery has occurred, and the cannula alone must be slowly pulled back until pulsatile flow returns. When that occurs, the cannula is advanced. When in a satisfactory position, the cannula is secured with sutures or adhesive tape and connected to a pressure transducer through which an infusion of heparinized 0.9% saline (500 u in 500 ml) provides continuous flushing. Care must be taken not to overload small babies with this fluid. We use a Teflon cannula with winged flanges on the hub which make suturing to the skin easier (Quik-Cath, Travenol Laboratories, Deerfield, IL, USA). Cannulas for children under about 4 years of age are 22 gauge and 2.5 cm long, while 20 gauge 2.3 cm long cannulas are used for older children, though 22 gauge are satisfactory even in adults. A transfixion technique is better for small arteries or in patients with a high haematocrit.

Complications related to percutaneous radial artery cannulation in children are rare. Although transient arterial occlusion or retrograde flow can often be detected by Doppler flow techniques, clinical arterial insufficiency to the hand was not detected in three studies of paediatric patients (Todres et al, 1975; Miyasaka et al, 1976; Marshall et al, 1984). The potential complications of retrograde and antegrade embolism can be avoided if meticulous cannula flushing techniques are observed (Lowenstein et al, 1971). Infection at the site of cannulation has not been a problem (Todres et al, 1975; Miyasaka et al, 1976). Arterial cannulas should be small enough to allow flow to continue distally.

When percutaneous radial artery cannulation fails, alternative approaches must be considered. Although other arteries (ulnar, brachial, axillary, femoral, dorsalis pedis, posterior tibialis or superficial temporal) have been successfully used, it is occasionally necessary to perform a cutdown. For radial artery cutdown, the artery is exposed through a 5 mm skin incision, cannulated under direct vision, and not ligated. The femoral artery can be cannulated 2 cm below the inguinal ligament using the Seldinger (1953) technique with a 3.0 Fr (20 gauge), 8 cm long cannula (Cook, Inc.) or by direct puncture with a 22 or 20 gauge cannula. Glenski et al

(1987) observed a 0.6% incidence of transient (no permanent) perfusion-related complications in children older than 1 month undergoing femoral artery cannulation for open heart surgery. Advantages may include fewer complications than with cutdown techniques (Glenski et al, 1987) and a more accurate reflection of central aortic pressure following cardiopulmonary bypass (Stern et al, 1985).

HEAT CONSERVATION

Heat loss

Most heat loss occurs through the body surface. Such loss occurs more rapidly in infants and neonates because their ratio of body surface area to mass is higher than that of older children and adults and is a problem in the operating theatre. Furthermore, the head, receiving a large fraction of cardiac output, comprises a disproportionate amount of the infant's body surface area.

Heat loss takes place by the mechanisms of radiation, conduction, convection, and evaporation (Figure 6.11; Brengelmann, 1973). Radiant heat loss occurs when the skin emits heat towards an object of lower temperature. More heat is lost when the object gaining the heat is of great mass; thus, the walls of the operating theatre are important recipients of radiant heat.

Conductive heat loss occurs by direct contact of the patient with an object of lower temperature. More heat is lost when the object gaining the heat is made of a material of high thermal conductance; thus, a metal operating table is a source of greater loss than is a plastic or cloth mattress.

Convection is loss of heat to air of lower temperature moving next to the body surface. More heat is lost with increasing velocity of the air.

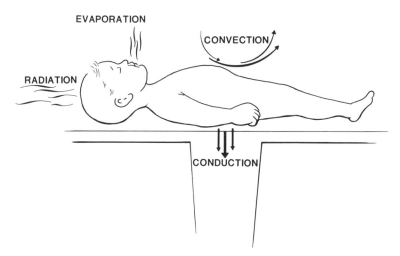

Figure 6.11. Mechanisms of heat loss in the operating theatre.

Evaporative heat loss occurs when heat is utilized to evaporate water on the body surface, such as sweat and cleansing solutions, or in the airway for humidification of gases. While 1 cal of heat is required to raise the temperature of 1 g of water by 1°C, 580 cal are utilized (and lost) to evaporate the same amount of water (Brengelmann, 1973).

Physiological response to cold

The infant responds to cold by attempting to conserve heat through cutaneous vasoconstriction and by increasing heat production. Sympathetically mediated vasoconstriction reduces the amount of heat at the body surface. While the vasoconstrictive response to cold is active in neonates, its effectiveness is limited by the relatively poor tissue insulation offered by their thin layer of subcutaneous fat and skin (Sinclair, 1972).

Heat production occurs by shivering and non-shivering thermogenesis. Shivering thermogenesis is the production of heat associated with vigorous contraction of many muscle groups. Neonates can shiver in response to severe cold, but more commonly accomplish shivering thermogenesis by a generalized increase in motor activity (Adamsons et al, 1965).

Non-shivering thermogenesis is the production of heat by increased metabolic activity, chiefly combustion of fatty acids and glucose (Britt, 1983). Non-shivering thermogenesis is stimulated by noradrenaline and occurs in several sites in the body, including brown adipose tissue, white adipose tissue, muscle, liver, and brain. Brown adipose tissue is rich in mitochondria, blood vessels, and sympathetic innervation, and is an important source of thermogenesis in hibernating mammals. It is present in the human neonate, continues to develop for a few weeks after birth, and recedes following infancy. Brown fat is poorly developed in the preterm neonate and is rapidly depleted during cold stress.

Both shivering and non-shivering thermogenesis significantly increase oxygen consumption. Lowering environmental temperature from 34 to 24°C increases the neonate's oxygen consumption by about 50% (Adamsons et al, 1965; Stern et al, 1965). In addition, cold shifts the oxyhaemoglobin dissociation curve to the left, limiting release of oxygen to the tissues. Thus, cold increases the infant's risk of hypoxia and is associated with poor growth and decreased survival in low birthweight neonates (Sinclair, 1972).

Heat conservation

Active measures must be taken to conserve heat when caring for an infant in the operating theatre. The room can be warmed to approach a thermal neutral environment for the patient, in which oxygen consumption is at basal rate during sleep. In 50% humidity, temperature ranges providing thermal neutrality are 32–34°C for the term neonate and 33–35°C for the preterm neonate (Hey and Katz, 1969, 1970). More than the room's air should be warmed—to reduce radiant heat loss, the room should be preheated long enough for the walls of the room to warm. Draughts should be eliminated to reduce convective heat loss.

Because an environment of thermal neutrality for an infant can be one of discomfort for operating theatre personnel, and only temperatures up to 24°C are tolerable, other heat-conserving measures can be used to supplement a lower room temperature. Insulating the baby with a stocking cap, clothing, blankets or surgical drapes will reduce heat loss and oxygen consumption (Hey and O'Connell, 1970) and aluminium foil around the limbs will reduce heat loss by radiation. Heat loss by evaporation of water in the airway is significantly less when heated humidified gases are used for ventilation (Fonkalsrud et al, 1980). Water-circulating heating blankets (Goudsouzian et al, 1973) and radiant heating lamps are valuable sources of heat which deserve routine use. A hot-air mattress (Howarth Air Engineering Ltd.) has proved extremely successful for temperature maintenance of very small babies during surgery.

The most common sites for thermistor probe placement in our practice are rectum, distal oesophagus, axilla, and nasopharynx.

Hyperthermia

Hyperthermia is associated with increases in respiratory rate, oxygen consumption, and evaporative water loss (Adamsons et al, 1965; Hey and Katz, 1969), and possibly with apnoea in preterm neonates (Daily et al, 1969). In the operating theatre, hyperthermia is most frequently caused by the prolonged use of a heating blanket under a patient covered by paper surgical drapes. It can be avoided by vigilant temperature-monitoring and judicious use of warming devices. Except with very prolonged surgery, heating devices are only required for children below 10 kg (Goudsouzian et al, 1973).

Malignant hyperthermia is discussed in Chapter 21.

INDUCTION OF ANAESTHESIA

Before anaesthesia is induced all equipment and connectors to be used are checked and all drugs drawn up into labelled syringes. Many drugs, for example relaxants, require dilution. Some units have a preoperative checklist which includes haematology and other laboratory data, details of premedication, consent form, time of starvation, loose teeth etc. so that mistakes cannot be made. The side of the operation, if this is relevant, should have been marked previously.

Inhalational induction

Inhalational induction is best achieved by drifting the gases from the cupped hand over the nose and mouth of the child, a mask being attached to the circuit only after the child is asleep. An induction with 50% cyclopropane with oxygen takes 30–40 s until loss of the eyelash reflex, after which the cyclopropane is discontinued as oxygen, nitrous oxide and halothane or isoflurane are introduced (Figure 6.12). Cyclopropane is of course highly explosive and its use is limited to areas where full antistatic precautions are in operation. The induction should not be prolonged beyond 30–40 s or an excessive quantity of cyclopropane will have been used. Halothane itself has excellent characteristics allowing a very smooth induction if the agent is gradually introduced. Isoflurane is less satisfactory as breath-holding, coughing and laryngeal spasm are common, though not necessarily related to the skill of the anaesthetist (Pandit et al, 1985). Induction is smoother if the child takes at least 10 breaths for each increased concentration of isoflurane—similar to an induction with ether. The application of distending pressure with a snug-fitting facemask, preferably with a cuff, and a tight bag overcome many minor respiratory complications during induction and also stridor during stimulating surgery such as anal dilatation.

Venous access can be established at this time and relaxant given if the patient is to be intubated. An alternative is to give a single bolus dose of, for example, suxamethonium, using a 25 G needle, into one of the small veins in the front of the wrist which are easily visible even in a fat child. The wrist is most satisfactorily held by the operator himself, the vein being distended and the skin stretched by holding the small wrist between index and middle fingers (Figure 6.13).

Intravenous induction

Intravenous induction is possible using, for example, thiopentone 2–5 mg/kg even in very small babies. EMLA cream may be used for local

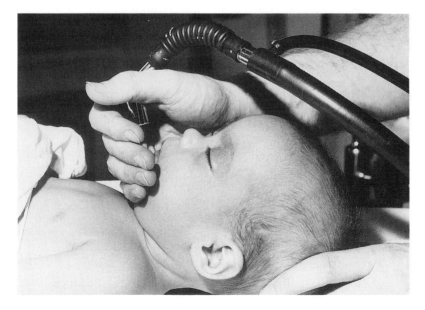

Figure 6.12. Inhalational induction at an early stage without a facemask.

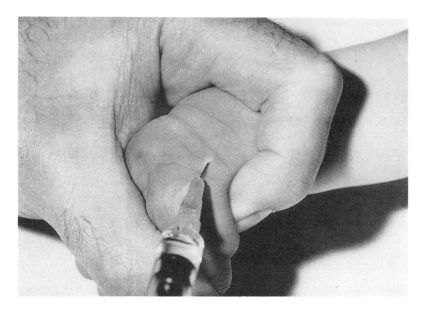

Figure 6.13. Technique of holding the wrist ' a bolus intravenous injection.

analgesia on the back of the hand; the cream is applied at the time of premedication. An older child can be distracted by being asked to cough at the moment of injection. The arm of a younger child who is being held may be taken over the shoulder of a parent or accompanying nurse and a vein on the back of the hand can be used with that hand firmly held out of sight. Ketamine is satisfactory as an agent for intravenous induction in a dose of 2 mg/kg, particularly for long operations when its hallucinogenic effects will be masked.

Rectal induction

The rectal route for induction of anaesthesia is popular in some centres, particularly those which have a patient-holding area within the operating department. It is a pleasant alternative for the apprehensive infant. Methohexitone 25 mg/kg may be given as 10% solution, or ketamine 10 mg/kg. Induction is slow and the infant must be closely watched as he or she falls asleep in case of respiratory obstruction.

TRACHEAL INTUBATION

Indications

Tracheal intubation for anaesthesia, pioneered in the late nineteenth century, was first applied to paediatric patients in the 1920s by Magill (Ayre, 1937a,b).

Its uses in anaesthetic practice are to establish and maintain a patent airway and to assist artificial ventilation of the patient.

Both patient factors and surgical considerations contribute indications for tracheal intubation. Patient factors include:

1. obstructed or difficult to maintain airway;
2. hypoventilation requiring mechanical ventilation;
3. full stomach accompanied by risk of pulmonary aspiration;
4. age.

The risk of cardiac arrest due to airway and ventilatory problems during anaesthesia is greater in infants than in older patients (Graff et al, 1960; Salem et al, 1975). Thus, infants under 5 kg or 4–6 months of age are usually intubated for all but the briefest surgical procedures.

Intubation is indicated when the surgical procedure:

1. requires control of ventilation, such as abdominal, thoracic, or neurological operations;
2. limits the anaesthetist's access to the airway, such as operations on the head, neck, or upper extremity, and those in the prone or sitting positions;
3. is of long duration (arbitrarily 1 hour).

Long-term nasotracheal intubation (>24 h) for children requiring intensive care has been well established since the 1960s (Allen and Steven, 1965; McDonald and Stocks, 1965). The most common indication for long-term tracheal intubation at the Children's Hospital, Denver is postoperative ventilatory support after cardiac or other major surgery (53%), followed by treatment of airway obstruction caused by laryngotracheobronchitis or epiglottitis (19%), neurological impairment (17%), respiratory failure (6%), and cardiovascular failure (5%).

Techniques

Intubation is usually performed after a relaxant has been given or with deep inhalational anaesthesia. Because the infant's larynx is relatively anterior and cephalad when compared to the older child or adult, a straight laryngoscope blade is preferred until the patient is about 2 years of age (Figure 6.14). Beyond infancy, when anatomical factors make direct laryngoscopy difficult, both blind nasotracheal intubation and intubation aided by indirect fibreoptic laryngoscopy (Rogers and Benumof, 1983) are useful.

In emergency situations when fasting time has been inadequate or gastric emptying has been delayed by stress, intravenous induction and paralysis, cricoid pressure, and intubation can proceed in rapid sequence following preoxygenation. Indications for possible awake intubation include the difficult airway, gastric outlet obstruction, and the moribund patient. The common practice of awake intubation for all neonates undergoing anaesthesia is often unwarranted; the accompanying changes in intracranial pressure may be deleterious (Friesen et al, 1987), especially for those at risk of intracranial haemorrhage.

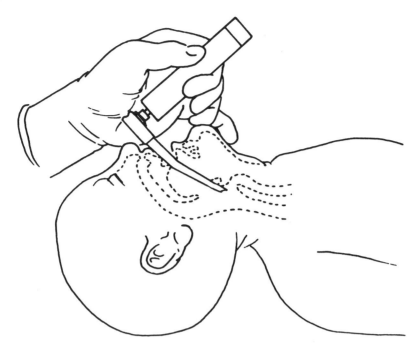

Figure 6.14. Laryngoscopy with a straight-bladed laryngoscope, facilitated by picking up the epiglottis.

Whichever type of tracheal tube and connector is used, the fixation must be very secure, after checking for the correct length and size. Auscultation is not necessarily a reliable means of detecting bronchial intubation, especially if the head is moved to a flexed or extended position for surgery. Centimetre marks on the concave surface of a tracheal tube make the placement much easier and at least 3 cm of the tube should always be in the trachea. If possible, there should be a secondary fixation, for example, of a catheter mount to the forehead, which prevents twisting and accidental extubation. An oral airway may be used alongside the tube in the mouth to minimize lateral movement (Figure 6.15).

Complications

Complications of tracheal intubation may manifest themselves while the tube is in place or after extubation. Disconnection of the tracheal tube from a mechanical ventilator can be life-threatening, so a pressure-sensitive disconnect alarm is important.

Displacement of the tracheal tube resulting in bronchial intubation or accidental extubation can occur. During long-term intubation, right main bronchial intubation occurred in about 4% of patients (Aass, 1975) and accidental extubation in about 2%. Such tube malpositions can be

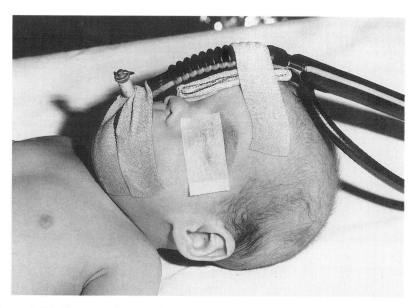

Figure 6.15. Fixation of an oral tracheal tube with a secondary fixation to the forehead.

minimized by confirming proper length of the tube after insertion, securing the tube adequately, sedating and restraining the patient, and reconfirming tube position at intervals by auscultation and radiographic examination.

Obstruction of the tube by inspissated secretions or clotted blood can occur. This can happen rather quickly during surgical procedures in which blood can enter the distal trachea, such as tracheo-oesophageal fistula repair. Capnography and airway pressure are useful monitors for this complication, but vigilance by the anaesthetist is of prime importance. Aass (1975) reported a 1.9% incidence of tube obstruction during long-term intubation. Humidification of inspired gases and frequent suctioning of the tracheal tube will reduce the risk of this complication.

Other complications manifest themselves after extubation of the trachea. Sore throat and hoarse voice are annoying but generally transient. Persistent hoarseness following long-term intubation (Lindholm, 1969) may indicate laryngeal damage.

Subglottic oedema, manifest as stridor, is a common and potentially serious complication of intubation in children. Following short-term intubation, its incidence is about 3% (Goddard et al, 1967; Jordan et al, 1970; Koka et al, 1977). Battersby et al (1977) showed that the incidence of postextubation stridor was not related to the duration of intubation; there was a lower incidence in long-term intubations (4%) than in those intubated and extubated within 24 h. Fearon et al (1966) reported an incidence greater than 10%.

Subglottic oedema is caused by pressure exerted on the tracheal mucosa by the tracheal tube. The pressure may be focal or circumferential, such as occurs when a tight-fitting tube is passed through the cricoid ring. When the pressure exerted by the tube exceeds the tracheal mucosa's capillary perfusion pressure of about 25 mmHg (about 32 cm H_2O), ischaemia of the mucosa results (hence the guideline to keep the air leak around the tracheal tube at a pressure less than 25 cm H_2O). Epithelial damage, demonstrated histologically within the first few hours of intubation, progresses to deep necrosis and cartilaginous excavation during 4 days of intubation in critically ill patients (Donnelly, 1969; Rasche and Kuhns, 1972).

In addition to duration of tracheal intubation, other factors correlate with development of postintubation stridor. Several factors are associated with the tracheal tube itself. Materials with which tubes are fabricated can cause tissue damage (Stetson and Guess, 1970); thus, the use of tubes made only of implantation-tested material is a standard which has led to a reduction in the incidence of postintubation tracheal damage. Movement of a tapered tube, such as the Cole tube, can result in the wide supraglottic portion of the tube being pushed into the glottis, causing ischaemia.

Pressure exerted on the tracheal mucosa by a large tube is a well documented factor associated with stridor in children (Allen and Stevens, 1965; Jordan et al, 1970; Koka et al, 1977). Thus, selecting a tube of proper diameter and confirming its fit by testing for air leak are important. Movement of the tube in the trachea causes mucosal irritation; changing the position of the head during surgical procedures, excessive coughing, movement of the agitated awake patient, and multiple intubation attempts are all associated with postintubation stridor.

Patient factors also contribute to the incidence of subglottic oedema. Peak incidence occurs between the ages of 1 and 3 years, when subglottic diameter is small, followed by a gradual decline as the patient grows until the age of 10 years, when it approaches zero (Jordan et al, 1970). Paradoxically, infants under 1 year of age have a relatively low incidence of postintubation stridor (Goddard et al, 1967; Jordan et al, 1970; Koka et al, 1977) and of glottic ulceration following long-term intubation (Lindholm, 1969), but there is a much higher incidence in Down's syndrome (Sherry, 1983).

A history of prior postintubation stridor or frequent viral laryngotracheobronchitis, perhaps indicative of subglottic stenosis, is associated with a higher incidence of postintubation stridor (Lee et al, 1980).

Laryngospasm following extubation is discussed later in this chapter (p. 145) and the management of postoperative stridor is further discussed in Chapter 10.

MAINTENANCE OF ANAESTHESIA

Spontaneous breathing with inhalational agents has limited use for the first 6 months of life, though anaesthesia with a facemask can be used successfully for short operations on babies over 4–5 kg body weight. Intubation is probably more satisfactory for longer procedures as it allows the anaesthetist more freedom to attend to the administration of fluids etc. The respiratory depressant effects of inhalational agents and the tendency of anaesthesia to reduce FRC and pulmonary compliance probably make spontaneous breathing techniques inappropriate for surgical procedures lasting for more than 30–40 min, even if the patient is intubated (Ewart et al, 1988). However, techniques which involve controlled ventilation for all patients may not be appropriate as there may be increased risks. The effects of equipment failure or a disconnection, for example, will be more catastrophic than if the patient is breathing spontaneously.

EXTUBATION

At the end of the procedure oxygen alone should be administered for a few minutes while the oropharynx is suctioned—also the trachea if secretions are present. Infants are usually extubated awake as the tracheal tube is well tolerated without coughing or straining, and the risk of laryngospasm is minimized. After suctioning the baby is well oxygenated again and the tube removed with positive pressure with the baby on his or her side. Some babies, for example those after intraocular surgery, are extubated deeply anaesthetized and allowed to recover very quietly. An increased inspired oxygen concentration is supplied until after the oral airway has been rejected.

Extubation at an intermediate stage is hazardous as laryngospasm and hypoxia may occur, particularly after halothane or isoflurane anaesthesia. Spasm usually breaks if the facemask is firmly applied together with distending pressure, but reintubation should not be delayed to the stage of bradycardia. Suxamethonium 1 mg/kg i.v. may be necessary if the child is to be reintubated.

REFERENCES

Aass AS (1975) Complications to tracheostomy and long-term intubation: a follow-up study. *Acta Anaesthesiologica Scandinavica* **19**: 127–133.

Adamsons K Jr, Gandy GM & James LS (1965) The influence of thermal factors upon oxygen consumption of the newborn human infant. *Journal of Pediatrics* **66**: 495–508.

Allen TH & Steven IM (1965) Prolonged endotracheal intubation in infants and children. *British Journal of Anaesthesia* **37**: 566–573.

Avery ME, Fletcher BD & Williams RG (1981) *The Lung and its Disorders in the Newborn Infant*. Philadelphia: WB Saunders.

Ayre P (1937a) Anaesthesia for intracranial operation. *Lancet* **i**: 561–563.

Ayre P (1937b) Endotracheal anaesthesia for babies: with special reference to hare-lip and cleft palate operations. *Anesthesia and Analgesia* **16**: 330–333.

Baraka A (1977) Functional classification of anaesthesia circuits. *Anaesthesia and Intensive Care* **5**: 172–178.

Battersby EF, Hatch DJ & Towey RM (1977) The effects of prolonged naso-endotracheal intubation in children. A study in infants and young children after cardiopulmonary bypass. *Anaesthesia* **32**: 154–157.

Blitt CD, Wright WA, Petty WC & Webster TA (1974) Central venous catheterization via the external jugular vein: a technique employing the J-wire. *Journal of the American Medical Association* **229**: 817–818.

Boulanger M, Delva E, Maillé JG & Paiement B (1976) Une nouvelle voie d'abord de la veine jugulaire interne. *Canadian Anaesthetists' Society Journal* **23**: 609–615.

Brengelmann G (1973) Temperature regulation. In Ruch TC & Patton HD (eds) *Physiology and Biophysics*, vol III, pp 105–135. Philadelphia: WB Saunders.

Britt BA (1983) Temperature regulation. In Gregory GA (ed) *Pediatric Anesthesia*, pp 253–314. New York: Churchill Livingstone.

Cote CJ, Petkau AJ, Ryan JF & Welch JP (1983) Wasted ventilation measured in vitro with eight anesthetic circuits with and without inline humidification. *Anesthesiology* **59**: 442–446.

Crone RK (1983) The respiratory system. In Gregory GA (ed) *Pediatric Anesthesia*, pp 35–62. New York: Churchill Livingstone.

Daily WJR, Klaus M & Meyer HBP (1969) Apnea in premature infants: monitoring, incidence, heart rate changes, and an effect of environmental temperature. *Pediatrics* **43**: 510–518.

Damen J (1987) Positive bacterial cultures and related risk factors associated with percutaneous internal jugular vein catheterization in pediatric cardiac patients. *Anesthesiology* **66**: 558–562.

Davidson JT, Bemhur N & Nathan H (1963) Subclavian venepuncture. *Lancet* **ii:** 1139–1140.

Donnelly WH (1969) Histopathology of endotracheal intubation. An autopsy study of 99 cases. *Archives of Pathology* **88**: 511–520.

Dorsch JA & Dorsch SE (1984) *Understanding Anesthesia Equipment*, 2nd edn, pp 182–196. Baltimore: Williams & Wilkins.

Dubick MN & Wright BD (1978) Comparison of laryngeal pathology following long-term oral and nasal endotracheal intubations. *Anesthesia and Analgesia* **57**: 663–668.

Duffin (1977) Fluidics and pneumatics: principles and applications in anaesthesia. *Canadian Anaesthetists' Society Journal* **24**: 126–141.

Edwards G, Morton HJV, Pask EA et al (1956) Deaths associated with anaesthesia: a report of 1000 cases. *Anaesthesia* **11**: 194–220.

English ICW, Frew RM, Pigott JF & Zaki M (1969) Percutaneous catheterisation of the internal jugular vein. *Anaesthesia* **24**: 521–531.

Ewart MC, Fletcher M, Davies C, Stocks J & Hatch DJ (1988) Comparison of total ventilation compliance during anaesthesia in spontaneously breathing and paralysed infants and young children. *British Journal of Anaesthesia* **60**: 320.

Fearon B, MacDonald RE, Smith C & Mitchell D (1966) Airway problems in children following prolonged endotracheal intubation. *Annals of Otology, Rhinology and Laryngology* **75**: 975–986.

Finholt DA, Henry DB & Raphaely RC (1985) Factors affecting leak around tracheal tubes in children. *Canadian Anaesthetists' Society Journal* **32**: 326–329.

Flynn PJ, Morris LE & Askill S (1984) Inspired humidity in anaesthesia breathing circuits: comparison and examination of Revell circulator. *Canadian Anaesthetists' Society Journal* **31**: 659–663.

Foëx P & Crampton Smith A (1977) A test for co-axial circuits. *Anaesthesia* **32**: 294.

Fonkalsrud EW, Calmes S, Barcliff LT & Barrett CT (1980) Reduction of operative heat loss and pulmonary secretions in neonates by use of heated and humidified anesthetic gases. *Journal of Thoracic and Cardiovascular Surgery* **80**: 718–723.

Friesen RH, Honda AT & Thieme RE (1987) Changes in anterior fontanel pressure in preterm neonates during tracheal intubation. *Anesthesia and Analgesia* **66**: 874–878.

Froese AB & Rose DK (1982) A detailed analysis of T-piece systems. In Stewart DJ (ed) *Aspects of Paediatric Anaesthesia*, pp 101–136. Amsterdam: Excerpta Medica.

Ghani GA (1984) Safety check for the Bain circuit. *Canadian Anaesthetists' Society Journal* **31**: 487–488.

Glenski JA, Beynen FM & Brady J (1987) A prospective evaluation of femoral artery monitoring in pediatric patients. *Anesthesiology* **66**: 227–229.

Goddard JE, Phillips OC & Marcy JH (1967) Betamethasone for prophylaxis of postintubation inflammation. A double-blind study. *Anesthesia and Analgesia* **46:** 348–353.

Goldsmith JP & Karotkin EH (1981) *Assisted Ventilation of the Neonate.* Philadelphia, Saunders.

Goudsouzian NG, Morris RH & Ryan JF (1973) The effects of a warming blanket on the maintenance of body temperatures in anesthetized infants and children. *Anesthesiology* **39:** 351–353.

Graff TD, Phillips OC, Benson DW & Kelley E (1960) Baltimore anesthesia study committee: factors in pediatric anesthesia mortality. *Anesthesia and Analgesia* **43:** 407–414.

Hatch DJ (1978) Tracheal tubes and connectors used in neonates—dimensions and resistance to breathing. *British Journal of Anaesthesia* **50:** 959–964.

Hatch DJ (1985) Paediatric anaesthetic equipment. *British Journal of Anaesthesia* **57:** 672–684.

Hatch DJ, Miles R & Wagstaff M (1980) An anaesthetic scavenging system for paediatric and adult use. *Anaesthesia* **35:** 496–498.

Hatch DJ & Sumner E (1986) *Neonatal Anaesthesia and Perioperative Care,* 2nd edn. London: Arnold.

Hatch DJ, Yates AP & Lindahl SGE (1987) Flow requirements and rebreathing during mechanically controlled ventilation in a T-piece (Mapleson E) system. *British Journal of Anaesthesia* **59:** 1533–1540.

Hey EN & Katz G (1969) Evaporative water loss in the newborn baby. *Journal of Physiology* **200:** 605–619.

Hey EN & Katz G (1970) The optimum thermal environment for naked babies. *Archives of Disease in Childhood* **45:** 328–334.

Hey EN & O'Connell B (1970) Oxygen consumption and heat balance in the cot-nursed baby. *Archives of Disease in Childhood* **45:** 335–343.

Humphrey D (1983) A new anaesthetic breathing system combining Mapleson A, D and E principles. *Anaesthesia* **38:** 361–372.

Humphrey D & Brock-Utne JG (1987) Suggested solutions to the problem of the T-piece anaesthetic breathing system. *Canadian Journal of Anaesthesia* **34:** S129–130.

Humphrey D, Brock-Utne JG & Downing JW (1986a) Single lever Humphrey ADE low flow universal anaesthetic breathing system. Part I: Comparison with dual lever ADE, Magill and Bain systems in spontaneously breathing adults. *Canadian Anaesthetists' Society Journal* **33:** 698–709.

Humphrey D, Brock-Utne JG & Downing JW (1986b) Single lever Humphrey ADE low flow universal anaesthetic breathing system. Part II: Comparison with Bain system in anaesthetized adults during controlled ventilation. *Canadian Anaesthetists' Society Journal* **33:** 710–718.

Jaeger MJ & Schultetus RR (1987) The effect of the Bain circuit on gas exchange. *Canadian Journal of Anaesthesia* **34:** 26–34.

Jernigan WR, Gardner WC, Mahr MM & Milburn JL (1970) Use of the internal jugular vein for placement of central venous catheter. *Surgery, Gynecology and Obstetrics* **130:** 520–524.

Jordan WS, Graves CL & Elwyn RA (1970) New therapy for postintubation laryngeal edema and tracheitis in children. *Journal of the American Medical Association* **212:** 585–588.

Kirby RR, Smith RA & Desautels DA (1985) *Mechanical Ventilation.* New York: Churchill Livingstone.

Koka BV, Jeon IS, Andre JM, MacKay I & Smith RM (1977) Postintubation croup in children. *Anesthesia and Analgesia* **56:** 501–505.

Lee KW, Templeton JJ & Dougal RM (1980) Tracheal tube size and postintubation croup in children. *Anesthesiology* **52:** S325.

Lindholm CE (1969) Prolonged endotracheal intubation. *Acta Anaesthesiologica Scandinavica* **(suppl 33):** 1–131.

Lowenstein E, Little JW III & Lo HH (1971) Prevention of cerebral embolization from flushing radial artery cannulas. *New England Journal of Medicine* **285:** 1414–1415.

Mansell A, Bryan C & Levison H (1972) Airway closure in children. *Journal of Applied Physiology* **33:** 711–714.

Mapleson WW (1954) The elimination of rebreathing in various semi-closed anaesthetic systems. *British Journal of Anaesthesia* **26:** 323–332.

Mapleson WW (1962) The effect of changes of lung characteristics on the functioning of automatic ventilators. *Anaesthesia* **17:** 300–314.

Marshall AG, Erwin DC, Wyse RKH & Hatch DJ (1984) Percutaneous arterial cannulation in children: concurrent and subsequent adequacy of blood flow at the wrist. *Anaesthesia* **39:** 27–31.

McDonald IH & Stocks JG (1965) Prolonged nasotracheal intubation. A review of its development in a paediatric hospital. *British Journal of Anaesthesia* **37:** 161–172.

McIntyre JWR (1986) Anaesthesia breathing circuits. *Canadian Anaesthetists' Society Journal* **33:** 98–105.

Miyasaka K, Edmonds JF & Conn AW (1976) Complications of radial artery lines in the paediatric patient. *Canadian Anaesthetists' Society Journal* **23:** 9–14.

Muller NL & Bryan AC (1979) Chest wall mechanics and respiratory muscles in infants. *Pediatric Clinics of North America* **26:** 503–516.

Mushin WW, Mapleson WW & Lunn JN (1962) Problems of automatic ventilation in infants and children. *British Journal of Anaesthesia* **34:** 514–522.

Mushin WW, Rendell-Baker L, Thompson P & Mapleson WW (1980) *Automatic Ventilation of the Lungs.* Oxford: Blackwell Scientific.

Newton NI, Hillman KM & Varley JG (1981) Automatic ventilation with the Ayre's T-piece. A modification of the Nuffield series 200 ventilator for neonatal and paediatric use. *Anaesthesia* **36:** 22–36.

Nunn JF (1977) *Applied Respiratory Physiology*, pp 232–233. London: Butterworths.

Pandit UA, Steude GM & Leach AB (1985) Induction and recovery characteristics of isoflurane and halothane anaesthesia for short operations in children. *Anaesthesia* **40:** 1226–1230.

Pethick SL (1975) Letter to the editor. *Canadian Anaesthetists' Society Journal* **22:** 115.

Pietak SP (1983) The anesthetic ventilator. *Canadian Anaesthetists' Society Journal* **30:** S42–45.

Podlesch I, Dudziak R & Zinganell K (1966) Inspiratory and expiratory carbon dioxide concentrations during halothane anesthesia in infants. *Anesthesiology* **27:** 823–828.

Prince SR, Sullivan RL & Hackel A (1976) Percutaneous catheterization of the internal jugular vein in infants and children. *Anesthesiology* **44:** 170–174.

Rao TLK, Wong AY & Salem MR (1977) A new approach to percutaneous catheterization of the internal jugular vein. *Anesthesiology* **46:** 362–364.

Rasche RFH & Kuhns LR (1972) Histopathologic changes in airway mucosa of infants after endotracheal intubation. *Pediatrics* **50:** 632–637.

Rayburn RL & Watson RL (1980) Humidity in children and adults using the controlled partial rebreathing anesthesia method. *Anesthesiology* **52:** 291–295.

Rees GJ (1950) Anaesthesia in the newborn. *British Medical Journal* **ii:** 1419–1422.

Rendell-Baker L & Soucek DM (1962) New paediatric facemasks and anaesthetic equipment. *British Medical Journal* **i:** 1960–1962.

Ring WH, Adair JC & Elwyn RA (1975) New pediatric endotracheal tube. *Anesthesia and Analgesia* **54:** 273–274.

Robinson S & Fisher DM (1983) Safety check for the CPRAM circuit. *Anesthesiology* **59:** 488–489.

Rogers SN & Benumof JL (1983) New and easy techniques for fiberoptic endoscopy-aided tracheal intubation. *Anesthesiology* **59:** 569–572.

Rose DK & Froese AB (1979) The regulation of P_aCO_2 during controlled ventilation of children with a T-Piece. *Canadian Anaesthetists' Society Journal* **26:** 104–113.

Salem MR, Bennett EJ, Schweiss JF et al (1975) Cardiac arrest related to anesthesia: contributing factors in infants and children. *Journal of the American Medical Association* **233:** 238–241.

Seldinger SI (1953) Catheter replacement of the needle in percutaneous arteriography. *Acta Radiologica* **39:** 368–376.

Sherry KM (1983) Postextubation stridor in Down's syndrome. *British Journal of Anaesthesia* **85:** 53–55.

Sinclair JC (1972) Thermal control in premature infants. *Annual Review of Medicine* **23:** 129–148.

Smallwood RW (1986) Ventilators: reported classifications and their usefulness. *Anaesthesia and Intensive Care* **14:** 252–257.

Stern L, Lees MH & Leduc J (1965) Environmental temperature, oxygen consumption, and catecholamine excretion in newborn infants. *Pediatrics* **36:** 367–373.

Stern DH, Gerson JI, Allen FB & Parker FB (1985) Can we trust the direct radial artery pressure immediately following cardiopulmonary bypass? *Anesthesiology* **62:** 557–561.

Stetson JB & Guess WL (1970) Causes of damage to tissues by polymers and elastomers used in the fabrication of tracheal devices. *Anesthesiology* **33:** 635–652.

Tocino IM & Watanabe A (1986) Impending catheter perforation of superior vena cava: radiographic recognition. *American Journal of Roentgenology* **146:** 487–490.

Todres ID, Rogers MC, Shannon DC, Moylan FMB & Ryan JF (1975) Percutaneous catheterization of the radial artery in the critically ill neonate. *Journal of Pediatrics* **87:** 273–275.

Toung TJK, Grayson R, Saklad J & Wang H (1985) Movement of the distal end of the endotracheal tube during flexion and extension of the neck. *Anesthesia and Analgesia* **64:** 1030–1032.

Tusiewicz K, Bryan AC & Froese AB (1977) Contributions of changing rib cage-diaphragm interactions to the ventilatory depression of halothane anesthesia. *Anesthesiology* **47:** 327–337.

Water DJ & Mapleson WW (1964) Exponentials and the anaesthetist. *Anaesthesia* **19:** 274–293.

Monitoring during paediatric anaesthesia

Monitoring is based on the need to enquire and advise in order not only to achieve the highest safety standards possible but to maintain the patient in theatre and return him or her from the recovery room in the optimum physiological condition. The need for this goes back to the very foundations of anaesthesia and is evidenced by the picture of Joseph Clover with his 'finger on the pulse' (Thomas, 1975). That we are currently failing always to apply a satisfactory standard of monitoring and that this contributes to mortality is evidenced by the survey of Lunn and Mushin (1982).

The information we seek and obtain from monitoring will vary considerably depending on such factors as the patient's age, general physical status, surgical pathology and the effects and duration of the surgery itself. The 'finger on the pulse' approach to monitoring has been rightly criticized because of the inability of anyone to pay full and continuing attention to all aspects of the clinical condition during a lengthy operation. In any individual patient the anaesthetist must decide how much monitoring is necessary in addition to basic clinical care because there is a limit to the quantity of information that can be assimilated. Monitors may be unreliable, alarms can be turned off and information can be misinterpreted. The anaesthetist should not devote so much attention to the monitors that he or she is distracted from adequate and direct observation of the patient. However, there is a basic level of monitoring which is now mandatory. The eventual well-being of the patient depends on the vigilance of the anaesthetist.

Infant and adult anaesthetic practices differ in their emphasis on monitoring because of differences in anatomy and physiology. For example, the newborn has a tendency to hypothermia, apnoea attacks and metabolic disturbances, which all have a deleterious effect on the quality of survival or even on survival itself. In the infant the emphasis is on the rapid onset of serious hypoxaemia if ventilation fails and the likelihood in this age group of hyperthermia. Routine monitoring should be directed to the early detection of those episodes which may be life-threatening and therefore will involve the supply of oxygen to the brain, or to detecting sudden circulatory failure. Unfortunately there is as yet no single, simple, safe and reliable monitor for early detection of such failure.

Monitoring ranges from clinical observation to specific appliance monitoring of respiration, circulation, temperature, neuromuscular, cerebral and metabolic function. An additional and important monitor is the trend-recording in graphical form on an anaesthetic record sheet of the main data.

This provides evidence that the information has been noted by the anaesthetist and relates changes to the overall management of the anaesthetic and operation.

CLINICAL MONITORING

Clinical monitoring involves tactile, visual and auditory observation of the patient and requires the close presence of the anaesthetist. 'Any damage to a patient which is accompanied by a failure to apply these senses continuously during the course of an anaesthetic is unlikely to be defendable in a court of law' (Green, 1987).

The important features are:

1. colour of mucous membranes, skin and operation site;
2. pulse rate and character;
3. peripheral circulation—capillary refill time in fingertips;
4. chest movement—magnitude and pattern;
5. noise of breathing and ventilator;
6. skin—colour, sweating, temperature of periphery;
7. eyes—lacrimation and pupil size;
8. limb position—muscle tone, movement.

These clinical observations should form the basis for continuous assessment of the patient's well-being. Information obtained from additional monitors should always be interpreted in relation to the clinical status.

INSTRUMENTAL MONITORING

Respiratory monitoring

Careful respiratory monitoring is mandatory during infant anaesthesia because of the high alveolar ventilation necessary to provide the oxygen requirement for the high metabolic rate. Minimal reduction in inspired oxygen concentration or alveolar ventilation may rapidly result in systemic hypoxaemia and if this is prolonged cerebral damage may result. Myocardial efficiency also falls but the ECG may remain normal for some time before showing bradycardia. By the time asystole occurs the brain will have been irreparably damaged.

Medico-legal experience suggests that the termination of anaesthesia and the first 10 min or so of recovery is the most likely time for damaging hypoxaemia to occur in infants. The cause is a combination of drug-induced central depression, airway obstruction, secretions and laryngospasm, and all general anaesthetic techniques can be incriminated. The most potent single factor is extubation of an infant with a suction catheter in the trachea so that the lungs become partially deflated and laryngospasm is stimulated. Hypoxia occurs almost instantaneously and in such circumstances laryngospasm is difficult to terminate. Very capable clinical monitoring of respiration must continue beyond anaesthesia until recovery is complete and the patient responds normally to auditory stimuli. Recovery to safe airway maintenance should be rapid, take place in close proximity to the theatre and be supervised by an experienced person on a one-to-one basis.

Prolonged postanaesthetic respiratory monitoring must occur in newborns below 44 weeks' postconceptual age as they are prone to apnoeic episodes. They must be nursed in hospital with an apnoea monitor for 24 h postanaesthetic.

Respiratory assessment in the operating room requires three aspects to be monitored:

1. inspiratory gas mixture;
2. airway patency and alveolar ventilation;
3. blood gas estimations.

Inspiratory gas mixture

There are a number of mechanisms for unexpected error in the inspired gas mixture. The uncommon but disastrous errors of crossed pipelines, mixed outlet hoses, or incorrect cylinders occur from time to time and may be fatal. They will continue to occur until hypoxic gas mixtures cease to be supplied. The occurrence of significantly hypoxic mixtures due to inaccurate or cracked flow meters or system leaks between the oxygen and nitrous oxide flow meters is more difficult to diagnose and therefore even more dangerous. Oxygen concentration should be measured just before the machine outlet by a simple inline oxygen analyser, although this may not indicate all instances of delivery of a hypoxic mixture (Sykes, 1987). All machines should be fitted with an independent audible oxygen pressure failure warning alarm. The delivery of a hypoxic inspiratory gas mixture, however acquired, must be considered negligent.

Monitoring airway patency and alveolar ventilation

The role of the stethoscope in the assessment of breath sounds, airway obstruction and correct tracheal tube placement cannot be over-estimated, and in spite of many advances in technology it is still an essential monitor involving minimal cost and effort.

In simple operations with spontaneous breathing it is adequate to observe the rate and movement of the reservoir bag in the anaesthetic system, and the magnitude and pattern of chest cage movement. Combined with auscultation this gives a satisfactory assessment of ventilation.

Changes in transthoracic impedance associated with changes in tidal volume can be used as an apnoea monitor or respiratory rate counter but not as a quantitative measure of ventilation. Because of cardiac or other artefact this method sometimes fails as an apnoea monitor to alarm within 20 s, and is not generally used in operating theatres.

During intermittent positive pressure ventilation (IPPV) in the operating theatre monitoring depends on the type of system used. Newborns are usually ventilated by hand, particularly in such operations as repair of tracheo-oesophageal fistula or diaphragmatic hernia where compliance may change rapidly. Airway obstruction from secretions or blood, or a major air leak from the fistula site may all occur suddenly. The advantages of hand ventilation are considerable, making it possible to recognize and treat such occurrences quickly. A preset overpressure valve should ideally be included so that excessive airway pressures cannot occur if the bag outlet is accidentally occluded.

When IPPV is carried out using some form of automatic ventilator, an aneroid pressure gauge in the inspiratory limb is an essential requirement. Excessive pressure suggests airway obstruction and low pressure suggests disconnection. A disconnection and overpressure alarm should be provided in all automatic ventilator systems and one based on a variable pressure cycling switch with a 15 s delay is suitable, but it cannot be used as a measure of adequacy of ventilation. Unfortunately fatal accidents still occur from unnoticed ventilator disconnection during IPPV.

Expired gas volumes should be measured either by a simple Wright's respirometer or a pneumotachograph. Some anaesthetic circuits such as the T-piece allow mixing of fresh and expired gas so that the effluent gas does not represent expired gas volume. In addition, if end expiratory positive pressure is maintained gas may be lost around a loose-fitting mask or tracheal tube. A pneumotachograph at the tracheal tube connection would overcome these problems, but it both increases dead space and resistance and is subject to calibration drift because of water vapour condensation on the mesh. Some intensive care unit (ICU) ventilators use a heated pneumotachograph in the expiratory limb to measure minute volume. The Wright's respirometer has been shown by Nunn and Ezi-Ashi (1962) and Conway et al (1974) to under-read at low volumes, but there is now a paediatric version accurate between tidal volumes of 15 and 200 ml (Hatch and Williams, 1988; Figure 7.1). Some ventilators will allow apparently acceptable chest movement despite inadequate fresh gas flow and significant rebreathing. Clinical assessment with correlation of chest cage movement, airway pressure, fresh gas flow and expired gas volume allows an experienced anaesthetist to feel confident that alveolar ventilation is within an acceptable range in fit patients. However, no anaesthetist can quantitatively assess ventilation. Malfunctioning, poorly designed or incorrectly used ventilation systems either for IPPV or spontaneous breathing may allow hypoxic or carbon dioxide-containing mixtures to occur as well as unpredictable quantities of inhalational agents. Great care should be taken to use simple, well maintained breathing systems whose method of functioning is well understood.

Arterial blood gas measurement

The only method currently available for the accurate measurement of arterial blood gas tensions intraoperatively in all circumstances is via an indwelling arterial pressure monitoring cannula. These lines may remain

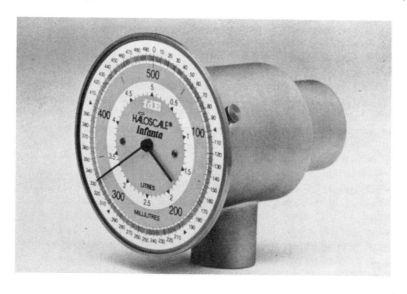

Figure 7.1. Paediatric Wright's Respirometer.

usable for 48–72 h but occasionally may last up to a week. Postoperatively, clinical assessment of failing spontaneous breathing becomes increasingly difficult the smaller the size of the patient, and earlier recourse to blood gas measurement is essential.

In the neonatal period it is particularly important to monitor oxygen and acid–base levels. The PaO_2 should be maintained between 50–70 mmHg (6.6–9.3 kPa) in the newborn of less than 44 weeks' postconceptual age as the retinal vessels may constrict at a PaO_2 above 100 mmHg (13.3 kPa) and retinopathy of prematurity may develop.

Flynn (1984) suggests that anaesthesia is unlikely to be a factor in the occurrence of this disorder, but more information is required.

Hypoxaemia and acidosis may cause the still reactive pulmonary vascular bed to constrict, increasing right-to-left shunting and further reducing the arterial oxygen tension. One of the essential aspects of a premature baby ICU is careful control of oxygen therapy on a continuous basis. Although this applies largely to newborns with respiratory distress syndrome there are an increasing number of surgical newborns who are premature, under-weight and ill, in whom the same problems apply.

Indwelling intravascular oxygen electrodes are available which continuously monitor oxygenation using a polarographic electrode. Newer catheters are heparin-coated to resist fibrin deposition but evidence suggests that platelet consumption continues when using long-term indwelling intravascular electrodes. Their use has declined because of the complications of infection, thromboembolism and vascular occlusion, and umbilical artery catheters are now used on a restricted basis. The development of miniature heparin-bonded fibreoptic sensors which have decreased drift and can measure PCO_2 and pH may cause some reversal of the above trend.

Transcutaneous gas measurement

Although there has been interest in skin oxygen measurements for many years it was not until 1972 that heated electrodes were used to 'arterialize' the skin. A Clark or Severinghaus-type electrode is sealed to the skin which is heated to 44°C. The electrode is moved every few hours to prevent skin damage. Eberhard et al (1976) reviewed the use of the Clark electrode. Numerous factors affect the cutaneous PO_2 ($PtcO_2$), including peripheral blood perfusion, skin properties, temperature, drift and calibration accuracy of the sensor and the ability to seal the sensor to the skin and avoid movement artefact.

Peabody et al (1978) found a good correlation between arterial and cutaneous PO_2 in most sick newborns over a wide range of conditions in the ICU. Cutaneous oxygen, however, was low in seriously hypotensive patients.

Hamilton et al (1985) reported a close correlation between $PtcO_2$ and PaO_2 in newborns under 8 weeks of age, but a variable and reducing relationship above this age with a mean ratio of about 0.83. A calibration time of 15–20 min limits the electrode's use in the operating theatre.

The $PtcO_2$ decreases considerably when the cardiac index falls below 2 l/min/m^2 (Tremper and Shoemaker, 1981). Attempts have been made to use heat output as a rough guide to the cardiac output. Measurement of $PtcO_2$ reflects changes in tissue oxygenation due to either hypoxaemia or reduced blood flow and is therefore a useful monitor of oxygen transport—it does not however measure arterial oxygenation.

Transcutaneous carbon dioxide ($PtcCO_2$) sensors do not correlate with $PaCO_2$ in low flow states but even when the cardiac output is normal there is marked individual variation in the $PtcCO_2$–$PaCO_2$ gradient (Tremper et al, 1981). In addition, local skin heating causes $PtcCO_2$ to be higher than $PaCO_2$ (Figure 7.2). Two-point calibration and reference to an arterial blood gas is

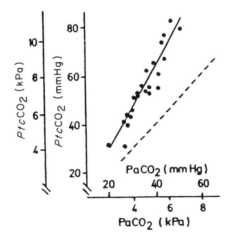

Figure 7.2. The relation between transcutaneous ($PtcCO_2$) and arterial ($PaCO_2$) 1 h after electrode placement (Marsden et al, 1985). The dashed line shows the line of identity.

required, which is time-consuming, but over the centre range a mean ratio of $PtcCO_2$:$PaCO_2$ of about 1.62:1.65 can be established and clinically useful data obtained (Marsden et al, 1985). In spite of inaccuracies in absolute values a great deal of information can be obtained from trends in $PtcO_2$ or $PtcCO_2$.

Transconjunctival gas measurement

A recent development is the measurement of transconjunctival oxygen ($PcjO_2$) using a miniature, non-heated Clark electrode and thermistor placed in contact with the tarsal portion of the palpebral vascular bed (Isenberg and Shoemaker, 1983). This monitor reflects changes in oxygen tension in the internal carotid artery and appears to be affected by the same factors that influence cerebral perfusion (Nisam et al, 1986). Miniaturized fibreoptic probes can also measure PCO_2 and pH. In haemodynamically stable states arterial CO_2 can be estimated from conjunctival CO_2, but in low flow states there is a closer relationship with venous or tissue measurements (Abraham et al, 1986). The role of conjunctival gas measurement needs further assessment but holds considerable promise in the management of states associated with cerebral oedema and underperfusion in both the ICU and the operating theatre. Although early reports suggest minimal conjunctival trauma, conjunctival gas measurement is unlikely to replace pulse oximetry as a universal everyday theatre monitor of oxygenation.

Mass spectrometry

The mass spectrometer allows rapid and very accurate measurement of respiratory gases and vapour concentrations during anaesthesia or in the ICU (Gillbe et al, 1981; Ozanne et al, 1981). Available machines have the facility to analyse up to 16 patients sequentially with a patient turnaround time of 2–3 min, but because of expense, size and maintenance problems, these machines are only appropriate to large operating theatre suites and ICU. The system operates by collecting respired gases using a fine nylon catheter and a variable sample suctioning rate, ranging from 200 ml/min down to 0.4–0.7 ml/s for newborns. Simultaneous measurement of minute gas samples takes place and wave forms representing the changes in concentration may be displayed for all gases and vapours. In addition, inspired and expired volumes can be measured by the use of inert tracer gases and hence oxygen uptake and carbon dioxide exchange can be calculated (Abbott et al, 1980).

The limiting factor in neonatal work is achieving a fast enough response time so that the end-tidal to alveolar gradient is minimal. Shortening the sample tubing will help but limits the number of beds monitored with this very expensive machine (Meny et al, 1985).

Measurement of gases and vapours in blood using gas-permeable membrane covered silastic catheters is still in the developmental phase (Brantigan et al, 1970).

Pulse oximetry

Until recently there has been no reliable non-invasive method of measuring arterial haemoglobin saturation as ear oximetry proved unreliable because of artefact from tissue and venous blood. This defect has been overcome by measuring light absorbance changes with arterial pulsation (Yelderman and New, 1983). Any pulsating arterial vascular bed is placed between a two-wavelength light source and detector. The transmitted light signal during diastole is used as a reference and the light absorbance signal produced by the arterial pulsation is analysed, so there is no artefact from surrounding venous blood or skin pigment. A microprocessor unit computes the haemo-globin saturation. The response time is rapid. Since light absorbance is measured at two wavelengths only, the pulse oximeter is unable to distin-guish three or more types of haemoglobin. Haemoglobin F has less effect on pulse oximeters than co-oximeters but bilirubin will cause under-reading of the true saturation as it absorbs light in the wavelengths used. There are minor differences in performance of different pulse oximeters, probably based on differences in the chosen light wavelength, the computation of the saturation and the design of the probes. The current status of pulse oximetry has been reviewed by Taylor and Whitwam (1986).

Pulse oximeters have been assessed in paediatric patients (Fanconi et al, 1985) and preterm infants (Deckhardt and Steward, 1984) and found to be safe and satisfactory. However, doubt continues to be expressed about the ability to control hyperoxia by pulse oximetry in the premature infant at risk of retinopathy, as oxygen tensions above 97.5 mmHg (13 kPa) have been associated with saturations as low as 92% (Southall et al, 1987; Wasunna and Whitelaw, 1987). This is an area where transcutaneous oxygen tension measurement is more sensitive than oxygen saturation because of the shape of the oxygen dissociation curve of haemoglobin F. Both measurements provide useful information but intermittent cross-reference with a direct arterial sample is still required.

Taylor and Whitwam (1988) compared the accuracy of five commercially available pulse oximeters and found that all underestimated arterial satu-ration by 2–3% in the 80–100% saturation range. Severinghaus and Naifeh (1987) tested the response of six pulse oximeters to sudden profound hy-poxia. Errors greater than 6% were found with a greater time lag on de-saturation than on resaturation. In some instances a nearly normal saturation was recorded when the real saturation was 40–70%. Some improvement occurred with modifications to some pulse oximeters.

Ridley (1988) reported increased inaccuracy of two pulse oximeters at low saturations in infants with cyanotic congenital heart disease who were chronically desaturated and polycythaemic. However, additional acute changes in saturation were accurately recorded. There is no doubt that in paediatric anaesthesia where desaturation occurs with frightening speed the pulse oximeter already has an established and proven place (Coté et al, 1988). Saturation is seen to be falling before clinical changes can be detected, and cyanosis is anyway an unreliable estimation of arterial desaturation (Comroe and Botelho, 1947). When the airway is shared, surgeons are also alerted to developing hypoxia at the same time as the anaesthetist so that arguments do not ensue and the hypoxaemia can be swiftly corrected.

During some periods of induction and recovery movement causes repeated probe displacement and the pulse oximeter is difficult to use, but these are areas where clinical observation should be maximal.

End-tidal carbon dioxide measurement

End-tidal CO_2 measurement using an infrared capnograph has been available for many years but until recently has not been widely used in the UK as a theatre monitor. This situation is now changing due to several factors:

1. Wide variations in arterial PCO_2 are no longer acceptable during anaesthesia because of the associated changes which may occur in myocardial function, cerebral blood flow, intracranial tension and some serum ionized electrolyte levels.
2. The need for very close moment-to-moment control of arterial CO_2 in intracranial operations and during some techniques in paediatric cardiac surgery.
3. The monitoring of intraoperative airway and ventilation errors (Coté et al, 1986).
4. The use of continuous end-tidal CO_2 monitoring in the early diagnosis of cerebral air embolism during intracranial surgery, especially in the sitting position.
5. The recent availability of high-quality rapid response time inline capnographs, such as the Hewlett Packard instrument.

End-tidal CO_2 measurement is ideally applicable in paediatric anaesthesia because of the lack of major pulmonary disease in the infant population. Lindahl et al (1987) have demonstrated the close relationship between arterial ($PaCO_2$) and end-tidal ($P_{ET}CO_2$) CO_2 in normal infants and children, and those with cardiac malformations resulting in overperfusion of the lung. A relationship of $PaCO_2 = 0.93 \times P_{ET}CO_2 + 3.1$ was found but with a maximum range of $P(a - ET)CO_2$ difference of about $\pm$ 5 mmHg (0.7 kPa). There was no difference between artificially ventilated and spontaneously breathing patients. The two exceptions were patients with severe pulmonary disease or cyanotic heart disease where the relationship was erratic. However, doubt has been expressed about the accuracy of end-tidal CO_2 measurement in neonates and small infants in clinical practice (Sasse, 1985). Difficulty may be attributable to the low tidal volume to equipment dead space ratio, rapid ventilatory rates and the high sampling rates required by capnographs. Badgwell et al (1987) found that even in very small infants a true end-tidal plateau could be obtained provided there was automatic interruption of fresh gas flow during expiration, so that undiluted alveolar gas was sampled. Where continuous flow circuits were in use a true end-tidal plateau was unlikely in infants under 8 kg weight. The Hewlett Packard infant capnograph has a response time of 0.05 s and measures directly through the window of low-volume inline cuvette. A continuous rapid response digital read-out records both inspired CO_2 and the end-tidal plateau level. With very rapid respiratory rates and low tidal volumes the monitor may fail to produce a reading.

CIRCULATORY MONITORING

Stethoscope

The stethoscope has an unchallenged place in paediatric anaesthesia and remains an essential monitor in spite of more recent and sophisticated equipment (Figures 7.3, 7.4). It provides reliable information about the intensity and character of heart sounds and mechanical heart rate, although this may frequently be too fast to count. Muffling of the heart sounds is an early indicator of hypovolaemia and may occur before there are easily detectable changes in systolic pressure or peripheral perfusion. The oesophageal stethoscope allows excellent monitoring of breath and heart sounds in the intubated patient, provided the balloon is situated in mid-oesophagus. There is the added advantage of less extraneous noise and less risk of displacement. Small oesophageal stethoscopes suitable for use in infants are now being produced (Portex Ltd).

Stethoscope tubing should be pliable enough to prevent the chest piece lifting but not so soft as to kink—the longer the tubing, the more attenuated the sound. Ertel et al (1966) reviewed the acoustics of the stethoscope and the relationship between design and function. A monaural moulded earpiece allows the anaesthetist to remain in contact with other activities in the operating room whilst monitoring heart and breath sounds continuously.

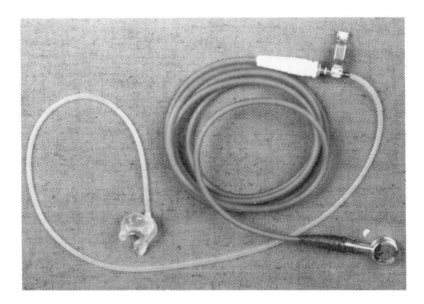

Figure 7.3. Precordial stethoscope with monaural earpiece. The chestpiece adheres to the skin with a double-sided sticky ring.

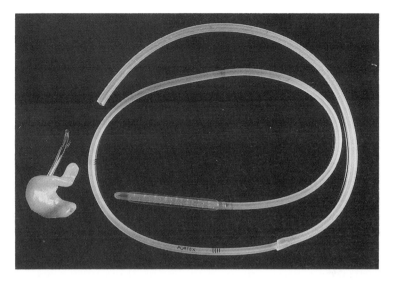

Figure 7.4. Oesophageal stethoscope with monaural earpiece

ECG

The ECG provides beat-to-beat information about the electrical activity of the heart, but it cannot be stressed too often that it provides no information about the pumping ability of the myocardium or the state of the peripheral circulation. The cardiac output can virtually cease well before there is any change in the ECG.

In the infant, lead 3 will usually provide the most pronounced R waves due to right axis deviation; otherwise lead 2 is likely to be the most useful lead for routine monitoring. Suitable ECG recorders for theatre use are expensive as they must have a filter system which allows unwanted signals to be suppressed. The most troublesome part of the monitor is the electrode–patient interface, but there is little problem if high-quality pre-gelled electrodes are used. The electric cautery must be adequately grounded to reduce interference and the risk of burns by earthing through ECG electrodes.

The ECG in paediatric practice should include a continuous digital display of heart rate, since fast apex and pulse rates are both difficult and distracting to count. A slow rate (below 100 beats/min) in infants may be the first sign of hypoxia. Vagal blocking premedication is not universally given in paediatric practice, but profound vagal slowing occurs readily in children from drugs such as succinylcholine, cyclopropane and newer agents such as fentanyl or vecuronium; or from traction on eye muscles or gut, cardiac and hilar dissection or adenoid curettage. Rapid cardiac rates may occur from excessive atropinization or, more frequently, an inadequate level of anaesthesia. While a normal rate is necessary for a satisfactory cardiac output (Table 7.1), rate is a relatively poor indicator of hypovolaemia in infancy. A soft bleep for the cardiac rate is useful for the background.

Table 7.1. Normal heart rate

Age	Average rate
Preterm	150 ± 20
Term	135 ± 20
1 month	160 ± 20
6 months	140 ± 20
1 year	120 ± 20
2 years	110 ± 20
5 years	90 ± 20
10 years	80 ± 20

The ECG also provides information about the existence of abnormal rhythms, most of which are benign in paediatric practice. They are usually associated with hypercapnia, high circulating adrenaline levels, the use of inhalational agents (particularly halothane), the presence of metabolic acidosis or electrolyte disturbance. Because of the limited lead selection available during surgery and the high electrical suppression for artefacts, ischaemic changes may be missed.

Measurement of blood pressure

The measurement of blood pressure is important in the small child (Table 7.2). During anaesthesia in the very young infant systolic arterial blood pressure seems to be closely related to circulating blood volume and arterial blood pressure is an excellent guide to the adequacy of blood replacement. Blood pressure is not, however, easy to measure accurately in the infant although most methods of measurement can be used. Kirkendall et al (1967) reported the importance of using the correct cuff size in blood pressure measurement in children and this was confirmed by Kimble et al (1981) in their assessment of the Dinamap in newborns. The cuff should be sufficient to cover two-thirds of the length of the patient's upper arm. At least one-half of the circumference of the arm should be covered by the bladder and the whole cuff should be applied firmly. A too narrow or too loosely applied cuff will give a falsely high reading.

Table 7.2. Normal blood pressure

Age	Blood pressure (mmHg)	Average range	
		Systolic (mmHg)	Diastolic (mmHg)
Newborn	80–50	80 ± 15	50 ± 15
6 months	90–60	90 ± 20	60 ± 10
1 year	95–65	95 ± 30	65 ± 20
2 years	100–65	100 ± 25	65 ± 25
5 years	95–55	95 ± 15	55 ± 10
10 years	110–60	110 ± 15	60 ± 10

Oscillometric method

This method employs an occlusive blood pressure cuff which is slowly deflated. Oscillation is produced in the cuff and transmitted to an aneroid gauge: as the cuff deflates the oscillation increases markedly about systolic pressure and then fades as diastolic pressure is reached. The maximum oscillation probably occurs around mean systemic pressure.

A major advance has been the development of an automated oscillometric monitor (for example, Dinamap, Applied Medical Research, Tampa, Florida, USA). A small microprocessor unit allows the monitor to run a variety of time cycles and provides a digital read-out of systolic and diastolic pressure and an integrated mean arterial pressure. Rate is also displayed. The machine automatically holds or terminates a cycle if artefact movement is too great, and high and low alarm systems are incorporated. Failure to empty the cuff completely between cycles causes both venous congestion of the arm and a low blood pressure measurement. One unit is suitable for all age groups, although a small adaptor is necessary for neonatal cuffs.

The accuracy of this method has been established by a number of workers both in adults (Silas et al, 1980; Borow and Newburger, 1982; Hutton et al 1984) and in the critically ill newborn and infant (Friesen and Lichtor, 1981; Kimble et al, 1981). In practice these machines are easy to use as the cuff position is not too critical; they have proved to be reliable and to require relatively little maintenance. The principal disadvantage is these monitors only measure blood pressure intermittently, but this is common to all equipment of this type. Automated oscillometric monitors form the basis of in-theatre blood pressure monitoring at the present time.

If the pulse rate provided by the automated blood pressure measuring device is not the same as that from the ECG or pulse oximeter, then the accuracy of the blood pressure reading should be questioned.

Ultrasonic detection of brachial artery flow

This system employs an occlusive cuff with an ultrasonic transducer over the brachial artery. Care must be taken to place the transducer directly over the artery and there must be protection from movement artefact. The transducer consists of an ultrasonic signal generator (usually 2–10 MHz) and a receiver. The change in frequency associated with blood flow in the artery is noted and by suitable filtering and amplification of the signal, systolic (commencing flow) and diastolic (continuous flow) pressures are recorded. This may be an audible signal, or on modern expensive automated machines a print-out may be produced at regular intervals.

This method has been found suitable in small infants (McLaughlin et al, 1971; Dweck et al, 1974). Poppers (1973) found a good correlation with arterial pressure in the newborn even in the presence of hypotension, using a 4 cm cuff and an 8 MHz signal generator. The Arteriosonde (Hoffman la Roche) uses an 8 MHz signal and has been found to be reasonably accurate (Reder et al, 1978).

Finger arterial pressure (the Finapres)

This device produces a calibrated arterial pressure wave on a beat-to-beat basis even in the presence of vasoconstriction (Dorlas et al, 1985). It depends on a small finger cuff which is modulated by a pumping mechanism so that plethysmographic excursions are kept to a minimum. As the transmural pressure remains almost zero, variations in cuff pressure are identical with finger arterial pressure pulsations. This device has been evaluated in adults and at present the technology is being modified for children. It offers the prospect of a non-invasive beat-to-beat monitor of arterial pressure.

Invasive blood pressure monitoring

This consists of an indwelling arterial cannula connected to a pressure transducer via a short length of rigid, fluid-filled, narrow-bore (1.5–3 mm diameter) recording line connected by a three-way stopcock. Amplification of electrical signals from the transducer produces a pressure trace on an oscilloscope or some other type of print-out. The characteristics of the pressure wave form can be seen in graphic form. A medium-scale oscilloscope display, which then averages several beats to produce a digital read-out of pressure, is most useful.

The main indications for intra-arterial pressure monitoring are:

1. anticipated massive shifts of blood or fluid;
2. actual or anticipated unstable blood pressure on a beat-to-beat basis or non-pulsatile flow;
3. induced hypotension of long duration or to a very low level;
4. very long duration surgery;
5. close blood gas supervision in theatre or postoperatively.

Clinical examples are: open and most closed heart or great vessel surgery; posterior fossa exploration; craniopharyngioma; clipping cerebral aneurysms; major craniofacial reconstructions; phaeochromocytoma and most neuroblastoma explorations; gastric interposition of the oesophagus; kidney and liver transplantation and many spinal fusions.

Intra-arterial pressure monitoring has two main requirements; the provision of a well maintained and calibrated system from transducer to print-out and the ability to insert and maintain a trouble-free sterile intra-arterial cannula.

The importance of correct calibration of the equipment cannot be overemphasized. Many modern monitors have 'push-button' zero and calibration but it is essential that this is periodically checked against a mercury column. In addition, the frequency response and harmonics of the tubing system may give an underdamped trace with considerable overshoot. The degree of damping required cannot be estimated by the appearance of the pressure wave form. Unless the dynamic response of a given recording system is known, an accurate pressure cannot be guaranteed. This subject has been fully reviewed by Gardner (1981). Various arteries, including radial, femoral, brachial, dorsalis pedis and superficial temporal, have been used for cannulation. In the neonate the umbilical artery may be used, although it should be noted that in the first days of life the distal aortic PaO_2 will be lower than in the carotid artery, due to right-to-left shunting at cardiac or ductus level. The difference will depend on the degree of shunting. The right radial artery is more representative of the carotid and retinal arterial PaO_2 and is preferred as a sampling site in premature newborns.

Sterility is essential at all times and a slow continuous flush of heparinized saline (1000 u heparin/l 0.9% saline) helps to prevent cannula blockage and embolism. In very small infants great care must be taken to limit and measure total fluid input and sodium content from indwelling cannulas as fluid overload occurs readily.

Central venous pressure (CVP)

A cannula sited in the lower superior vena cava (SVC) or right atrium measures right atrial filling pressure and this can be used to reflect circulating blood volume provided that other aspects of the circulation, such as left ventricular function, pulmonary vascular resistance and peripheral vascular capacitance are considered. In addition it provides a reasonably accurate sampling site for the measurement of acid–base status if an arterial line is not present. In the small fat infant it may be the optimum venous access for rapid blood replacement. The main indications for an intraoperative CVP cannula are:

1. rapid massive volume loss or replacement;
2. long duration surgery with continuous small volume loss which becomes progressively more difficult to assess;
3. rapid changes in vascular capacitance, such as in phaeochromocytoma, neuroblastoma, or in some patients when induced hypotension is used;
4. unstable circulations, such as in congenital heart disease.

The most commonly used vein for CVP measurement is the internal jugular vein, though the subclavian vein is also used. Long-line cannulas from the antecubital fossa are difficult to insert percutaneously under 4 years of age and femoral vein cannulas have an increased risk of thromboembolism and may not read an accurate CVP.

The internal jugular vein is the access of choice in the infant and is a reliable and easy cannulation, provided great care is taken to define the landmarks (English et al, 1969; Prince et al, 1976). Subclavian vein puncture is relatively easy in the small infant using the infraclavicular approach (Davidson et al, 1963), but it is extremely difficult to persuade a reasonable-sized i.v. cannula safely to enter the SVC from the right side. The cannulation is best performed using a guide-wire and flexible cannula and so requires a full surgical aseptic technique. It is a more suitable technique for the ICU than the operating theatre. The guide-wire sets produced by Vygon (Leader Cath 115, Vygon, Ecouen, France) are very satisfactory in the under 2-year age group. Double- and triple-lumen catheters are also available. Ever-present dangers with central venous lines are the risks of air embolism, sepsis, thromboembolism and perforation leading to cardiac tamponade, haemothorax or pleural fluid. Careful placement and good nursing can reduce these risks to a minimum. The use of internal jugular CVP lines has been one of the major advances in the management of infants undergoing major surgery over the last decade.

Left atrial pressure

Left atrial pressure measurement is essential following the repair of some of the more complex congenital heart lesions when left-sided function may be impaired. This is easily measured by the insertion of a recording line via the right upper pulmonary vein into the left atrium at the time of operation, and such lines have proved to be reliable and trouble-free. Following non-cardiac operations pulmonary wedge pressure may be measured by the use of a Swan–Ganz catheter inserted via the right internal jugular or right subclavian veins. In the small infant this is a difficult technique and the procedure has the potential for major complications. There are few indications for the measurement of left atrial or pulmonary wedge pressure outside cardiac surgery in paediatric surgical practice. Difficulties are much more likely to occur from changes in pulmonary vascular resistance and right heart function.

Pulmonary artery pressure

Pulmonary artery pressure or right ventricular pressure is an essential measurement in many babies after cardiac surgery (see Chapter 13). Here a recording catheter is left in the pulmonary artery either through the right ventricular wall or via an internal jugular cannula. Infants who have had a high pulmonary blood flow from lesions such as truncus arteriosus or total anomalous pulmonary venous drainage are prone to develop pulmonary vascular hypertensive crises after repair of the defect, as the infant pulmonary vascular bed becomes excessively reactive. Diagnosis and treatment of such episodes is markedly helped by pulmonary artery pressure measurement, which may be necessary for periods of a week or more. The use of a recording catheter placed in the pulmonary artery or right ventricle via a central vein is an essential but very invasive monitor. Problems of infection and thromboembolism to the pulmonary vascular bed are ever-present and this is not a technique to be undertaken lightly or without experienced and competent staff. In newborns who develop a transitional circulation in association with such problems as prematurity, congenital diaphragmatic hernia or meconium aspiration, pulmonary artery pressure measurement would be helpful. However, this is a difficult technique in this age group and may in itself predispose to a continuation of the transitional circulation. In clinical management it is often better to assess the response to treatment and reversibility of the right-to-left shunt by measuring changes in arterial PO_2 and transcutaneous PO_2, especially the difference between pre- and postductal PaO_2.

Close monitoring of the PaO_2 is essential in sick preterm babies in order to avoid a prolonged high PO_2 in the retinal arteries.

An essential requirement of this group of newborns is biochemical and blood gas stability and lack of peripheral stimulation. Invasive monitoring must not aggravate the situation.

Cardiac output

There are currently no methods for measuring cardiac output in general operating theatres in children, and no prospect of doing so in the near future. Cardiac output measurement by the Fick and dye dilution methods are not suitable for repeated use in most ICU practice. Although a correlation coefficient of 0.95 was found between these techniques, 25% of measurements show a substantial error. There are now methods which can be used in the ICU.

Thermodilution

This method requires a pulmonary artery catheter and meticulous attention to detail and its repeated use may lead to fluid overload in small children. Comparison with the dye dilution method in adults gives a correlation coefficient of 0.96 with a maximal error of $\pm 16\%$, but minor changes in the injection technique can produce over-estimates of up to 50%.

Doppler ultrasound

This entirely non-invasive method uses the Doppler frequency shift between emitted and received ultrasound signals to measure a blood flow velocity-flow time for a single beat. Measurement of cross-sectional area at the point of flow can be measured by echocardiography and this allows stroke volume to be computed. Stroke volume and cardiac rate allow cardiac output to be calculated. As aortic flow is measured the coronary artery component of the cardiac output is not included and the angle between the direction of flow and ultrasound signal has to be assumed, but provided it is less than 20° the error is under 6%. There are a number of potential errors with this method but in the hands of an experienced and skilled investigator the technique produces results which compare as favourably with the standard techniques as these do among themselves (Schuster and Nanda, 1984). The percentage change on sequential measurements is more reliable than the absolute value.

Transcutaneous aortovelography

This technique uses Doppler ultrasound to measure an aortic blood velocity. Cross-sectional area is not measured by echocardiography as this requires

considerable skill and is a major source of error, which is likely to increase
with small-sized vessels. Once a normal range of values is established aortic
blood velocity measurements may be used by themselves to assess cardiac
output without conversion to a volumetric measurement or correction for
body size (Haites et al, 1985). Reproducibility is good, with a deviation of
about 6–7% between estimations. Sequential estimates of cardiac output are
satisfactory and the technique is suitable for ICU use.

Thoracic electrical impedance

This method has produced results which were not comparable with those
produced by thermodilution and it has been regarded as not clinically useful
because of lack of precision and technical difficulties (Donovan et al, 1986).
There is some hope that this situation may eventually change with improved
equipment but its role in children is uncertain.

Blood loss and replacement (see also p. 188)

Adequate replacement of blood loss is essential in the infant patient, and
this is an area which frequently causes concern to the anaesthetist who is
inexperienced in the management of small babies. It is essential that the
anaesthetist calculates an acceptable volume loss and notes the haemoglobin level for each patient at the commencement of anaesthesia so that the
probable need to replace blood or colloid may be predicted early (Table 7.3).

Table 7.3. Average blood volume

Age	Blood volume (ml kg^{-1})
Newborn	80–85
6 weeks to 2 years	75–80
2 years to 15 years	70–75

Intraoperative blood loss of under 10% of the circulating blood volume
can be replaced with crystalloid fluid; losses over 20% will usually require
blood. Adequate crystalloid fluid must always be given (see Chapter 8).

Monitoring of blood loss should be simple, reasonably accurate, and
practised routinely. This is achieved by weighing small numbers of swabs
before drying out occurs, and maintaining a regular cumulative total. Allowance is made for loss on drapes and for additions of non-blood fluids such as
cerebrospinal fluid, urine, or irrigating fluid. Suction bottle loss is measured
directly. The great advantage of swab-weighing is that it is quick, reliable,
and can be checked against the anaesthetist's own estimate.

The alternative to swab-weighing involves washing swabs in a standard
volume of fluid and measuring the haemoglobin content colorimetrically

and hence calculating blood loss. As with weighing, loss on drapes and gowns can only be measured retrospectively.

Errors in blood loss measurement by any technique will be cumulative, and with long-duration surgery will be significant. At best, measurement can only act as a guideline but it should always form the basis of a blood transfusion blood loss balance sheet which must be kept routinely for any but the most trivial surgery. The final assessment of the adequacy of the circulating volume must always be clinical and is based on the following:

1. *Blood pressure*: peak systolic pressure and its trend, diastolic pressure and pulse pressure. A falling systolic pressure with a rising diastolic pressure indicates significant volume depletion with constriction of the peripheral circulation.
2. *Auscultation of chest sounds*: reduced intensity and lack of crispness of apex sounds suggest volume depletion and a low cardiac output in small infants.
3. *Peripheral circulation*: capillary refill time should be rapid and the extremities pink and warm. Prolonged refill time and increased core–peripheral gradient are important clinical signs suggesting volume depletion or low cardiac output from other causes.
4. *Pulse*: pulse rate rises with volume depletion but in the small infant this is not a reliable guide to hypovolaemia. With volume depletion the pulse pressure narrows, thus making the peripheral pulse less easy to feel.
5. *Central venous pressure*: this is an essential trend monitor for volume assessment in major surgery. There may be a significant reduction in the quality of the peripheral circulation, with little reduction in CVP in the early stages of blood loss due to vasoconstriction. If hypotension and a poor peripheral circulation persist then volume expansion must commence until the peripheral circulation improves or a CVP measurement of 12 mmHg (16 cm H_2O) is reached. Cardiac output increases directly with increasing right atrial filling pressure until a certain point, around 12–14 mmHg, when no further increase in cardiac output occurs. Failure of the peripheral circulation to improve by this point implies other problems, such as erroneous CVP readings due to malplacement of the catheter, compromised cardiac function or local peripheral circulatory problems.

Blood is now infrequently used in less major surgery because of the risks involved in donor transfusion. Major volume loss should be replaced with blood products but it is frequently technically difficult to maintain a normal haematocrit in a small baby because of the wide and unknown variations in the haematocrit of the blood transfusion products currently supplied. Later adjustment to the haematocrit may be difficult and the extremes of haematocrit may seriously impede oxygen transport.

When massive transfusion is required over a short time, monitoring of acid–base status and coagulation indices should commence. Coagulation indices should include:

1. Platelet count. Levels below $60\,000/mm^3$ should initiate a request for platelet-rich plasma as bleeding is likely if the count falls further.

2. Prothrombin time and partial thromboplastin time.
3. Tests for fibrinolysis (estimation of fibrin degradation products), especially if the patient has been severely shocked, hypothermic or septicaemic.

Platelets should be given if the count falls below 40 000/mm^3 and fresh frozen plasma if the prothrombin time and partial thromboplastin time are prolonged by more than 25%.

These factors should continue to be monitored and deficiencies treated every 50% additional blood volume loss or until adequate levels are achieved.

After major surgery the haematocrit should be monitored regularly over the next 24–48 h and volume replaced as whole blood, packed cells or plasma, so that a haematocrit of 35–40% is maintained.

Temperature monitoring (see also p. 136)

Temperature should always be monitored in newborns and small infants, who show instability of body temperature over the relatively short periods of time involved in surgery. They are particularly susceptible to the adverse environmental temperature conditions often present in modern air-conditioned operating theatres.

Other reasons for routine temperature monitoring during straightforward surgery are the unlikely occurrence of the malignant hyperpyrexia syndrome and the overall benefits to any patient of maintaining normothermia during surgery (Vale, 1973).

Shanks (1975) reviewed the relationships between the temperature measured at differing sites in the surgical patient. Routine monitoring should be simple, reliable and safe. The most suitable measuring site for core temperature in infants is the mid-oesophagus if intubated, and over the axillary artery in the closed axilla in non-intubated patients. This will read a temperature about 0.5°C below true core temperature. Rectal temperature is unreliable and there is the danger of rectal perforation. The nasopharynx will read a low temperature if there is an air leak around the tracheal tube, and the wedged nasal temperature may be difficult to achieve. There is the risk of nasal mucosal damage and bleeding. Thermistor probes should be flexible, atraumatic and easily sterilized or disposable.

During the operation heat may be added to the patient by the use of humidified and heated inspiratory gas (Shanks, 1974). Some form of warming mattress is mandatory. Electric blankets, water and hot air mattresses have all been used. Any form of heating appliance has the potential to overheat and cause burns and must therefore be provided with its own thermometer, a safety cut-out thermostat in case of overheating, and a high-level alarm. The most efficient, clean and safe form of heating appliance is an air mattress, which provides a hot microclimate around the body under the drapes. Small newborns undergoing major and lengthy surgery will maintain and even gain temperature when this is used.

The need to maintain temperature in the newborn has been so widely preached for many years that it has led to over-enthusiastic heating of older infants. The 1- to 4-year-old has a high metabolic rate, and may readily become pyrexial (38–39°C) if placed on an efficient heating appliance; in addition, anaesthetic techniques involving the use of suxamethonium or halothane may increase body temperature. Hence all newborns and infants should have their temperature monitored for any but the most trivial surgery, and it is mandatory if heating appliances are being used.

Neuromuscular function monitoring

The routine intraoperative monitoring of neuromuscular function has not been widely practised in the UK, although some centres have used sophisticated neuromuscular function measurements in the assessment of muscle relaxants. In paediatric practice the extreme predictability of the most commonly used relaxant, d-tubocurarine, and the lack of readily available nerve stimulators fostered this attitude. There are now important reasons why attitudes should change.

Newer muscle relaxants, such as atracurium and vecuronium, seem to have significant advantages in some areas of paediatric practice. Their pharmacokinetics make them suitable agents to be given by continuous slow infusion and there may be advantages in this approach. To be satisfactory in routine clinical practice neuromuscular function must be monitored. Viby-Mogensen (1982) reviewed in detail the clinical assessments of neuromuscular transmission and stressed the need for supramaximal stimulation. In a recent review of some nerve stimulators used in adult practice Kopman and Lawson (1984) found that several currently available battery-operated stimulators when used with pre-gelled electrodes were unable to deliver a supramaximal stimulus at all frequencies. Indeed, there was considerable variation in the milliamperage required for supramaximal stimulation, probably because of variation in depth and position of the nerve and therefore of electrode placement. The authors recommended the need for stimulators to be able to achieve and display an output of 50–60 mA at all frequencies.

Mylrea et al (1984) discussed the relationship between stimulators and the errors in assessing neuromuscular blockade. Several currently available stimulators were not satisfactory. In contrast, the Bard Stimulator (Bard Biomedical, CR Bard Inc., Westmont, IL, USA) has a variety of stimulation modes, produces a 50–60 mA output at maximal stimulation, and displays the milliamperage. It is easy to use and requires little maintenance.

Lam et al (1981) reported on the design and use of a monitor for use in paediatric practice. This involves the stimulation of the median nerve at the wrist. A thenar muscle electromyogram (EMG) is rectified and integrated electronically to produce a meter display of the degree of neuromuscular block. The routine use of such equipment seems essential with the use of newer muscle relaxants and the increasing duration of major surgery.

The Datex Relaxograph provides continuous assessment of neuromuscular block by train-of-four stimulation of a peripheral nerve and both measurement and display on hard copy of the integrated EMG response by the use of five surface electrodes. The machine calibrates automatically at the start by finding the optimum signal levels and supramaximal current.

Every 20 s it calculates the percentage of the first twitch to the reference twitch as well as the train-of-four. Carter et al (1986) demonstrated reliable correlation with a force transducer system. Its use in small and relatively obese children is limited by the difficulty of positioning the stimulating electrode to obtain a supramaximal current as well as problems with the size and siting of the recording electrodes.

Sensory-evoked potentials

The use in the operating theatre of sensory-evoked potentials has recently been reviewed by Lam (1987). The amplitude of a sensory-evoked potential is small so computer summation and averaging are required to extract a useful signal. Increasing experience with this technique during the last few years has provided information about monitoring the integrity of neuronal function during carotid endarterectomy and spinal cord function during aortic cross-clamping and scoliosis surgery. At present the role of sensory-evoked potentials as a theatre monitor is unclear as the technique is complicated and interpretation difficult. However, with special expertise it is proving to be a useful monitor of cord function during scoliosis surgery. Further evaluation is required.

The cerebral function analysing monitor (CFAM) may be of value in monitoring depth of anaesthesia (Prior and Maynard, 1986).

Metabolic monitoring

The infant's high metabolic rate and oxygen consumption create a high carbohydrate and water turnover so that prolonged water and carbohydrate deprivation are not well tolerated. Preoperative starvation should be kept to a minimum and the time of the last food and fluid noted before the induction of anaesthesia.

In the newborn, glucose levels will fall after the initial depletion of body glycogen stores. The peak incidence of hypoglycaemia is 24–72 h post-delivery in babies who are premature or small-for-dates and therefore have limited carbohydrate reserves. Prolonged interference with feeding will increase the severity of hypoglycaemia. The glucose level may fall to 1.1–1.7 mmol/l (20–30 mg%). If the level remains below 1.7 mmol/l for several hours in full-term neonates, severe cortical neuronal damage is likely and non-specific central nervous system symptoms such as fits, twitching and apnoea may occur. Very premature babies may also readily develop hyperglycaemia. Glucose levels require monitoring at least 6-hourly in patients at risk and it is important that the laboratory measures glucose and not total reducing substances. Dextrostix should be available in every paediatric operating theatre and ICU.

Ware and Osborne (1976) reported postoperative hypoglycaemia in infants who had prolonged preoperative starvation. With shorter preoperative starvation, the more liberal use of i.v. fluid therapy and more rapid postoperative fluid intake, hypoglycaemia is unlikely.

Juvenile diabetics and patients with glycogen storage disorders create particular problems and glucose levels must be monitored intraoperatively.

The level of ionized calcium falls during the first week of life with a slow rise to adult levels during the second week. Low birthweight infants may show a greater fall and present with non-specific central nervous system symptoms similar to those of hypoglycaemia. The normal level during the first week of life is 2.03–2.30 mmol/l (8.12–9.2 mg%). Calcium levels should be monitored in newborns undergoing surgery and levels below 1.75 mmol/l must be treated by the slow intravenous injection of 30 mg/kg calcium gluconate. This may need to be repeated, or calcium gluconate added to the i.v. infusion.

In the immediate postnatal period there is an increase in red cell breakdown. Excessive haemolysis may occur if there is rhesus incompatibility and drugs given in the neonatal period may displace protein-bound bilirubin from plasma protein-binding sites. Anaesthesia may depress liver function and with the associated reduction in water turnover bilirubin excretion may be reduced. High levels of unconjugated bilirubin may result in kernicterus with permanent damage to the basal ganglia, but the dangerous level is variable due to multiple factors. Those at greatest risk are underweight, fluid-depleted infants who frequently come to surgery for correction of gut malformations. Kernicterus may occur with an unconjugated bilirubin well below 340 μmol/l (20 mg%) in poor-risk patients. The presence of jaundice means that bilirubin levels (conjugated and unconjugated) must be monitored.

Coagulation disorders may occur due to low levels of vitamin K-dependent factors (factor II—prothrombin—VII, IX and X). These reach their lowest level about the third day of life and then slowly rise to adult levels over the next few weeks. Prothrombin time and partial thromboplastin time should be measured.

In sick, hypoxic, acidotic and hypothermic newborns tests for fibrinolysis and intravascular coagulation should be monitored. This includes an assay of fibrin degradation products and evidence of platelet consumption.

MANDATORY MONITORING

This consists of those activities which should be regarded as the minimum necessary in a fit patient (ASA Grades 1 and 2) to ensure an adequate flow of oxygenated blood to the brain and so preserve the integrity of the central nervous system. Hypoxia plays a significant role in the aetiology of cardiac arrest. Anaesthesia can be given with only clinical monitoring and there may be situations where this is necessary and acceptable. However, unwillingness to acquire and use the information from the proven basic monitors now available raises the question of the degree of responsibility being shown to our patients (Cohen et al, 1988).

Induction

Induction of anaesthesia in infants should always take place in the presence of a competent assistant who may be an operating department assistant, nurse, or another doctor, because serious hypoxia develops fast if technical problems are encountered. Familiarity with and knowledge of equipment are essential. During periods which are distracting to the anaesthetist, such as induction, intubation and siting an i.v. infusion, the assistant must directly monitor colour and chest movement and palpate a peripheral pulse. A precordial stethoscope should be applied as soon as practicable.

Maintenance

During surgery lasting for any period beyond a few minutes, the following should be used routinely: inspired oxygen analyser, precordial stethoscope, ECG, automated blood pressure monitor and pulse oximeter. If the patient is paralysed and ventilated a ventilator disconnection alarm must be fitted. All operating theatres must have this equipment and there is little excuse for failing to connect it to the patient.

Termination of anaesthesia

This is the highest risk period in an infant anaesthetic. The pulse oximeter should be maintained until movement precludes its use. The ECG should continue until muscle relaxant reversal drugs are effective and movement artefact interferes with the recording. Close individual experienced supervision must continue until the infant is awake and crying or responding sensibly to the spoken word. Breathing, airway, colour and peripheral pulse must be constantly observed by someone trained to recognize and treat airway obstruction and apnoea. Anaesthetic personnel should be available in close proximity. Infants should not be removed partially recovered from the theatre to a distant recovery area. If these criteria for recovery cannot be fulfilled then the operating list should be interrupted until full recovery has taken place.

Poor-risk patients and those undergoing major surgery may require a variety of additional monitors to help maintain optimum conditions.

REFERENCES

Abbott TR, Goodwin B, Clark G & Rees GJ (1980) Mass spectrometer measurement of oxygen uptake and carbon dioxide exchange during cardiopulmonary bypass. *British Journal of Anaesthesia* **52:** 29–40.

Abraham E, Marke DR, Pinholster G & Fink SE (1986) Non-invasive measurement of conjunctival PCO_2 with a fibreoptic sensor. *Critical Care Medicine* **14:** 138–141.

Badgwell JM, Heavner JE, May WS, Goldthorn JF & Lerman J (1987) End-tidal PCO_2 monitoring in infants and children ventilated with either a partial rebreathing or a non rebreathing circuit. *Anesthesiology* **66:** 405–410.

Borow KM & Newburger JW (1982) Non invasive estimation of central aortic pressure using the oscillometric method for analysing systemic artery pulsatile flow: comparative study of indirect systolic, diastolic and mean brachial artery pressure with simultaneous direct ascending aortic pressure measurements. *American Heart Journal* **103**: 879–886.

Brantigan JW, Gott VL, Vestal ML, Ferguson GJ & Johnson WH (1970) A non thrombogenic diffusion membrane for continuous in vivo measurement of blood gases by mass spectrometry. *Journal of Applied Physiology* **28**: 375–377.

Carter JA, Arnold R, Yates PM et al (1986) Assessment of the Datex Relaxograph during anaesthesia and atracurium induced neuromuscular blockade. *British Journal of Anaesthesia* **58**: 1447–1452.

Cohen DE, Downes JJ & Raphaely RC (1988) What difference does pulse oximetry make? *Anesthesiology* **68**: 181–183.

Comroe JH & Botelho S (1947) The unreliability of cyanosis in the recognition of arterial anoxaemia. *American Journal of Medical Sciences* **214**: 1–6.

Conway CM, Leigh JM, Preston TD, Walters FJM & Webb DA (1974) An assessment of three electronic respirometers. *British Journal of Anaesthesia* **46**: 885–891.

Cote CJ, Liu LMP, Szyfelbein SK et al (1986) Intraoperative events diagnosed by expired carbon dioxide monitoring in children. *Canadian Anaesthetists' Society Journal* **33**: 315–319.

Cote CJ, Goldstein EA, Cote MA, Hoaglin DC & Ryan JF (1988) A single-blind study of pulse oximetry in children. *Anesthesiology* **68**: 184–188.

Davidson JT, Benhur N & Nathan H (1963) Subclavian venepuncture. *Lancet* **ii**: 1139–1140.

Deckhardt R & Steward DJ (1984) Noninvasive arterial haemoglobin saturation versus transcutaneous oxygen tension monitoring in the preterm infant. *Critical Care Medicine* **12**: 935–939.

Donovan KD, Dobb GJ, Woods WPD & Hockings BE (1986) Comparison of trans-thoracic electrical impedance and thermodilution methods for measuring cardiac output. *Critical Care Medicine* **14**: 1038–1044.

Dorlas JC, Nijboer JA, Butijn WT, Van Der Hoeven GMA, Settels JJ & Wesseling KH (1985) Effects of peripheral vasoconstriction on the blood pressure in the finger, measured continuously by a new noninvasive method (the Finapres). *Anesthesiology* **62**: 342–345.

Dweck HS, Reynolds DW & Cassady G (1974) Indirect blood pressure measurement in newborns. *American Journal of Diseases of Children* **127**: 492–494.

Eberhard P, Mindt W & Kreuzer F (1976) Cutaneous oxygen monitoring in the newborn. *Paediatrician* **5**: 335–369.

English ICW, Frew RM, Pigott JF & Zaki M (1969) Percutaneous catheterisation of the internal jugular vein. *Anaesthesia* **24**: 521–531.

Ertel PY, Lawrence M, Brown RK & Stern AM (1966) Stethoscope acoustics: II. Transmission and filtration patterns. *Circulation* **34**: 899–909.

Fanconi S, Doherty P, Edmonds JF, Barker GA & Bohn DJ (1985) Pulse oximetry in paediatric intensive care: comparison with measured saturations and trans-cutaneous oxygen tension. *Journal of Pediatrics* **107**: 362–366.

Flynn JT (1984) Oxygen and retrolental fibroplasia: update and challenge. *Anesthesiology* **60**: 397–399.

Friesen RH & Lichtor JL (1981) Indirect measurement of blood pressure in neonates and infants utilizing an automatic non-invasive oscillometric monitor. *Anesthesia and Analgesia* **60**: 742–745.

Gardner RM (1981) Direct blood pressure measurement—dynamic response require-ments. *Anesthesiology* **54**: 227–236.

Gillbe CE, Heneghan CPH & Branthwaite MA (1981) Respiratory mass spectrometry during general anaesthesia. *British Journal of Anaesthesia* **53**: 103–109.

Green RA (1987) Medico-legal aspects of anaesthesia. In Kaufman L (ed) *Anaesthesia Review*, vol 4, pp 147–158. Edinburgh: Churchill Livingstone.

Haites NE, McLennan FM, Mowat DHR & Rawles JM (1985) Assessment of cardiac output by the Doppler ultrasound technique alone. *British Heart Journal* **53**: 123–129.

Hamilton PA, Whitehead MD & Reynolds EOR (1985) Underestimation of arterial oxygen tension by transcutaneous electrode with increasing age in infants. *Archives of Disease in Childhood* **60**: 1162–1165.

Hatch DJ & Williams GME (1988) The Haloscale 'Infanta' Wright respirometer. An in vivo and in vitro assessment. *British Journal of Anaesthesia* **60**: 232–238.

Hutton P, Dye J & Prys-Roberts C (1984) Assessment of the Dinamap 845. *Anaesthesia* **39**: 261–267.

Isenberg SJ & Shoemaker WC (1983) The transconjunctival oxygen monitor. *American Journal of Ophthalmology* **95**: 803–806.

Kimble KJ, Darnall RA, Yelderman M, Ariagno RL & Ream AK (1981) An automated oscillometric technique for estimating mean arterial pressure in critically ill newborns. *Anesthesiology* **54**: 423–425.

Kirkendall WM, Burton AC, Epstein PH & Freis ED (1967) American Heart Association recommendations for human blood pressure determination by sphygmomanometer. *Circulation* **36**: 980–988.

Kopman AF & Lawson D (1984) Milliamperage requirements for supramaximal stimulation of the ulnar nerve with surface electrodes. *Anesthesiology* **61**: 83–85.

Lam AM (1987) Do evoked potentials have any value in anaesthesia? *Canadian Journal of Anaesthesia* **34**: S32–S36.

Lam HS, Cass NM & Ng KC (1981) Electromyographic monitoring of neuromuscular block. *British Journal of Anaesthesia* **53**: 1351–1357.

Lindahl SGE, Yates AP & Hatch DJ (1987) Relationship between invasive and non invasive measurements of gas exchange in anaesthetized infants and children. *Anesthesiology* **66**: 168–175.

Lunn JN & Mushin WW (1982) *Mortality Associated with Anaesthesia*. London: Nuffield Provincial Hospitals Trust.

Marsden D, Chiu MC, Paky F & Helms P (1985) Transcutaneous oxygen and carbon dioxide monitoring in intensive care. *Archives of Disease in Childhood* **60**: 1158–1161.

McLaughlin GW, Kirby RR, Kemmerer WT & de Lemos RA (1971) Indirect measurement of blood pressure in infants utilizing Doppler ultrasound. *Journal of Pediatrics* **79**: 300–303.

Meny RG, Bhat AM & Aranas E (1985) Mass spectrometer monitoring of expired carbon dioxide in critically ill neonates. *Critical Care Medicine* **13**: 1064–1066.

Mylrea KC, Hameroff SR, Calkins JM, Blitt CD & Humphrey LL (1984) Evaluation of peripheral nerve stimulators and relationship to possible errors in assessing neuromuscular blockade. *Anesthesiology* **60**: 464–466.

Nisam M, Albertson TE, Panacek E, Rutherford W & Fisher CJ (1986) Effects of hyperventilation on conjunctival oxygen tension in humans. *Critical Care Medicine* **14**: 12–15.

Nunn JF & Ezi-Ashi TI (1962) The accuracy of the respirometer and ventigrator. *British Journal of Anaesthesia* **34**: 422–432.

Ozanne GM, Young WG, Mazzie WJ & Severinghaus JW (1981) Multipatient anesthetic mass spectrometry. *Anesthesiology* **55**: 62–70.

Peabody JL, Gregory GA, Willis MM & Tooley WH (1978) Transcutaneous oxygen tension in sick infants. *American Review of Respiratory Disease* **118**: 83–87.

Poppers PJ (1973) Controlled evaluation of ultrasonic measurement of systolic and diastolic blood pressures in pediatric patients. *Anesthesiology* **38**: 187.

Prince SR, Sullivan RL & Hackel A (1976) Percutaneous catheterization of the internal jugular vein in infants and children. *Anesthesiology* **44**: 170–174.

Prior PF & Maynard DE (1986) *Monitoring Cerebral Function*. Amsterdam: Elsevier.

Reder RF, Dimich I, Cohen ML & Steinfeld C (1978) Evaluating indirect blood pressure measurement techniques: a comparison of three systems in infants and children. *Paediatrics* **62**: 326–330.

Ridley SA (1988) A comparison of two pulse oximeters. Assessment of accuracy at low arterial saturation in paediatric surgical patients. *Anaesthesia* **43**: 136–140.

Sasse FJ (1985) Can we trust end-tidal carbon dioxide measurements in infants? *Journal of Clinical Monitoring* **1:** 147–148.

Schuster AH & Nanda NC (1984) Doppler echocardiographic measurement of cardiac output: comparison with a non-golden standard. *American Journal of Cardiology* **53:** 257–259.

Severinghaus JW & Naifeh KH (1987) Accuracy of response of six pulse oximeters to profound hypoxia. *Anesthesiology* **67:** 551–558.

Shanks CA (1974) Humidification and loss of body heat during anaesthesia. II. Effects in surgical patients. *British Journal of Anaesthesia* **46:** 863–866.

Shanks CA (1975) Mean skin temperature during anaesthesia: an assessment of formulae in the supine surgical patient. *British Journal of Anaesthesia* **47:** 871–875.

Silas JH, Barker AT & Ramsay LE (1980) Clinical evaluation of Dinamap 845 automated blood pressure recorder. *British Heart Journal* **43:** 202–205.

Southall DP, Bignall S, Stebbens VA, Alexander JR, Rivers RPA & Lissauer T (1987) Pulse oximeter and transcutaneous arterial oxygen measurements in neonatal and paediatric intensive care. *Archives of Disease in Childhood* **62:** 882–888.

Sykes MK (1987) Essential monitoring. *British Journal of Anaesthesia* **59:** 901–912.

Taylor MB & Whitwam JG (1986) The current status of pulse oximetry. Clinical value of continuous non invasive oxygen saturation monitoring. *Anaesthesia* **41:** 943–949.

Taylor MB & Whitwam JG (1988) The accuracy of pulse oximeters. A comparative clinical evaluation of five pulse oximeters. *Anaesthesia* **43:** 229–232.

Thomas KB (1975) *The Development of Anaesthetic Apparatus. A History Based on the Charles King Collection of the Association of Anaesthetists of Great Britain and Ireland*, p 15. Oxford: Blackwell Scientific Publications.

Tremper KK & Shoemaker WC (1981) Transcutaneous oxygen monitoring of critically ill adults with and without low flow shock. *Critical Care Medicine* **9:** 706–709.

Tremper KK, Shoemaker WC, Shippy CR & Nolan LS (1981) Transcutaneous PCO_2 monitoring on adult patients in the ICU and the operating room. *Critical Care Medicine* **9:** 752–755.

Vale RJ (1973) Normothermia—its place in operative and postoperative care. *Anaesthesia* **28:** 241–245.

Viby-Mogensen J (1982) Clinical assessment of neuromuscular transmission. *British Journal of Anaesthesia* **54:** 209–223.

Ware S & Osborne JP (1976) Postoperative hypoglycaemia in small children. *British Medical Journal* **ii:** 499–501.

Wasunna A & Whitelaw AGL (1987) Pulse oximetry in preterm infants. *Archives of Disease in Childhood* **62:** 957–971.

Yelderman M & New W (1983) Evaluation of pulse oximetry. *Anesthesiology* **59:** 349–352.

Fluid and electrolyte balance

INTRODUCTION

A person can survive for 1 or 2 weeks without water, but the operating theatre is not the place for this fact to be put to the test! Yet there is still a prejudice against the administration of salt and water to the paediatric patient, a lingering fear of so-called 'salt intolerance'. The result is that an infant can arrive in the operating theatre in a somewhat dehydrated state. Comparison of morbidity is difficult as there are many other variables including of course the length of surgery. However, it is accepted that the morbidity of a second operation, a second stress, will be less if there is no deficiency of volume resulting from the first stress.

A newborn infant can survive an anaesthetic without an intravenous infusion, but in these days of longer, more complex operations, increased postoperative problems and the increase in the actual number of procedures for one patient, the establishment of a line preoperatively is regarded as essential. Frequently, the acquisition of this line is a difficult part of the care, and most difficult when most needed.

Other complicating practical factors have to be addressed: in the assessment of fluid balance, laboratory data, which are liable to errors of sampling technique, storage and laboratory determination, must always also be interpreted along with the history and physical examination of the patient.

There is also the impossibility of communication with the really young, and consequent reliance on a third person to provide and probably interpret vital information.

There are also many occasions, especially if the surgery is urgent and the infant is sick, when the first real examination by anyone on the operating team is immediately before the operation, without an opportunity to observe the baby for a few days while the diagnosis is being made. Rapid assessment and treatment will then occur, and this is not the ideal approach.

EVALUATION OF PATIENT (Bennett, 1975a)

A careful history should obtain information regarding recent feeding habits, incidence of vomiting and diarrhoea, and urine output. The degree of weight loss is important in assessing dehydration. Acute changes are reflected in weight loss and the volume of fluids to be given can be fairly accurately determined by the decrease in weight associated with the current illness, especially when vomiting or diarrhoea are present. An exception would be intussusception when enemas may have been given.

Physical examination should take particular note of the following signs:

1. *Body temperature*. In a critically ill infant, the temperature may be subnormal. It should be restored to normal by placing the infant in a heated incubator before final evaluation is made or anaesthesia is begun. A core–peripheral temperature gradient greater than 2°C strongly suggests fluid depletion.

2. *Skin turgor*. Loss of elasticity and a wizened appearance are definitive signs of dehydration.

3. *Pitting oedema*. The presence of this sign indicates that there has been inadequate replacement of electrolyte solutions, that is, dextrose and water rather than saline have been given.

4. *Thirst*. This is not always easy to determine at this age, but if from the history thirst is suggested, there is usually some indication that it is present. Although thirst is sensory, it is diagnostic of hypertonic dehydration. It implies an absolute or relative water lack, and perhaps a reduction in body water totally. Two stimuli appear to be potent in the production of thirst—the effective osmolarity as this reflects an intracellular water deficit, and a decrease in volume, commonly of all the compartments. Cellular dehydration is usually caused by an increase in the effective extracellular osmotic pressure rather than total osmotic pressure. This hypertonicity of the extracellular fluid may be from contracted extracellular water due to a lack of intake, or it may be due to a hypertonic expansion of the extracellular space. In a comparison of hypertonic glucose with saline solutions, saline is much more potent, as in the short term, glucose diffuses into the cell. It then is the effective rather than the total osmolarity which is the real stimulus.

   The absence of thirst is also useful, but this will not mean that fluids are unnecessary. It implies that the effective osmolarity of the extracellular fluid is low, or of hypotonicity whether expanded or contracted in volume. If from the history, sodium deficiency is indicated, as it will be with vomiting, diarrhoea, sweating or fistulous states, then water and sodium must be administered. The presence of a dry tongue and depression of the fontanelles are evidence of dehydration.

5. *Veins*. Fullness of the veins in the scalp and hands is a sign that the blood volume is probably adequate. The veins of the scalp, hands and feet, on both dorsal and ventral aspects, can be seen easily. These veins reflect early changes in blood volume and cardiac output. They are well seen when volume is normal, are tense and distended with both water and sodium excesses, and are thin and small when dehydration or sodium deficits are present. The colour of the veins, especially those on the ventral aspect of the wrist, will reflect cardiac output. If they are small and dark, arterial oxygenation is poor, cardiac output is low, the local distribution of blood is compromised, or tissue extraction of oxygen is high. In most cases, it is the cardiac output that is low. If the veins are blue, full and easily seen, the reverse is indicated.

6. *General behaviour.* A quiet, non-responsive, inactive baby should alert one to the probability of electrolyte depletion, particularly alkalosis.
7. *Pulse rate.* A rapid, thready pulse usually indicates an inadequate circulating blood volume and/or sodium deficit.
8. *Blood pressure.* Hypotension readily occurs with reduction in circulating blood volume.
9. *The clinical picture* of a fluid and electrolyte overload is one of full bounding pulse, sweating, salivation, hypertension and rapid deep respirations at a high functional residual capacity.

Laboratory studies should include:

1. haemoglobin and haematocrit determinations;
2. serum electrolytes;
3. urinalysis (specific gravity, pH, volume and electrolytes);
4. creatinine or blood urea nitrogen;
5. arterial blood gases (pH, $PaCO_2$, base excess);
6. ECG;
7. osmolality of urine and blood.

In the preoperative period, fluid, electrolyte and blood replacement should be such as to bring blood volume and serum electrolyte values within the normal range and to establish an adequate urine flow.

INTRAVENOUS ACCESS AND THERAPY

Many infants can survive without intravenous fluids for routine minor procedures. But the acquisition of a suitable intravenous route is of importance for access, proper hydration, rapid drug administration and possible resuscitation.

Materials

Scalp vein needles and plastic cannulas are both satisfactory for neonatal and infant use though 26, 24 and 22 G Teflon cannulas have largely replaced scalp vein needles. It is relatively easy to place a plastic cannula percutaneously into a vein on the dorsum of the hand or foot. These are much more stable than scalp vein needles. The use of a scalp vein needle is only acceptable if attention is paid to securing the needle and the hand properly and major blood loss is not expected. Jugular and subclavian punctures are claimed to be easy to perform by some practitioners and are acceptable if indicated, but there is always the risk of perforation of the vena cava or of a pneumothorax (see Chapter 6).

In general, the intravenous route and the operative field should be on opposite sides of the heart, and in the lateral position; the dependent arm should be a second choice for the intravenous site. Care should be taken in the choice of site for intravenous infusions. Patients with abdominal tumours, for example, in whom the inferior vena cava may be damaged, should have venous access in the arm.

There does not seem to be the same risk of phlebitis in the newborn and the infant when the long saphenous vein is chosen for the intravenous site as there is in the adult patient. Swelling and oedema are common at the puncture site especially after 48–72 h, but the likely causes are the use of hypertonic fluids, the addition of various drugs, irritants or even retraction of the vein wall from around the catheter where the wall had been providing a seal rather than infection or phlebitis. Many recommend a change in the intravenous site at regular intervals of 24–48 h. For very long-term intravenous alimentation, especially when the solution to be used will be full strength, placement of the catheter in a central vein is desirable and either Hickman or Broviac is suitable.

Microdrips and volume devices

Both of these are safeguards against an overload of fluid being given accidentally. While these are satisfactory when fluid is to be given slowly, as in the ward, sometimes there are drawbacks to their use in the operating room. In the rapid administration of fluids to these small patients, usually by syringe injection, it is very difficult to prevent the minute air bubbles associated with microdrips from being drawn into the venous line. Many of these infants, where rapid administration is required, have congenital heart disease and the risk of air reaching the left side of the heart in these cases is increased. They are otherwise difficult to pressurize for rapid transfusion. For this reason, some prefer the regular adult set even for the newborn for use during operative procedures, and a change to the microdrip in the postoperative period. There are also special low-volume sets for infants and neonates, where the capacity is as low as 2 ml in the extension set and where there are no side injection ports, which can be difficult to rid of air. When drugs are to be injected, these low-volume sets reduce the amount of fluid which must be given to ensure that the drug is in the patient and not still in the intravenous line. All connections should be thoroughly secured and, if possible, visible at all times. All solutions should preferably be warmed to body temperature. Accurate measurements must be available as proper charting of the fluids administered during the operation is mandatory.

VOLUME CHANGES

Volume changes may involve all the compartments or they may be selective and these changes may be of expansion or of contraction, isotonic, hypertonic, or hypotonic type.

1. *Isotonic expansion* is due to the administration of an excess of isotonic, and therefore, probably a physiological salt solution. This will not lead to osmolal gradients between the interior and the exterior of the cell, and there is no shift of water between compartments. But the blood is diluted, the haemoglobin falls, serum proteins and oncotic pressure diminish,

and this isotonic solution will expand both the intravascular and the interstitial spaces.

2. *Isotonic contraction* is the reverse of isotonic expansion. There is no change in extracellular osmolality, and therefore no shifts of water in relation to the cell. There is contraction of both the blood and the interstitial volumes. Serum sodium remains normal.

3. *Hypertonic expansion* is caused by the intravenous administration of a solution of hypertonic saline. The volume and osmolality of the extracellular fluid are increased, resulting in a water shift from the cells until both compartments are iso-osmolal again.

4. *Hypertonic contraction* is caused by a loss of water with a relatively smaller loss of salt. The osmolality of the extracellular water increases, water flows from the cells, and cellular dehydration occurs.

5. *Hypotonic expansion* occurs when the gain in volume in the extracellular space is predominantly of water. Water, being freely diffusible, enters the cells and so all the compartments are increased in volume. At iso-osmolality, however, there is a decrease in osmotic pressure.

6. *Hypotonic contraction* is due to the loss of salt and water, but relatively more of salt. There is a diminution in extracellular osmolality and a water shift into the cells, but, while the extracellular compartment is decreased, the intracellular water content increases until osmolality is equilibrated (Kerrigan, 1963).

THE RESPONSE TO DEHYDRATION

The infant protects him- or herself from the effects of water deprivation by a series of steps involving a great reduction in the excretion of sodium and a greatly increased tubular reabsorption of water. This water reabsorption is limited by the filtered solute load, which is a metabolic function. But the reabsorption of sodium, which is almost complete, reduces this solute load and allows the reabsorption of relatively greater amounts of water (Winters, 1973).

The increase in extracellular sodium raises the extracellular osmotic pressure and water shifts from the cells to protect the extracellular and plasma volumes; this movement provides more water for the excretion of waste products. This water shift produces *thirst* and increases antidiuretic hormone and the tubular reabsorption of water.

The response to dehydration can be seen in water deprivation and in any decrease in body liquid volumes whether by vomiting, diarrhoea, sweating, fistulous losses or other causes. Sodium has priority over water in this process since it can be almost completely reabsorbed from tubules, whereas water is limited by the solutes requiring excretion (including sodium, when necessary).

RECOGNITION AND CORRECTION OF DEFICITS IN WATER AND ELECTROLYTES (Driscoll and Heird, 1973)

Water deficiency, hypertonic dehydration, hyperosmolality

Thirst is the principal symptom of hypertonic dehydration. Unfortunately, in an infant its presence must commonly be deduced by guesswork. Weight loss is proportional to water loss, and the converse is also true. When death occurs, it is due to the intense rise in osmotic pressure and ensuing respiratory arrest. Signs of dehydration may not appear until 5% has been lost, are obvious at 10% and become severe at 15% loss of total body water. Death is said to occur at about 25% of total body water loss and takes 5–10 days to occur. These figures will vary with the acuteness of the deprivation. Thirst, however, occurs at about 2% deficit. Dehydration (10% loss) in the infant represents 75 ml/kg water.

Calculation

Amount = % dehydration × TBW = litres of dextrose 5% in water + (normal maintenance + K^+ as KCl); where % dehydration is assessed clinically and from the weight loss, and TBW is the total body water prior to the illness (newborn 75–80%; infant 70% of the body weight).

Sodium deficiency or decrease in extracellular water volume

This deficiency can be clinically divided into two groups: firstly, where the concentration of extracellular sodium is low but total body sodium is normal or high, and secondly, where the total body stores of sodium are low. Hyponatraemia reflects a relative or absolute increase in the ratio of water to sodium ions and indicates that the intracellular water is expanded and diluted. This is a frequent deficiency, not only because losses of sodium via sweat and kidney are commonly unreplaced, but also because all the secretions of the gastrointestinal tract contain sodium in significant quantities. The sodium content of these fluids is influenced by aldosterone, but the volume of fluid secreted is not affected. Regulation is not necessarily in accordance with the body's needs. Tubes and suction devices frequently augment the losses. In sodium depletion, the cause is usually loss of the body's own electrolyte-containing solutions, rather than a lack of intake. The clinical syndrome is that of an infant with a large, rapid weight loss. Thirst is not a feature.

Information derived from a small portion of a small compartment, such as serum sodium, can be projected only in terms of the contents of other compartments, or the concentrations of electrolytes contained in them. The interpretation of laboratory values for serum sodium may be complex. A decrease in serum sodium may be absolute or relative, or it may represent displacement by fat, glucose, or urea. Hyponatraemia, or indeed hypernatraemia, may be real or relative. A change in the serum sodium may represent distribution or concentration. It is the ratio of sodium ions to water molecules that is important; this determines the osmolality of the extracellular fluid. Hyponatraemia indicates a relative or absolute increase in the ratio of water to solutes. Hypernatraemia reflects a relative or absolute deficit of water. Sodium concentration, by itself, cannot be used to determine the state of hydration, since expanded or contracted volumes of total body water can be accompanied by high, normal, or low levels of serum sodium. A normal serum concentration indicates a normal ratio between solutes and water, whether volume is high, normal, or low. The osmolality in the extracellular fluid is normal, therefore the volume of the intracellular water is normal. Hyponatraemia, on the other hand, indicates an expanded and hypotonic intracellular fluid. Hypernatraemia reflects a contracted and hypertonic intracellular fluid. Both may be associated with variable states of hydration.

The interpretation that a normal ratio of sodium ions to water molecules in the extracellular fluid indicates a normal intracellular volume has important implications. The production of antidiuretic hormone and aldosterone is increased or decreased by changes in intracellular osmolality and volume, and aldosterone is also influenced by extracellular osmolality and volume.

Calculation (hyponatraemia)

Amount of Na^+ required = $(Na_n^+ - Na_p^+) \times TBW$ = mmol Na^+ as NaCl (isotonic or hypertonic) + (normal maintenance + KCl); where Na_n^+ is the normal serum Na^+, and Na_p^+ is the present concentration. TBW represents the total body water prior to the present illness.

Potassium

Just as sodium is the important extracellular cation, potassium is the important intracellular cation with 98% of the total body potassium present in the cells. Serum potassium concentrations more often reflect the pH. Other factors, of which there are many, affect the distribution of intracellular to extracellular potassium. Potassium is extremely important to the newborn and the infant as the commonest operative procedures mainly relate to the gastrointestinal tract or heart, when gastric suction or diuretics respectively are involved. Both of these are associated with hypokalaemia. The stress response (cortisol and/or adrenalin) is associated with hyperkalaemia (Bennett, 1975a).

After the administration of adrenal hormones, together with the initial glycogenolysis, there is an early shift of K^+ and H^+ from the cell in exchange for Na^+ and H_2O (Cooke's effect). Maximum postoperative losses begin on the first day and continue for 2 or 3 days. Without any additional losses, for example, from gastric aspiration, these losses amount to 2–4 mmol/kg for the first day and 0.5–2 mmol for subsequent days. Protein breakdown involves a loss of about 4 mmol of K^+ per gram of protein catabolized.

Of the many electrolyte abnormalities, hypokalaemic alkalosis is the most vulnerable to additional stress. The infant is sicker than is usually recognized. The administration of saline, without replacing K^+, will lower the already reduced K^+, and cortisol release will further increase the intracellular deficit. K^+ deficiency limits the renal ability to excrete an acid load. Diarrhoea, diuresis, and diabetes mellitus are potent potassium-depleting lesions.

A respiratory alkalosis affects potassium balance and accentuates an incipient hypokalaemia. A decrease in 10 mmHg $PaCO_2$ lowers the serum K^+ by 0.6 mmol/l. This may become important with anaesthesia or mechanical ventilation where some degree of alkalosis is achieved. The restoration of spontaneous respiration may not occur until the alkalosis has been corrected and K^+ balance has been established. Borderline digitalis intoxication may become manifest.

Calculation

Amount of K^+ required = 1–3 mmol/kg/day for each mmol that the serum potassium is below normal. This is because the ratio of potassium on the inside of the cell to that on the outside is 30:1, and the ratio of intracellular fluid to extracellular fluid (ICF:ECF) is 2:1 in the older infant. This dosage of potassium should never be administered without certain safeguards, namely that it should be administered slowly; rarely should potassium be administered at a rate greater than 3 mmol/kg/day; also with adequate urine output and ECG control.

Occasionally, during cardiac procedures in the infant on digitalis or diuretics, perhaps with pulmonary hypertension or some other entity where arrhythmias are common, it becomes obvious that potassium must be given; no particular dose can be specified for rapid administration, but the slow intravenous administration of increments of 0.5–1 mmol K^+ as KCl seems safe (see pp. 209 and 334).

Calcium

The importance in calcium homeostasis lies in sudden corrections of salt and water imbalances, with fluids containing high sodium and low potassium concentrations; for example, the abrupt administration of sodium to correct a water intoxication can lead to tetany. Tetany is rare, however, in the infant even though hypocalcaemia may be present. Calcium exists in three forms: 46% bound to serum albumin; 50% in an ionized diffusible state (Ca^{2+}), and 4% non-ionized but soluble. Its importance in the regulation of cellular irritability has been stressed. The balance of calcium ions with potassium and magnesium ions is well appreciated. There is a strong relationship to toxic effects associated with digitalis administration and potassium deficiencies.

The serum calcium ion-selective electrode is altering the appreciation of the levels of ionized serum calcium necessary for the proper function of some body mechanisms. Levels of 0.3 mmol/l of ionized calcium are adequate for the clotting mechanism, and 0.5 mmol/l appears to be an adequate level for efficient myocardial contractility. It is possible that most of the signs of calcium changes are due to other ionic shifts that occur simultaneously. A Ca^{2+} intoxication will cause a diuresis.

Magnesium (Stowens, 1973)

The normal serum Mg^{2+} is 0.75–1.2 mmol/l; about one-third is bound to serum proteins and the rest is ionized and diffusible. The distribution of Mg^{2+} is similar to K^+ but 50–60% of Mg^{2+} is present in bone where it forms a magnesium reserve that can be readily mobilized. The ion is primarily intracellular, and the intra- to extracellular ratio is 15:1. It is active in intracellular enzymatic activity, nerve impulse conduction, and muscle contraction. The movements of the ion are influenced by the same factors that affect Ca^{2+}.

Hypermagnesaemia is a rare but potentially fatal syndrome. It can occur from magnesium sulphate enemas, from an acute diabetic acidosis, or from renal failure. The symptoms are weakness, lethargy and hypotension. Diminished tendon reflexes and ECG changes of hypermagnesaemia occur late and treatment is the administration of Ca^{2+} salts. However, with renal failure, dialysis may be necessary to reduce the serum concentrations of magnesium.

Hypomagnesaemia, likewise, is uncommon. It occurs when patients are on prolonged magnesium-free diets, such as when fluids are administered parenterally during a period of prolonged gastric suction. It can also occur with severe diarrhoea, malabsorption syndromes, the late stages of cirrhosis, and burns. The problem in the management of hypomagnesaemia is not so much one of treatment but of recognition, with its ill-defined symptoms in the presence of other electrolyte disturbances. Treatment, when it has been decided to administer Mg^{2+}, consists of oral or parenteral administration of magnesium sulphate in the amount necessary to provide 0.25–0.5 mmol/kg/day. Frequent serum determinations are necessary and great care must be exercised, especially if there is any evidence of renal failure.

It has been suggested that magnesium toxicity is related to the respiratory syndrome of the newborn when the mother has been treated with $MgSO_4$ for toxaemia of pregnancy; other reports detailing high levels of Mg^{2+} in the newborn do not support this hypothesis.

It is difficult to give a specific dose since the cation is also predominantly intracellular. A diagnosis of hypomagnesaemia will be made more commonly if the possibility is kept in mind that it can occur. It appears that 0.25 mmol Mg^{2+}/kg given by slow intravenous administration over 24 h is well tolerated.

Chloride

Chloride (Bennett, 1975a) is the principal anion of the body. At birth, the chloride content of the body is relatively greater than in the adult, but proportionately this may be related to the relative increases in volume of the extracellular compartment in the newborn. The Cl^- space, like the Na^+ space, represents the functional extracellular fluid space.

In a high intestinal obstruction, Cl^- loss predominates, resulting in a hypochloraemic, hypokalaemic alkalosis. In a low intestinal obstruction, the ionic components of the intestinal secretions approximate to those of plasma, and there will be less tendency for pH alterations. Cl^- excretion occurs mainly by way of the kidney. Like Na^+, Cl^- is filtered through the glomerulus, and 80% is reabsorbed in the proximal convoluted tubule along with the other ions. Much of the remainder is absorbed with Na^+ in the distal tubule under the control of aldosterone. When bicarbonate is being reabsorbed, chloride can undergo interchange. The sweat chloride of the newborn is normally 20–30 mmol/l.

Hypochloraemia is usually associated with some degree of hyponatraemia. It occurs in most depletion states, in most dilutional states, in cardiac failure treated with digitalis or diuretics, and in all conditions associated with vomiting in infants, especially pyloric stenosis. The symptomatology, apart from the pallor of the infant, is intimately bound to that of the primary disturbance, and usually has no direct stigmata which will implicate shifts in either the concentration or the distribution of the chloride ion.

Calculation (chloride replacement)

Amount of Cl^- required $= (Cl_n^- - Cl_p^-) \times TBW =$ mmol Cl^- as NH_4Cl or $NaCl$ + (normal maintenance + K^+ as KCl); where Cl_n^- is the Cl^- normally in the serum, and Cl_p^- is that currently present. TBW is the total body water prior to this illness.

BLOOD (Oh et al, 1966; Bennett, 1975a; Furman et al, 1975)

The blood volume of an infant is usually estimated as 80–85 ml/kg. There are no extravascular reserves of red blood cells, such as exist for platelets and white blood cells. There is an intravascular excess of haemoglobin under normal circumstances. However, plasma volume has been accurately measured. Five per cent of the total body weight (50 ml/kg) is usually accepted as the normal, both in the infant and the newborn. The blood volume of the newborn, on the other hand, is more variable. The range for normality is 60–129 ml/kg. But, with this wide range for the normal and the inaccuracies involved, any guide to the intraoperative blood replacement which is based upon a percentage of the blood volume that has been lost can only be of limited use unless some value can be accepted for the normal. If the plasma volume of the newborn and the infant is accepted as 5% (50 ml/kg) of body weight, the use of a figure based upon the haematocrit (hct) is reasonable. Then the formula 50 + hct as ml/kg will be of benefit as it allows percentage guides to be used as a rule of thumb, and those babies with low haematocrits prior to operation will receive blood earlier and at the point of less loss than those with a high haematocrit. Infants with a high haematocrit, for instance above 70%, would not be transfused until a much later time. Where the operative procedure is to reduce the need for these high haematocrits (e.g. in cyanotic heart disease and shunt procedures) blood loss up to 20% of blood volume may be replaced with plasma.

There is some basis for the retention of percentage blood loss as the guide for blood replacement. Traditionally the infant has been classed as an individual in whom shock is said to be precipitous. More probably, it is the reduced blood volume and the infant's ability to compensate that maintains the vital signs until compensation suddenly fails. Replacing blood loss at relatively fixed percentages has reduced the incidence of this former intraoperative catastrophe.

It is appreciated that 2,3-diphosphoglycerate (2,3-DPG, a metabolic product) materially alters the ability of oxygenated haemoglobin to give up its oxygen, and in the process to accept H^+ ions. With high levels of 2,3-DPG in the cell, its oxygen affinity is low. When 2,3-DPG levels fall, as in stored blood, oxygen affinity rises, and a shift to the left occurs in the oxyhaemoglobin dissociation curve (the Valtis–Kennedy effect). Blood pH also affects the haemoglobin oxygen affinity. A change of 0.01 pH unit causes a 5% change in 2,3-DPG in the opposite direction. A change in 2,3-DPG of 5% alters the P_{50} (partial pressure at 50% saturation) by 1.0 mmHg in the same direction. All these physical characteristics are advantageous to the infant in whom tissue perfusion may be compromised and potential hypoxia at the cellular level may occur (Macdonald, 1977). In the newborn, the increased affinity is not due to 2,3-DPG deficiency. It has been related to the lowered sensitivity of haemoglobin F to 2,3-DPG, but recently it has been suggested that the thickness of the red cell membrane is the critical factor. In infants, other factors can alter the 2,3-DPG levels:

1. cyanotic heart disease where mean levels are almost double the normal;
2. chronic respiratory disease where hypoxia is prominent;
3. cardiac failure—cyanotic or non-cyanotic;
4. anaemia;
5. sickle cell disease, which can appear in the infant at about 6 months of age.

The anaemia of infancy has a 2,3-DPG level that is high, and this compensates for a defect in oxygen delivery to the cells by a reduced affinity for haemoglobin. This high 2,3-DPG has also been attributed to the high phosphate content of the milk diet at this age. The importance of 2,3-DPG to transfusion relates to the fact that under storage conditions using acid citrate dextrose as the preservative anticoagulant, red cells rapidly deplete the 2,3-DPG (in 4 days). With citrate phosphate dextrose as the preservative anticoagulant, the time is nearer 7 days for the storage defect to be severe.

For administration, it is apparent that warming the blood is the essential step. The administration of sodium bicarbonate, calcium chloride or gluconate, is not recommended unless there are specific indications for their use. Whether the infant has anaemia or hypovolaemia, the oxygen-carrying capacity should be restored preoperatively. If it is anaemia, packed cells in some form are preferred but not immediately preoperatively; if it is hypovolaemia, whole blood is preferable. There are still risks in the administration of blood and blood products which may weigh against this decision.

Correction of anaemia (Bennett, 1975a)

If packed cells are used (of a haematocrit of approximately 70%), a guide to the quantity required can be obtained from the following equation: ml of packed cells = 1.5 ml of packed cells for each % point the haematocrit needs to be raised per kg body weight = 1.5 ml/%hct/kg. For whole blood, the factor would be 2.5 as the haematocrit of whole blood is approximately 40%. For frozen red cells, 1.1 ml of frozen red cells should raise the haematocrit 1%/kg, the cells being resuspended in a small amount of either crystalloid or colloid.

Intraoperative replacement measurement

The accurate measurement of blood loss is vital to any replacement regimen. The volumes to be measured will be small and yet must be as accurate as possible. Many methods are advocated: weighing sponges, haemoglobin-ometry, calibrated suction bottles (for infants), and visual estimation. Most people, realizing the potential danger of inaccurate estimation will err on the high side. Some add an arbitrary 25%.

Blood losses over 10% of estimated blood volume should be replaced, and when losses of this order are anticipated, transfusion should be considered at an early stage. Replacement will vary with the clinical condition, circumstances, and type of operation. Once a decision has been made to replace blood, it should be completely replaced, ml for ml, and some would add 5 ml/kg. This leaves the infant at a disadvantage if earlier in the operation blood has been replaced with a crystalloid (or colloid) solution, as this requires two to three times the volume because of its distribution intra- and extravascularly. An electrolyte solution in place of blood is not recommended for the infant. Of course, if the infant's condition is deteriorating from loss of blood, blood is necessary, promptly and fully. If frozen red cells are used intraoperatively, it should not be forgotten that, reconstituted with an electrolyte solution, there is no protein, and there are no clotting factors in the perfusate; these have to be added whenever relatively large volumes are to be given.

For acute replacement of a large blood loss the infant should be intubated with controlled ventilation and supplemental oxygen, and the blood should be warmed with a suitable system. Relatively fresh blood is preferable. It should be firstly, syringed for accurate replacement (remembering that the first syringe of blood will be at room temperature); secondly, filtered (the older the blood the more it needs filtering), and lastly, measured and recorded accurately.

The advisability of sodium bicarbonate, calcium ions etc. is a matter of individual preference. Potassium does not return intracellularly just by rewarming. Most of the acidosis (CO_2 elevation) will be eliminated by the controlled ventilation, the metabolic component by proper perfusion of the liver and the kidneys. Physiological salt solution (lactated Ringer's, Normosol, Hartmann's, etc.) is added in an amount of 0.5–2.0 ml/ml of blood given. This reduces the incidence of postoperative pulmonary complications and corrects for the extracellular fluid loss due to the initial hypotension.

Haemodilution (Furman et al, 1975)

This is a method of blood or red cell replacement using arterial haematocrits for red cell mass and calculating the ability of the patient to supply oxygen to the tissues as blood is lost. It relies on calculation to determine a safe level of haematocrit and blood loss before replacement. This method assumes that there is a uniform blood volume and that the haematocrit falls linearly with the blood loss. These assumptions are false.

Albumin or dextran (Bennett, 1975a)

Substitute blood therapy is also used in neonates and infants. There are no determinations as to how much can be given to this group. If we compare albumin and dextran, albumin can be given in unlimited amounts, and there is no interference with cross-matching. It is not allergenic, but it is costly and the supply is limited. Dextran has the reverse characteristics. Some specific indications for each are:

1. *Albumin*. Indicated in special conditions where serum albumin is low due either to loss or low production (renal or hepatic disease); in an emergency or to replace a specific loss; to reconstitute packed or frozen cells; in exchange transfusions; for plasmapheresis, or for cardiac surgery.
2. *Dextran* (hetastarch; Hespan). Indicated where rheology has been compromised by high haematocrits, 'sludging', shock; in cyanotic heart disease; or for surgery where the reduction of agglutination, rouleaux formation, and microthrombi is beneficial; perhaps in sickle cell states, and questionably in emergency situations.

Amounts

Albumin. As a 5% solution in lactated Ringer's solution; dose: 10–20 ml/kg; this amounts to 0.5–1.0 g albumin/kg body weight.

Dextran. Molecular weight 8000+, LMWD (low molecular weight dextran) 75 000; as a 6% solution, with or without saline; dose: 7–15 ml/kg.

Albumin has been the subject of some concern recently. The rapid restoration of blood volume (and cardiac output) in an episode of hypotension reduces the clinical manifestations of shock and will reduce the morbidity. There is evidence that shock treated by albumin can result in acute respiratory failure in the postoperative period and many prefer to treat shock with crystalloid and/or blood. Hypotension, on the other hand, does not always correlate with shock. The tissue hypoxia and capillary damage of shock may be responsible for the albumin leakage. In the absence of capillary wall damage, it seems that albumin incurs a risk in volume replacement.

THE NEONATE (Bennett and Salem, 1974; Bennett, 1975a, 1975b, 1977; Hatch and Sumner, 1986)

The newborn and infant are at the age when even small differences in fluid balance may assume great importance. In addition, in this period the child is undergoing rapid physiological alterations, which by themselves produce significant derangements. A serious drawback to studies in the newborn and infant are the difficulties, even the impossibility, of carrying out those determinations which might serve to increase our knowledge; this may be for either technical or ethical reasons. Unfortunately, much of our information in newborn physiology is limited to inferences, casual observations, or experimental results obtained under conditions that do not withstand proper scrutiny. The size and relative inactivity of the newborn and infant offer the prospect for accurate measurement, but these very same factors create serious difficulties.

Normal values

The precise dimensions of the various body compartments and their exact composition in the newborn and infant are not known. Tables 8.1 and 8.2 provide some general values in comparing the adult and the neonate. Body surface area is commonly used in the measurement of these values. It should be appreciated that the surface area:weight ratio is increased in the neonate. Table 8.3 defines the maximum daily fluid losses by secretions in the infant and newborn.

Certain of these values deserve special mention. The newborn has more Na^+ and Cl^- per kg body weight than does the adult, presumably because the extracellular fluid space is proportionally larger in the former. Serum potassium is also significantly higher in the newborn, perhaps related to the acidaemia. Serum phosphorus is characteristically higher in those infants fed cows' milk, which contains a higher concentration of this element than

Table 8.1. Normal values for body compartments and their components

	Neonate	Adult
Extracellular fluid	40%	20%
H_2O turnover per day	15%	9%
Blood urea nitrogen	1.7–2.5 mmol/l	3.4–4.2 mmol/l
Urinary Na^+	50 mmol/l	30 mmol/l
Urine specific gravity	1005–1020	1005–1035
Serum Na^+	136–143 mmol/l	135–140 mmol/l
HCO_3	20 mmol/l	25 mmol/l
Blood volume	60–129 ml/kg	70 ml/kg
Haemoglobin	18–25 g/dl	15 g/dl
Haematocrit	50–60%	45%
Insensible H_2O loss	400 ml/m²/day	variable
Intracellular water	35%	40%
Solutes in urine	10–30 mosmol/kg/day	

Table 8.2. Body water compartments as percentage of body weight

Space	Newborn	Infant	Child
Intracellular fluid	35	25	20
Extracellular fluid	40	40	40
Blood volume	6.5–12.9	8.0	7.5
Plasma volume	5	5	5

Table 8.3. Maximum losses from secretions/kg/24 h

	H_2O (ml)	Na^+ (mmol)
Sweat	200	36
Saliva	20	2
Gastric juice (tube) (suction)	125	7–18
Pancreatic juice (fistula)	10	2
Intestinal juices (fistula)	40	4
Bile (fistula)	7	2
Vomiting	100	15
Diarrhoea	100	15

human milk. The high levels of phosphate may in turn act as a diuretic and result in a low urine concentration. The total body water of the infant is greater whether calculated by body weight or by surface area. However, this does not mean that the infant has an excess volume of water. In fact, water turnover is much greater in the infant than in the adult, and the infant is more susceptible to dehydration. The ratio of extracellular to intracellular fluid begins to decline soon after birth, and approaches the adult ratio by 2 years of age. An infant deprived of water may deplete his extracellular fluid space within 5 days, whereas an adult may take twice as long to reach a similar state.

The fetal kidney clears inulin in amniotic fluid, the inference being that the fetal kidney has excretory capacity. Capacities for clearing inulin, creatinine and urea are the same as or less than those in the adult. Creatinine clearance depends upon muscle mass, and body weight may provide a better basis for its measurement in the newborn. The neonate's ability to excrete acid and produce ammonia suggests that he or she can cope with the fixed acids. A greater metabolic rate also implies an increased ability to produce H^+, and it thus follows that use of adult nomograms to assess neonatal base deficits is not satisfactory. Nomograms for use in the newborn have been designed.

The infant has less albumin and less globulin than do older children. The resultant lower osmotic pressure encourages a rapid transfer of fluids into the tissues, including the glomeruli. In all, 65% of the body's albumin is extravascular and available for use. A significant albumin loss is necessary to affect the osmotic pressure gradients, but administration of albumin or other protein solutions should be considered when there is serious albumin deficiency. In other situations, blood can be reconstituted from packed or frozen cells, and administered with lactated Ringer's solution.

Blood volume (Oh et al, 1966; Bennett, 1975a)

The blood volume of a neonate with a normal haemoglobin is estimated to be 80–85 ml/kg. For the premature infant, a higher figure, perhaps equal to 100 ml/kg, has been suggested. There have been few investigations of blood volume in the normal infant, and figures have not been accurately derived.

The normal range for blood volume is 60–129 ml/kg. Placental transfusion, and the position of the baby at birth relative to the placenta, may influence blood volume in the newborn.

The newborn kidney (Bennett, 1975a)

The administration of fluids and electrolytes to the neonate has been strongly influenced by the traditional concept that the neonatal kidney is immature, that it is unable to excrete sodium, and that it is unable to concentrate urine (Rickham, 1957; Rickham and Johnson, 1969). Because of these views, and because the neonate can normally exist on a sodium intake of 1–2 mmol/kg/day, some authors have put primary emphasis on the administration of 5–10% dextrose in water, plasma, blood or no fluids at all (Rickham, 1957). The immaturity of the renal function is usually determined by calculations utilizing body weight. However, if other criteria such as extracellular fluid or total body water are used, there may be no real difference in renal function in the first 7 days of life.

Concentration is mainly a function of solute load. It represents the ability to excrete and conserve water, sodium and urea. Urea forms one of the principal solutes for concentration and is low in the neonate. The ability of the newborn to excrete a dilute urine is a normal event. The neonate is usually unable to concentrate urine to a specific gravity of more than 1020, representing about 800 mosmol/l when compared with serum osmolality. However, all the appropriate mechanisms are present. The volume and concentration of urine are a result of facultative absorption in the distal tubules and the net result of the amounts of solute and solvent presented. The production of concentrated urine depends upon the development of a high concentration of sodium in the interstitial fluid of the renal medulla as a consequence of active transport of sodium out of the ascending limb of Henle's loop to the interstitium, as well as the countercurrent pattern of flow between the loops and the medullary capillaries. Any process that disturbs the function of the medulla produces an early marked impairment of this concentrating ability. Urine-concentrating ability is further reduced by starvation, by a low-protein diet, or by overhydration. Urea is necessary for the concentration of urine, and the ability of an individual kept on a protein-free diet to excrete hypertonic urine is diminished. It can be restored by giving urea. The newborn, who uses nitrogen primarily for growth, has a blood urea of 1.7–2.5 mmol/l. Therefore, he or she does not have the same ability to concentrate urine. Urine-concentrating ability may be further lowered by a solute load such as mannitol or by a saline infusion. The decrease in maximum urinary osmolality that characterizes renal damage is ascribed to a solute diuresis, provoked by the concentration of urea in the glomerular filtrate and the resulting increase in solute load per individual nephron. Urea, in these circumstances, increases its excretion by an increase of the blood urea concentration.

The newborn kidney differs from that of the older child. It has fewer nephrons, and the loops of Henle, the distal convoluted tubules, and the collecting ducts have not yet reached adult stage. The loops—cortical rather than medullary—are shorter, and there is less convolution of the distal tubules. There is thus less physical ability to concentrate and therefore to conserve. The mechanisms by which these activities are performed, i.e. countercurrent systems and active reabsorption, are compromised. There will be a tendency to develop diuresis, whether water, electrolyte or osmotic in origin.

Sodium conservation

Normal neonates may appear to conserve sodium, in that they exist on a sodium intake of less than 1–2 mmol/kg/day. This represents an absolute figure and does not take into account the negative sodium balance of the first few days of life. During this period the 40% extracellular fluid volume, present at birth, is reduced towards the 20% volume of the infant. It is interesting that this figure of sodium intake is about twice that recommended for the adult with supposedly mature renal function. There is abundant evidence that the neonatal kidney can excrete a high level of water, phosphates, chlorides, bicarbonate, urea and acid. However, in the presence of sodium and potassium deficiencies, as in alkalosis, there may be a dilute urine with an alkaline pH, in contrast to the infant who is conserving sodium and therefore excreting acidic urine.

Excretory ability appears to be adequate, but there is a tendency to hyponatraemia in the presence of sodium deficiency. Balance studies of 57 newborns have demonstrated that revised concepts of neonatal renal function and administration of fluids to the neonatal surgical patient are in order. These studies have shown that the functional capacity of the neonatal kidney is limited by factors such as solvent quantities and solute loads.

The neonatal kidney is capable of concentrating urine, and the problem is that of conserving rather than failure to excrete sodium (Bennett et al, 1970). Aldosterone excretion rate has been measured and related to mean sodium, blood urea, and urinary specific gravity (Bennett et al, 1971). As mean serum sodium decreased from 140 to 125 mmol/l aldosterone increased. This would indicate a response of the newborn to a low serum sodium with an increase in aldosterone in an attempt to retain sodium. Similarly, aldosterone release occurred as blood urea nitrogen increased. This could be an indication of the value of the blood urea nitrogen as a measure of hydration or renal blood flow.

The urinary specific gravity is reflected in the aldosterone level and could be an index of a decrease in the renal blood flow, dehydration, or sodium loss. These three stimuli physiologically increase the production of aldosterone, namely, flow, osmolality and volume.

It may be concluded that:

1. the newborn can produce aldosterone, and there appears to be an effective action in that sodium/potassium exchange occurs with sodium deficiency;
2. there is also a correlation between aldosterone and serum sodium;
3. there is further correlation between the state of hydration as evidenced by blood urea nitrogen and urinary specific gravity and the level of aldosterone as measured by the aldosterone excretion rate.

The effects of surgery upon sodium metabolism and the aldosterone secretion rate in children have been studied. In a herniorrhaphy group, there was no change in aldosterone secretion rate, suggesting that no sodium retention occurs in the infant (Weldon et al, 1967; Bryan, 1971). However, in a further group of five patients, these investigations found a significant increase in aldosterone secretion rate and a tendency to retain sodium. Four of these five operations were Duhamel procedures, requiring extensive bowel preparations, and it is quite possible that sodium was needed to a greater extent, in that postoperative urinary losses actually increased in three infants.

The apparent sodium retention is open to interpretation. In the absence of sufficient water, renal blood flow decreases, glomerular filtration rate becomes low, and a relative renal shutdown occurs. Owing to continued hypotonic fluid losses, serum sodium increases and relative hypernatraemia occurs. In reality this represents hypertonic dehydration. It has been shown that serum sodium is the significant independent variable with the aldosterone secretion rate in neonates (Breivik, 1969; Irvin, 1972; Siegel et al, 1974).

The general conclusions are that the neonate requires water and electrolytes during operations and in the postoperative period, and that there is no difficulty in excreting sodium within wide limits. The urine-concentrating ability and the ability to excrete a dilute urine are relatively normal. Recognizing that surgery is a major stress, further stress should not be added to the patient by withholding fluid or electrolytes. All abnormal losses, for example from the stomach, should be replaced with equal volumes of isotonic saline solutions. The newborn can respond to a sodium deficiency with an increase in aldosterone secretion rate. The neonate can also respond to this hormone by reabsorption of sodium from the urine, depending upon the quantities available. The low concentrations of sodium in the urine may in some cases result from the hypotonic quality of the fluids administered and the large quantity of urine resulting. An osmotic diuresis, from the characteristic low newborn renal threshold for glucose, is possible, and may occur as a result of an excess amount of 10% glucose solution. However, if the newborn is given only small amounts of fluid, then the free water from metabolism is utilized as a maintenance solution. Both of these possibilities offer cogent reasons for the administration of balanced salt solutions. The newborn and the small infant do not follow the adult patterns of salt losses, and the newborn continues to secrete a dilute urine-containing sodium. The gastric secretion rate does not diminish, and the newborn has the ability to produce a gastric secretion that contains as much as 165 mmol/l sodium (Gutierrez et al, 1960; Wangel and Callender, 1968). This loss of fluid will produce a hypo-osmotic state. When other losses occur, such as insensible losses that are normally hypotonic, the newborn may have an iso-osmotic contraction of the extracellular space. Since the usual influences on antidiuretic hormone and aldosterone are absent, the newborn continues to excrete urine of normal volume and content. This is in sharp contrast to the adult, whose gastric secretion contains less sodium (60–90 mmol/l), and in whom a hypotonic loss results in hypertonic dehydration and appropriate hormonal production (Table 8.4).

Table 8.4. Usual losses for newborns

Insensible water loss	30–80 ml/kg/day
Na^+ insensible water	2–5 mmol/day
Urine Na^+	0.75–2.25 mmol/day
Gastric aspirate (Na^-)	115–165 mmol/l

Potassium replacement is necessary in the postoperative period, especially if an aldosterone mechanism is indicated (Heird et al, 1973). There is no correlation between the weight, and presumably the maturity, of the newborn and the range for aldosterone. There is also no difference between the potassium requirements of the mature and the premature neonate.

FLUIDS FOR ANAESTHESIA AND SURGERY

Any preoperative deficit of fluids and electrolytes has to be made up at some time in the perioperative period. Ideally, this should be before, but in most instances it will be during the operation. It is necessary to develop some rational scheme towards the volume and the content of this replacement.

Operative fluids

Before the requirements of the infant, the newborn, and the child for fluids and electrolytes are considered, three aspects need to be mentioned—the reasons for the administration of glucose, the benefits to be derived from the administration of a physiological salt solution, and the fact that the infant receives nil by mouth for several hours at least.

Glucose (Bennett, 1975b)

The metabolic rate of infants, the oxygen consumption, and the infant's ability to produce hydrogen ion are almost double that of the adult. Because of this metabolic rate, almost all solutions administered to the infant should contain 5% dextrose, with the exception of large volumes of replacement solutions. The advantages of administering glucose are:

1. it prevents hypoglycaemia, a major problem in newborns, especially if premature;
2. it supplies metabolic needs;
3. it encourages neoglucogenesis and is protein-sparing;
4. it limits glycogenolysis;
5. the limitation of glycogenolysis and the effect this has on protein-sparing reduce the degree of potassium loss in the surgical infant.

Metabolic requirements of glucose at this age are 5 g/kg/day. Since the water requirements are 100 ml/kg/day, it becomes obvious that glucose has to be added, at least to all maintenance fluids, in a 4 or 5% solution. In preterm neonates, higher concentrations may be required.

While recognizing that there are disputes associated with the use of these names, the expressions 'a physiological salt solution' and a 'balanced salt solution' are here used synonymously. With either of these terms is implied an electrolyte solution, the components of which approximate the components of the fluid which surrounds the cell, the interstitial fluid, or the ultrafiltrate of blood. While it is admitted that there are slight variations between the numerous commercially prepared solutions, for all practical purposes these variations are not significant. Therefore, in this context, physiological salt solution, balanced salt solution, lactated Ringer's solution, Hartmann's solution, Normosol etc. are deemed to be interchangeable.

Lactated Ringer's solution (Bennett, 1975a)

The intraoperative use of a solution such as lactated Ringer's has many advantages:

1. the maintenance of renal haemodynamics as opposed to the reported depression of renal blood flow and glomerular filtration rates of 40–80% in the pre-salt infusion era;
2. the prevention of postoperative acute renal shutdown, a complication that carries a high mortality rate (70% in the surgical patient);
3. the avoidance of postoperative acute water retention;
4. a marked decrease in the incidence of significant intra- and postoperative hypotension;
5. a decrease in the morbidity associated with vascular surgery;
6. a decrease in the need for blood transfusion;
7. the fact that, physiologically, these solutions are similar to that of the interstitial space;
8. the possible reduction of the risk of pulmonary emboli.

It lacks, however, the buffering capacity of the interstitial water, somewhere about one-fifth of that of the plasma, and the oncotic pressure of 5 mmHg (principally from the 1% albumin content of the interstitial fluid).

There are certain conditions where a lactated solution (bicarbonate, acetate, or other alkali-containing fluid) is not the recommended replacement. These are:

1. In metabolic alkalosis, for example, pyloric stenosis. In this condition, the bicarbonate in plasma is already high and the need is for H^+. Saline acts as an H^+ donor and does not contribute to the bicarbonate load. Saline is the preferable solution.
2. In cardiac surgery where excessive amounts of sodium may be administered. This is usually in an attempt to correct metabolic acidosis after a period of cardiac arrest. When this can be anticipated, it may be better to use a non-sodium solution—dextrose and water—rather than complete the operation with an extracellular hyperosmolar sodium state due to the amount of sodium bicarbonate administered during the procedure.
3. In chronic respiratory disease, where the bicarbonate of the plasma is already high. Once again, a chloride solution, such as saline, is preferable.
4. In those (rare) conditions where chloride is specifically indicated. Here hypochloraemia requires saline rather than a lactated solution.

Intraoperative fluids (Table 8.5)

The considerations are as follows:

Normal maintenance

This amounts to 1–1.5 l/m^2/day for the hospitalized neonate and infant. This figure is based upon an insensible water loss of 700–800 ml/m^2/day to which

Table 8.5. Intraoperative fluid and electrolyte requirements

Dextrose 5% in lactated Ringer's solution *or* 4% glucose in 0.18% NaCl	4–15 ml/kg/h (2–3 h); (simple operations 3–4; abdominal 8–10; thoracic 4–6; neurosurgical 4–6 ml/kg/h)
Saline (NaCl), isotonic	Volume equal to the losses; to correct or replace preoperative needs
Sodium bicarbonate (mmol/ml)	According to the acidosis in 10 ml amounts or derived from the blood gas data
Albumin 5% in lactated Ringer's solution	Where indicated
Blood Under 10% Over 20% Between 10 and 20%	No replacement Must be replaced (with 5 ml/kg extra) The situation will suggest whether or not to replace blood loss, but some colloid is nearly always required

must be added solvent water for the urinary excretion of waste products. The figure 1–1.5 l/m^2/day is based on the fact that the active well child in hospital requires as much water as the active well child outside of hospital. This would be reduced by an inactivity associated with illness, but the catabolism of the stress response, the increased requirements from fever, hyperventilation or acidosis will materially increase the normal maintenance amount. Insensible water loss is of two forms: firstly, an invisible loss from the skin, a fluid the composition of which is closely related to N/3 saline; and secondly, from the respiratory tract, water only. Visible sweating, such as that associated with fever, would increase both the water and the electrolyte needs. Insensible losses increase in premature babies and those nursed with overhead heaters.

The normal maintenance under anaesthesia is then: 1–1.5 l/m^2/day = 70–100 ml/kg/day = 3–4 ml/kg/h of a solution of 5% dextrose in water with one-fifth of the amount as dextrose 5% in lactated Ringer's solution. However, during the operation, it is not convenient to be constantly changing the type of solution, and since other losses are of a more concentrated nature, the recommended maintenance under anaesthesia is dextrose 5% in lactated Ringer's solution.

Anaesthetic system

Even though Ayre's T-piece (or a variation) is becoming more frequently used for anaesthesia, closed or semi-closed (semi-open) systems are also in vogue. Whichever system is employed, dry cold gases leave the anaesthesia machine and before reaching the alveoli, will be warmed and humidified. If this occurs in the infant's respiratory tract, it represents an obligatory water loss, depending upon the minute ventilation, the fresh gas flow into the system, the relative humidity in the system and the ambient temperature. During controlled ventilation with the T-piece, relatively low fresh gas flows with some rebreathing are commonly used, significantly reducing this water loss.

Fluid requirements have been measured when an ultrasonic nebulizer has been employed in the anaesthetic circuit and have shown that the normal maintenance requirements would be reduced by 1–2 ml/kg/h if the inspired gases were 100% humidified (Swenson and Egan, 1969). Additionally, measurements of infants have shown that the use of an ultrasonic nebulizer has resulted in a water gain of 2 ml/kg/h or 2 g/kg/h as water. In a circle system, the flow rates commonly used make them virtually non-rebreathing.

For the anaesthetic system utilized (if an ultrasonic nebulizer is not employed within the circuit), up to 1 ml/l of minute ventilation per hour on a closed circuit and up to 2.5 ml/l per minute ventilation per hour in a non-rebreathing system may be needed. This water loss contains no electrolytes, but it represents a quantity that cannot be ignored.

Translocation at the site of surgery

This broad category includes the changes related to chemical reactions, trauma, surgical manipulation in and around the operative site, and those occurring at the cellular level. In the infant, the relative amounts of greater omentum and peritoneal surface are less than in the adult because of the small greater omentum. The response to injury at the operative site includes the translocation of extracellular fluid into the area where it is removed from the effective circulation for several days (third space).

Whether this fluid can be equilibrated in a period of time with a tracer substance is immaterial. If there is a relative reduction in the extracellular fluid, it has to be replaced. At the cellular level, whether because of alterations in the circulation or the effects of hydrostatic pressure, stress or stagnation of tissue perfusion, or perhaps even because of regional tissue hypoxia or acidosis, there is an interchange across the cell membrane of ions: K^+ and H^+ for Na^+ and H_2O. This ionic shift is accompanied by a net water shift into the cells. It lasts for several days, but it does remove available fluid from the extracellular fluid compartment.

The amounts considered are extremely variable. Of course, they depend upon the severity of the injury, the site, the time element, and the compensation that is possible. There is no way to determine the amount with any accuracy; it is a matter of judgement. Obviously, the amount will be less for limited superficial procedures than for those procedures involving the upper part of the peritoneal cavity. The usual figures involved are from 1 to 10 ml/kg/h; the high amount is that associated with upper peritoneal 'burns'. This translocation cannot continue indefinitely. It is considerably diminished after 2–3 h. Therefore, the amount for this third space deficit is 1–10 ml/kg for the first 2–3 h of the surgical procedure.

Changes in extracellular fluid volume associated with blood loss

This is the net result of hydrostatic–oncotic pressure gradients. Conventional Starling forces will withdraw fluid from the interstitial space as the blood volume falls from blood loss or vasodilation. Hypotension results, independently of whether it is a real or relative decrease in the effective volume. The body protects itself against hypovolaemia, but there are no known volume sensors of the extravascular compartment. If blood loss continues without replacement until shock supervenes, the interstitial fluid will be utilized for the replacement of blood volume. To regain the proper volume status of the various compartments, more will obviously be needed if blood is given later rather than earlier. The usual administration is to allow 0.5–2.0 ml/ml blood loss given as a salt solution, depending upon the timing of the replacement.

Changes associated with the anaesthetic agent or methods

These can be very complex. They may be those associated with the following:

1. Venodilation, vasodilation, cardiac depression. All anaesthetic agents are cardiac depressants and will cause some compensatory response

from the body if function is to remain unaltered. With halogenated agents, for 1–2 h after administration, the blood volume increases at the expense of the interstitial volume.
2. Hypothermia, associated with water and electrolyte shifts internally into the cell, and with a cold diuresis; both have a hypotensive effect.
3. Hyperthermia, which requires large volumes of fluid to replace the increased losses from the lungs and skin.
4. Hypercarbia, associated with a transfer across vascular and cellular membranes of HCO_3^- for Cl^- and, with this, water. The endothelium of the capillary allows a greater transfer of fluid to the interstitial compartment. This is a Bohr type of effect; although there has been no external loss of fluids, large quantities of an iso-osmolal electrolyte solution may be necessary to maintain blood pressure.
5. Induced hypotension, which involves a shift similar to that with halothane. Whether this influences fluid administration depends on the particular technique used to produce the hypotension.

Changes associated with pathophysiology of the disease or the preparation of the patient

In the perioperative period, any deficiency of fluids and electrolytes has to be replaced. The losses that occur because of the disease, for example those of an intestinal obstruction, or those due to the pathophysiology accompanying the illness—vomiting, diarrhoea, fistulous drainages, exudations, protein or blood losses of infarcted bowel etc.—should be replaced, ideally by an equal volume of a fluid of similar composition to that lost. In most instances this is impractical. Generally, the fluids most suitable are saline as an isotonic solution if the fluid contains a high proportion of H^+; if not, a lactated Ringer's solution.

It is necessary to correct effects, overloads or deficits, untreated or improperly treated, of various illnesses. Once again, this is better done preoperatively, but often it will be either an urgent measure or during the procedure. The most important of these effects are those of gastric or colonic lavage.

Volume and content of the intraoperative fluids

It would be both impossible and impractical to derive a fluid of which the exact nature corresponded to the individual requirements of a specific infant. For simplicity a solution is used which is of suitable composition for the majority of patients.

For simple surgery, it is not necessary to give much more than the normal maintenance requirements, 3–4 ml/kg/h dextrose 5% in lactated Ringer's solution or 4% dextrose in 0.18% NaCl. Those who prefer to be more precise, when there are no other needs, will use a one-fifth strength salt solution. For major surgery, usually upper abdominal type, the amount varies according to the site and severity of the operation: 5–15 ml/kg/h of dextrose 5% in lactated Ringer's solution for 2–3 h, and then a reduced amount according to the physical condition of the infant. For infants without a central venous pressure manometer or a catheter in the bladder to measure urine output, this will be at best no more than an intelligent guess. The usual amounts are of the order of 8–10 ml/kg/h. For non-cardiac, thoracic, neuro-surgical, and other operations in general, 4–6 ml/kg/h of dextrose 5% in lactated Ringer's solution is usually sufficient. Using the adult-type drip, 8 ml/kg/h is one half-drop/kg/min.

There are several acute conditions in the neonate where there is a need to replace or to maintain the intravascular volume, not because of blood loss, but because of a sudden translocation of fluid from the vascular compartment. Such conditions are: acute respiratory acidosis; congenital diaphragmatic hernia; congenital lobar emphysema, and intraoperative bowel washouts with agents such as n-acetylcysteine. If a balanced salt solution was used, it would distribute at this age in the ratio of 3 or 4:1 as regards interstitial to intravascular compartment; an overwhelming amount would then be employed. But if colloid is also given (albumin as a 5% solution in lactated Ringer's solution) a much smaller volume achieves the same effect. Hypotension from these causes listed can be quite rapid and alarming.

In cardiac surgery, the replacement of blood loss in conditions associated with a high haematocrit with crystalloid can also mean that two to three times as much salt solution would be given as with the judicious use of colloid.

Table 8.5 summarizes these facts. The figures given are for common procedures where no other criteria are to be considered.

PREMATURE BABIES

There are certain differences in compartment volumes for the premature or low birthweight infant. The water content may be as high as 80% or more, with the increase mainly in the extracellular fluid space. Albumin is normally less than 3 g%. Urine output is 0.3–0.5 ml/kg/h. Blood volume also tends to be higher—100 ml/kg. With heart disease, which is common in this group, especially patent ductus arteriosus, blood volume can be expected to be greater than 100 ml/kg.

Some of these babies, when they arrive in the operating room, are receiving hyperalimentation solutions. These may be given by a peripheral vein rather than centrally, and in these cases, the fluid is dilute and the volume of the order of 200 ml/kg/day. A constant drug administration, such as prosta-glandin E_1 or E_2, given as a continuous drip, may be present. For these reasons, the premature baby rarely arrives in a volume-deficient state or dehydrated. It is more likely that overhydration may be present. The types of operation and the exudates that result make the measurement of blood loss difficult, and yet shock is to be avoided as far as possible. High-concentration dextrose solutions should be stopped preoperatively because serious hyperglycaemia associated with the stress of surgery is a real danger.

Premature babies easily develop pulmonary oedema as the transudation pressure in the pulmonary capillaries is 15 mmHg, which is low compared with the older child. Since shock manifests itself as bradycardia, hypotension and pallor and since bradycardia has a major effect on cardiac output, the tendency should be to maintain blood volume and to replace red cell mass as early as possible. If there is a choice, it is better to overload the baby and risk pulmonary oedema rather than to risk a shock syndrome. Nevertheless, preterm neonates in general have a great venous distensibility and capacity and can tolerate fluid loads well. The amounts necessary are small and are preferably given by syringe. The capacity of i.v. apparatus will be critical.

Clinical assessment of normovolaemia in the preterm baby is difficult and since the results of dehydration may be catastrophic, it is wise to err on the side of slight overhydration. Serious overhydration in this age group can lead to reopening of a patent ductus and left-to-right shunting.

Intussusception

Like congenital hypertrophic pyloric stenosis (see p. 442), this condition usually occurs in infants who were fit and healthy prior to this illness. However there may be an underlying chronic or acute cause for the intussusception. In this disease, several problem areas need to be considered:

1. Bloody diarrhoea always occurs, causing severe hypovolaemia, protein loss, anaemia and electrolyte disturbances. Signs of shock may be present and there is still a mortality from inadequate volume replacement.
2. Vomiting is also common, and therefore dehydration, hyponatraemia, hypokalaemia, hypochloraemia and alkalosis may be present.
3. Enemas (of tap water or saline) as part of the non-operative routine may have been used in an attempt to reduce the intussusception. The absorption of this fluid can result in water intoxication, though severe volume depletion is more common.

Before surgery is contemplated, resuscitation is required, though venous access may be poor. The preoperative requirements of resuscitation are colloid and crystalloid; blood—preferably, if available—or albumin (5% solution of albumin in saline 0.9%, 10–20 ml/kg initially) being given fairly rapidly and continued until the peripheral circulation improves. Crystalloid is given after initial colloid resuscitation and saline is logical since this will have been lost with vomiting. If there is time, 4–8 mmol K^+ as KCl can also be given slowly.

During the operation, the type and amount of solution to be given will vary according to the ease with which the intussusception can be reduced. Usually, if there is strangulated oedematous gut, an easy reduction is prevented. Further losses of blood and protein from manipulation may occur into the bowel wall and will need replacement with blood and plasma. The same reservations apply to replacing intravascular colloid with lactated Ringer's solution as in other circumstances; the danger here is one of overload in that the distribution of colloid and crystalloid are not the same. A bowel resection may be necessary and due to the manipulations that will have preceded this decision, the needs are greater than for a usual bowel resection.

Average quantities required during surgery are 8–10 ml/kg/h of dextrose 5% in a balanced salt solution. Diarrhoea or the rapid correction of deficits in sodium may lead to a magnesium deficiency, or a disturbance in the Ca^{2+}/Mg^{2+} ratio, and require postoperative management.

Acute appendicitis

This condition is uncommon in infancy, so the diagnosis tends to be made late in the illness. It also tends to be a somewhat difficult diagnosis to make as it may be confused with gastroenteritis. The triad of fever, dehydration, and acidosis is frequently part of the clinical picture. Vomiting and anorexia may have been present for some time and severe fluid deficits may be present. Unlike older children, infants with acute appendicitis need somewhat larger volumes of water and electrolytes for preparation. During the procedure, the normal amounts of 6–8 ml/kg/h will suffice if the preoperative requirements have been met.

Colostomy, colostomy closure, abdominoperineal resections and Duhamel procedures

All infants and neonates with diseases where these may be the elective procedures present similar problems, namely that all have probably received bowel preparations in the form of enemas or antibiotics, locally or orally. The antibiotics are neomycin or kanamycin in type and have been known to be absorbed in sufficient quantities to cause neuromuscular problems from the supposedly intact bowel mucosa. The enemas can be saline, water, magnesium sulphate or others.

Therefore, the newborn or infant may show changes associated with water intoxication, hyponatraemia with or without deficiency of total body sodium, hypokalaemia, or even hypermagnesaemia. The low sodium may be a dilutional effect or may be due to the loss of sodium into the bowel lumen. These deficiencies of sodium may be severe, up to 20 mmol/l or more.

Repeated enemas may cause gross hypovolaemia, and the hypovolaemic, hyponatraemic infant is at an increased risk from anaesthesia, especially on induction. Intravenous routes may be difficult to obtain.

High colostomies and ileostomies may also have had a chronic diarrhoea, perhaps since the original procedure was done. Electrolytes in general, and specifically magnesium, may be low. Anaemia occurs frequently.

Blood loss during the operation is usually of a significant amount and will often have to be replaced.

A careful examination on arrival in the operating area is essential. Special notice should be made of any of the criteria of water intoxication. The pallid infant with moist mucous membranes and good well filled veins may be on the verge of convulsions from water overload. On the other hand, an examination should be made for any evidence of hyponatraemia and/or hypovolaemia. Haemoglobin, blood urea nitrogen or serum creatinine done serially should be compared and the timing of these studies noted. Any discrepancy between what is reported and what may be anticipated from the history or physical examination is a warning of some inadvertent complication.

Postoperatively, there is usually some measurable loss of a serosanguinous discharge; the loss may consist of blood, serum, proteins, water and electrolytes, including potassium. These should be assessed and if necessary replaced.

Intraoperatively, 6–8 ml/kg/h of dextrose 5% in lactated Ringer's solution for 2–3 h with appropriate blood replacement is usually adequate. Hypertonic saline, as a 3 or 5% solution, may be necessary to correct a low extracellular osmolarity or a definite hyponatraemia. Eventually, in water intoxication, the free water will be excreted, causing extra losses of electrolyte which should be replaced.

SHOCK (Bennett 1975a) (see also p. 434)

The treatment of shock in general follows the usual lines of replacement of the circulating blood volume as rapidly as possible, then correction of the other fluid and electrolyte defects, treatment of any acidosis, and isolation and treatment of the underlying cause. If this underlying cause is known when shock is recognized (for example, postoperative bleeding) then the proper fluid is whole blood or reconstituted red cells with lactated Ringer's solution. But, as a guide, it is recommended that:

1. As rapidly as possible 300 ml/m^2 of the most readily available colloid or isotonic crystalloid solution should be given intravenously. To an infant this represents 20 ml/kg of blood, plasma, 5% solution of albumin in saline, lactated Ringer's solution, or others. If dextran is chosen, it should be remembered that dextran interferes with blood cross-matching techniques, and a sample of blood should be acquired before the administration of this agent. This may not be such a problem when transfusion practices resort to non-specific blood or frozen, washed or packed red cells.
2. Dextrose 5% in lactated Ringer's solution 3500 ml/m^2, the equivalent of 200 ml/kg should be given fairly rapidly to maintain vital signs and to improve the circulating dynamics. The actual rate of administration will depend upon the patient's response at the time.
3. A multi-electrolyte solution, such as Darrow's solution, with a higher K$^+$ content, 3500 ml/m^2, after urine formation has occurred, should be administered, not quite as rapidly as the first two solutions but with ECG monitoring.
4. Specific fluid and electrolyte therapy should be given at any time as required, with the usual restrictions on potassium administration.
5. Glucose is necessary to avoid complicating the clinical picture with hypoglycaemia.

POSTOPERATIVE FLUID AND ELECTROLYTE REQUIREMENTS
(Fisher, 1977; Table 8.6)

Excluding cardiac and certain specific procedures in the newborn and infant, recommendations for postoperative fluid therapy encompass the following points.

Table 8.6. Postoperative fluid and electrolyte requirements

Volume	1–1.5 l/m²/day = 70–100 ml/kg/day
Content	Dextrose 5% in water—one-fifth to two-fifths of the daily volume to be dextrose 5% in a lactated Ringer's solution. Abnormal losses to be replaced with isotonic saline solution in an equal quantity
	Potassium as KCl—4–20 mmol of solution infused
	Colloid, blood—as required

Maintenance fluid therapy

Maintenance fluid therapy for the postoperative period closely parallels the parameters already described for maintenance operative fluid therapy. The minimal requirements of infants in the postoperative period have been studied and the volume of fluid required to maintain a stable body weight at this time was 765 ± 154 ml/m²/day (55 ± 10 ml/kg/day; Swenson and Egan, 1969). It was stressed that these requirements are the minimal possible 'since a loss of effective blood volume as a consequence of internal fluid shifts would indicate a need for additional fluid for plasma volume expansion'.

The value of humidification and nebulization of the environment in reducing the fluid needs has been mentioned. It has been suggested that the presence or absence of humidity in the atmosphere surrounding the infant has an impact on his or her daily water requirement. In an incubator this may be so. However, the trend is to use the type of microenvironment that is infrared heat-controlled for the newborn and the infant, and this type of neonatal care will increase insensible fluid losses. Insensible water loss for the normal well neonate has been found to be 235 ml/m²/day (17 ml/kg/day). The ill newborn can lose up to 80 ml/kg/day from insensible losses. The maintenance fluid needs to have an electrolyte composition about that of N/5 saline because respiratory losses of water contain no electrolyte. The composition of sweat is influenced by aldosterone, reducing the sodium and increasing the potassium concentration present in the fluid. Antidiuretic hormone is also known to affect the sweat glands, which respond like micronephrons. This fluid requirement will increase with fever, sweating, hyperventilation, acidosis, the use of infrared heaters for neonatal warmth and phototherapy units. The sodium losses from this extra fluid are also increased, but not necessarily the concentrations; normally sweat is about two-thirds saline.

The postoperative fluid requirements are: $1–1.5 \, l/m^2/day = 70–100 \, ml/kg/day = 3–4 \, ml/kg/h$ of dextrose 5% in water, one-fifth of the daily volume to be given as dextrose 5% in lactated Ringer's solution. In the presence of fever, hyperventilation, sweating, acidosis, and other variations from the normal, two-fifths of the daily volume should be dextrose 5% in lactated Ringer's solution.

Replacement

This category of postoperative requirements includes the correction of laboratory-measured deficits of sodium and potassium, acidaemia, and so on. It also involves those secretions, discharges, and exudates which together constitute the usual postoperative losses, but which are average quantities not usually measured for volume or content. These include urine, stools, moderate gastric aspirations, effusions, and others where the amount is not excessive. These losses of fluids that are isotonic (or nearly so) with the interstitial compartment should be replaced with an equal volume of isotonic saline. Hypotonic saline is not recommended as the extra water can compound the renal losses of both water and electrolyte. Specific defects should be corrected by a calculated volume of an appropriate fluid.

Abnormal losses

This refers to those losses, gastric aspirations, effusions, fistulous drainage, diarrhoeas, discharges, and so on, where the volume is abnormally high. Because these fluids are isotonic, the losses would result in a depletion of water and electrolytes (and possibly also proteins and red cells). If gastric secretion is taken as the prime example: in the newborn with nasogastric tube in place the volume can reach 125 ml/kg/day (normally 20–40 ml/kg/day); the Na^+ content may be as high as 165 mmol/l (usually 115–165 mmol/l), and the H^+ content reaches adult proportions within 24 h of birth (Gutierrez et al, 1960; Table 8.4). These quantities of water and electrolyte would rapidly deplete the neonate and infant. Careful attention should be paid to this quantity and the volume should be promptly replaced with an equal volume of isotonic saline (unless the sodium content has been measured and found to be other than that estimated). Gastric secretion is also under the influence of aldosterone to some extent but the effect of anti-diuretic hormone or aldosterone may be minimized by the presence of mechanical or pathological stimuli (such as nasogastric tubes).

Potassium

Potassium losses or requirements have been recognized as being increased in this postoperative period as a result of stress; hormonal influences such as steroids, aldosterone, or antidiuretic hormones; from the usual potassium content of gastric and intestinal secretions and acid–base changes; from catabolism, glycogenolysis, neoglucogenesis, and others. The amount required is extremely variable. Normally, 0.5–1.0 mmol/kg/day will suffice. This figure may be based on caloric or water needs for the surgical newborn, as may all the other electrolyte needs. Normally, the newborn needs: metabolic 100 cal/kg/day; water 55 ml/100 cal (minimum); and Na^+, K^+, Cl^- 1–3 mmol/kg/day. This amount will provide for the insensible losses and for urine excretion with an osmolality of 450–500 mosmol/l. In the presence of large losses of hydrogen ion, alkalosis (respiratory or metabolic), large sodium deficits, diuretic effects (whether water or chemical), these potassium requirements may increase five to six times in order to supply the proper amounts for potassium balance. Potassium supplementation is necessary postoperatively in the newborn and the infant in amounts which vary from 4 to 20 mmol of K^+, as KCl for each litre of solution that is given each day. The larger amount would be given as compensation for gastric secretions or for alkalosis. Rarely should potassium be given at a rate greater than 3 mmol/kg/24 h, and preferably with adequate urine formation or ECG control and by a slow intravenous drip.

Colloid

Exudates, transudates, and discharges may all contain protein and this loss may have to be replaced to maintain serum oncotic pressure. Albumin, being the main contributor to this, is the replacement to be preferred, but plasma is almost as good. Table 8.3 indicates the postoperative considerations for the neonate and infant. There are contraindications to the administration of sodium lactate solution in the postoperative period similar to those with intraoperative fluids (see above).

Glucose

Due to the metabolic requirements at this age dextrose 5%, sometimes even 10%, needs to be added to almost all solutions given except in the case of large abnormal losses. The renal threshold for glucose of an infant is relatively low and an osmotic diuresis may appear earlier than in a similar situation in the older child.

Osmolality

This has been suggested as the index for water and electrolyte needs in the postoperative period. Urinary and serum osmolality should be followed and the ratio should be kept in the vicinity of 1.5:1. Urinary osmolality is then about 450 mosmol/l.

Insensible water and electrolyte losses may produce hypertonic dehydration in the neonate and small infant, but this may be balanced by their ability to secrete a hypertonic fluid from the stomach. This group would then be much more the subject of an isotonic contraction and dehydration of the extracellular fluid space, but being isotonic, the interior of the cells would not be affected and a hormonal response (of aldosterone and anti-diuretic hormone) may not occur. Urine formation, gastric secretion, sweat and other body fluids normally affected by these hormones may continue as if the body was not deficient in these elements, even if dehydration was severe. Consequently no effort may be made to conserve volume or sodium—a dangerous state indeed, especially in abdominal surgery.

Urinary volume

If the other parameters that alter the formation of urine can be eliminated, the volume may be useful as a guide to fluid administration. The amount of urine that is considered adequate and reflecting proper hydration is 0.3–0.5 ml/kg/h for the newborn and 0.5–1.0 ml/kg/h for older children (Bennett, 1975a).

Fluids and electrolytes should be those considered necessary and appropriate and in the correct concentrations, and the approach should not be 'give him plenty of all the ingredients, and let him work it out for himself'.

REFERENCES

Bennett EJ (1975a) *Fluids for Anesthesia and Surgery in the Newborn and the Infant.* Springfield, Illinois: Charles C Thomas.
Bennett EJ (1975b) Fluid balance in the newborn. *Anesthesiology* **43:** 210–224.
Bennett EJ (1977) Anesthetic management of emergency neonatal problems. In Aladjem S & Brown AK (eds) *Perinatal Intensive Care,* pp 348–369. St Louis: CV Mosby.
Bennett EJ & Salem MR (1974) Pediatric anesthesia. In Nyhus LM (ed) *Surgery Annual,* p 17. New York: Appleton-Century-Crofts.
Bennett EJ, Daugherty MJ & Jenkins MT (1970) Some controversial aspects of fluids for the anesthetized neonate. *Anesthesia and Analgesia: Current Researches* **49:** 478.
Bennett EJ, Bowyer DE & Jenkins MT (1971) Studies in aldosterone excretion of the neonate undergoing anesthesia and surgery. *Anesthesia and Analgesia* **50:** 638.
Breivik H (1969) Preoperative hydration with lactated Ringer's versus a salt free restrictive program. *Acta Anaesthesica Scandinavica* **13:** 113.
Bryan GT (1971) Aldosterone secretion rates in children with normal adrenal function. *Pediatrics* **47:** 587.
Driscoll JM & Heird WC (1973) Maintenance fluid therapy during neonatal period. In Winters RW (ed) *The Body Fluids in Pediatrics,* p 265. Boston: Little, Brown.
Fisher MM (1977) Postoperative intravenous therapy. *Anaesthesia and Intensive Care* **5:** 187.
Furman EB, Roman DG, Lemmer LAS et al (1975) Specific therapy in water, electrolyte and blood-volume replacement during pediatric surgery. *Anesthesiology* **42:** 187–193.
Gutierrez IZ, Sukarochana K & Kiesewetter WB (1960) Electrolyte replacement of gastric drainage in pediatric surgery patients. *Surgery* **48:** 610.
Hatch DJ & Sumner E (1986) *Neonatal Anaesthesia and Perioperative Care.* London: Arnold.

Heird WC, Grebin B & Winters RW (1973) The stabilization of disorders of water, electrolyte and acid–base metabolism in newborn infants under intensive care. In Abramson H (ed) *Resuscitation of the Newborn Infant.* St Louis: CV Mosby.

Irvin TT (1972) Plasma volume deficits and salt and water excretion after surgery. *Lancet* **ii**: 1159.

Kerrigan GA (1963) Water and electrolyte metabolism in pediatrics. In Bland JH (ed) *Clinical Metabolism of Body Water and Electrolytes,* pp 263–386. Philadelphia: WB Saunders.

Macdonald R (1977) Red-cell 2,3-diphosphoglycerate and oxygen affinity. *Anaesthesia* **32**: 544.

Oh W, Blankenship W & Lind J (1966) Further study of neonatal blood volume in relation to placental transfusion. *Annals of Pediatrics* **207**: 147.

Rickham PP (1957) *The Metabolic Response to Neonatal Surgery.* Cambridge, MA: Harvard Press.

Rickham PP & Johnson JH (1969) *Neonatal Surgery,* pp. 49, 53 and 103. New York: Appleton-Century-Crofts.

Siegel SR, Fisher DA & Oh W (1974) Serum aldosterone concentrations related to sodium balance in the newborn infant. *Pediatrics* **53**: 410.

Stowens D (1973) Magnesium toxicity. *Journal of the American Medical Association* **225**: 751.

Swenson O & Egan TJ (1969) Measurement of postoperative water requirements in infants. *Journal of Pediatrics* **4**: 133.

Wangel AG & Callender ST (1968) Gastric secretion in the premature infant. *Gut* **9**: 249.

Weldon VV, Kowarski A & Migon CJ (1967) Aldosterone secretion rates in normal subjects from infancy to adulthood. *Pediatrics* **39**: 713.

Winters RW (1973) *The Body Fluids in Pediatrics.* Boston: Little, Brown.

Regional anaesthesia

THE DEVELOPMENT OF PAEDIATRIC REGIONAL ANAESTHESIA

Koller discovered the local anaesthetic properties of cocaine in 1884, after which the practice of regional anaesthesia and peripheral nerve block developed very rapidly. Virtually all the techniques in use today in adults had been described within 20 years of this date, and local anaesthesia had also been used in children. Bier, in his original paper on spinal anaesthesia published in 1899, referred to the effects of cocaine in an 11-year-old boy (Faulconer and Keys, 1965), and reports of spinal anaesthesia in children between the ages of 3 months and 6 years had appeared by 1901 (Bainbridge, 1901).

Regional anaesthesia in children did not become popular however, possibly because it was assumed that the criteria for its use were the same as for adults. Whereas the main advantage of regional block in adults was that general anaesthesia could be avoided in patients who were medically unfit, children for the most part tolerated general anaesthesia well, so there was little to be gained from using regional block for the surgery itself, and general anaesthesia was in any case necessary in most children if the block was to be performed easily, safely and effectively.

Little further progress was made until long-acting local anaesthetic agents became available. It was then found that regional block, performed after the induction of general anaesthesia, had some advantages. It allowed light planes of general anaesthesia to be used during the operation, and this was particularly useful at a time when day-stay surgery was becoming increasingly popular for children. A combination of light general anaesthesia and regional block was ideal for these cases (Armitage et al, 1975). Long-acting agents also provided analgesia extending several hours into the postoperative period, and this feature is chiefly responsible for the recent renewal of interest in local anaesthesia in children.

Regional anaesthesia now has an established place in many paediatric anaesthetic regimens. The block, performed under general anaesthesia before the start of surgery, provides a painless postoperative recovery for the many paediatric procedures which can be completed within an hour or so, and if necessary it can be repeated at the end of the longer cases. This pain-free interval provides an ideal psychological environment for the recovering child, and since the duration of action of most regional blocks is fairly predictable, subsequent analgesia can be specifically timed so that it is effective when the block begins to regress. If intramuscular analgesia is likely to be required, it can be given painlessly within the anatomical area of the block. When prolonged and continuous analgesia is needed, a catheter technique may sometimes be indicated.

CHOICE OF BLOCK

Although blocks which are commonly used in adults are not always suitable for children, the converse is also true and some are particularly useful in children. Three factors should be taken into account when paediatric regional block is being considered:

1. A child under general anaesthesia is unable to report paraesthesiae when a needle is advanced towards a nerve, and neural damage due to needle trauma is therefore a possible hazard when peripheral nerve blocks are attempted. Although this is not an absolute contraindication to their use in children—indeed many anaesthetists find them safe and successful—it is better, where possible, to use central blocks such as a caudal in which success does not depend on the proximity of needle to nerve. Where small, peripheral lesions are to be removed, local infiltration is preferable to peripheral nerve block for the same reason. When peripheral nerve block is the method of choice, a nerve stimulator may help to ensure that the needle is correctly placed.
2. Some central blocks in children may be effective over a wider area than in adults. A caudal, for example, can provide analgesia not only for circumcision and hypospadias repair, but also for lower limb surgery, inguinal herniotomy and orchidopexy.
3. Some regional blocks are easier to perform in children. As technical procedures are usually more difficult than in adults, anaesthetists are sometimes surprised to find that a caudal, which is often difficult and occasionally impossible in adults, is very easy in a child.

LOCAL ANAESTHETIC DRUGS IN CHILDREN

Infants and children differ from adults anatomically, physiologically and metabolically, and local anaesthetics, like any other drug, may therefore produce effects which differ from the expected adult pattern.

The time and the minimum concentration of drug required to produce a block both depend on the diameter and degree of myelination of the nerve fibre. The nerves of infants are smaller and less myelinated than their adult equivalents so it is not surprising to find that, in general, onset times are shorter and blocks can be obtained with somewhat lower concentrations of drug. The infant's epidural space contains less fat than the adult's and since the fat globules are less densely packed, local anaesthetic solution can spread more easily. This is the anatomical basis for the fact that a paediatric caudal can affect the thoracic dermatomes and provide anaesthesia for abdominal surgery.

Three factors are mainly responsible for the pharmacokinetic behaviour of a local anaesthetic drug in infants:

1. the rate of absorption, which is rapid;
2. the volume of distribution, which is very much larger than in adults;
3. the serum protein concentrations, which are lower than in adults.

Local anaesthetic drugs are bound in the serum to two proteins—albumin and alpha₁ acid glycoprotein (AAG). AAG has a high affinity for the drug and is responsible for its initial binding and for preventing high concentrations of the free fraction of drug and the systemic toxicity which they cause. However, it soon becomes saturated. Albumin, on the other hand, has a low affinity for local anaesthetics, but a very much larger capacity for them. At birth, the concentration of albumin is 60–80% of the adult value, and that of AAG is only 50%. Adult concentrations are not reached until 6–12 months of age. Bilirubin tends to inhibit the binding of local anaesthetics to albumin—a point which should be borne in mind when local anaesthesia is being considered in an infant with neonatal jaundice.

The peak concentration of a local anaesthetic also depends upon whether the drug is administered as a single injection, or as an infusion or a series of injections. In the former case, the rate of absorption and the volume of distribution are important, and clearance plays very little part. In the latter case, however, clearance is the most important factor.

There are differences not only in the infant's ability to metabolize local anaesthetics of the ester and amide groups, but also in its metabolism of drugs in the same group. The concentration of cytochrome P-450—the enzyme involved in the metabolism of the amide drugs—is the same in infants and adults, but only lignocaine is metabolized similarly in both age groups (Blankenbaker et al, 1975). The neonate has a very limited capacity for metabolizing mepivacaine (Brown et al, 1975), and it cannot perform the process of N-dealkylation required for the metabolism of bupivacaine for some hours after birth (Di Fazio, 1979). Ester drugs, such as procaine, are metabolized slower in the neonate than in the adult.

The first stage in the metabolism of prilocaine is hydrolysis to ortho-toluidine whose hydroxylated products can cause methaemoglobinaemia. In adults, this complication only occurs after excessive doses of prilocaine, but there is evidence that in infants it may occur with doses within the therapeutic range as fetal haemoglobin is sensitive to transformation to methaemoglobin (Duncan and Kobrinski, 1983). The use of prilocaine in this age group is therefore best avoided. In other respects, the drug is a very safe local anaesthetic.

Adrenaline is sometimes administered with local anaesthetic drugs in order to limit systemic absorption of the drug, to prolong its effects and, in the case of local infiltration anaesthesia, to reduce bleeding at the site of surgery. The possibility of myocardial sensitization in a child undergoing halothane anaesthesia was considered by Maze and Denson (1983) who found no adverse effects when the dose of adrenaline was limited to 1 ml/kg of the 1:200 000 solution.

CENTRAL BLOCKS

Caudal block

This is a most useful block, as it is widely applicable and technically simple. It can provide analgesia for surgery up to and including the umbilicus, and has even been advocated for upper abdominal surgery though, not surprisingly, the large doses required to anaesthetize the higher abdominal dermatomes have occasionally caused complications (McGown, 1982).

Dosage

When deciding upon suitable dosage, the anaesthetist should keep two points in mind:

1. A caudal is usually a single injection and if surgery has commenced under general anaesthesia, as is common practice, an additional dose cannot easily be given if the first one proves inadequate. The initial dose must therefore be large enough to provide the required level of analgesia in all cases.
2. Although it is possible to obtain surgical anaesthesia and perform the surgery with the caudal as the sole agent, this is an ordeal for the child and general anaesthesia should be induced first and maintained throughout the surgical procedure. The function of the caudal is therefore to provide analgesia only and strong concentrations of local anaesthetic are unnecessary for this. Indeed they should be avoided because they induce lower limb motor block which can cause the child much distress. The exception to this is the use of the caudal as the sole agent in newborns for operations such as anoplasty or urethral valves.

Schulte-Steinberg and Rahlfs (1970) investigated the spread of analgesia in children between the ages of 7 weeks and 11+ years and found that the dose–response correlated best with age, although there was also good correlation with weight and height. The equation derived by these workers (Schulte-Steinberg and Rahlfs, 1977) has been simplified by Hain (1978): volume of drug = (age in years + 2 ml) divided by 10, per segment to be blocked, using lignocaine or bupivacaine. Since this work was carried out, however, advances in obstetric and neonatal care have resulted in an increasing number of babies surviving elective delivery several weeks preterm. Chronological age in these cases is obviously misleading, so weight is now generally used as a predictor for spread of analgesia.

Several dose regimens have been recommended, but since they give the mass or volume of drug required to anaesthetize one segment, it is not always easy to calculate the volume of solution needed for different operations in children of different weights. The regimen shown in Table 9.1 is an attempt to simplify paediatric caudal dosage. It defines three areas—lumbosacral, thoracolumbar and mid-thoracic—and the doses given for each area produce analgesia in virtually every case. A 20 kg boy receives

Table 9.1. Paediatric caudal dosage*

Area	Dose (ml/kg)
Lumbosacral	0.5
Thoracolumbar	1
Mid-thoracic	1.25

* Drug concentrations: 0.25% plain bupivacaine for volumes up to 20 ml; 0.19% plain bupivacaine for volumes over 20 ml.

10 ml of 0.25% bupivacaine for a circumcision, and 20 ml for an inguinal herniotomy. If large volumes of 0.25% bupivacaine are given, motor block is common, so when the calculated volume exceeds 20 ml, one part of water or saline is added to three parts of 0.25% bupivacaine, resulting in a concentration of 0.19%. A 20 kg child therefore receives 25 ml of 0.19% bupivacaine for an orchidopexy or repair of an umbilical hernia.

When applying any dose regimen, it is important to take into account not only the innervation of the skin incision, but also the innervation of the structures which will be stimulated during surgery. For example, the testis, which derives its nerve supply from the 10th thoracic segment, is handled and stimulated during orchidopexy and the mid-thoracic dose is therefore given, although the incised skin, like that for inguinal herniotomy, receives its innervation from the 12th thoracic segment.

Duration of action

Jensen (1981), using 0.25% bupivacaine in a dose of 0.5 ml/kg for circumcision and the repair of hypospadias, found that analgesia lasted 4–8+ h. For thoracolumbar and mid-thoracic blocks, the duration is shorter, but is rarely less than 3 h.

Plasma concentrations

Doses based on regimens similar to Table 9.1 have proved satisfactory clinically, and are in common use. They are, however, comparable with doses used for caudals and epidurals in adults, and interest has centred around the plasma concentrations of local anaesthetic which they produce in children. Reynolds (1971) has suggested that in adults even the mildest signs of local anaesthetic toxicity are unlikely to appear at plasma bupivacaine concentrations less than 1.6 μg/ml, but this figure should be treated merely as a guide. The plasma concentration is not the only factor determining the appearance of toxic symptoms. Scott (1975) has shown that symptoms appear at lower concentrations when the drug has been given rapidly. Furthermore, plasma concentrations are often measured on venous samples, whereas it is the arterial concentration which determines the onset of toxic symptoms.

Eyres et al (1978) gave 2 mg bupivacaine per kg body weight— intermediate between the lumbosacral and thoracolumbar doses in Table 9.1—to children aged 5 days to 15 years, and recorded mean venous plasma concentrations well below 1 µg/ml (Figure 9.1). In a later study (Eyres et al, 1983), they gave 3 mg/kg, which corresponds almost exactly to the mid-thoracic dose in Table 9.1. The highest concentration obtained was 2 µg/ml, but the mean values were less than 1.4 µg/ml and are shown in Figure 9.2. In this series, simultaneous arterial and venous samples were taken from some of the patients (Figure 9.3).

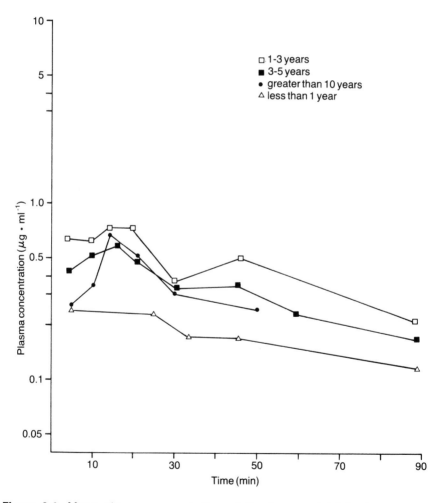

Figure 9.1. Mean plasma concentrations following caudal injection of bupivacaine 2 mg/kg in children. From Eyres et al (1978), with permission.

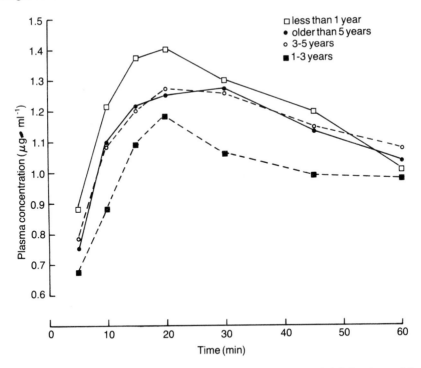

Figure 9.2. Mean plasma concentrations following caudal injection of bupivacaine 3 mg/kg in children. From Eyres et al (1983), with permission.

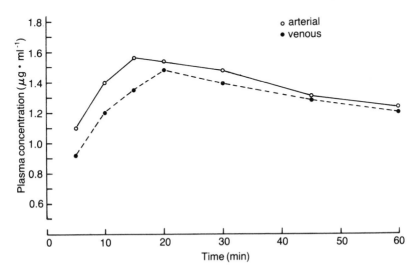

Figure 9.3. Mean arterial and venous plasma bupivacaine concentrations after caudal injection of 3 mg/kg in children. From Eyres et al (1983), with permission.

Complications

Caudal block in children is notable for its simplicity, safety and effectiveness, and complications are uncommon.

Hypotension.   This is a hallmark of central blocks in adults but it is rare in children. McGown (1982) measured the blood pressure in 465 cases and found that it remained within 25% of the precaudal value in all but 11 cases. In one case, the hypotension was attributed to blood loss during the operation, and responded to intravenous infusion, as did two other cases. None of the others required treatment, and vasopressors were never used.

Urinary retention.   This is very rare indeed provided that the concentration of local anaesthetic is sufficient only for analgesia and does not produce motor block. It is important that the child is not made unduly anxious about passing urine as this can in itself predispose to retention. Only two of the author's cases have developed retention serious enough for their discharge from hospital to be delayed.

Intravenous needle insertion.   The occasional puncture of a blood vessel is inevitable with any blind technique, but in paediatric caudal block, the diagnosis is not always obvious and there is no doubt that even when blood has not appeared at the needle hub, the subsequent injection can be wholly or partly intravascular (Figure 9.4). This is probably because, with the patient in the left lateral position with the buttocks raised, the sacrum is higher than the right atrium and blood will only appear at the needle hub if some factor such as partial respiratory obstruction causes an increase in venous pressure. Similarly, aspiration is unreliable as a test, since blood is not always seen when aspiration is attempted from flaccid veins.
   The incidence of intravascular needle placement has been conservatively estimated as 10–15% (McGown, 1982), but the chances of actual intravascular injection can be minimized by adhering to three points of technique:

1. A 23 G needle should be inserted at an angle of about 40° to the skin. The tip then avoids the anterior part of the sacrum where epidural veins are plentiful.
2. The needle should not be advanced more than 2–3 mm after it has penetrated the sacrococcygeal ligament.
3. Aspiration should be carried out gently after the initial injection of up to 1 ml of solution. If the needle lies in a vein, the latter will be temporarily distended and the aspiration test is more likely to be positive.

Dural puncture.   The incidence is very much less than the anaesthetist's anxiety about it. The caudal block must, of course, be correctly performed if this complication is to be avoided, and the needle must not be advanced into the sacral cavity up to the hub after penetration of the sacrococcygeal ligament, as is commonly done in adults. Particular care must be taken in the newborn. Seven dural taps in six patients, occurring over a wide age range and including adults, are known to the author during

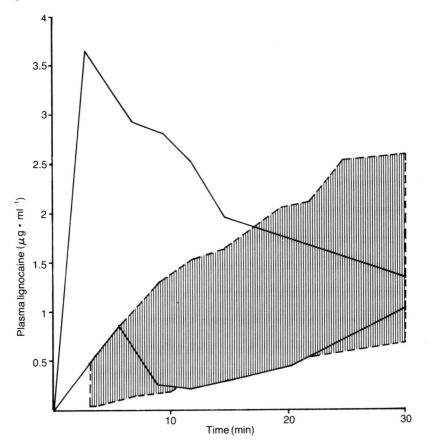

Figure 9.4. Intravascular and partial intravascular injection of lignocaine during caudal block in two patients (solid lines). The range of lignocaine concentrations at each time interval for the other patients in this series is shown by the shaded area.

the course of over 4000 caudals. In six of these, no attempt was made to induce a block, but the seventh case required a second operation and when penetration of the sacrococcygeal ligament again produced cerebrospinal fluid (CSF), a spinal block was performed, but was unsuccessful, giving inadequate analgesia. It is possible therefore that these cases may have caudally placed loculi of CSF, connected to the theca above by a narrow channel, rather than a theca which extends to the base of the sacrum.

Disadvantages

Motor block and paraesthesiae. These unwanted side-effects are sometimes put forward as a reason for preferring a peripheral nerve block to a caudal, but they are only troublesome if needlessly strong solutions, such as 0.5% bupivacaine, are used. Very few children complain spontaneously of motor symptoms if the dose and dilution regimen in Table 9.1 is used, though many admit to paraesthesiae on direct questioning.

Caudal catheters.   Although the epidural space has a good blood supply and an excellent record of defence against infection, most anaesthetists are unwilling to insert a caudal catheter so near to the anus because it is very difficult to ensure that the catheter dressing stays intact and the area remains clean. The presence of a catheter, acting as a foreign body, invites infection under these circumstances. Caudal block is therefore generally regarded as a single injection technique. If long-term postoperative analgesia is required, it can be supplied through a catheter inserted by the lumbar or lower thoracic route, since this area is much easier to keep sterile. However, some workers (Bland et al, 1985; Schulte-Steinberg et al, in press) have used the caudal route to pass catheters to the lumbar and lower thoracic regions, and have encountered no complications; Busoni and Sarti (1987) have taken advantage of the fact that fusion of the sacral vertebrae does not occur until early adult life and have passed a needle and catheter between S2 and S3 into the sacral epidural space.

Lumbar and thoracic epidural block

In adults, epidural anaesthesia has several advantages in addition to the obvious one of pain control. For example, it is possible to avoid general anaesthesia in patients who would tolerate it badly, such as those with severe chronic respiratory disease. In cases where an epidural catheter has been left in place, postoperative management is greatly facilitated since unsedated, alert and pain-free patients can cough effectively and move freely. Epidural anaesthesia provides prophylaxis against deep vein thrombosis, does not cause gastric stasis, encourages intestinal motility and reduces the incidence and severity of paralytic ileus.

In children, however, general anaesthesia is almost always required if the epidural and the operation are to be performed under satisfactory conditions, and deep vein thrombosis and chronic respiratory disease with sputum retention are not common paediatric problems. Even if perfect epidural analgesia is obtained in the postoperative period, additional sedation is usually required, especially in younger children. Epidural block is therefore of limited value, though it does have a place for children undergoing major surgery of the chest and abdomen and some orthopaedic procedures, in which the need for really effective long-term analgesia is sufficient to justify its use.

Technique and equipment

The smaller the patient, the narrower the epidural space, and modifications of standard methods and equipment are required if the epidural needle and catheter are to be safely and accurately placed and dural puncture avoided. The paediatric needle illustrated in Figure 9.5 has been used satisfactorily by

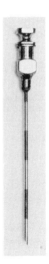

Figure 9.5. Paediatric epidural needle. Needle Industries Ltd, Redditch, UK.

the author for several years. The shaft is 5 cm long, graduated in centimetres, is thin-walled and accepts an 18 gauge epidural catheter. The bevel is short, but of conventional design and the stilette prevents tissue-coring. More recently, Portex Ltd have marketed a 19 gauge Tuohy needle with a 21 gauge nylon catheter. The shaft is 5 cm long, but it is graduated every 0.5 cm and the bevel is rounded (Desparmet, 1986).

Approach to the epidural space

A needle introduced at right angles to the skin by the traditional midline approach takes the shortest path across the epidural space and is therefore more likely to puncture the dura than a needle introduced obliquely. Puncture may also occur with the catheter when the midline approach is used because the catheter tip, after emerging from the needle, impinges on the dura even when a Huber-pointed needle is used.

The paramedian approach is more satisfactory because the angle of needle insertion is independent of the distance between the vertebral spines. The needle can therefore be inserted with cephalad inclination, and this has three advantages:

1. the needle traverses the epidural space obliquely, so the distance between its point of entry into the space and the dura is increased (Figure 9.6) and the likelihood of dural puncture is diminished;
2. the catheter passes very easily up the epidural space because it can slide parallel to the dura instead of striking it at right angles;
3. a specially contoured needle tip is unnecessary.

Anterior-facing bevel. The bevel of a needle introduced into the

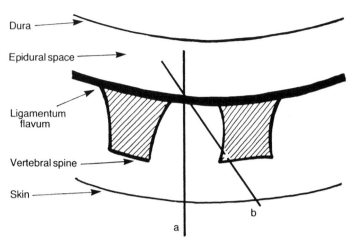

Figure 9.6. Insertion of epidural needle. Needle (a), inserted by the midline approach, encounters the dura before needle (b), inserted the same distance by the paramedian approach with cephalad inclination.

epidural space is usually directed so that it faces cephalad, and the length of the bevel therefore occupies part of the width of the space. As the angle of cephalad inclination is increased, the bevel faces posteriorly towards the anaesthetist, but it still lies across the epidural space and in children its length may be a sizeable proportion of it (Figure 9.7). On the other hand, if the needle is introduced so that the bevel faces anteriorly, away from the anaesthetist, it lies in the longitudinal plane of the space instead of across it, and the risk of dural puncture is reduced. These remarks apply to bevels of conventional design (Figure 9.5)—a rounded bevel facing anteriorly would direct the catheter towards the dura rather than parallel to it.

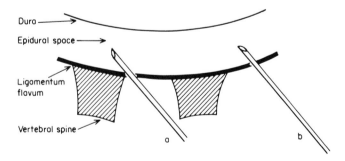

Figure 9.7. Insertion of epidural catheter. Both needles are inserted by the paramedian route and are directed cephalad. The bevel of needle (a) lies across the epidural space. The bevel of needle (b) faces anteriorly and its plane is parallel to the long axis of the epidural space.

Position of the catheter.   The catheter tip should be placed as close as possible to the spinal nerves supplying the cephalad end of the surgical field. This ensures that all the field is analgesic since gravity carries the local anaesthetic solution to the caudad segments when the child is sitting up in the postoperative period. A catheter placed in the segmental midpoint of the surgical field may be satisfactory if analgesia is achieved with bolus top-ups, but is unsatisfactory if a local anaesthetic infusion is used because the cephalad segments tend to remain unanaesthetized. If a catheter proves to be lying too far cephalad, it can easily be withdrawn until it is correctly placed, whereas a catheter which is too caudad cannot be further advanced unless the whole epidural procedure is repeated and the catheter inserted afresh.

Dosage

The test dose.   It is important for the anaesthetist to be clear about the reasons for performing a test dose and the information being sought from it. A test dose is usually given with the intention of excluding intravascular and subarachnoid placement of the needle or catheter, and four criteria must be satisfied if it is to be valid:

1. the test solution must be capable of producing unequivocal and easily observable evidence of these mishaps within a reasonably short time;
2. the test dose itself should be unlikely to produce any detectable effect if injected into the right place;
3. the cardiovascular state of the child must be stable before the injection;
4. the anaesthetist must allow sufficient time for the test effect to become apparent before injecting the full dose (Wildsmith and Armitage, 1987).

Lignocaine (2%) with adrenaline 1 in 200 000 is a suitable test solution because the adrenaline will produce a significant rise in blood pressure and increase in pulse rate within 1 min of intravascular injection in conscious or anaesthetized children. Lignocaine 2% given intrathecally will produce dense sensory and motor block within 5 min, but in the anaesthetized child it is impossible to determine whether this has occurred. It is therefore unrealistic to expect that subarachnoid injection can be excluded during the perioperative period, though test doses may have a place postoperatively when the necessary neurological information can be obtained from the conscious child.

Since only the test for intravascular injection is applicable under all circumstances and since a positive result is observable within a minute, there is a good case for the monitoring of a slow injection of an adrenaline-containing solution rather than the administration of a formal test dose, which has been described as more of a ritual than a practical exercise (Scott, 1983).

Peroperative.   The dose and concentration of local anaesthetic depends on whether both muscle relaxation and analgesia are required or analgesia alone. The author uses the epidural to obtain analgesia, for which a concentration of 0.25% bupivacaine is sufficient, and prefers to obtain muscle relaxation with neuromuscular blocking drugs. The dose of local anaesthetic depends on factors such as the extent of surgery and the type of incision (vertical or horizontal), as well as the position of the epidural catheter, but 0.5–0.75 ml/kg body weight for the initial dose and half this volume for subsequent top-ups is usually adequate.

Ecoffey and colleagues (1986) gave a general anaesthetic maintained with nitrous oxide, phenoperidine, pancuronium and intermittent positive pressure ventilation and followed this with an epidural using 0.5% bupivacaine with adrenaline in a dose of 0.75 ml/kg. Murat and colleagues (1987) also used bupivacaine with adrenaline, but in a concentration of 0.25% for children less than 8 years of age. Stronger solutions (0.37 or 0.5%) were used for older children when abdominal relaxation was required. These authors gave an initial dose of 0.75 ml/kg to children weighing less than 20 kg, and 1 ml/10 cm height to children taller than 100 cm. Half these volumes were given for subsequent top-up doses.

Postoperative.   Analgesia in the postoperative period may be continued either by intermittent top-ups or by giving an infusion. The former gives excellent results provided that the quality and extent of the analgesia are regularly and expertly assessed and a top-up given at the earliest sign that the block is wearing off. The top-up should be given by the anaesthetist who inserted the catheter or by a skilled medical deputy. These requirements are often difficult to meet and it is likely that at some stage a top-up will be given too late. A continuous infusion may therefore be more practical. With the child in a stable and pain-free state, 0.1% bupivacaine is delivered from an infusion pump at an initial rate of 1 ml/h/year of age. A continuous infusion, however, rarely results in truly continuous analgesia unless some adjustments are made and at the above flow rate, there will be some regression of the block over a period of hours. A top-up is then needed before the pump is reset at a higher infusion rate. Thus, clinical assessment is still necessary, albeit at longer intervals than with the intermittent top-up method. The anaesthetist should be aware that an epidural infusion may produce motor block even when a low concentration of drug is used. This occurs, usually with high flow rates, because continuous irrigation of the epidural space allows the eventual diffusion of solution into the relatively resistant, heavily myelinated motor fibres. A disadvantage of the infusion method is that 0.1% bupivacaine is not commercially available and has therefore to be prepared locally.

Murat and colleagues continued their intermittent top-up regime into the postoperative period, that is, they gave bupivacaine with adrenaline in a dose of 0.37 ml/kg to children weighing less than 20 kg, and 0.5 ml/10 cm height to children taller than 100 cm.

Plasma concentrations

Information about the plasma concentrations of local anaesthetic during epidural anaesthesia in children is limited. The dose and concentration of bupivacaine used by Ecoffey and colleagues (1986) produced maximum plasma concentrations 20 min after injection. These authors studied 10 infants and, with the exception of one in whom a value of 2.2 µg/ml was found, all had concentrations less than 1.8 µg/ml.

Armitage (1985) gave 0.25% plain bupivacaine in a dose of 0.5 ml/kg to a 24 kg boy of 6½ years. The injection was given in three increments over a period of 10 min. A peak plasma concentration of 0.6 µg/ml was recorded 30 min after the last increment. A top-up of 6 ml, given 80 min later when the clinical effects were judged to be wearing off, produced a plasma concentration of 0.8 µg/ml within 20 min. It is possible, therefore, that higher values may be seen after top-ups than after the initial, larger loading dose.

Complications

Hypotension. There is general agreement that epidural block in children rarely results in hypotension. Arthur (1980) used it in children undergoing surgery for coarctation of the aorta in an attempt to control the undesirable hypertension which often persists into the postoperative period. Hypotension did not occur even though the block was high and large doses were given.

Urinary retention. Children undergoing operations for which epidurals are indicated usually require a urinary catheter for surgical reasons. This is perhaps fortunate, because retention would otherwise be considered a disadvantage and it would of course be very likely to occur, particularly if motor block had developed during the course of the epidural infusion.

Pressure sores. There is a danger that lack of sensation together with any immobility caused by motor block may result in damage to a child's delicate skin, and the author has seen such a case. The epidural infusion should be controlled so that motor block is minimal, pressure areas regularly treated and the child encouraged to be mobile in bed.

Spinal (subarachnoid) block

Until recently there has been virtually no place for spinal anaesthesia in children because it takes longer to prepare for and perform than caudal block, has no advantage over it for shorter procedures and is less suitable than the epidural technique for long-term postoperative analgesia. However, it is now being advocated for surgery in premature and formerly premature infants who have been treated for the respiratory distress syndrome (RDS) (Abajian et al, 1984; Harnik et al, 1986). These infants continue to suffer from bronchopulmonary dysplasia for several months after recovery from RDS, and Steward (1982) has shown that they are more prone to complications following general anaesthesia than full-term babies of the same weight. Spinal anaesthesia has been found to be a safe alternative when surgery is required for conditions such as inguinal hernia. This block, with the caudal in the newborns, is the only form of paediatric regional anaesthesia in which the block is routinely performed and the operation carried out on a conscious patient, and in which the block acts as a substitute for general anaesthesia rather than as an adjunct to it.

Abajian et al (1984) and Harnik et al (1986) use 0.5% amethocaine in 5% dextrose, and the author has found both 0.25% cinchocaine in 3% dextrose and 0.25% bupivacaine in 4% dextrose to be satisfactory. Harnik et al recommend a dose of 0.13 ml/kg for inguinal herniotomy in infants weighing less than 4 kg, and 0.07 ml/kg for larger infants. The dead space of a 22 g, 3.5 cm paediatric lumbar puncture needle is approximately 0.04 ml and this should be taken into account when the dose is being calculated and drawn up. The subarachnoid puncture should be made caudad to the third lumbar vertebra to avoid possible damage to the spinal cord, and the procedure is facilitated if the skin and underlying tissues are infiltrated with 1% procaine. It is important to time the operation in relation to the baby's feeding regimen, since the crying of a hungry baby renders hernia repair much more difficult. A dummy, or the anaesthetist's finger, usually keeps the baby quiet, but is inadequate if a feed has to be long delayed. The upper limbs should be lightly immobilized.

PERIPHERAL NERVE BLOCKS

Central blocks produce anaesthesia over a comparatively wide area, only a small part of which may be involved in the surgery. Peripheral nerve blocks have the advantage that they provide a more localized area of anaesthesia which may still be perfectly adequate for some operations. They may also be feasible when a central block is contraindicated due to anatomical abnormality or local infection. There are virtually no side-effects, generalized motor block of the lower limbs is avoided, and the dose is usually smaller than that required for a caudal block.

On the other hand, there are serious disadvantages. The failure rate is comparatively high. Success depends on the solution being deposited close to the nerve, and some of the best methods of ensuring this are either inappropriate or hazardous. For instance, paraesthesiae cannot be elicited in anaesthetized patients, and a nerve stimulator is only helpful if the nerve to be anaesthetized contains motor fibres. The danger of needle trauma to the nerve, inherent when peripheral nerve blocks are attempted in anaesthetized patients, has already been mentioned. Ischaemia and necrosis of distal tissues may result if digital ring blocks or blocks of the dorsal nerves of the penis are accidentally performed with local anaesthetic solutions containing adrenaline, whereas such solutions may safely be used for central blocks. In spite of these disadvantages, successful peripheral nerve blocks have an elegance and specificity which many anaesthetists find attractive, and their use in paediatric practice is increasing. Blunted or short bevelled needles allow different tissue planes to be appreciated more readily.

Ilioinguinal and iliohypogastric block

The ilioinguinal and iliohypogastric nerves run deep to the aponeurosis of the external oblique muscle from a point medial and caudad to the anterior superior iliac spine. Block of these nerves produces anaesthesia over the groin region and is therefore suitable for inguinal herniotomy. There is resistance to a blunted 23 G needle when it meets the aponeurosis, and loss of resistance when it penetrates it.

Smith and Jones (1982) recommended that the injection should be directed laterally towards the iliac crest and mediocaudally towards the inguinal ligament, and they used 0.5% bupivacaine in a dose of 0.5 ml/year of age. They assessed the effects in children undergoing inguinal herniotomy as day cases. Five out of 58 required additional analgesia within 4 hours of the end of surgery, but the authors concluded that the technique was simple, safe and effective.

Block of dorsal nerves of penis (penile block)

Operations on the prepuce and penis are common in children and block of the dorsal nerves of the penis provides satisfactory analgesia for these procedures. The dorsal nerves lie to the left and right, superficial and deep to Buck's fascia (the fascia penis). Local anaesthetic solution injected through a 23 G needle inserted at the base of the penis deep to Buck's fascia spreads to both sides and anaesthetizes the deep nerves. Entering the skin slightly lateral to the midline reduces the incidence of haematoma. The superficial nerves are anaesthetized by withdrawing the needle superficial to Buck's fascia and injecting the solution subcutaneously to left and right.

White and colleagues (1983) used 0.5% plain bupivacaine in a dose of 0.2 ml/kg. After performing an aspiration test, they injected two-thirds of the volume deep to Buck's fascia and the remainder superficially. The mean duration of analgesia was more than 12 h.

Yeoman and colleagues (1983) compared penile block with caudal block and found that the analgesia began to wane after 3–4 h, but 40% of children in both groups were pain-free more than 6 h after operation. Their technique for penile block differed from that of White et al (1983). The needle was advanced on to the lower surface of the symphysis pubis and then redirected 2 mm inferior to it. They gave 0.5% plain bupivacaine in a dose of 1 ml for boys up to 3 years of age and 0.3 ml/year of age thereafter at this one site, and they had one failure in 19 patients.

The penis is a highly vascular organ, and needle insertion carries a risk of damage to blood vessels and the corpora cavernosa. White et al (1983) reported two small haematomas at the base of the penis in their series of 27 cases. It is, of course, vital that adrenalin-free local anaesthetic solutions are used.

Very occasionally a midline septum prevents free diffusion of solution deep to Buck's fascia. In such cases, the block is incomplete and a second paramedian injection is required.

Lower limb blocks

McNicol (1985) has described block of the sciatic nerve by the anterior approach in children. The technique, similar to that used in adults, involves locating the femur and then redirecting the needle medial to it. Loss of resistance is felt as the needle passes into the neurovascular compartment deep to the adductor muscles. Bupivacaine (0.5%) with adrenalin is given in a dose of 1 mg/kg, that is, 0.2 ml/kg.

McNicol (1986) has also described combined block of the lateral cutaneous nerve of the thigh and the femoral nerve, for which he uses the same drug in a dose of 0.5–1 mg/kg (0.1–0.2 ml/kg).

Perhaps the most original application of individual nerve blocks in the lower limb is the work of Kempthorne and Brown (1984). They blocked the tibial and common peroneal nerves in head-injured children with severe extensor spasm and deformity. This improved the effectiveness of physiotherapy and facilitated rehabilitation.

Axillary block

Axillary block, unlike the other peripheral blocks mentioned, does not have to stand comparison with central blocks, since the latter are inappropriate for anaesthesia of the upper limb. It may be used for operations involving deep tissues of the hand and forearm for which local infiltration would be impractical or inadequate. Bupivacaine (0.25%) with adrenaline, injected into the axillary sheath in a dose of 0.3 ml/kg, produces analgesia lasting several hours. A 25 G, 16 mm needle is directed towards the axillary artery. Resistance as the needle enters the sheath and the 'click' as it pierces it are not always felt in children, but oscillation of the needle hub due to transmitted pulsation of the artery is an indication that the needle is correctly placed, and when this sign has been observed, a successful block usually results. Aspiration tests should be carried out before and during the injection. Movement of the needle, with the risk of accidental intra-arterial injection, can be minimized by using the remote injection technique in which the needle hub is distanced from the syringe by a length of flexible tubing.

Intercostal block

This block is frequently undertaken by surgeons during thoracotomy when 1 ml 0.25% bupivacaine per rib is infiltrated close to the posterior angle. There is a significant risk of pneumothorax if this block is performed with the chest closed.

Local infiltration

Children often present for the removal of superficial lesions such as cysts, moles and naevi. The anaesthetist may be reluctant to perform central or peripheral nerve blocks if the lesions are small, but he or she should remember that local infiltration can contribute greatly to patient comfort after their removal. Bupivacaine (0.25%) with adrenaline should be injected in a <

shape from two points on each side so that the lesion is enclosed within a diamond-shaped band of solution (Figure 9.8). The lines of infiltration must not be so close to the lesion that it is distorted or obliterated by injected fluid.

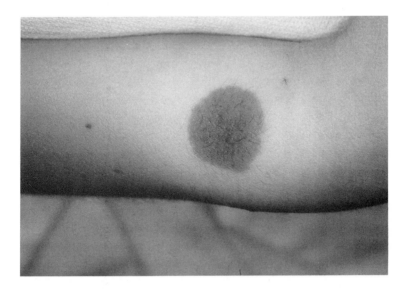

Figure 9.8. The skin surrounding a hairy mole has been infiltrated with 0.25% bupivacaine with adrenaline 1 in 200 000 from two infection sites. The site at '2 o'clock' is clearly visible; the other is diametrically opposite. Skin blanching, caused by the adrenaline, indicates the extent of anaesthesia.

Other techniques

It must not be assumed that the techniques considered here are the only ones suitable for use in children. Others may be used, with appropriate modifications, provided that the anaesthetist has experience with the particular block in adults and provided also that it can be successfully and safely performed in anaesthetized subjects.

REFERENCES

Abajian JC, Mellish RWP, Browne AF, Perkins FM, Lambert DH & Mazuzan JE Jr (1984) Spinal anesthesia for surgery in the high-risk infant. *Anesthesia and Analgesia* **63:** 359–362.

Armitage EN (1985) Regional anaesthesia in paediatrics. In Sumner E & Hatch DJ (eds) *Clinics in Anaesthesiology: Paediatric Anaesthesia.* London: W. B. Saunders.

Armitage EN, Howat JM & Long FW (1975) A day-surgery programme for children incorporating anaesthetic outpatient clinic. *Lancet* **ii:** 21–23.

Arthur DS (1980) Postoperative thoracic epidural analgesia in children. *Anaesthesia* **35:** 1131.

Bainbridge W (1901) Report on 12 operations on infants and young children under spinal anesthesia. *Archives of Pediatrics* **1**: 510.

Bland BAR, Schulte-Steinberg O & Bosenberg AT (1985) Paediatric thoracic epidural anaesthesia via the caudal route: anatomical and radiological considerations in human infant and child cadavers and piglets. Abstract of paper presented at Annual Scientific Meeting of the Association of Paediatric Anaesthetists.

Blankenbaker WL, Di Fazio CA & Berry FA (1975) Lidocaine and its metabolites in the newborn. *Anesthesiology* **42**: 325–330.

Brown WU, Bell GC, Lurie AO, Weiss JB, Scanlon JW & Alper MH (1975) Newborn blood levels of lidocaine and mepivacaine in the first postnatal day following maternal epidural anesthesia. *Anesthesiology* **42**: 698–707.

Busoni P & Sarti A (1987) Sacral intervertebral epidural block. *Anesthesiology* **67**: 993–995.

Desparmet J (1986) Equipment for paediatric epidurals. *Anaesthesia* **41**: 337–338.

Di Fazio CA (1979) Metabolism of local anaesthetics in the foetus, newborn and adult. *British Journal of Anaesthesia* **51**: 29–34S.

Duncan PG & Kobrinski N (1983) Prilocaine-induced methaemoglobinemia in a newborn infant. *Anesthesiology* **59**: 75–76.

Ecoffey C, Dubousset A-M & Samii K (1986) Lumbar and thoracic epidural anesthesia for urologic and upper abdominal surgery in infants and children. *Anesthesiology* **65**: 87–90.

Eyres RL, Kidd J, Oppenheim RC & Brown TCK (1978) Local anaesthetic plasma levels in children. *Anaesthesia and Intensive Care* **6**: 243–247.

Eyres RL, Bishop W, Oppenheim RC & Brown TCK (1983) Plasma bupivacaine concentrations in children during caudal epidural analgesia. *Anaesthesia and Intensive Care* **11**: 20–22.

Faulconer A & Keys TE (1965) *Foundations of Anesthesiology*, vol. 2, p 853. Springfield, Illinois: Charles C Thomas.

Hain WR (1978) Anaesthetic doses for extradural anaesthesia in children. *British Journal of Anaesthesia* **50**: 303.

Harnik EV, Hoy GR, Potolicchio S, Stewart DR & Siegelman RE (1986) *Anesthesiology* **64**: 95–99.

Jensen BH (1981) Caudal block for postoperative pain relief in children after genital operations. A comparison between bupivacaine and morphine. *Acta Anaesthesiologica Scandinavica* **25**: 373–375.

Kempthorne PM & Brown TCK (1984) Nerve blocks around the knee in children. *Anaesthesia and Intensive Care* **12**: 14–17.

Maze M & Denson DM Jr (1983) Aetiology and treatment of halothane-induced arrhythmias. *Clinics in Anaesthesiology* **1**: 301–321.

McGown RG (1982) Caudal analgesia in children. Five hundred cases for procedures below the diaphragm. *Anaesthesia* **37**: 806–818.

McNicol LR (1985) Sciatic nerve block for children. Sciatic nerve block by the anterior approach for postoperative pain relief. *Anaesthesia* **40**: 410–414.

McNicol LR (1986) Lower limb blocks for children. Lateral cutaneous and femoral nerve blocks for postoperative pain relief in paediatric practice. *Anaesthesia* **41**: 27–31.

Murat I, Delleur MM, Esteve C, Egu JF, Raynaud P & Saint-Maurice C (1987) Continuous extradural anaesthesia in children. Clinical and haemodynamic implications. *British Journal of Anaesthesia* **69**: 1441–1450.

Reynolds FA (1971) A comparison of the potential toxicity of bupivacaine, lignocaine and mepivacaine during epidural blockade for surgery. *British Journal of Anaesthesia* **43**: 567–571.

Schulte-Steinberg O & Rahlfs VW (1970) Caudal anaesthesia in children and spread of 1% lignocaine. *British Journal of Anaesthesia* **42**: 1093–1099.

Schulte-Steinberg O & Rahlfs VW (1977) Spread of extradural analgesia following caudal injection in children. A statistical study. *British Journal of Anaesthesia* **49**: 1027–1034.

Schulte-Steinberg O, Bland BAR & Downing JW (1988) Thoracic epidural anaesthesia via the caudal route in infants and children (in press).

Scott DB (1975) Evaluation of the clinical tolerance of local anaesthetic agents. *British Journal of Anaesthesia* **47**: 328–333.

Scott DB (1983) Abdominal and perineal surgery. In Henderson JJ & Nimmo WS (eds) *Practical Regional Anaesthesia*, p 226. Oxford: Blackwell Scientific Publications.

Smith BAC & Jones SEF (1982 Analgesia after herniotomy in a paediatric day unit. *British National Journal* **285**: 1466.

Steward DJ (1982) Preterm infants are more prone to complications following minor surgery than term infants. *Anesthesiology* **56**: 304–306.

White J, Harrison B, Richmond P, Procter A & Curran J (1983) Postoperative analgesia for circumcision. *British Medical Journal* **286**: 1934.

Wildsmith JAW & Armitage EN (1987) *Principles and Practice of Regional Anaesthesia*, pp 50, 87. Edinburgh: Churchill Livingstone.

Yeoman PM, Cooke R & Hain WR (1983) Penile block for circumcision? A comparison with caudal blockade. *Anaesthesia* **38**: 862–866.

The postoperative period

The postoperative period commences on completion of the surgical procedure and encompasses the periods of recovery in the operating theatre, recovery room, ward and when appropriate the intensive care unit. This chapter will examine the ways in which the infant and child differ in their metabolic response to surgery, and the physiological factors that render them at risk during this period. It will also discuss the common postoperative complications of anaesthesia and surgery and the various techniques that are employed for postoperative pain relief.

Complex neonatal and paediatric surgery should only be performed in hospitals with appropriate resources to cater for all perioperative needs. Children often have more than one congenital malformation and the timing of various surgical procedures requires detailed planning and multidisciplinary consultation. Such patients are best operated on in paediatric hospitals by paediatric surgeons and anaesthetists with subspecialist availability. It can be anticipated that some infants and children undergoing surgery will require admission to an intensive care unit for closer monitoring and nursing surveillance, the performance of special procedures and the delivery of advanced cardiorespiratory support. Surgery that is likely to require such back-up should only be performed in a hospital with an appropriately staffed and equipped neonatal and paediatric intensive care unit.

METABOLIC RESPONSE TO SURGERY

Following surgery or major injury, the healthy adult undergoes a three-phase metabolic response—a catabolic phase lasting from 3–7 days; an early anabolic phase lasting weeks and a late anabolic phase lasting a period of months. The healthy neonate undergoes a similar, albeit attenuated response immediately following delivery (Wilkinson et al, 1962). During phase one, which lasts 1–3 days, the neonate receives minimal intake and significant weight loss occurs as a result of negative balance for water, calories, nitrogen and electrolytes. During phase two, fluid and caloric intake increase but weight loss continues as a result of a negative water balance. Phase three, one of anabolism and rapid weight gain, begins when full oral intake is established. It is believed that this three-phase metabolic response occurs throughout all age groups.

Neonatal stress responses have been found to be three to five times greater than in adults, although the duration is shorter (Anand, 1986). Preterm and full-term infants undergoing surgery with minimal anaesthesia exhibit a marked release of catecholamines (Anand et al, 1985a), growth hormone (Milne et al, 1986), glycogen (Anand et al, 1985a), glucocorticoids and aldosterone (Obara et al, 1984; Srinivasan et al, 1986) as well as inhibition of insulin secretion (Anand et al, 1985b).

Hormonal and metabolic stress response can be attenuated by adequate depth of anaesthesia (Anand, 1986; Anand and Hickey, 1987a; Anand et al, 1987a, b, 1988). It has been suggested that the pathological stress response of neonates under light anaesthesia may be associated with increased postoperative morbidity and mortality.

As the infant has double the metabolic rate of the adult, accelerated weight loss occurs in the face of reduced intake. After uncomplicated surgery, the newborn infant has less tendency to sodium and water retention and weight gain (Colle and Paulsen, 1959). Fortunately, postoperative ileus is uncommon or short-lived and a normal intake and positive nitrogen balance are rapidly achieved in most patients. The responses of the older child and adolescent are probably similar to those of the adult.

The normal metabolic response to surgery may be prolonged and exaggerated by greater degrees of surgical stress or by complications such as sepsis or circulatory shock. Maintenance volumes of dextrose/saline solutions do not provide maintenance calories. The newborn infant, particularly if premature, has minimal energy stores and readily exhibits signs of protein–calorie malnutrition if starvation is permitted to continue. If enteral feeding is not feasible, parenteral nutrition should be commenced early. It has been estimated that whereas an adult has the energy reserves to survive for about a year on 3 litres of 10% dextrose a day, a small preterm infant will survive only 11 days on 75 ml/kg/day of 10% dextrose (Heird et al, 1972).

RESPIRATORY FUNCTION (see also p. 256)

Physiologically and anatomically, the infant has limited respiratory reserves and is poorly situated to deal with an increased respiratory load. This accounts for the high incidence of respiratory failure after surgery in the first 2 years of life. Postoperatively, the infant may be embarrassed by pain, abdominal distension, circulatory instability or disturbances of body temperature. In the neonate, these factors may be superimposed on the processes of adaptation to extrauterine life.

Metabolic rate and oxygen consumption in the neonate are approximately twice that of the adult, and when tissue hypoxia occurs anaerobic metabolism generates lactic acidosis at double the rate. For the same reason, apnoea or alveolar hypoventilation from any cause leads to an increase in $Pa\mathrm{CO_2}$ at approximately twice the rate of the adult. In the face of cardiorespiratory failure, a combined metabolic and respiratory acidosis occurs with alarming rapidity, leading to further depression of function. Any deviation of environmental temperature outside the thermoneutral range may lead to cold stress or heat stress with an increased metabolic demand.

Other factors limiting postoperative respiratory reserve include the immaturity of the chest wall (Muller and Bryan, 1979), dependence on diaphragmatic function, the tendency to small airways closure, and fatiguability of diaphragmatic muscle (Keens et al, 1978).

The airways of the infant are relatively large when compared with those of the adult. The trachea of a 3 kg infant, for instance, is approximately one-third the diameter of that of a 60 kg adult and the bronchioles are half the diameter of those of the same adult. In absolute terms, however, the airways of the infant are small and more prone to obstruction by mucus, blood or other debris.

Respiratory reserve may be further compromised by developmental defects or disease processes such as kyphoscoliosis, muscular dystrophy, cystic fibrosis, congenital heart lesions and many other problems. In these situations, the need for postoperative respiratory support following elective surgery can often be anticipated.

CARDIOVASCULAR SYSTEM (see also p. 258)

Compared with the adult heart, fetal and neonatal hearts contain less contractile tissue. It has been shown that this histological difference is functionally important in that the fetal myocardium develops greater tension at rest and less active tension during contraction (Friedman, 1973). It is a less compliant heart with limited stroke volume and cardiac output is therefore extremely rate-dependent. Bradycardia associated with hypoxaemia or vagal stimulation is associated with signs of inadequate cardiac output. In addition the neonatal myocardium may be less responsive to inotropic agents such as dopamine.

In the newborn, episodes of reduced tissue perfusion or tissue hypoxia are associated with marked third space fluid extravasation. Volume expanders form an important part of most resuscitation protocols.

NORMAL RECOVERY

In the operating theatre

Patients should usually remain in the operating theatre until spontaneous ventilation is judged adequate and protective reflexes have returned. The stomach should be decompressed prior to extubation if considered appropriate, thereby reducing the risk of vomiting and aspiration.

On occasions, it may be desirable to transfer the intubated patient to the recovery room and to perform the extubation at a later time. Patients in whom respiratory function is compromised preoperatively or in whom postoperative intubation, ventilation or cardiovascular support is required are transferred directly to the intensive care unit. Most neonates undergoing major surgery require immediate postoperative care in the intensive care unit.

The likely requirements for postoperative analgesia should be assessed towards the conclusion of the anaesthetic. Prevention of pain is usually considered more effective than attempts to abolish it after its onset. The techniques of pain relief that may be employed are discussed later in this chapter.

In the recovery room

Following anaesthesia and surgery, patients should be transferred to a properly designed recovery room where consciousness can be regained and cardiopulmonary stability established (Anonymous, 1983). The recovery room should have an adequate number of beds and nursing staff to provide the necessary surveillance of all patients returning from the theatre suite. It has been recommended that between 1.5 and 3 spaces should be provided per operating theatre (Anonymous, 1983). All basic resuscitation equipment and drugs should be available to this area. Each bed must have suction apparatus conforming with the appropriate standards and an oxygen outlet for use with a range of oxygen catheters, masks and headboxes suitable to deliver oxygen therapy to all age groups.

Routine oxygen therapy has not been recommended for infants and children with healthy lungs. Recent evidence from pulse oximetry however suggests that a significant number of healthy children become moderately desaturated (SaO_2 74–93%) in the immediate postoperative period and that this is unpredictable and not always evident on clinical observation (Glazener and Motoyama, 1984; Tomkins et al, 1988). A case can be advanced for routine oxygen therapy until consciousness is fully regained and perhaps for the first 30 min after operation.

Oxygen therapy should always be administered if cyanosis is evident, for which the cause must be sought, after major cardiothoracic, abdominal and intracranial surgery and when oxygen consumption is increased by shivering, muscle rigidity or pyrexia.

The risk of retrolental fibroplasia in premature infants receiving oxygen therapy should be considered and oxygen concentrations prescribed according to blood gas estimation, pulse oximetry or transcutaneous oxygen monitoring. The latter technique is of limited value when skin perfusion is decreased, as may occur after prolonged operative procedures.

A means of inflating the lungs with oxygen, e.g. modified Ayre's T-piece, Bain circuit or self-inflating bag (e.g. Ambu), must be provided at each bed. In a paediatric recovery room, equipment should be available to cater for patients of all sizes. A tilting trolley with a firm base and mattress is essential equipment, although neonates and infants will often be nursed in incubators or cots. Medical lighting meeting an approved standard should be installed to guarantee optimal observation conditions (Hood, 1977). Recovery room nursing staff should have facilities for rapid communication with theatre personnel. An intercom system is appropriate for this need. Medical staff must be immediately available to deal with sudden, unexpected anaesthetic or surgical complications.

The time that a child remains in the recovery room will usually be determined by the type of anaesthesia delivered and the nature and duration of the surgery performed. The majority remain for a period between 30 and 60 min or until such time as stability is achieved. Close observation is necessary to detect bleeding, airway obstruction or other surgical or anaesthetic complications. A specially designed record of recovery room observations and therapy should be kept. In order to guarantee continuity of care, all patients must be handed over to ward staff with detailed information regarding the surgery performed, the recovery room course and any complications that have been encountered.

COMMON PROBLEMS IN THE IMMEDIATE POSTOPERATIVE PERIOD

Postoperative pain

Pain is the inevitable result of most surgical procedures and frequently results in detrimental physiological and behavioural changes. Pain may lead to tachycardia, hypertension and bleeding and the restless child may interfere with dressings and surgical wounds such as burn grafts or plastic surgical procedures. Analgesia can prevent harmful stress responses and may reduce postoperative morbidity and mortality.

The problem of pain relief in the neonate is particularly vexing. In the past some found it convenient to hold the belief that the human neonate was not capable of perceiving pain. In this way it was possible to avoid the difficulties associated with opiate administration. It is now clear that the neonate possesses all of the anatomical and neurochemical systems necessary for pain perception and exhibits characteristic physiological and behavioural changes in response to pain (Anand and Hickey, 1987b). The humane approach, therefore, is to take all possible steps to alleviate pain in our patients.

Postoperative analgesia may be a residual benefit of the form of anaesthesia provided as the use of intraoperative narcotics, local blocks or regional techniques may extend into the postoperative period. It is the impression of many that recovery is smoother and the pain less intense if discomfort is prevented by a prophylactic approach to the early postoperative period. In long surgical procedures, it may be necessary to supplement the local blockade prior to completion of anaesthesia.

TECHNIQUES OF PAIN RELIEF

Continuous intravenous narcotics

Intramuscular injections are painful, have a slow onset of action and their absorption is variable, particularly in the presence of poor peripheral perfusion. By avoiding the peaks and troughs of plasma levels associated with intermittent injection, continuous morphine or other opiate infusions can provide constant, adequate analgesia without respiratory depression and with a reduced incidence of nausea and vomiting. The total dose of drug required is approximately half that of intermittent injection and analgesia is less dependent on the availability and subjective impressions of nursing staff.

Whilst narcotics are freely employed in children, their use has in the past been restricted in infants under 12 months of age (though a single dose of codeine phosphate 1 mg/kg i.m. has proved satisfactory for newborns (Purcell-Jones et al, 1987). This has stemmed from several reports of sensitivity to the drugs with resulting respiratory depression or apnoea. Respiratory depression may be due to either different pharmacokinetics or to increased sensitivity to the respiratory-depressant effects of narcotics, i.e. shift of CO_2 response curve to the left.

Beyond the neonatal period morphine pharmacokinetics vary little with age (Dahlstrom et al, 1979). Morphine infusions should, however, be used with caution in the neonatal period as elimination half-life (13.9 ± 6.4 h) is significantly longer than in older children and adults (about 2 h; Koren et al, 1985). The same workers found that morphine concentrations in neonates receiving 20 µg/kg/h for 24 h were three times higher than in older children receiving the same schedule. They also reported that two infants receiving higher dosages, 32 and 40 µg/kg/h, developed generalized seizures (see also p. 268).

Continuous infusions of morphine can be safely employed in unventilated neonates and infants provided that liver function is not compromised and that very close surveillance of respiratory function is available in the postoperative intensive care ward. The infusion dose range of morphine in infants and children is 10–50 µg/kg/h. In view of the pharmacokinetic data and potential complications it would seem advisable not to exceed 20 µg/kg/h in the neonatal period. It should be noted that the highest dose (50 µg/kg/h) provides the same total dose of morphine as that provided by the recommended intramuscular dosage (i.e. 0.2 mg/kg 4-hourly). An initial intravenous bolus of morphine 0.1 mg/kg should be administered for rapid achievement of a steady state plasma concentration.

Drugs may be infused via either syringe pumps or volumetric infusion pumps. The former are very suitable for use in small children because of their accuracy at lower infusion rates and the constraints placed on fluid volumes. Other narcotic drugs have been employed in children. Fentanyl has been shown to be haemodynamically stable in neonates although its elimination half-life is prolonged (317 compared with 129 min in adults; Johnson et al, 1984; Koehntop et al, 1986). It appeared from the study by Koehntop et al that neonates are more sensitive to the respiratory-depressant effects of a given plasma level of fentanyl than adults.

The infusion dose of fentanyl in children is 2–4 µg/kg/h. A loading dose of 1–2 µg/kg should be administered in unventilated patients (see also p. 80).

Local anaesthetic techniques (see also Chapter 9)

Until recent years, there has been little application of neural blockade techniques in paediatric anaesthesia and the use of local anaesthetic agents has been restricted to local infiltration and topical techniques. An upsurge of interest in central and peripheral neural blockade has followed the availability of longer-acting local anaesthetic agents, greater understanding of the physiological effects and pharmacokinetics and more detailed knowledge of the anatomy of various blocks in children.

Neural blockade is technically more difficult in small children because the anatomical site is smaller. The closer proximity of structures that can potentially be damaged, such as the pleura, dura and blood vessels, increases the risk of complications. Most techniques are combined with light general anaesthesia as patient co-operation may be difficult to obtain. This latter fact limits their use in the postoperative period.

Bupivacaine is the most popular and useful long-acting local anaesthetic agent currently available. Bupivacaine, without adrenaline, provides analgesia lasting 3–5 h when employed in the epidural space. Much longer periods of analgesia, lasting 12–24 h, may occur when bupivacaine is used for peripheral nerve blockade. Adrenaline is used for local infiltration techniques other than for blocks of fingers, toes or other poorly perfused tissues. It is useful for multiple intercostal blockade where large doses of local anaesthetic agent must be used. A total dose of 3 mg/kg bupivacaine via the epidural route without adrenaline has been shown to achieve safe plasma levels in children (Eyres et al, 1983, 1986).

In a large percentage of paediatric surgery, the duration of the procedure is short and the analgesia provided by neural blockade extends into the postoperative period. This allows a smooth reawakening and more controlled period in the recovery room. A more prolonged period of postoperative analgesia can be guaranteed by a top-up immediately prior to completion of general anaesthesia. Careful monitoring is required during the recovery period when cardiorespiratory instability may occur. Half the initial dose of local anaesthetic agent is recommended for top-ups.

In most centres, the routine use of top-ups in the postoperative period has not been widely practised apart from the occasional use of intercostal blocks or femoral nerve blockade. The use of 50% nitrous oxide (Entonox) may facilitate administration of the block.

Any of the neural blockade techniques applicable to adults can be performed in children and their details are found elsewhere in this and other standard textbooks (Cousins and Bridenbaugh, 1980). All techniques may confer a period of postoperative analgesia and it is likely that we will see an increased application of neural blockade in children in the future. The following techniques are those most commonly employed.

Epidural blockade

Thoracic, lumbar and caudal epidural techniques have been described in infants and children, although the caudal approach is by far the most commonly employed (Schulte-Steinberg, 1980). The small epidural space and the caudad extension of the dural sac make dural puncture and total spinal anaesthesia more likely. Dural puncture is somewhat more difficult to detect in the small child. Less cardiovascular disturbance is seen with epidural blockade in children compared with adults although the same precautions should be taken. The volume of local anaesthetic agent for lumbar and caudal blockade is approximately 0.1 ml/segment/year (Schulte-Steinberg, 1980). Bupivacaine 0.25–0.5% solutions are the most commonly used for prolonged analgesia. The total dose of local anaesthetic agent in mg/kg must be calculated if toxicity is to be avoided.

Thoracic epidural blockade is rarely used, the most common application being bilateral thoracotomy for malignancy. In this situation, it has the advantage of reducing the total dosage of local anaesthetic agent which would otherwise be required for bilateral intercostal blockade. Thoracic epidural blockade may be considered in older children with major chest trauma. Lumbar epidural blockade provides excellent operating conditions and is used for prolonged intra-abdominal surgery of a major nature and postoperative analgesia becomes an added benefit.

The use of continuous thoracic and lumbar blockade is limited by the size of needle required. A 19 gauge Tuohy needle is the smallest through which an epidural catheter can be passed and its use is therefore restricted to children over 12 years of age.

Caudal epidural blockade is widely practised for surgery below the umbilicus, such as circumcision, hypospadias repair and perianal procedures (Lourey and McDonald, 1973). It not only simplifies the anaesthesia but facilitates a smooth, pain-free postoperative period. Blockade to the level of T10 can be achieved with larger volumes of local anaesthetic agent. The risk of dural puncture is low if care is exercised.

Intercostal blockade

Intercostal nerve block provides a simple and safe method of providing analgesia of the thoracic wall and upper abdomen without sympathetic blockade. It may be performed either intraoperatively by the surgeon under direct vision through the thoracotomy wound or postoperatively by the anaesthetist. The safety margin for the technique is increased by the presence of a chest drain, as the major complication relates to pneumothorax. In small children the pleura is very close to the skin and the needle should not be inserted more than 2 mm beyond the rib. Unless a chest drain is in place, blockade should not be performed medial to the angle of the rib as the pleura is unprotected by internal intercostal muscles at this site. Particular care must also be taken when large intercostal collateral vessels are present, such as occurs with coarctation of the aorta. Bilateral intercostal blockade is required for midline upper abdominal incisions and care must be taken not to exceed the total safe dosage of bupivacaine (3 mg/kg) when multiple intercostal spaces are blocked. Analgesia may last from 12 to 24 h and this period is prolonged by the use of adrenaline. Motor blockade may occur and paradoxical movement of a segment of chest wall may be evident. The technique is also useful following chest trauma.

Brachial plexus blockade

Axillary, supraclavicular and interscalene approaches have been used in children to provide analgesia for the upper extremity for reduction of fore-arm fractures, creation of arteriovenous fistulae for haemodialysis and other procedures. The principles of the techniques are identical to those used in adults. The safety of the axillary approach offers an advantage. Pneumothorax is the principal risk of the supraclavicular approach. Repeated blockade for postoperative pain is easily performed, particularly when using the axillary technique as adequate co-operation is readily obtained.

Femoral nerve blockade

The technique of femoral nerve blockade is simple and safe and can readily be repeated in a ward setting (Khoo and Brown, 1983). It provides excellent anaesthesia to the anterior aspect of the thigh and is therefore useful for burns grafting. The donor site may cause severe postoperative discomfort, leading the restless child to disturb the dressings. Effective analgesia can be provided for fractured shaft of femur and this may reduce restlessness that can be deleterious with multiple injuries (Berry, 1977). In children with craniocerebral trauma, pain may induce muscular spasms and increased intracranial pressure. This can be prevented by effective analgesia.

Intravenous regional anaesthesia (Bier block)

This technique provides adequate operating conditions for simple procedures on the hand or reduction of arm fractures (FitzGerald, 1976). The analgesia persists for several hours following release of the tourniquet. If the block is to be used in children basic rules should be followed—venous access established, resuscitation facilities readily available, lignocaine or prilocaine the agents of choice.

Ankle block

Ankle blocks are used for operations on the feet, such as wedge resection for ingrown toenails or plantar warts. The analgesia commonly persists for a period of 10 h or longer. Details of other blocks are to be found in Chapter 9.

RESPIRATORY PROBLEMS

Upper airway obstruction

Postoperative upper airway obstruction may occur as a result of underlying disease or deformity of the airway, as a result of the surgery performed, as a complication of intubation or due to alteration of conscious state. The syndromes and diseases most commonly associated with airway problems are listed in Table 10.1; see also p. 481).

Table 10.1. Syndromes and diseases associated with airway difficulties

Angio-oedema	Down's syndrome
Apert's syndrome	Goldenhar syndrome
Beckwith's syndrome	Hurler's syndrome
Behçet's syndrome	Klippel–Feil syndrome
Cherubism	Marfan's syndrome
Cleft palate	Pierre Robin syndrome
Collagen diseases	Scleroderma
Cri du chat syndrome	Treacher Collins' syndrome
Crouzon's syndrome	

Upper airway obstruction may result directly from surgery such as cleft palate repair, palatoplasty, tongue resection, resection of cystic hygroma and other airway lesions or adenotonsillectomy, particularly when the latter is performed for obstructive sleep apnoea.

Tongue resection in the infant with Beckwith's syndrome is usually complicated by massive swelling and a nasotracheal tube is best left in situ until oedema resolves. Following adenotonsillectomy the pharynx should be inspected with a laryngoscope to exclude blood clot or foreign body such as packing gauze. In the recovery period, retronasal clot may migrate into the hypopharynx causing complete airway obstruction. Major adenoidal haemorrhage is difficult to control and may necessitate postnasal packing. Such children may need to be left intubated and sedated until the pack is removed after about 24 h.

A well positioned nasopharyngeal tube will relieve supraglottic airway obstruction such as that occurring after major craniofacial surgery and in infants with Pierre Robin syndrome. The length of the tube is critical (Heaf et al, 1982).

A tight tracheal tube or traumatic intubation may cause subglottic oedema and postintubation group (see p. 142). Children with Down's syndrome frequently have subglottic narrowing and are particularly at risk from this complication (Sherry, 1983). Symptoms including stridor and retraction are usually evident within 30 min of extubation and may be progressive to a point where relief of airway obstruction becomes necessary. A similar situation occurs more frequently after bronchoscopy in infancy. The inhalation of racemic adrenaline (2.25% solution) as used in the management of viral croup has also proven to be beneficial for postintubation subglottic oedema (Jordan et al, 1970). If used, it will virtually eliminate the need for reintubation. Racemic adrenaline is nebulized with oxygen and delivered by mask or intermittent positive pressure breathing (Fogel et al, 1982). The somewhat empirical dosage is 0.05 ml/kg diluted to 2 ml with normal saline. Airway obstruction recedes within minutes and the effect (unlike its effect when used in viral croup) is often sustained. Circumoral pallor may occur but complications such as tachycardia or tachyarrhythmias are rare. Dexamethasone 0.25 mg/kg i.v. may also be helpful for this type of stridor (Deming & Oech, 1961; Biller et al, 1970). An alternative approach is the application of continuous positive airway pressure by nasal prongs or a single nasal cannula. The zero pressure point at which extrathoracic airway collapse occurs is moved down the trachea, and again the improvement is often dramatic. With both therapies, the need for further trauma to the subglottic area is avoided. Close observation is required and gentle reintubation is recommended if severe airway obstruction persists. If this is necessary it is wise to choose a tracheal tube of smaller diameter than that used in the first instance.

Airway obstruction related to altered conscious state demands meticulous maintenance of the airway and posturing of the patient until recovery occurs. If narcotics are implicated, small titrated doses of the opiate antagonist naloxone may prove useful. In general, children with airway abnormalities must regain consciousness completely before they will cope with extubation.

In cases where obstruction is present prior to surgery and where aggravation of the obstruction is likely, it may be elected to leave the child intubated, and a transfer to the intensive care unit for postoperative management should be arranged.

Laryngospasm may occur during emergence from halothane anaesthesia. This may take place in the recovery room in patients transferred from the operating theatre whilst still anaesthetized. Most respond to oxygen administration under positive pressure although occasionally suxamethonium may be necessary to produce relaxation.

Apnoeic episodes

Periodic breathing or recurrent apnoeic attacks lasting 20 s or longer are common in otherwise normal premature infants. Such attacks may be compounded by cyanosis, bradycardia and hypertension followed by hypotension if the attack is prolonged. Apnoeic attacks are more common during rapid eye movement (REM) sleep. The frequency of apnoeic attacks gradually decreases with postnatal age and they usually disappear by the time term is reached. Even after apnoeic attacks have resolved, premature infants or ex-premature infants who develop an intercurrent illness or who are submitted to anaesthesia or surgical stress may revert to their more primitive behaviour and once again develop recurrent apnoeic attacks. This behaviour should be anticipated in infants with a conceptual age less than 46 weeks who have a preanaesthetic history of idiopathic apnoea (Liu et al, 1983). The exact cause is unknown and may well be multifactorial (Gregory and Steward, 1983). The problem may occur following relatively minor surgery such as herniotomy and the episodes usually resolve within 3 or 4 days. Theophylline acts as a respiratory stimulant and may abolish episodes of apnoea (Kuzemko and Paala, 1973). It can be administered in the recovery room as soon as the problem becomes evident and its use has reduced the need for respiratory support in such babies. A loading dose of theophylline of 8 mg/kg by slow intravenous injection should be given and an increase in pulse rate, respiratory rate and general activity is usually seen. Maintenance therapy is often unnecessary but, if required, should be given in a dose of 5 mg/kg/dose at 12-hourly intervals. If continued therapy is necessary, monitoring of theophylline levels is mandatory. The therapeutic range is 40–80 µmol/l. In infants where recurrent apnoea persists despite theophylline loading, continuous positive airway pressure (CPAP), either nasopharyngeal or tracheal, will often regularize ventilation (Kattwinkel et al, 1975; Martin et al, 1977). Intermittent mandatory ventilation (IMV) or continuous positive pressure ventilation (CPPV) may be necessary in some refractory cases. CPAP, IMV and CPPV require transfer to the intensive care unit, and weaning from respiratory support may take several days. Infants considered predisposed to recurrent apnoea who are undergoing major surgery, particularly involving the gastrointestinal tract, should be considered for elective postoperative ventilation.

RESPIRATORY FAILURE

Signs of respiratory failure in the immediate postoperative period may be misinterpreted because of the persisting effects of anaesthetic agents and changes in perfusion associated with surgical stress and body temperature alterations.

The diagnosis is particularly difficult in infancy. Cyanosis is a delayed sign in the presence of anaemia, including the physiological anaemia of infancy. Hypoxaemia and acidosis should be suspected in the presence of lethargy or restlessness, pallor, poor respiratory effort, poor perfusion, bradycardia and hypotension. Respiratory distress marked by tachypnoea, chest wall retraction and grunting are signs for concern. A high index of suspicion and early blood gas analysis are required if respiratory failure is to be recognized.

Clinical examination of the thorax, while providing some useful information, may be misleading in infants as breath sounds are evenly transmitted. Clinical observation of respiratory effort, the chest X-ray and blood gas analysis hold the key to the acute assessment of respiratory status. Pulse oximetry provides a useful guide to adequacy of oxygenation on a continual basis.

Postoperative respiratory failure may relate to preoperative respiratory impairment or to surgical and anaesthetic complications. The common causes of postoperative respiratory embarrassment are listed in Table 10.2. A detailed history of events will usually provide the correct diagnosis. For example, a child with restrictive lung disease due to kyphoscoliosis undergoing corrective spinal surgery will readily develop respiratory failure with excessive narcotic administration, pneumothorax or sputum retention and atelectasis. Transfer to the intensive care unit for observation and mechanical ventilation is necessary when respiratory failure occurs.

HYPOTENSION AND HYPOPERFUSION

Poor peripheral perfusion may reflect either reduced cardiac output or peripheral vasoconstriction, or both. Peripheral vasoconstriction and mottling may reflect shock but is also seen with prolonged surgical stress and hypothermia. The management of any poor perfusion state is based on the principles of particular attention to ventricular preload, contractility and afterload.

Table 10.2. Causes of postoperative respiratory failure.

1. Preoperative respiratory impairment
2. Postoperative surgical and anaesthetic complications
   Upper airway obstruction
   Depressed respiratory drive
      Volatile anaesthetics
      Narcotics
      Prematurity
      Hypothermia
   Pain—thoracic and upper abdominal incisions
   Persisting effects of muscle relaxants
   Atelectasis/consolidation
      Aspiration
      Impaired cough
   Pneumothorax
   Reduced lung compliance—pulmonary oedema
   Diaphragmatic palsy
   Increased intra-abdominal pressure

Excluding children with heart disease, the commonest cause of reduced cardiac output is hypovolaemia (reduced preload) associated with blood loss, inadequate correction of dehydration states and third space losses. In the newborn, in particular, episodes of reduced tissue perfusion, hypoxia and sepsis are associated with marked third space fluid extravasation. Rewarming after hypothermia increases circulatory capacitance and may unmask hypovolaemia.

The child compensates well for volume depletion, and hypotension is a relatively late feature. Volume expansion is the first manoeuvre in any hypotensive, hypoperfused child, particularly if myocardial function is known to be normal. If the cause is not immediately obvious, hypoxia and acidosis must be excluded by blood gas analysis and treated if present. Suitable volume expanders include blood, plasma protein solutions, or if these are not available, crystalloid solutions. The response to a 10 ml/kg bolus should be assessed and if favourable, the bolus repeated. Hypotension due to hypovolaemia will usually represent a blood volume deficit of at least 30 ml/kg.

In children with congenital heart disease undergoing cardiac catheterization, cardiac surgery or incidental surgery, evidence of poor cardiac output may represent impaired myocardial function. Hypoxia and acidosis may also compound the issue. The early use of dopamine 5–10 µg/kg/min by continuous infusion is recommended whilst attention is directed towards oxygenation, ventilation, volume status and acid–base balance. Such children with cardiovascular instability are usually best monitored and supported in the paediatric intensive care unit.

Postoperative vomiting

Despite improvements in anaesthetic agents and anaesthetic technique, the incidence of postoperative vomiting in children remains unacceptably high.

It is distressing to the child and may have undesirable consequences due to the mechanical effects on wound healing or fluid loss. The risk of aspiration of gastric contents is high if the conscious state is impaired, particularly when local anaesthetic agent has been applied to the larynx. Patients who have a full stomach or are considered at risk of vomiting should have their stomach emptied under anaesthesia and postoperatively the airway should be protected with a tracheal tube until protective reflexes have returned. Antacids may be administered if the gastric pH is less than 5 to reduce the risk of chemical pneumonitis should aspiration occur.

The incidence of vomiting is closely related to the type of premedication administered (Rowley and Brown, 1982). Papaveretum and hyoscine premedication is associated with a 54% incidence of postoperative vomiting compared with 25% of other types of premedication or no premedication. The incidence of postoperative vomiting associated with the use of opiates is not surprising, as these agents stimulate the chemoreceptor trigger zone. A lower incidence of vomiting is found when reduced dosages of morphine are used (Riding, 1960). This is an argument in favour of the continuous infusion of opiates for postoperative pain relief. Local and regional blockades are also associated with a reduced incidence of vomiting, presumably because they minimize the use of volatile anaesthetic agents and opiate analgesics.

Children also find the pain of injection unpleasant. Consideration should therefore be given to using alternative types and routes of premedication. Oral benzodiazepines administered approximately 2 h before surgery provide adequate sedation for many cases.

Postoperative vomiting depends on many variables including the patient, the type and duration of anaesthesia and the nature of the operation. Postoperative factors such as movement, drugs and oral intake are also important. The choice of premedication should take these factors into account. Antiemetics should be prescribed routinely for situations where the incidence of vomiting is high, i.e. following strabismus surgery, ear and upper abdominal surgery. Metoclopramide is a useful antiemetic, particularly as it also hastens gastric emptying. The dosage is 0.12 mg/kg, administered not more than 6-hourly.

DELAYED RECOVERY FROM ANAESTHESIA

Most children have normal pulmonary, hepatic and renal function and recovery from anaesthesia is rapid and smooth. When this is not the case it is first necessary to distinguish failure to regain consciousness from persistent neuromuscular blockade. The latter is best evaluated using a peripheral nerve stimulator.

Failure to regain consciousness

This is most commonly due to the residual effects of premedication and anaesthetic agents. It may be due to overdosage or to failure to metabolize or excrete the agents employed. Delayed recovery may follow prolonged use of volatile inhalational agents particularly if cardiac output and minute ventilation are depressed. Correction of these factors will hasten recovery. Narcotic depression of conscious state (and respiration) may occur when excessive doses are used to produce anaesthesia, in neonates and when the hepatic glucuronidase system is impaired. If narcotic depression is suspected a trial of naloxone (10 μg/kg) may prove extremely useful.

Metabolic disturbances such as hyponatraemia, CO_2 narcosis and acidosis from other causes may lead to prolonged depression. The interaction between respiratory depression, hypercarbia and anaesthetic agents is obvious.

The possibility of various central nervous catastrophes must be entertained in specific forms of surgery and if complications occur during anaesthesia. Some considerations include postictal states, hypoxic injury, air or other embolism and intracranial hypertension.

Prolonged neuromuscular blockade

Prolonged paralysis may follow the use of succinylcholine in patients with abnormal plasma pseudocholinesterase. Diagnosis rests with the clinical history of prolonged paralysis after a standard dose of succinylcholine and is supported by assessing the plasma pseudocholinesterase inhibition by dibucaine.

Prolonged action of non-depolarizing muscle relaxants may be due to age (increased sensitivity in neonates), excessive dosage, hypothermia, acidosis, hypokalaemia, liver and renal disease and concurrent administration of aminoglycoside antibiotics. Children with myasthenia gravis, muscular dystrophies and myotonia congenita all have increased sensitivity to non-depolarizing relaxants.

Residual neuromuscular blockade can be demonstrated with a peripheral nerve stimulator. The features of non-depolarizing block include poorly sustained response to tetanic stimulation, diminished response to a train-of-four stimuli and post-tetanic facilitation. Anticholinesterases will improve muscle tone in such cases. Artificial ventilation should be continued until recovery is complete.

DISTURBANCES OF BODY TEMPERATURE

Hyperthermia or hypothermia may occur during anaesthesia and both may be associated with increased metabolism and increased demands for oxygen and alveolar ventilation. Whilst hypothermia itself is associated with reduced metabolism, any attempt by the body to restore temperature to normal is asssociated with a marked increase in metabolism as a result of shivering or non-shivering thermogenesis (oxidation of brown fat). Decompensation may occur if cold stress or heat stress are superimposed on the cardiorespiratory instability of the early postoperative period.

The newborn is most vulnerable to cold stress (Heim, 1981). Metabolic rate is minimal when ambient temperature and body temperature are maintained in a narrow thermoneutral zone. Most heat loss occurs as a result of radiation, and body temperature can be maintained by nursing infants in double-walled incubators or with servo-controlled radiant heaters in the pre- and postoperative period.

Hypothermia is most likely to occur during prolonged procedures in small infants with a large surface area, particularly when the use of heating apparatus is restricted, e.g. cardiac catheterization, burns surgery. It may delay the recovery from anaesthetic agents. Body temperature should be recorded on return to the recovery room and the patient should not be returned to the ward until core temperature is greater than 36°C. A heated incubator should be prepared for the immediate use of infants following surgery.

Hyperthermia may occur due to overheating (operating room, warming blanket, humidifier), anticholinergic overdose, sepsis, malignant hyperthermia and when sweating is impaired (cystic fibrosis, Riley–Day syndrome, spinal cord injury). Malignant hyperthermia may occur in susceptible individuals (usually with a subclinical familial myopathy), and in association with central core disease, Duchenne's muscular dystrophy and myotonia congenita. Malignant hyperthermia may first manifest in the postoperative period and contingencies to deal with it must be available (see p. 528).

AWAKENING RESPONSES

Anticholinergic poisoning

Excessive anticholinergic administration may produce a spectrum of central nervous system effects varying from depression to excitement, restlessness and delirium. This is much more likely to occur with scopolamine than atropine. Depending on the timing of premedication in relation to surgery, features of anticholinergic poisoning may be present preoperatively. Postoperative delirium is most likely to occur after surgery of short duration, although the action of scopolamine may be very prolonged. The response to scopolamine is variable, and features of poisoning may occur with normal doses. Physostigmine, unlike neostigmine, crosses the blood–brain barrier and can reverse the delirium (Greene, 1971). The dosage of physostigmine is 0.02 mg/kg intravenously every 5 min until the desired response is obtained (maximum dose 0.2 mg/kg). The half-life of physostigmine is short and if symptoms return and persist, an infusion can be commenced at a rate of 1–10 μg/kg/min.

Shivering and rigidity

Shivering and muscle rigidity are most likely to occur during emergence from prolonged halothane anaesthesia, but may occur following any prolonged procedure associated with a fall in body temperature. Whilst induction and recovery times are shorter with enflurane, the incidence of excitement phenomena is greater. Oxygen therapy may be warranted to enable the child to cope with a marked increase in oxygen consumption.

Disorientation, hyperactivity and excitability

Children are prone to disorientation, hallucinations and at times uncontrollable activity during emergence from anaesthesia. This may sometimes be related to the form of anaesthesia—ketamine is the most commonly incriminated. Delirium may also occur on recovery from barbiturate or halothane anaesthesia. Other reversible causes should be sought. Hypoxia and pain are common causes of restlessness and the former must be excluded. Narcotic analgesics are dangerous therapy for restlessness due to hypoxia. Sensory deprivation from eye bandages, the foreign environment of the recovery room and a sedated state may explain the behavioural disturbance in some cases. In such circumstances, the presence of the parent in the recovery room may be of major therapeutic benefit.

POSTOPERATIVE INTENSIVE CARE

The need for sudden, unexpected transfer from the recovery room to the intensive care unit after surgery should be rare. In most instances, the requirement for postoperative support in the intensive care unit can be anticipated from the preoperative status of the patient, the nature of the surgery to be performed and the likely postoperative course. Unplanned admission is most commonly related to upper airway obstruction (post-bronchoscopy, cleft palate surgery, adenotonsillectomy) and cardiorespiratory failure in neonates and infants after cardiac catheterization.

Increasingly, many sick infants are admitted to the intensive care unit from the ward or emergency room preoperatively for institution of cardiorespiratory support, including ventilation and inotropic therapy prior to surgery. This is particularly important for infants with cardiorespiratory failure secondary to congenital heart disease or other conditions such as urgent diaphragmatic hernia. The improvement in physical status that can be demonstrated in some conditions has undoubtedly contributed to improved surgical results (Jones et al, 1985). This approach has the advantage of introducing a valuable time interval between the induction of anaesthesia and institution of invasive monitoring and the commencement of the surgical insult. These children are invariably returned to the intensive care unit postoperatively for continued supportive care and close monitoring.

REFERENCES

Anand KJS (1986) Hormonal and metabolic functions of neonates and infants undergoing surgery. *Current Opinions in Cardiology* **1**: 681–689.

Anand KJS & Hickey PR (1987a) Randomized trial of high dose sufentanil anesthesia in neonates undergoing cardiac surgery: effects on metabolic stress response. *Anesthesiology* **67**: A502.

Anand KJS & Hickey PR (1987b) Pain and its effects in the human neonate and fetus. *New England Journal of Medicine* **317**: 1321–1329.

Anand KJS, Brown MJ, Bloom SR & Aynsley-Green A (1985a) Studies on the hormonal regulation of fuel metabolism in the human newborn infant undergoing anesthesia and surgery. *Hormone Research* **22:** 115–128.

Anand KJS, Brown MJ, Causon RC, Christofides ND, Bloom SR & Aynsley-Green A (1985b) Can the human neonate mount an endocrine and metabolic response to surgery? *Journal of Pediatric Surgery* **20:** 41–48.

Anand KJS, Sippell WG & Aynsley-Green A (1987a) Randomized trial of fentanyl anaesthesia in preterm infants undergoing surgery: effects on the stress response. *Lancet* **i:** 243–248.

Anand KJS, Carr DB & Hickey PR (1987b) Randomized trial of high-dose sufentanil anesthesia in neonates undergoing cardiac surgery: hormonal and hemodynamic stress responses. *Anesthesiology* **67:** A501.

Anand KJS, Sippell WG & Schofield NM (1988) Does halothane anaesthesia decrease the metabolic and endocrine stress responses of newborn infants undergoing operation? *British Medical Journal* **296:** 668–672.

Anonymous (1983) Guidelines for the care of patients recovering from anaesthesia. *Royal Australasian College of Surgeons Bulletin* **3:** 24–25.

Berry FR (1977) Analgesia in patients with fractured shaft of femur. *Anaesthesia* **32:** 576–577.

Biller HF, Bone RC, Harvey JE et al (1970) Laryngeal edema. An experimental study. *Annals of Otology, Rhinology and Laryngology* **79:** 1084–1087.

Colle E & Paulsen EP (1959) Response of the newborn infant to major surgery. *Pediatrics* **23:** 1063–1084.

Cousins MJ & Bridenbaugh PO (1980) *Neural Blockade in Clinical Anesthesia and Management of Pain.* Philadelphia: JB Lippincott.

Dahlstrom B, Bolme P & Feychting J (1979) Morphine pharmacokinetics in children. *Clinical Pharmacology and Therapeutics* **26:** 354–365.

Deming MJ & Oech SR (1961) Steroid and antihistamine therapy for postintubation subglottic edema in infants and children. *Anesthesiology* **22:** 933–936.

Eyres RL, Bishop W, Oppenheim RC & Brown TCK (1983) Plasma bupivacaine concentrations in children during caudal epidural analgesia. *Anaesthesia and Intensive Care* **11:** 20–22.

Eyres RL, Hastings C, Brown TCK & Oppenheim RC (1986) Plasma bupivacaine levels following lumbar epidural anaesthesia in children. *Anaesthesia and Intensive Care* **14:** 131–134.

FitzGerald B (1976) Intravenous regional anaesthesia in children. *British Journal of Anaesthesia* **48:** 485–486.

Fogel JM, Berg IJ, Gerber MA & Sherter CB (1982) Racemic epinephrine in the treatment of croup: nebulisation alone versus nebulisation with positive pressure breathing. *Journal of Pediatrics* **101:** 1028–1031.

Friedman WF (1973) The intrinsic physiologic properties of the developing heart. In Friedman WF, Lesch M & Sonnenblick E (eds) *Neonatal Heart Disease,* pp 21–49. New York: Grune & Stratton.

Glazener C, Motoyama EK (1984) Hypoxemia in children following general anesthesia. *Anesthesiology* **61 (suppl):** A416.

Greene LT (1971) Physostigmine treatment of anticholinergic-drug depression in postoperative patients. *Anesthesia and Analgesia* **50:** 222–226.

Gregory GA & Steward DJ (1983) Editorial: Life threatening perioperative apnoea in the ex-'premie'. *Anesthesiology* **59:** 495–498.

Heaf DP, Helms PJ, Dinwiddie MB & Mathew DJ (1982) Nasopharyngeal airways in Pierre Robin syndrome. *Journal of Pediatrics* **100:** 698–703.

Heim T (1981) Homeothermy and its metabolic cost. In Davis JA & Dobbing J (eds) *Scientific Foundations of Paediatrics,* 2nd edn, pp 91–128. London: Heinemann.

Heird WC, Driscoll JM, Schullinger JN, Grebin B & Winters RW (1972) Intravenous alimentation in paediatric patients. *Journal of Pediatrics* **80:** 351–372.

Hood JW (1977) Application of the new Australian standard for clinical lighting. *Anaesthesia and Intensive Care* **5**: 51–55.

Johnson KL, Erickson JP, Holley FO & Scott JC (1984) *Anesthesiology* **61**: A441.

Jones RDM, Duncan AW & Mee RBB (1985) Perioperative management of neonatal aortic isthmic coarctation. *Anaesthesia and Intensive Care* **13**: 311–318.

Jordan WS, Graves CL & Elwyn RA (1970) New therapy for post-intubation laryngeal oedema and tracheitis in children. *Journal of the American Medical Association* **212**: 585–588.

Kattwinkel J, Nearman HS, Fanaroff AA, Katona PG & Klaus MH (1975) Apnea of prematurity. *Journal of Pediatrics* **86**: 588–592.

Keens TG, Bryan AC, Levison H & Ianuzzo CD (1978) Developmental pattern of muscle fiber types in human ventilatory muscles. *Journal of Applied Physiology: Respiratory, Environmental and Exercise Physiology* **44**: 909–913.

Khoo ST & Brown TCK (1983) Femoral nerve block—the anatomical basis for a single injection technique. *Anaesthesia and Intensive Care* **11**: 40–42.

Koehntop DE, Rodman JH, Brundage DM, Hegland MG & Buckley JJ (1986) Pharmacokinetics of fentanyl in neonates. *Anesthesia and Analgesia* **65**: 227–232.

Koren G, Butt W, Chinyanga H, Soldin S, Tan Y-K & Pape K (1985) Postoperative morphine infusion in newborn infants: assessment of disposition, characteristics and safety. *Journal of Pediatrics* **107**: 963–967.

Kuzemko JA & Paala J (1973) Apneic attacks in the newborn treated with aminophylline. *Archives of Diseases in Childhood* **48**: 404–406.

Liu LMP, Cote CJ, Goudsouzian NG et al (1983) Life threatening apnea in infants recovering from anaesthesia. *Anesthesiology* **559**: 506–510.

Lourey CJ & McDonald IM (1973) Caudal anaesthesia in infants and children. *Anaesthesia and Intensive Care* **1**: 547–548.

Martin RJ, Nearman HS, Katona PG & Klaus MH (1977) The effect of low continuous positive airway pressure on the reflex control of respiration in the preterm infant. *Journal of Pediatrics* **90**: 976–981.

Milne EMG, Elliott MJ, Pearson DT, Holden MP, Orskov H & Alberti KGMM (1986) The effect of intermediary metabolism of open-heart surgery with deep hypothermia and circulatory arrest in infants of less than 10 kilograms body weight. *Perfusion* **1**: 29–40.

Muller NL & Bryan AC (1979) Chest wall mechanics and respiratory muscles in infants. *Pediatric Clinics in North America* **26**: 503–526.

Obara H, Sugiyama D, Maekawa N et al (1984) Plasma cortisol levels in paediatric anaesthesia. *Canadian Anaesthetists' Society Journal* **31**: 24–27.

Purcell-Jones G, Dorman F & Sumner E (1987) The use of opioids in neonates. A retrospective study of 933 cases. *Anesthesia* **42**: 1316–1320.

Riding JE (1960) Postoperative vomiting. *Proceedings of the Royal Society of Medicine* **53**: 671–677.

Rowley MP & Brown TCK (1982) Postoperative vomiting in children. *Anaesthesia and Intensive Care* **10**: 309–313.

Schulte-Steinberg O (1980) Neural blockade for paediatric surgery. In Cousins MJ & Bridenbaugh PO (eds) *Neural Blockade in Clinical Anaesthesia and Management of Pain*, pp 503–523. Philadelphia: JB Lippincott.

Sherry KM (1983) Postextubation stridor in Down syndrome. *British Journal of Anaesthesia* **85**: 53–55.

Srinivasan G, Jain R, Pildes RS & Kannan CR (1986) Glucose homeostasis during anaesthesia and surgery in infants. *Journal of Paediatric Surgery* **21**: 718–721.

Tomkins DP, Gaukroger PB & Bentley MW (1988) Hypoxia in children following general anaesthesia. *Anaesthesia and Intensive Care* **16**: 177–181.

Wilkinson AW, Stevens LH & Hughes EA (1962) Metabolic changes in the newborn. *Lancet* **i**: 983–987.

Neonatal physiology and anaesthesia

Neonatal surgery is increasingly performed in specialized centres, each serving a population of 2–3 million. This policy allows the infant to be treated in a paediatric environment by trained paediatric surgeons, physicians, anaesthetists and nursing staff and where the pathology and radiology services are appropriate for the needs of the infant patient (Leading article, 1978). Though transfer in utero is recommended whenever possible, the transport of sick newborn babies over great distances by surface or air is now safe even for those intubated and ventilated.

The neonatal period is defined as the first 28 days of extrauterine life and by the end of this time many physiological systems have started to mature in the healthy term baby. However, with babies surviving from gestational periods as short as 26 weeks with birthweights as low as 600 g, the immaturities of the neonatal period can be expected to extend well beyond the defined 4 weeks in this group of babies. An accurate assessment of postconceptual age is important because physiological differences between infants who are small for gestational age and those whose weight is appropriate cause an increased morbidity and mortality in the small-for-dates group (Figure 11.1; Saigal et al, 1984). The neonatal period should thus be considered to extend until at least 44 weeks postconception.

In developed countries infant mortality is 7–12 per 1000 live births with mortality declining more rapidly in the newborn than in the neonatal group. A further limited reduction is possible but this can only be achieved at much greater expense (Bloom, 1984). The mortality in the group of 500–600 g birthweight may be as high as 90%.

Most surgery is performed on newborns to correct congenital abnormalities, some of which may be immediately life-threatening. It should be remembered that such abnormalities may be multiple, and coexisting conditions may have profound implications for the anaesthetist—for example, 30% of patients with oesophageal atresia have congenital heart disease.

It is possible to diagnose with increasing accuracy conditions such as hydrocephalus, abdominal wall defects, tracheo-oesophageal fistula, congenital diaphragmatic hernia and certain obstructive conditions of the urinary tract using ultrasound examinations in the antenatal period (Gauderer et al, 1984). Fetal surgery for conditions such as hydronephrosis is already a practical possibility (Spielman et al, 1984) and is now frequently undertaken (Da Luca, 1987). Antenatal diagnosis poses both medical and ethical problems, but it does allow the delivery of the baby to be close to a

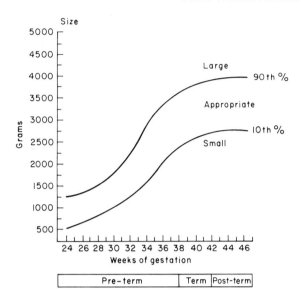

Figure 11.1. The 10th and 90th percentile lines for babies of varying gestational ages. From Lubchenco (1976), with permission.

regional paediatric surgical unit and also at an optimal time for surgery to take place.

The differences between anaesthesia for newborns and the older child are related to differences in anatomy and physiology—differences which are greatest in the very young. Techniques must be based on a sound knowledge of neonatal physiology and the reactions of immature systems to various stresses related to anaesthesia and surgery. Pre- and postoperative monitoring must involve detection of apnoea or hypoxia, changes in blood volume and maintenance of body temperature and blood sugar levels.

PHYSIOLOGICAL DIFFERENCES

Respiration

Newborns have poor respiratory reserves, which means that respiratory failure, and hence the need for respiratory support, is a common sequel to pathology in any system (Hislop and Reid, 1981).

At birth the total pulmonary resistance at 25 cm $H_2O/l/s$ is five times that of the adult so that the work of breathing is greater. In the first week of life the lungs are relatively stiff (compliance 6 ml/cm H_2O) but after that the specific compliance is similar to the adult. The compliance of the chest wall at birth is five times that of the adult, and is even higher in the preterm baby, so that if the lung compliance falls further (for example, with surfactant deficiency or pulmonary oedema), lung volumes will not be maintained.

The high compliance of the chest wall also means that intercostal retraction occurs if the work of breathing increases or if there is respiratory obstruction. The closing volume in the lungs occurs within tidal breathing and although the physiological intrapulmonary right-to-left shunt is not greatly increased from the adult level after the first week of life, there will be a large increase with a minor reduction in the functional residual capacity (FRC). Because of this, the response to constant distending pressure in the form of continuous positive airway pressure (CPAP) is strikingly beneficial in improving oxygenation and reducing the work of breathing in this age group (Figure 11.2; Cogswell et al, 1975).

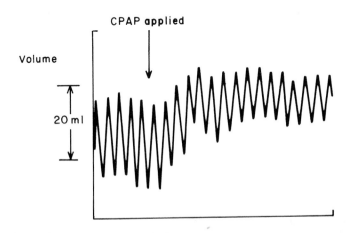

Figure 11.2. The effect of increasing continuous positive airway pressure (CPAP) on functional residual capacity. From Hatch (1981), with permission.

Oxygen consumption at neutral thermal environment is approximately 7 ml/kg/min, which is twice that of the adult. Tidal ventilation does not greatly differ (on a weight basis) from the adult, and as the infant's oxygen consumption is double, the resting respiratory rate is also twice that of the adult. Infants rely mainly on the function of the diaphragm, which means that if this is prejudiced, for example by severe abdominal distension, or a phrenic palsy from birth injury, or following thoracic surgery with mediastinal dissection, respiratory failure rapidly ensues. The 'bucket handle' effect of the downward sloping ribs to increase intrathoracic volume begins in the first year of life, so that the tidal volume is relatively fixed and increases in alveolar ventilation only come from increasing respiratory rate; such increases are an excellent sign of impending respiratory failure. The diaphragm will easily fatigue as the proportion of high oxidative type I fibres is low. A term baby has 25% of these fibres compared with 55% in the adult, whereas a preterm baby may have as few as 10% (Keens et al, 1978). Newborns are obligatory nose-breathers and use may be made of this phenomenon in the application of CPAP via one nasal prong. Nasal resistance is 45% of the total airways resistance and this is a relatively lower value than the adult. Further inroads into respiratory reserve are caused by the tendency to apnoea, especially in preterm babies. This tendency is increased with general anaesthesia and systemic conditions such as sepsis, pneumonia or intraventricular haemorrhage. The attacks are pathological if they extend beyond 15 s or involve bradycardia or cyanosis. Moderate apnoea will respond to constant distending pressure, which increases firing from chest wall stretch receptors, and also to theophylline therapy (Murat et al, 1981; Miller et al, 1985).

Circulation

Fetal myocardium develops less active tension during isometric contraction and whereas 60% of the adult myocardium is contractile mass, only 30% of that of the infant takes part in contraction. The infant has a poor capacity to increase the stroke volume, so that to increase the cardiac output the rate must increase. The output can be expected to increase with rates of up to 200 beats/min. Conversely, bradycardia will cause a fall in cardiac output and this together with apnoea produces a very dangerous situation. The average systolic blood pressure of the term baby is no more than 75–80 mmHg. Tachycardia is the response to acute blood loss, mediated by carotid sinus baroreceptors, but the mechanism is immature, as full compensation for a fall in blood pressure does not occur. Peripheral vasoconstriction occurs very readily in the skin, muscles, liver, intestines and kidneys and may be difficult to reverse. The pulmonary vascular resistance (PVR) of the newborn is labile, so in conditions such as hypoxia and acidosis the pulmonary resistance increases, causing a right-to-left shunt through a patent ductus arteriosus and/or patent foramen ovale (Figure 11.3). This state of transitional circulation may cause critical hypoxaemia unless treatment is directed towards reducing the PVR. Until the ductus is closed by fibrosis after 3–4 weeks of life it may reopen if exposed to hypoxia or fluid overload.

Attempts to close the ductus are made using the prostaglandin synthetase inhibitor, indomethacin; conversely, prostaglandin E_1 or E_2 may be infused intravenously to maintain ductal patency where this is essential, for example, in newborns with pulmonary atresia with intact septum or preductal coarctation of the aorta, until surgery can take place (Mott, 1980). The lability of the pulmonary vasculature is caused by an abundance of smooth muscle, which extends more peripherally than later in life and is a failure of normal regression of the muscle in the first few hours of life (Haworth and Hislop, 1981; Haworth, 1986).

Transitional circulation commonly occurs in babies with hyaline membrane disease, diaphragmatic hernia and meconium aspiration syndrome, and may also occur for no obvious reason. These babies die with hypoxia and falling cardiac output unless the reversible component of the PVR is treated with high fraction of inspired oxygen, hyperventilation, correction of acidosis and the use of the pulmonary vasodilating agent tolozoline in bolus doses of 1–2 mg/kg or prostacyclin 4–20 ng/kg/min (Fox and Duara, 1983).

The normal newborn has autoregulation of cerebral blood flow to maintain a constant flow with changes of systemic blood pressure between 60 and

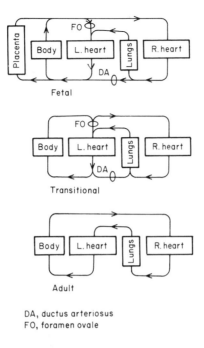

DA, ductus arteriosus
FO, foramen ovale

Figure 11.3. The transitional circulation—transitional between the fetal and adult circulations. From Dawes (1968), with permission.

130 mmHg. This mechanism may be disturbed after periods of hypoxia, so that surges of arterial or venous pressure may cause rupture of delicate intracerebral capillaries and intraventricular haemorrhage (Milligan, 1980). This has very serious consequences for handicap in later life, and is unfortunately a relatively common occurrence in sick preterm babies.

Temperature (see also p. 136)

Newborns attempt to maintain core temperature at 37°C, but may not achieve this because of the large surface:weight ratio, immature sweat function and low basal metabolic rate for the first few hours of life; neither can they protest about, or move from, adverse thermal conditions. The trigeminal area of the face contains superficial thermoreceptors and a cold stimulus causes a sympathetically mediated increase in heat production from the metabolism of triglycerides in brown fat, with a consequent increase in oxygen consumption which is likely to make worse any pre-existing hypoxia. Brown fat is found over the back and acts as thermal lagging around the great thoracic vessels (Hey, 1972). Babies are nursed in open or enclosed incubators with servo temperature control in the neutral thermal environment at which oxygen demands are minimal (Figure 11.4). A better definition of neutral thermal environment has been suggested by Sauer et al (1984); the ambient temperature at which the core temperature of the infant at rest is between 36.7 and 37.3°C and the core and skin temperatures are changing less than 0.2 and 0.3°C per hour, respectively.

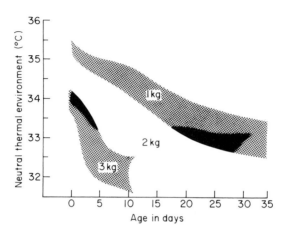

Figure 11.4. Changes in the neutral environment with birthweight and age. From Hey and Katz (1970), with permission.

Neutral thermal environment may be 31°C for a clothed 3 kg baby, but up to 36°C for a naked low birthweight preterm baby. There is increased morbidity and mortality if a baby cools, with increased tendency to hypoxia, acidosis, coagulopathy and intraventricular haemorrhage, and the subsequent brain growth will be slower. Heat loss by radiation to the surroundings is reduced by a heat shield within the incubator. If the journey to an operating department is difficult and body temperature may not be maintained, it has been suggested that surgery for conditions such as necrotizing enterocolitis in very preterm babies could take place in an open incubator in the intensive care unit. Other advantages include decreased handling of the baby, no interruption of vital monitoring and a reduced risk of displacement of the tracheal tube, venous and arterial lines (Besag et al, 1984).

Liver function

Before birth most of the functions of the liver are taken over by the placenta and the maternal liver. Many aspects of liver function are immature at birth, such as detoxication and carbohydrate metabolism, though the enzyme systems mature rapidly and function at adult levels by 10–12 weeks of life. The carbohydrate reserves of the newborn are relatively low and because most glycogen is stored between 36 and 40 weeks' gestation, preterm babies have very poor reserves. Blood sugar levels average 2.7–3.3 mmol/l (50–60 mg/100 ml). Because only severe hypoglycaemia is symptomatic, all newborns require 4-hourly testing of blood sugar (e.g. BM-Test sticks) and levels below 1.6 mmol/l (30 mg/100 ml) are treated with an i.v. infusion of 10% dextrose, though higher concentrations may often be necessary. Until the liver is mature, synthesis of the vitamin K-dependent factors II, VII, IX and X is suboptimal, with lowest levels occurring on the second and third days of life. The routine administration of vitamin K_1 to all newborns (1 mg i.m.) partially prevents this haemorrhagic condition of the newborn.

Preterm babies have poor prothrombin activity even after vitamin K because of even greater immaturity of the liver than term infants. Hepatic immaturity also means that drugs such as barbiturates and opioids which undergo oxidation in the liver will have a prolonged and profound effect and should be used with extreme caution or avoided altogether. The conjugation of bilirubin is less efficient, with low activity of the uridine diphosphoglucuronyl transferase system; uncoupling of at least one of the two molecules may occur with hypoxia or acidosis or one molecule may be displaced by certain drugs such as sulphonamides. This may increase the concentration of unbound bilirubin which, being lipid-soluble, increases the possibility of brain damage. Levels of up to 340 μmol/l (20 mg/100 ml) of unconjugated bilirubin may be dangerous, but lower levels can also cause damage in the preterm baby who may also be hypoxic or acidotic. The tendency to apnoea is increased or the baby may just be very sleepy. Phototherapy, using light of 425–475 nm, is used to decompose unconjugated bilirubin in the skin and has markedly reduced the number of exchange transfusions performed (McDonagh, 1981; Robertson, 1986) (Figure 11.5).

Haemoglobin

At the moment of birth, the mean haemoglobin (Hb) in the umbilical cord averages 18 g/dl. The Hb concentration rises by 1–2 g in the first days of life because the extracellular fluid volume decreases and the fluid intake is low. Thereafter the Hb level declines, causing the physiological anaemia of infancy. Preterm babies have a greater fall which lasts longer because of a lower red cell survival and poorer production of red cells (Chessells, 1979). A Hb less than 10 g/dl is always abnormal and investigation of its cause is necessary, though surgery should not be delayed for levels just below 10 g/dl (Figure 11.6).

Transportation

The establishment of regional centres for neonatal surgical care, together with intensive care, has necessitated the development of sophisticated transport systems. These systems provide as high a degree of monitoring and support as the baby would have if he or she was already in the regional centre (Hackel, 1975). The apparatus which is used for the transport is based

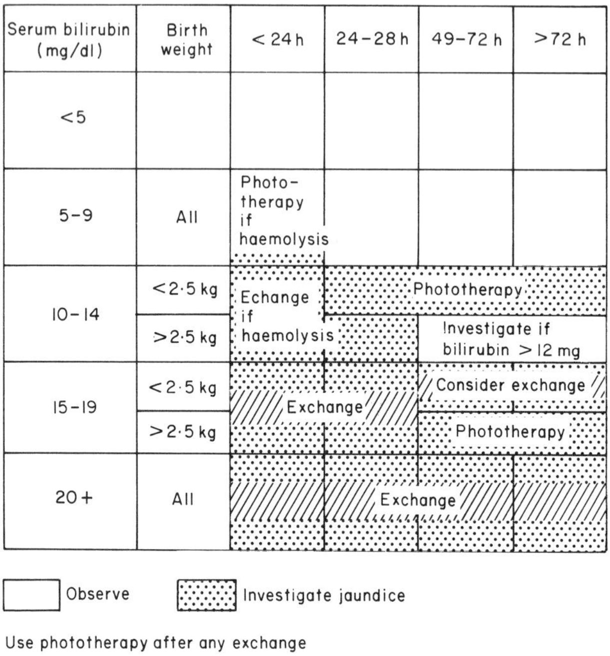

Serum bilirubin (mg/dl)	Birth weight	< 24 h	24–28 h	49–72 h	>72 h
<5					
5–9	All	Photo-therapy if haemolysis			
10–14	<2·5 kg	Echange if haemolysis	Phototherapy		
	>2·5 kg			Investigate if bilirubin > 12 mg	
15–19	<2·5 kg	Exchange		Consider exchange	
	>2·5 kg			Phototherapy	
20+	All		Exchange		

▢ Observe   ▨ Investigate jaundice

Use phototherapy after any exchange

Figure 11.5. The management of hyperbilirubinaemia in newborn infants. Guidelines are based on serum bilirubin concentration, birthweight, age and clinical status of the patient. In the presence of (1) perinatal asphyxia; (2) respiratory distress; (3) metabolic acidosis (pH 7.25 or below); (4) hypothermia (temperature below 35°C); (5) low serum protein (5 g/dl or less); (6) birthweight below 1.5 kg, or (7) signs of clinical or central nervous system deterioration: treat as in next higher bilirubin category. Reproduced from Maisels (1975), with permission.

on one of the commercial transport incubators (for example, Vickers) and it is common practice for the receiving centre to send out a small team of doctor and trained nurse to collect such critically sick infants from peripheral hospitals. The advantage of this system is that the babies can be assessed and prepared for the journey by the team which is more familiar with techniques of transportation. Very few commercial transport incubators are completely suitable and it is usual for one to be mounted on a larger trolley suitable for moving into an ambulance. This provides increased space for batteries, oxygen and air cylinders, monitoring and suction apparatus.

Incubators must provide a neutral thermal environment often achieved using a heat storage principle, have good visibility with adequate illumination and allow easy access to the baby for suctioning or other nursing procedures. The temperature within the ambulance must be maintained at least at 24°C. All electrical apparatus is mains- and battery-driven and an air compressor or oxygen concentrator can provide the gases necessary for respiratory support. If gases are from cylinders, then spares should be carried.

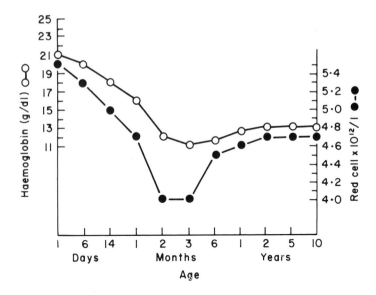

Figure 11.6. Changes in haemoglobin concentration and red cell count in the first 10 years of life. From Davenport (1980), with permission.

Approximately 50% of neonates transported in this way require respiratory support so most transport incubators provide a neonatal ventilator based on the T-piece occluding principle, which is a more basic variety of that used in modern neonatal intensive care units (for example, Bourn BP 200). The ventilator must be capable of delivering 21–100% oxygen and have the facility for intermittent positive pressure ventilation, intermittent mandatory ventilation and CPAP. It is usual to wrap the infants in special aluminium foil to give some protection against loss of heat, and monitoring should include ECG, blood pressure using one of the automated measurement systems, core temperature and transcutaneous oxygen and CO_2 monitoring, especially if the baby requires an increased inspired oxygen concentration. Modern pulse oximetry has been a great advance in the monitoring of small babies during transportation. Maintenance intravenous fluids are administered using a battery-driven syringe pump. The fluids should contain dextrose and if necessary a blood sugar estimation should be performed on the journey.

Before the collection team sets off, the baby should be resuscitated and where necessary acidosis corrected, the intravenous line being very firmly secured with tape and an arm splint. It is a good idea to take a Polaroid photograph of the baby for the mother to have until she is fit enough to join the baby at a later stage.

Before transfer a nasogastric tube should be passed in all sick babies as gastric dilatation may occur in any baby, but especially in those with suspected intestinal obstruction, or diaphragmatic hernia, where intestinal gas may prejudice respiratory function. If in doubt, tracheal intubation should take place before departure as intubation on the journey is not easy. Secure fixation of the tube is necessary and regular suctioning is necessary to prevent blockage of the tube during transit. A chest drain may also be required.

The transport equipment also includes a prepacked kit of equipment such as intravenous cannulas, a self-inflating manual bag system, for example Ambu, apparatus for intubation and for placement of a chest drain as well as drugs for resuscitation. Blake et al (1975) presented a group of 222 patients transported over distances as great as 50 miles. The condition of 4% of the patients deteriorated, but 56% were stable and 40% actually improved during the journey.

Basic principles of neonatal anaesthesia

The baby is brought to the prepared operating theatre in the neutral thermal environment in a heated incubator. Anaesthesia is induced on the operating table with warm coverings and though some heat loss is inevitable at this stage, it should be minimized by using aluminium foil to the limbs and head to reflect radiant heat, a heated mattress, preferably of the hot-air type (Figure 11.7), an overhead heater for induction of anaesthesia and insertion of venous and other lines, an ambient temperature of 24°C without draughts, and heated, humidified inspired gases.

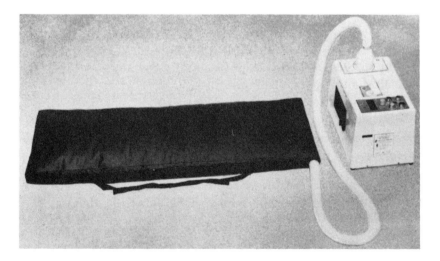

Figure 11.7. Warm air mattress for the operating table (Howorth Air Engineering).

These precautions to minimize loss of heat are especially important for the preterm baby (Neuman and Hansen, 1980). Preparation of the skin by the surgeons should not be prolonged and should utilize warm solutions. During the operation, the incubator should be kept switched on so that the baby may go back to the ward in a heated atmosphere.

General anaesthesia for newborns always involves intubation, even for minor surgical procedures. The airway may be difficult to maintain using a facemask and inhalational anaesthetic agents cause marked respiratory depression and a reduction in the FRC, so that controlled ventilation should always be used. Because the compliance of the chest is lower than that of the abdomen and gastric distension occurs with assisted ventilation using a facemask, tracheal intubation is essential.

It is nowadays generally accepted that intubation should take place after induction of anaesthesia, as with older patients. However, for anaesthetists in training, before they are confident at intubating newborns, it may be safer to intubate babies awake below 10–14 days of age. Awake intubation is easily performed without trauma if the head is firmly held and the shoulders are not allowed to rise from the table. If intubation difficulties, such as tracheal stenosis, are encountered there is less difficulty in maintaining full oxygenation of the infant while a smaller tracheal tube is inserted. The converse of this is that there may be great difficulty in maintaining the airway and oxygenation after a muscle relaxant has been given and before the trachea is intubated. A pressure transducer placed over the anterior fontanelle during awake intubation shows a marked rise in intracranial pressure (ICP), though such a rise is not as great as that seen during normal crying. Clinical fontanometry is now a much more accurate means of assessing ICP in infants using non-invasive means (Mehta et al, 1988). The rise in ICP may be a significant factor if the baby is at risk from intraventricular haemorrhage because of prematurity, or already has raised ICP, or a coagulopathy, and in these cases intubation under anaesthesia with muscle relaxation should be considered. It is necessary to weigh up the various risks before deciding which course of action to take and the anaesthetist must be confident that he or she can intubate the baby without causing hypoxia. A small Guedel airway in the mouth alongside the tube prevents lateral movement and a secondary fixation of a catheter mount to the forehead prevents the tube from twisting. Perfect sizing and fixation of the tracheal tube is essential in neonatal anaesthesia.

Venous access is routinely established preoperatively and induction of anaesthesia achieved using thiopentone 2 mg/kg; alternatively, an inhalational induction is possible with cyclopropane and oxygen or oxygen, nitrous oxide and halothane, enflurane or isoflurane. This is followed by a muscle relaxant, suxamethonium 1 mg/kg, atracurium 0.5 mg/kg or vecuronium 0.1 mg/kg intravenously. It is generally agreed that some sensitivity to non-depolarizing muscle relaxants exists for the first 7–10 days of life, though there is a wide variation in response. It is usual to give the drugs in a diluted form—except for atracurium—incrementally until the desired result is obtained. For example, increments of 0.25 mg of tubocurarine may be given to gain control of the ventilation without exceeding an initial total dose of 1 mg for the term baby and possibly half this figure for the preterm. Newborns, especially those born prematurely, are particularly sensitive to both intravenous and inhalational agents and excessive doses cause severe depression of the cardiovascular, respiratory and central nervous systems. However, every attempt should be made to provide adequate anaesthesia and analgesia for the baby undergoing surgery; otherwise there is a harmful stress response with damaging catabolic metabolism postoperatively (Anand et al, 1988).

Careful, controlled ventilation is the technique of choice for all neonatal anaesthetics, even for those where this is a theoretical disadvantage, such as tracheo-oesophageal fistula, lobar emphysema or lung cysts. Adequate alveolar ventilation is assured and some positive end expiratory pressure helps to maintain an adequate lung volume. Most paediatric anaesthetists prefer to ventilate newborns by hand, particularly during thoracic surgery when rapidly changing lung compliance and respiratory obstruction can be detected and compensations made. T-occluding ventilators for the operating theatres, such as the Nuffield 200 series or Sheffield, are convenient, but are not routinely used except where a steady state is particularly desirable, such as neurosurgery or open heart surgery. These machines may actually be dangerous during a thoracotomy where great falls in pulmonary compliance will result in severe hypoventilation unless the operator is exercising extreme vigilance. For those unused to hand ventilation, a manometer incorporated in the T-piece, or other circuit, will show the pressures which are delivered to the airway. A respiratory rate of 30–40 breaths/min is used, with pressures of up to 25 cm H_2O and a fresh gas flow of 4 l. A positive end expiratory pressure of 5 cm H_2O is easy to obtain during hand ventilation. The aim is to produce mild hyperventilation, but particular care should be taken with tracheo-oesophageal fistula not to cause gastric distension or the further distension of lung cysts. Controlled ventilation is, however, not contraindicated in these conditions.

The inspired gases should be warmed to 33°C and fully humidified to preserve mucociliary function and to prevent heat loss from the baby. A heated water bath-type of humidifier is satisfactory.

For fit term babies, maintenance of anaesthesia with intermittent halothane or isoflurane 0.25–0.5% with 50% oxygen and 50% nitrous oxide gives ideal results and allows lower doses of relaxants. If no increment of relaxant or halothane is given within 20 min of the end of surgery, reversal should be easy and the patient should be fully awake after the relaxant has been reversed. Enflurane does not have any particular advantages over halothane in this age group, though it may cause fewer dysrhythmias. The reductive metabolism of halothane which may cause hepatic sensitization in postpubertal patients occurs only very rarely in children (Wark, 1983). Halothane preserves the blood flow to the liver better than other agents so should not be contraindicated in patients with liver disease.

Intravenous analgesics such as fentanyl and alfentanil are long established as suitable agents for paediatric anaesthesia. However, their use in neonatal anaesthesia is controversial since even small doses of fentanyl (2 µg/kg) will cause postoperative respiratory difficulties such as apnoea and hypoventilation in a significant number of babies. Those patients who require mechanical ventilation postoperatively, such as after cardiac surgery or with conditions such as congenital diaphragmatic hernia or gastroschisis, may be safely given opioid analgesics intravenously as part of an anaesthetic technique. Newborns have smaller fat deposits and a less well developed blood–brain barrier. The markedly increased sensitivity to the effects of opioid analgesics may be a result not only of larger quantities of the drug crossing the blood–brain barrier, but also of the increased sensitivity of specific cerebral receptors related to poorer myelination of the central nervous system. In addition to this, reduced hepatic and renal function together with the increased volume of distribution will cause prolonged and unpredictable activity of these drugs. For sick patients who need mechanical ventilation postoperatively a very satisfactory technique is to use fentanyl 2–10 μg/kg, relaxant and controlled ventilation with oxygen–nitrous oxide or oxygen–air mixtures.

When very accurate volumes of fluid are to be administered, it is wise to use a syringe and three-way stopcock. Accurate infusions should be given using either an electronically controlled gravity feed giving set or an infusion pump. If the latter is used the cannulation site should be checked regularly for extravasation into the tissues. When accuracy of volume administration is less critical, a standard paediatric burette with 30–100 ml chamber is adequate. When blood is administered rapidly or in large volumes it should be warmed and filtered as for an adult. Blood loss should be carefully measured using scales for swab-weighing and surgical suction apparatus which allows small volumes of blood to be measured accurately.

After the surgery has been completed atropine and neostigmine are given (atropine 0.02 mg/kg, or glycopyrrolate 0.01 mg/kg and neostigmine 0.05 mg/kg) and controlled ventilation with high fraction of inspired oxygen continued until full spontaneous ventilation has been re-established and the baby is fully awake, opening his or her eyes and moving all his or her limbs. Before extubation the nostrils should be carefully suctioned with a soft suction catheter.

A newborn is an obligatory nose-breather and may become obstructed if the nasal resistance is increased. This may occur with secretions, too large a nasogastric tube or congenital choanal atresia.

The baby is extubated and returned, covered with warm wrappings, to a preheated incubator when the respiratory effort is judged to be fully adequate in terms of depth, rate and absence of signs of respiratory distress or obstruction such as intercostal or suprasternal recession and nasal flaring. The tube is withdrawn during compression of the T-piece bag so that the baby coughs as soon as the tube leaves the trachea and expels any secretions.

Poor respiratory function postoperatively is not uncommon. The dose of relaxant may be excessive or an increment given too late, or the effects of normal doses potentiated by high doses of halothane or diazepam transferred via the placenta from the maternal circulation. There will be respiratory difficulty if the function of the diaphragm is prejudiced by severe abdominal distension or phrenic palsy after thoracic surgery. Difficulty in reversing the non-depolarizing relaxant is possible if the patient is hypothermic, acidotic, has a low ionized Ca^{2+}, is very preterm or has a low cardiac output. Facilities for mechanical ventilation and intensive monitoring postoperatively must be ready for any baby operated on in the neonatal period. In some centres a period of mechanical ventilation is routine postoperatively. In other units, respiratory support is given only to those patients who show signs of respiratory distress when surgery is completed. Respiratory support which employs ventilators specifically designed for use in infants, based on the T-piece occluding principle, such as Bourn BP 200, is now both safe and routine. Ventilation takes place via a nasal tracheal tube, though constant distending pressure in the form of CPAP can be administered via one nasal prong with great effect.

Analgesia

Analgesia for babies weighing less than 5 kg continues to pose problems of assessment and administration. Immature metabolic systems cause changes in pharmacokinetics; for example, older children and adults have an elimination half-life of morphine of 2 h, but Koren et al (1985) showed that the mean elimination half-life of morphine is 13.9 h for newborns with a very wide range, so that infusions may be cumulative and multiple doses dangerous. There is a tendency to apnoea, intensified by stress, especially of anaesthesia and surgery, and not related to the type of anaesthetic. Respiratory arrest has been described by Purcell-Jones et al (1987) after injudicious use of opioids in newborns postoperatively. Drug effects may be unpredictable and because of dilutional factors and mild hepatic dysfunction can cause the morphine half-life to extend to over 28 h.

Analgesics may have depressant effects on an immature cardiovascular system, causing hypotension and bradycardia, leading to severe falls in cardiac output, especially if the baby is hypovolaemic.

An immature central nervous system with poor myelination of large sections of the brain gives greater sensitivity to opioid analgesics for a given dose. Moss et al (1982) have shown sustained higher levels of endogenous β-endorphin after birth and with a less well developed blood–brain barrier these may have a greater central depressant effect. The high levels are not merely from placental transfer from the mother because of the high rate of turnover of these substances. A further problem of assessment is that as newborns develop, so do their reactions to a painful stimulus and twice as much electrical stimulation is required to produce a response in a 1-day-old infant as in a 3-month-old baby (Gross and Gardiner, 1980). All newborns also have normal periods of sleeping and crying even postoperatively, and cry for a variety of reasons even when not in pain.

Newborns do feel pain which must be obtunded both intra- and postoperatively (Berry and Gregory, 1987). Though the detection of pain is not easy, there is overwhelming evidence of appreciation of pain in newborns. The evidence includes changes in skin conduction levels which increases with pinpricks which do not cause withdrawal. Williamson and Williamson (1983) showed that physiological variables such as heart rate, respiratory rate, length of time spent crying and fall in PaO_2 are all significantly changed by circumcision performed on infants with no anaesthesia compared with those having it carried out with dorsal nerve block of the penis, indicating a significant response to pain.

Anand et al (1987) demonstrated that 10 µg/kg fentanyl in addition to $50:50\ N_2O:O_2$ anaesthesia obtunds undesirable metabolic responses. Catecholamines, other stress hormones and catabolic metabolism with endogenous protein breakdown which is most sensitively shown by the urinary 3 methyl histidine:creatinine ratio are blocked by inhalational agents or opioids. Postoperative complications are probably less in neonates given fentanyl.

Voice spectrographic analysis clearly identifies the type of cry associated with pain, though a parent or a well trained staff nurse may be equally certain (Levine and Gordon, 1982).

Clearly, adequate anaesthesia over-rides all other considerations and everything possible should be done to give neonates the same standard of care of anaesthesia and analgesia as any patient. A mixture of $50:50\ N_2O:O_2$ alone is insufficient; the pulse oximeter allows more confident use of more nitrous oxide. Local blocks, wound infiltration, nerve and regional blocks (caudals and spinal) should be used whenever possible as the effects will last well into the postoperative period. Volatile agents are probably safer than opioids because of their more rapid clearance, and as effective, though it should be remembered that minimum alveolar concentration falls with decreasing postconceptual age, e.g. isoflurane 1.8% at 45 weeks, 1.4% at 35 weeks and 1.25% at 32 weeks (Ledez and Lerman, 1987). Opioids are normally given if respiratory support is planned for the postoperative period and large doses of fentanyl, for example 10–20 µg/kg, are well tolerated. Smaller doses of fentanyl (2–3 µg/kg) will occasionally cause respiratory depression postoperatively and all babies given such doses require close monitoring after surgery if they are breathing spontaneously. There is a greater clearance of fentanyl in older infants, but these infants display a secondary peak in plasma levels. In newborns the elimination half-life of fentanyl is at least two and a half times that of the older child (Koehntop et al, 1986).

Not all babies require postoperative analgesia if they have been adequately anaesthetized, but they do require individual assessment. Warmth, swaddling, early feeding if possible, and local blocks reduce the need for opioid analgesics. Single, small doses of analgesics are effective, for example codeine phosphate 1 mg/kg i.m.; this will not cause respiratory depression. This agent should not be given intravenously as it occasionally causes a profound fall in cardiac output.

Continuous infusions have theoretical advantages and no cases of respiratory difficulties have been reported in spontaneously breathing newborns given 5–10 µg/kg/h of morphine (one-quarter to one-half the older child dose). However, the technique is vulnerable to dilutional errors or mechanical failure of the infusion pump. Such infusions should be confined to high-dependence areas where equipment for monitoring, resuscitation and respiratory support is available, and given only to those babies considered suitable after major abdominal or thoracic surgery.

The preterm baby

Many aspects of preterm physiology and anaesthetic management have already been covered. With increasing survival of babies born prematurely there is an increased need for surgery for conditions such as necrotizing enterocolitis, hydrocephalus and patent ductus arteriosus. Preterm babies are especially likely to develop inguinal hernia. The risks of anaesthesia are increased in this age group, with even less efficient control of ventilation than the term baby (Steward, 1982). There is also the additional possibility of residual lung damage from intubation and mechanical ventilation earlier in life. This mild bronchopulmonary dysplasia causes oxygen dependence, reduced lung compliance and tachypnoea at rest with an increased risk of postoperative respiratory failure. Such is the risk of general anaesthesia that techniques involving only caudal or spinal analgesia are widely advocated where applicable (Abajian et al, 1984; see Chapter 9).

It is likely that preterm babies, before the retina has become fully vascularized at about 42 weeks postconceptual age, are at risk of developing retinopathy of prematurity which may be caused by a high PaO_2 even during anaesthesia (Betts et al, 1977). Though other factors are probably involved, such as $PaCO_2$ and concentration of haemoglobin A, it is wise to limit the inspired oxygen concentration to give a PaO_2 between 50 and 75 mmHg (7–10 kPa). A satisfactory monitor is a transcutaneous oxygen electrode, which is a good guide to PaO_2, even though it may take up to 20 min to stabilize and may be affected in a non-linear fashion by anaesthetic gases. Oxygen saturation should be maintained between 90 and 92% on the pulse oximeter. The incidence of retinopathy is rising in spite of advances in the delivery and monitoring of oxygenation. Major surgery with general anaesthesia does not contribute to the risk, but it is assumed that the cicatricial form is caused by several factors, such as changes in PaO_2 and $PaCO_2$ (Flynn, 1984).

Some preterm babies may be so sensitive to anaesthetic agents that even nitrous oxide is unsuitable; for such babies it may be necessary to use air:oxygen mixtures to give the required fraction of oxygen concentration. Small doses of halothane or isoflurane will be needed intermittently.

The diaphragm is likely to fatigue easily and is a further factor causing reduced respiratory reserve. Animal work shows that halothane depresses the minute ventilation and FRC during spontaneous breathing in newborn lambs and doubles the $PaCO_2$. Even nitrous oxide may have some of these effects in preterm babies. The units of gas exchange are smaller in the preterm lung (75 μm diameter) compared with the adult (250 μm) and thus have a greater tendency to collapse, but the FRC is partly maintained by the high respiratory rate so that there is little time for the gas to escape and the FRC to fall. If the respiratory rate does fall, the FRC is reduced and during apnoea it may fall to very low levels (Gregory and Steward, 1983). At least 30% of premature babies have apnoea during the first few weeks of life, a tendency worsened by changes in temperature and with general anaesthesia. It is not uncommon for apnoea to occur during induction of anaesthesia but what is more disturbing is the tendency to apnoea in the postoperative period for up to 12 h after surgery. The infants most at risk are preterm babies in the age group up to 46 weeks postconceptual age; especially those with a history of previous apnoeic spells. Infants in this group are treated only for essential surgery and not on a day-stay basis; they are carefully monitored for apnoea for the first 24 h postoperatively. Theophylline 8 mg/kg i.v. may be given before the end of surgery in babies who have previously suffered from apnoeic episodes.

Intraventricular cerebral haemorrhage is the commonest serious neurological disorder of the neonatal period as it affects 40–50% of all infants below 35 weeks postconceptual age (Volpe, 1981), increasing in incidence as gestational age is shorter. Haemorrhage is associated with respiratory distress syndrome, hypoxia, acidosis, high ventilatory requirements, as well as coagulation abnormalities (Levene et al, 1982; McDonald et al, 1984).

If autoregulation of cerebral blood flow has failed with systemic hypotension and maximal cerebral vasodilatation, any sudden rise in cerebral blood flow may rupture the fragile, unsupported vascular matrix. This may occur after rapid infusion of blood volume expanders or with hyperosmolar solutions of glucose or sodium bicarbonate. There is an acute rise in blood pressure as a patent ductus is being ligated and this should be performed gently in the preterm baby.

Intraventricular cerebral haemorrhage can be detected via the anterior fontanelle by ultrasound imaging and this investigation is routine in all patients at risk. The degree of haemorrhage is graded I–IV, which helps with prognosis of severity of subsequent neurodevelopmental handicap. Grade I bleeding is confined to the periventricular germinal matrix, but if it ruptures into the ventricles there is a worse prognosis. Hydrocephalus commonly follows intraventricular haemorrhage; this may be managed conservatively or may require a ventriculo-peritoneal shunt at a later date.

Preterm newborns are very susceptible to infections and early signs of sepsis are subtle, including increasing apnoea and difficulty in maintaining temperature. Physical, humoral and cellular mechanisms of immunity have reduced efficiency in the newborn and there may be a relative hypogamma-globulinaemia falling to 10% of normal in the preterm baby. Neonatal anaesthesia involves invasive manoeuvres such as intubation and vascular access which provide a route for infection. The skin of the preterm baby is very delicate and easily becomes infected. Every care should be taken to use as sterile a technique as possible for all anaesthetic procedures.

REFERENCES

Abajian JC, Mellish RWP, Browne AF et al (1984) Spinal anesthesia for surgery in the high risk infant. *Anesthesia and Analgesia* **63**: 359–362.

Anand KJS, Sippell WG & Aynsley-Green A (1987) Randomized trial of fentanyl anaesthesia in preterm babies undergoing surgery: effect on the stress response. *Lancet* **i**: 243–248.

Anand KJS, Sippell WG & Schofield NM (1988) Does halothane anaesthesia decrease the metabolic and endocrine stress responses of newborn infants undergoing operation? *British Medical Journal* **296**: 668–672.

Berry FA & Gregory GA (1987) Do premature infants require anesthesia for surgery? *Anesthesiology* **67**: 291–293.

Besag FMC, Singh MP & Whitelaw AGL (1984) Surgery of the ill, extremely low birth weight infant: should transfer to the operating theatre be avoided? *Acta Paediatrica Scandinavica* **73**: 594–595.

Betts EK, Downes JJ, Schaffer DB et al (1977) Retrolental fibroplasia and oxygen administration during general anesthesia. *Anesthesiology* **47**: 518–520.

Blake AM, McIntosh N, Reynolds EOR et al (1975) Transport of newborn infants for intensive care. *British Medical Journal* **4**: 13–17.

Bloom BS (1984) Changing infant mortality: the need to spend more while getting less. *Pediatrics* **73**: 862–866.

Chessells JM (1979) Blood formation in infancy. *Archives of Disease in Childhood* **54**: 831–834.

Cogswell JJ, Hatch DJ, Kerr AA et al (1975) Effects of continuous positive airway pressure on lung mechanics of babies after operation for congenital heart disease. *Archives of Disease in Childhood* **50**: 799–804.

DaLuca FG (1987) The status of prenatal diagnosis and fetal surgery. *Pediatric Surgery International* **2**: 259–266.

Davenport HT (1980) *Paediatric Anaesthesia*, 3rd edn. London: Heinemann.

Dawes GS (1968) *Fetal and Neonatal Physiology*. Chicago: Year Book Medical Publishers.

Flynn JT (1984) Oxygen and retrolental fibroplasia: update and challenge. *Anesthesiology* **60:** 397–399.

Fox WW & Duara S (1983) Persistent pulmonary hypertension in the neonate: diagnosis and management. *Journal of Pediatrics* **103:** 505–514.

Gauderer MWL, Jassani MN & Izant RJ Jr (1984) Ultrasonographic antenatal diagnosis: will it change the spectrum of neonatal surgery? *Journal of Pediatric Surgery* **19:** 404–407.

Gregory GA & Steward DJ (1983) Life threatening perioperative apnea in the ex 'premie'. *Anesthesiology* **59:** 495–498.

Gross SC & Gardiner GG (1980) *Child Pain: Treatment Approaches in Pain: Meaning and Management*, pp 127–142. New York: JPMS Books.

Hackel A (1975) A medical transport system for the neonate. *Anesthesiology* **43:** 258–267.

Hatch DJ (1981) Respiratory measurement in infancy. In Gray TC and Rees GJ (eds) *Paediatric Anaesthesia*, pp 27–40. London: Butterworths.

Hatch DJ & Sumner E (1986) *Neonatal Anaesthesia and Perioperative Care*, 2nd edn. London: Arnold.

Haworth SG (1986) Lung biopsies in congenital heart disease: computer assisted correlations between structural and hemodynamic abnormalities. In: Doyle EF, Engle MA, Gersony WM et al (eds) *Pediatric Cardiology*, pp 942–945. New York: Springer-Verlag.

Haworth SG & Hislop AA (1981) Normal structural and functional adaptation to extrauterine life. *Journal of Pediatrics* **98:** 915–918

Hey EN (1972) Thermal regulation in the newborn. *British Journal of Hospital Medicine* **8:** 51–64.

Hey EN & Katz G (1970) The optimum thermal environment for naked babies. *Archives of Disease in Childhood* **45:** 328–334.

Hislop AA & Reid L (1981) Growth and development of the respiratory system: anatomical development. In Davis JA & Dobbing J (eds) *Scientific Foundations of Paediatrics*, 2nd edn, pp 390–431. London: Heinemann.

Keens TG, Bryan AL, Levison H et al (1978) Development pattern of muscle fiber types in human ventilatory muscles. *Journal of Applied Physiology* **44:** 909–913.

Koehntop DE, Rodman JH, Brundage DM et al (1986) Pharmacokinetics of fentanyl in neonates. *Anesthesia and Analgesia* **65:** 227–232.

Koren G, Butt W, Chinyonga H et al (1985) Postoperative morphine infusion in newborn infants: assessment of disposition characteristics and safety. *Journal of Pediatrics* **107:** 963–967.

Leading article (1978) Paediatric anaesthesia. *British Medical Journal* **ii:** 717–718.

LeDez KM & Lerman J (1987) Minimum alveolar concentration (MAC) of isoflurane in preterm infants. *Anesthesiology* **67:** 301–307.

Levene MI, Fawer C-L & Lamont RF (1982) Risk factors in the development of intraventricular haemorrhage in the preterm neonate. *Archives of Disease in Childhood* **57:** 410–417.

Levine JD & Gordon GA (1982) Pain in prelingual children and its evaluation by pain-induced vocalisation. *Pain* **14:** 85–93.

Lubchenco LO (1976) *The High Risk Infant*. Philadelphia: Saunders.

McDonagh AF (1981) Phototherapy: a new twist to bilirubin. *Journal of Pediatrics* **99:** 909–911.

McDonald MM, Johnson ML, Rumack CM et al (1984) Role of coagulopathy in newborn intracranial hemorrhage. *Pediatrics* **74:** 26–31.

Mehta A, Wright BM & Shore C (1988) Clinical fontanometry in the newborn. *Lancet* **i:** 754–756.

Miller MJ, Carlo WA & Martin RJ (1985) Continuous positive airway pressure selectively reduces obstructive apnea in preterm infants. *Journal of Pediatrics* **106:** 91–94.

Milligan DWA (1980) Failure of autoregulation and intraventricular haemorrhage in preterm infants. *Lancet* **i**: 896–898.

Moss IR, Conner H, Yee WFH et al (1982) Human β-endorphin-like immunoreactivity in the perinatal/neonatal period. *Journal of Pediatrics* **101**: 443–446.

Mott JC (1980) Patent ductus arteriosus: experimental aspects. *Archives of Disease in Childhood* **55**: 99–105.

Murat I, Moriette G, Blin MC et al (1981) The efficacy of caffeine in the treatment of recurrent idiopathic apnea in premature infants. *Journal of Pediatrics* **99**: 984–989.

Neuman GG & Hansen DD (1980) The anaesthetic management of preterm infants undergoing ligation of patent ductus arteriosus. *Canadian Anaesthetists' Society Journal* **27**: 248–253.

Purcell-Jones G, Dormon F & Sumner E (1987) The use of opioids in neonates. A retrospective study of 933 cases. *Anaesthesia* **42**: 1316–1320.

Roberton NRC (1986) Neonatal jaundice. In Meadow R (ed) *Recent Advances in Paediatrics No 8*. Edinburgh: Churchill Livingstone.

Saigal S, Rosenbaum P, Stoskopf B et al (1984) Outcome in infants 501–1000 g birth weight delivered to residents of the McMaster Health Region. *Journal of Pediatrics* **105**: 969–976.

Sauer PJJ, Dane HJ & Visser HKA (1984) New standards for neutral thermal environment of healthy very low birth weight infants in 1 week of life. *Archives of Disease in Childhood* **59**: 18–22.

Spielman FT, Seeds JW & Corke BC (1984) Anaesthesia for fetal surgery. *Anaesthesia* **39**: 756–759.

Steward DJ (1982) Preterm infants are more prone to complications following minor surgery than are term infants. *Anesthesiology* **56**: 304–306.

Volpe JJ (1981) Neonatal intraventricular hemorrhage. *New England Journal of Medicine* **304**: 886–891.

Wark HJ (1983) Postoperative jaundice in children—the influence of halothane. *Anaesthesia* **38**: 237–242.

Williamson PS & Williamson RN (1983) Physiologic stress reduction by a local anesthetic during newborn circumcision. *Pediatrics* **71**: 36–40.

Anaesthesia for paediatric surgery

OPHTHALMIC SURGERY

General principles

Since few children are able to tolerate eye surgery under topical analgesia, general anaesthesia is usually required. The majority of children presenting for ophthalmic surgery are in ASA categories I or II, but congenital or acquired medical problems occur in a significant number of cases, so that careful preoperative assessment is always essential. The presence of serious associated anomalies may act as a contraindication to even minor surgery being performed on a day-stay basis.

Tracheal intubation is required for most ophthalmic procedures, and preformed tubes such as the RAE (Ring et al, 1975) are very satisfactory for most cases. Succinylcholine should be avoided in children at risk from malignant hyperpyrexia, in those with myotonia, where prolonged muscle contraction may occur, and when it is necessary to avoid an increase in intraocular pressure. Anaesthesia may be maintained using controlled or spontaneous respiration, the former being preferable for all but the most trivial operations in the first 6 months of life. Smooth induction, maintenance and recovery are extremely important, especially for intraocular surgery.

As with all branches of paediatric anaesthesia, careful and meticulous continuous monitoring is essential, with particular importance being given to the ECG because of the high incidence of cardiac irregularities which arise during ophthalmic surgery.

Associated anomalies

It is important to remember that congenital defects are often multiple, so that a child presenting with one congenital anomaly, however trivial, may have other congenital problems such as renal or cardiac disease which may be more significant to the anaesthetist. Ophthalmic problems form part of a number of well recognized syndromes (Table 12.1), but other anomalies which do not fit into any of these syndromes may also occur.

Table 12.1. Syndromes with anaesthetic implications for
ophthalmic surgery

Syndrome	Principle anomalies
Conradi–Hunermann	*Cataracts*
	Dyschondroplasia, dwarfism
	Intubation problems
	Poor veins
Freeman–Sheldon	*Strabismus*
(whistling face)	Microstomia—sometimes extreme
Hallerman–Streiff	*Cataract, microphthalmia*
	Mandibular hypoplasia
Homocystinuria	*Dislocated lenses*
	Skeletal and cardiac anomalies
	Coagulation defects, hypoglycaemia
Laurence–Moon–Biedl	*Retinitis pigmentosa*
	Obesity
	Renal failure
Lowe	*Cataract, glaucoma*
	Severe mental retardation
	Hypotonia
	Renal tubular dysfunction
Marfan's	*Dislocated lenses*
	Skeletal anomalies
	Cardiac anomalies
Mucopolysaccharidoses	
Morquio (IV)	*Corneal opacities*
	Intubation problems
	Kyphoscoliosis
	Cardiorespiratory failure
Maroteaux–Lamy (VI)	*Atlanto-occipital dislocation*
Myopathies and	*Squint*
muscular disorders	Respiratory problems
	Malignant hyperpyrexia
	Cardiac conduction defects
Rubella syndrome	*Cataract*
	Deafness
	Interstitial pneumonia
	Cardiac anomalies
Smith–Lemli–Opitz	*Squint*
	Microcephaly
	Micrognathia
Stickler	*Retinal detachment, strabismus*
	Micrognathia
	Cleft palate

Ophthalmic problems may be secondary to other medical problems, as in
the case of retinopathy of prematurity following a period of hyperoxia. In
addition, there is the possibility of medical problems arising as a consequence of the ophthalmic lesion itself, as in the case of retinoblastoma.

Malignant hyperpyrexia

A high incidence of malignant hyperpyrexia has been reported during squint and ptosis surgery, confirming the impression that malignant hyperpyrexia-susceptible individuals often demonstrate musculoskeletal abnormalities. This subject is fully discussed in Chapter 21.

Intraocular surgery

The control of intraocular pressure (IOP) is the main problem facing the anaesthetist during intraocular surgery. IOP represents a balance between the formation of aqueous humour and its drainage through the canal of Schlemm into the aqueous veins and periocular venous system. The most marked increases in IOP occur during coughing, straining and vomiting, so that the need for smooth induction, maintenance and recovery from anaesthesia is clear. Laryngoscopy and tracheal intubation have also been shown to raise IOP, though the increase is transient and IOP returns to normal within a few minutes, so that it is of no great significance in elective surgery. Of the drugs affecting IOP (Table 12.2), succinylcholine has been shown to cause the most marked increase, with conflicting results being reported for ketamine. The effect of succinylcholine can possibly be minimized by pretreatment with a small dose of non-depolarizing relaxant, though Meyers et al (1978) have expressed doubts about the efficacy of this pretreatment. The intravenous administration of lignocaine (1.5 mg/kg) has also been suggested as pretreatment to minimize the rise in IOP caused by succinylcholine.

Table 12.2. Drugs affecting intraocular pressure (IOP) (modified from France, 1983)

Drug	Effect on IOP
Succinylcholine	+
Ketamine	+ or 0
Pancuronium	0 or −
Atracurium	0
Vecuronium	0
Tubocurarine	−
Halothane	0 or −
Isoflurane	0 or −
Other general anaesthetics, hypnotics and sedatives	−
Carbonic anhydrase inhibitors	−
Osmotic diuretics	−
Topical ophthalmic drugs	
Adrenaline	−
Ecothiopate	−
Pilocarpine	−
Timolol maleate	−

Tubocurarine causes a consistent fall in IOP, as do most general anaesthetics, sedatives and hypnotics, and a range of topically applied ophthalmic drugs. Some studies have suggested that halothane and isoflurane reduce IOP, while others have found no significant effect.

Increases in IOP may cause damage to the contents of the globe, such as herniation of the vitreous into the anterior chamber, or even extrusion of the contents of the open eye. In operations for cataract the increase in IOP which may occur with crying and coughing in the postoperative period can also prejudice the success of the surgery, so the child should be kept as calm as possible during this period.

Falls in IOP are probably less important than increases, but may lead to falsely low diagnostic measurements being made in borderline glaucoma. In these cases IOP measurements should probably be made shortly after induction of anaesthesia, before tracheal intubation. A short period of inhalational anaesthesia has been shown not to lower IOP significantly (Dear et al, 1987).

The commonest intraocular operations in children are those for glaucoma and cataract. Intraocular tumours are relatively rare, but severe oculocardiac reflex dysrhythmics may occur during enucleation. Extreme care must be taken to ensure that the operation is performed on the correct eye.

Glaucoma

The common pressure-relieving operations in glaucoma are goniotomy, iridectomy and trabeculectomy, and these require smooth general anaesthesia along the lines described below. Succinylcholine is contraindicated if ecothiopate has been used in the previous 4–6 weeks, since prolonged block will occur. Ecothiopate (Phospholine) iodide is, however, seldom used in the treatment of glaucoma nowadays. Atropine-resistant bradycardia has been reported following the use of timolol maleate, a non-selective beta-blocker.

Cataract

Early surgery in the treatment of cataract gives the best chance of satisfactory vision, so these patients often require anaesthesia in the first few weeks of life. It is therefore important for the anaesthetist to be aware of the general problems of neonatal anaesthesia outlined elsewhere in this book, and for these operations to be performed whenever possible in paediatric centres. Approximately half of all cataracts in children are congenital, the rest being due to specific causes like Marfan's syndrome or infections such as toxoplasmosis, cytomegalic inclusion disease and herpes simplex. Drug-induced cataracts may develop following steroid therapy.

The specific requirements for cataract surgery are smooth anaesthesia in a completely still patient, with minimal change in IOP either during or for the first few hours following surgery. Duration of anaesthesia is unpredictable, making the use of infusions of the newer non-depolarizing muscle relaxants, atracurium (8 µg/kg/min) or vecuronium (1.5 µg/kg/min), monitored by peripheral nerve stimulation, ideally suitable. It has recently been shown (Bonsu et al, 1987; Ridley and Hatch, 1988) that the post-tetanic count is a more sensitive monitor of the degree of relaxation with this technique than the train-of-four. Nitrous oxide is not contraindicated in these children, since although air is introduced into the anterior chamber of the eye, the effect of nitrous oxide on its volume does not appear to be clinically significant. Supplementary inhalational or intravenous agents may be used, though intravenous narcotics must be administered with caution in the first year of life because of the increased sensitivity of the respiratory centre to their depressant effects. Laryngospasm can be prevented by delaying extubation until the child is virtually awake, though coughing on the tube must be avoided. Intramuscular codeine phosphate (1 mg/kg) provides safe postoperative analgesia in infants, though it's half-life is prolonged in the very young.

Penetrating eye injury

Much has been written about the avoidance of increases in IOP in cases of penetrating eye injury, particularly with reference to the use of succinylcholine. In some of these cases, however, the eye is clearly irretrievably damaged, and in others iris prolapse may have sealed the wound, effectively preventing further loss of intraocular contents. There are, however, a small number of patients in whom any increase of IOP may cause serious disruption of the eye leading to avoidable loss of vision. It is thus important to discuss the situation with the surgeon since the avoidance of succinylcholine increases the risk of aspiration of gastric contents, and the balance of relative risks must be assessed. A suggested anaesthetic technique for this situation is described on p. 451.

Extraocular surgery

Squint

The main concern for the anaesthetist during squint (strabismus) surgery is the ease with which the oculocardiac reflex can be elicited by the surgeon when traction is applied to the extraocular muscles, particularly the medial or lateral rectus. The reflex also sometimes occurs during enucleation of the eye. The afferent limb of the reflex arc is formed by the oculomotor branch of the trigeminal nerve, and the efferent limb by the vagus. Bradycardia is the commonest reflex change to occur, but other arrhythmias are also occasionally produced, including bigemini, ventricular ectopic beats and even ventricular fibrillation. The incidence is said to be as high as 90% in non-atropinized patients. The arrhythmia can be very severe, but usually disappears as soon as the muscle traction is discontinued. Atropine 0.02 mg/kg or glycopyrrolate 0.01 mg/kg intravenously are equally effective in blocking the reflex, and it is sound practice to administer this routinely following induction in these cases.

Drugs which are sometimes used topically to produce vasoconstriction of the conjunctival vessels may cause problems for the anaesthetist. Hypertension has been reported following topical instillation of adrenaline or phenylephrine, and arrhythmias can occur, particularly in association with halothane. Enflurane has the highest threshold for the production of arrhythmias in the presence of adrenaline, but problems seldom arise even with halothane if not more than one drop of 1 in 1000 solution is instilled into each eye. Patients with strabismus are sometimes treated with ecothiopate (Phosphaline) iodide and if this drug has been used in the previous 4–6 weeks succinylcholine is contraindicated, since prolonged block will occur.

Nausea and vomiting are more frequent following squint surgery than many other types of surgery in children, but are seldom persistent and usually respond to simple antiemetic therapy such as prochlorperazine 0.2 mg/kg (maximum dose 12.5 mg). Droperidol has also been used effectively (0.075 mg/kg intravenously) in the treatment of postanaesthetic vomiting in children (Lerman et al, 1986).

Strabismus operations are not particularly painful, and many children require no postoperative analgesia. For those who do, a mild analgesic is usually sufficient.

The risk of malignant hyperpyrexia is only significant in secondary strabismus, when it forms part of a generalized muscular disorder. Strabismus may also be secondary to cerebral palsy.

Nasolachrymal duct obstruction

Obstruction of the nasolachrymal duct in children is usually relieved without difficulty by syringing and probing under general anaesthesia. Although simple probing has been carried out without tracheal intubation this is not an entirely safe practice, since the procedure can cause bleeding into the pharynx. Intubation with packing of the oropharynx is therefore recommended for this procedure in every case. In a small percentage of cases syringing and probing fails to cure the problem, and these patients require insertion of silastic tubes into the tear ducts for several weeks. In cases of persistent obstruction, dacryocystorhinostomy may be required. Blood loss during this procedure may be considerable, and can be reduced by topical vasoconstriction of the nasal mucosa. Induced hypotension is used in some centres.

Surgery to the eyelids

Surgery to the eyelids is often of a minor nature, for removal of dermoid cysts and similar lesions, or may be more major, for ptosis or major deformities of the lids. Ptosis correction may involve elevation of the lid using a fascia lata sling. These procedures are fairly lengthy, and may involve moderately severe blood loss. If performed for myasthenia gravis the well documented anaesthetic problems posed by this condition will require attention.

GENITOURINARY SURGERY

Preoperative assessment

Children presenting for genitourinary surgery need particularly careful preoperative assessment, since they may have impaired renal function, secondary disturbances of body chemistry and fluid balance, or other significant congenital anomalies.

Haemoglobin levels are often low, either as a result of chronic infection, or as a secondary effect of the disease process, as with Wilm's tumour, for example. A moderate reduction in haemoglobin should not necessarily be regarded as an indication for postponing surgery, though children with levels below 7 g/100 ml should not be accepted for anaesthesia unless the surgery is urgent.

Children in acute renal failure seldom require genitourinary surgery, except in the newborn period for obstructive lesions such as posterior urethral valves. The blood chemistry at birth reflects that of the mother, so that urea and creatinine values may be relatively normal at first, as may serum electrolyte levels. Normal urine output should be at least 0.5 ml/kg. When the underlying cause of the acute renal failure is reversible and treatment is instituted early, chances of recovery are good, though the recovery phase with polyuria requires careful management.

It is much more common to be presented with a child in chronic renal failure, and in this case it is necessary to assess whether renal function is adequate to stand the additional stress of anaesthesia and surgery. With reduction in glomerular filtration rate (GFR), plasma urea and creatinine levels rise, though the catabolic effect of growth may mask this to some degree, and normal values vary with age (Barratt and Baillod, 1982). The effect of chronic renal failure on water and electrolyte balance depends largely on the aetiology. In chronic obstructive renal disease the renal medullary concentrating mechanism is mainly affected, with the production of relatively large volumes of dilute urine which is low in sodium. In chronic glomerulonephritis the reduction in GFR usually exceeds the reduction in tubular reabsorption, so that sodium and water retention develop. Diseases such as chronic pyelonephritis tend mainly to affect sodium reabsorption, with the loss of significant amounts of sodium in the urine and a tendency to hyponatraemia. Careful recording of intake and output, together with serum and urinary osmolality and electrolyte levels, is therefore essential for the safe management of these cases, together with clinical evaluation of the state of hydration. Metabolic acidosis is common, making the child more vulnerable to any further metabolic upset.

A detailed account of fluid and electrolyte management can be found in Chapter 8.

Hypertension may be secondary to renovascular disease or in rare cases may suggest the presence of a catecholamine-secreting tumour. If the hypertension has been of long standing, a careful check should be made for signs of hypertensive cardiovascular disease (Dillon, 1982).

Renal patients may be receiving a number of drugs of significance to the anaesthetist. These include diuretics, antihypertensives and steroids.

Preoperative assessment should always include a check for the presence of other associated congenital anomalies, which may or may not be directly related to the renal problem.

Congenital renal anomalies

The main syndromes affecting renal function have been listed elsewhere in this book (see Chapter 21). Renal anomalies also frequently occur, however, either in isolation or in association with other congenital defects, in a non-specific manner. They may be associated with obvious external defects, such as anomalies of the limbs or face, but are not infrequently found in association with internal anomalies, particularly those of the cardiovascular, pulmonary or gastrointestinal systems. The urogenital anomaly may affect the kidney or urinary tract, or may appear as an external defect, such as exstrophy or hypospadias.

Kidney

Congenital anomalies of the kidney vary from minor defects of little or no clinical significance, through conditions with impaired renal function such as polycystic kidneys, to complete renal agenesis with oligohydramnios, secondary pulmonary hypoplasia and compression defects as seen in Potter's syndrome. Varying degrees of maldevelopment of the renal parenchyma—renal dysplasia—may occur, either as the primary anomaly or secondary to urinary tract obstruction.

Renovascular anomalies such as renal artery stenosis may cause severe hypertension, and anomalous renal vessels may obstruct urine flow, as may other renal anomalies such as supernumerary or ectopic kidneys, malrotations and duplications. Horseshoe kidneys are vulnerable to trauma because of their location and relative immobility.

Urinary tract

Congenital anomalies of the urinary tract may cause intrauterine urinary obstruction leading to secondary renal dysplasia or hydronephrosis as well as oligohydramnios and its sequelae. Distal urinary tract obstruction, causing severe bladder distension, is now thought to interfere with the development of surrounding structures, causing the condition now referred to as the urethral obstruction malformation complex. This may include deficiences in abdominal wall musculature—prune belly syndrome—malrotation, cryptorchidism and lower limb anomalies (Pagon et al, 1979; Nakayama et al, 1984). The commonest causes are posterior urethral valves, urethral strictures or diverticuli.

A combination of urinary tract obstruction and infection may cause ureteric reflux, with secondary renal parenchymal damage leading later to the development of hypertension in some cases. Patients with reflux may present for diagnostic cystoscopy, retrograde pyelogram, urodynamic studies or reimplantation of the ureters.

Prune belly syndrome (Figure 12.1).   The prune belly syndrome occurs in 1 in 40 000 births, almost exclusively in males. The role of lower urinary tract obstruction in the aetiology of the condition has been referred to above, but other congenital anomalies may occur in association. These include cryptorchidism, volvulus, pulmonary stenosis, deafness and men-

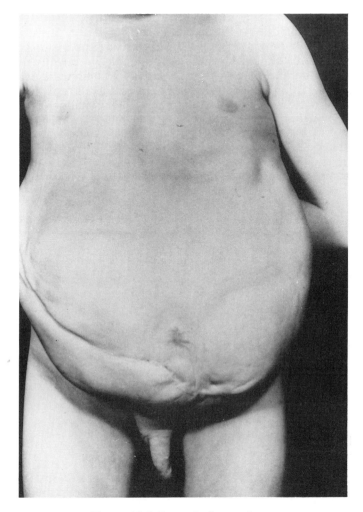

Figure 12.1. Prune belly syndrome.

tal retardation. The severity of the muscular defect varies, as does the degree of renal dysplasia. The skin over the abdomen is classically wrinkled like a prune, and the testes are undescended. Lack of abdominal musculature often makes coughing and clearing of respiratory secretions ineffective, which leads to a high incidence of chest infections, especially if there is associated pulmonary hypoplasia. Renal function may be seriously impaired, and 20% of babies are stillborn or die from renal or pulmonary failure within the neonatal period. Many children require operations to improve urinary drainage and prevent further renal damage.

Anaesthesia should aim to avoid aspiration of gastric contents, either by awake intubation in the newborn or by rapid sequence induction with cricoid pressure. Anaesthesia can however be conducted satisfactorily with spontaneous or controlled ventilation, and normal doses of muscle relaxants can be used. In a recent review of 133 anaesthetics in 36 children with prune belly syndrome (Henderson et al, 1987), minor postoperative chest infections posed the greatest problems. Pre- and postoperative chest physiotherapy and antibiotic cover may reduce the incidence of respiratory complications, and postoperative ventilation is seldom required.

Posterior urethral valves.   As well as possibly leading to the urethral obstruction malformation complex mentioned above, posterior urethral valves cause acute urinary obstruction at birth. Uraemia, dehydration, acidosis, hyperkalaemia, hyponatraemia and sepsis may all be present and require correction before surgery can be carried out. This is carried out either by urethral or suprapubic catheterization. In the immediate period after relief of the obstruction a massive diuresis may occur. As much as 1 l of fluid may be required in the first 12 h after surgery, together with potassium supplements. Surgical correction is usually obtained by cystoscopic fulguration of the valves via the urethra. The long-term results depend on the degree of renal damage, with many children developing chronic renal failure by the time they reach puberty.

Bladder exstrophy

This major congenital defect has an incidence of between 1 in 10 000 and 1 in 50 000 live births, with males being affected six times as frequently as females. The defect arises because of failure of the infraumbilical mesenchyme to migrate into the area of the cloacal membrane, preventing the midline fusion of the infraumbilical anterior abdominal wall. The mucosa of the posterior bladder wall and ureteric orifices remains exposed, and there is complete epispadias. Infection is inevitable, and the ureteric orifices become fibrosed, leading to urinary obstruction. The bladder mucosa undergoes squamous metaplasia, and adenocarcinoma may develop. Early surgical closure in the newborn period may minimize these complications (Johnston, 1982a), and can usually be accomplished without iliac osteotomies. If repair is delayed beyond the first few days of life, bilateral iliac osteotomies are necessary, and these are performed with the infant in the prone position before the baby is turned supine for formal closure of the bladder. Considerable blood loss should be expected, and central and peripheral venous cannulas should be inserted.

Even after early closure, however, problems of incontinence, bladder capacity and abnormalities of the urinary tract may remain. Repeated anaesthetics may be required for assessment of the degree of upper urinary tract dilatation, for continence and bladder enhancement operations (ileocystoplasty or colocystoplasty) or for creation of artificial sphincters. Most of these procedures are major, many requiring full arterial and central venous monitoring, as induced hypotension may be necessary to minimize blood loss.

Caudal analgesia is a useful adjunct to general anaesthesia for bladder exstrophy surgery.

Hypospadias

Many operations have been performed over the years for this common anomaly, with varying degrees of success. Those most commonly performed for mild or moderate degrees of hypospadias do not present the anaesthetist with any particular problems, and techniques using spontaneous or controlled ventilation can be employed. Intra- and postoperative pain relief can be effectively provided by caudal analgesia or dorsal nerve block of the penis. These blocks are described in detail in Chapter 9.

In recent years, more major operations such as the Duckett procedure or bladder mucosal graft operations have been carried out. The Duckett procedure is fairly lengthy and many anaesthetists would use controlled ventilation for this reason. Bladder mucosal graft operations involve laparotomy and hence always require muscle relaxation and controlled ventilation, and blood loss may be considerable.

Though hypospadias may be associated with hernia, hydrocoele and undescended testis, other anomalies of the urinary tract are rare.

Orchidopexy

Undescended testis (cryptorchidism) occurs in 1% of full-term infants, and more commonly in prematurity. Orchidopexy is usually performed in early childhood to minimize the risks of infertility and testicular malignancy, and to repair the associated inguinal hernia. Traction on the spermatic cord is a powerful vagal stimulant, and may induce severe laryngospasm in the non-intubated patient unless deeply anaesthetized or protected by adequate local nerve block. Effective regional analgesia can be produced with caudal or ilioinguinal–iliohypogastric nerve blocks, described fully on p. 228.

Circumcision

Anaesthesia for circumcision can be conducted with spontaneous or controlled ventilation. If spontaneous ventilation is employed using a facemask, relatively deep anaesthesia is required to avoid laryngeal spasm when the foreskin is clamped unless effective local analgesia is obtained. Caudal anaesthesia using 0.25% bupivacaine (0.5 ml/kg) or dorsal nerve block of the penis with 0.5% bupivacaine *without adrenaline* (0.2 ml/kg) provides a useful adjunct to general anaesthesia, and also gives good postoperative pain relief. These techniques are described in detail in Chapter 9.

There is no medical indication for circumcision in the newborn baby, and the practice of performing this procedure soon after birth, often without anaesthesia, should be abandoned.

Adrenogenital syndrome

Deficiency of C-21 hydroxylase activity causes masculinization in the female, and if complete also leads to severe salt loss from impairment of aldosterone secretion. C-11 hydroxylase deficiency, a rarer anomaly, is associated with hypertension. Treatment with cortisone suppresses adrenocorticotrophic hormone production, but malformation of the external genitalia requires surgical genitoplasty. This is usually performed at about 6 months of age. Careful preoperative evaluation of fluid and electrolyte state is necessary, and steroid cover is required in doses of hydrocortisone 25 mg below 10 kg; 50 mg at 10–30 kg and 100 mg over 30 kg body weight. These children are usually fat, and venous access may be difficult. Considerable blood loss can occur, so that a reliable venous line is essential. Caudal analgesia is helpful in reducing blood loss as well as providing good postoperative analgesia. Hydrocortisone is given immediately postoperatively, but fludrocortisone is restarted when the patient has been re-established on oral feeding.

Tumours

Tumours arising in the renal area, even when they are not renal in origin, may affect renal function either by their size or by compression of renal vessels or ureter.

Nephroblastoma (Wilm's tumour)

This is the commonest abdominal tumour in childhood, usually presenting between 6 months and 5 years of age. In about 5% of cases bilateral tumours are found, and there is an association with other renal anomalies, including hypoplastic or horseshoe kidney, duplications and hypospadias. Preoperative anaemia may exist, and hypertension may result either from renal artery compression or secretion of renin by the tumour. The lungs and liver are common sites for metastases. Treatment is by surgical resection, followed by radiotherapy or chemotherapy.

The anaesthetist is faced with a number of problems. The tumour may be large enough to splint the diaphragm and restrict respiration, and will also increase the risk of regurgitation of gastric contents, so that rapid sequence induction with cricoid pressure is advisable. The tumour may infiltrate into the inferior vena cava or renal vein, and venous return may be compromised during surgical manipulation. Blood loss can be massive in an already anaemic patient, so transfusion should be started early. Venous access should be into the upper part of the body, and central venous pressure should be measured by the internal jugular or subclavian route. Direct arterial cannulation may be helpful, but is not essential. Third space losses are usually high, and volume replacement should bear this in mind. Renal function may be defective, especially if there are associated anomalies in the remaining kidney.

In the case of bilateral tumours the kidneys are sometimes packed with ice to preserve renal function. This is especially useful when surgical removal of tumour mass by partial nephrectomy is required. It is important to avoid systemic hypothermia by keeping the child well covered and on a warming mattress, by warming and humidifying the inspired gases, and by using warm fluids for volume replacement. Occasionally 'bench surgery' is undertaken, in which the kidney is removed, the tumour is dissected from it, and then the kidney is replaced.

Anaesthesia may be required for radiotherapy or for subsequent surgery, when the adverse effects of chemotherapy, particularly on the cardiovascular system, must be borne in mind. Ketamine is a useful agent for radiotherapy in children.

Neuroblastoma

This retroperitoneal tumour, which arises from the adrenal medulla or paravertebral ganglia, is found more commonly in females than males (Johnston, 1982b). Derived from neural crest tissue, it may invade the spinal canal, causing cord compression, and can also be found in the mediastinum. The common sites of metastasis are bone marrow, liver and brain. The problems facing the anaesthetist are similar to those in Wilm's tumour, related largely to the size of the tumour, blood loss and compression of surrounding structures. Hypertension may develop either from renal artery stenosis or as a result of catecholamine secretion. Approximately 80% of cases have raised VMA (vanillylmandelic acid) but only 10–15% have symptoms of catecholamine secretion. These should be treated as for phaeochromocytoma.

Phaeochromocytoma

This is a rare tumour arising from chromaffin cells derived from the neural crest. Tumours may be single or multiple, and are found anywhere along the sympathetic chain from the base of the skull to the lower abdomen, though the majority arise within the adrenal glands. Multiple tumours may occur. The most striking feature of these tumours is the secretion of catecholamines, often in large quantities. This is particularly hazardous if the undiagnosed patient presents for unrelated surgery, since careful preoperative preparation is essential for a successful outcome. Adrenaline is usually the main catecholamine produced by intra-adrenal tumours, with noradrenaline produced by those sited elsewhere. Extra-adrenal sites are commoner in children than in adults, and in one paediatric series 70% were bilateral (Kaufman et al, 1983).

The presence of high levels of circulating catecholamine in the bloodstream produces physiological changes which must be understood by the anaesthetist. When the main catecholamine is noradrenaline, severe and prolonged peripheral vasoconstriction leads to marked reduction of circulating blood volume. Administration of general anaesthesia in the unprepared patient leads to a sudden and dramatic vasodilatation effectively producing a massive hypovolaemia which can be catastrophic. Preoperative α-adrenergic blockade (e.g. phenoxybenzamine orally) must be instituted a week or so before surgery, to allow time for restoration of a normal circulating blood volume. Tumours secreting mainly adrenaline are associated with tachycardia and tachyarrhythmias requiring preoperative β-blockade, but with less peripheral vasoconstriction. In most cases of phaeochromocytoma the α effect predominates (Hull, 1986).

Diagnostic tests include estimation of urinary catecholamine metabolites. Intermediate metanephrines have proved more reliable diagnostic pointers than hydroxy-methoxy-mandelic acid (HMMA), also referred to as vanillyl-mandelic acid (VMA), but false negatives are not uncommon. Plasma catecholamine levels provide the best indicator, but may be raised in other causes of hypertension.

Preoperative preparation.   Phenoxybenzamine is the most commonly used α-adrenergic blocking agent in the preoperative preparation of these patients for elective surgery. This long-acting drug must be used with caution (1–2 mg/kg twice daily orally) at first, since it blocks not only postsynaptic α_1 receptors, but also presynaptic α_2 receptors, leading to an increase in noradrenaline release by loss of negative feedback. Postural hypotension may also occur. When effective α-blockade has been achieved, tachycardia may be controlled by β-blocking agents. β-Blockade should never be used before α-blockade has been established, since vasoconstriction may be worsened. Recently, pretreatment with the calcium influx blocker, nifedipine (0.5 mg/kg/day, orally) has been used successfully in some centres (Serfas et al, 1983; Landers et al, 1985).

Volume loading in the immediate preoperative period is not thought to be necessary if effective α-blockade has been established over a long enough period, since spontaneous correction of blood volume occurs. Patients presenting for emergency surgery, however, do require preoperative volume loading, monitored by invasive arterial and central venous pressure measurement. In these cases, preoperative adrenergic blockade is best performed with an infusion of labetalol starting at 1 mg/kg/h, and even then the risk of anaesthesia is substantially increased. Serum electrolytes, creatinine and blood sugar should be checked, and ECG should be performed to exclude cardiac ischaemia and evaluate any arrhythmias.

Anaesthetic management should be aimed at avoiding those drugs which stimulate catecholamine release, either directly or indirectly, suppressing the adrenergic response to surgical stimulation and minimizing the response to tumour handling. Sedative or narcotic premedication is likely to be helpful in reducing anxiety and hence catecholamine levels. Fentanyl and vecuronium would appear to be logical drugs to use, since neither causes histamine release. Alfentanil has also been advocated, since it has good vasodilating properties and a short elimination half-life. Enflurane is probably the volatile inhalational agent of choice because of its relative lack of myocardial sensitivity in the presence of catecholamines (Johnston et al, 1976). Intravenous access should be established before induction of anaesthesia, and ECG, arterial and central venous pressures must be monitored throughout the operation and immediate postoperative period. Periods of hypertension occurring during surgery can be controlled with an infusion of sodium nitroprusside. Phentolamine is less satisfactory because of the tachycardia and tachyphylaxis which occur. Ventricular arrhythmias, if they arise, are treated with lignocaine. Amiodarone has been reported to be effective in controlling supraventricular tachycardia (Solares et al, 1986). If β-blockers are used, they should be cardioselective, but in the presence of cardiomyopathy may cause cardiac failure.

Anaesthesia for renal transplantation

Renal transplantation is being increasingly performed for end-stage renal failure in children (Fernando, 1982; Potter et al, 1986). Preoperative clinical assessment of the recipient must be undertaken to ensure that the child is fit for surgery, and to decide whether preoperative dialysis is required. Preoperative investigations should include full blood count, electrolytes, calcium, urea and creatinine estimations, and chest X-ray. An average of 4–6 units of blood should be cross-matched, depending on the age of the child.

Particular note should be taken of any drug therapy which the child has recently received, including steroids, which may require additional cover for the perioperative period. Recipients of their first grafts with no history or cytotoxic antibodies will receive immunosuppressant drugs, including steroids, before surgery. β-Blockade should be discontinued, and β-sympathetic drive can best be enhanced if necessary with an infusion of dobutamine (2–10 μg/kg/min according to response).

Premedication may be prescribed, though reduced doses may be required. Respiratory depression has been reported after the use of narcotic analgesics in anuric patients. Antibiotic cover for cadaver graft recipients should commence with the premedication, continuing for at least 48 h.

The main anaesthetic problems which may arise, apart from any relating to the general condition of the recipient, are those of potential major blood loss. Transplantation of a donor kidney from an adult or large child into a small recipient requires anastomoses to the aorta and inferior vena cava, with cross-clamping, rather than to the iliac vessels. Reliable peripheral, central venous and arterial lines should therefore be inserted into the upper part of the body. In children who have had previous arteriovenous shunts, sites for arterial cannulation may be limited. It has been suggested that an existing shunt can be disconnected so that the arterial end can be used to monitor blood pressure and sample arterial blood, and the venous end for infusion (Cramolini, 1987), but extreme care must be taken to avoid infection.

Acidosis may develop during the period of aortic cross-clamping, and potassium toxicity has been reported from the transfusion of cadaver kidney preservation fluid into the circulation. A large kidney may absorb a considerable proportion of the child's cardiac output so that significant hypotension may occur on removal of the arterial clamps. Transfusion to a reasonably high central venous pressure before release of the clamps will minimize this problem. Transplanting a large kidney into a small infant may require maximal muscle relaxation during closure, which can be obtained using a drug like atracurium which does not rely on renal excretion for its elimination. Venous return may be compromised during abdominal closure.

A high urine output (at least 2 ml/kg/h) is desirable, and this should be continued into the postoperative period. Mannitol (0.5 g/kg) may be given in theatre before release of the clamps, and dopamine infusion in a renal dose (2 μg/kg/min) should be started on return to the postoperative ward. Serum and urinary electrolytes and osmolalities should be checked regularly, and fluid replacement adjusted as appropriate. Postoperative hypovolaemia should be avoided by clinical observation of the peripheral circulation and maintaining a central venous pressure of between 8 and 10 cm/H_2O, using blood or plasma according to the haematocrit. Postoperative hypertension can be controlled with hydralazine 1 mg/kg/day or labetalol. Drugs used in the control of acute hypertensive crises in children are shown in Table 12.3.

Anaesthetic agents in renal disease

Most studies have shown that changes in renal function during anaesthesia, particularly reduction in urine flow, are more commonly due to extrarenal factors such as fluid deprivation and the stress response to surgery than to primary renal factors. Light levels of anaesthesia (1 MAC (minimum alveolar concentration)) do not appear to interfere with renal function or autoregulation of renal blood flow, and even at 2 MAC there is rapid recovery of any transient decrease in renal function caused by fall in cardiac output if the patient is well hydrated (Berry, 1983). It is however well known that anaesthetic agents which release inorganic fluoride during their biotransformation are potentially nephrotoxic, especially if used in combination with drugs such as the aminoglycosides. The problem was first demonstrated with methoxyflurane, which was shown to cause an inability to concentrate the urine in some patients, and this has been one of the main factors leading to the virtual abandonment of this agent in most countries.

The newer inhalational agents, enflurane and isoflurane, both release inorganic fluoride during their metabolism, but they are biotransformed to a much smaller degree than methoxyflurane. There is now clear evidence that enflurane can lead to loss of concentrating power in the kidney, particularly after prolonged use or in patients with pre-existing renal disease. Isoflurane, however, is only metabolized to a very small degree in humans, and nephrotoxicity has not yet been reported despite extensive clinical use. Inhalational agents are likely to remain popular in renal disease since their uptake and elimination are independent of renal function.

The pharmacokinetics and pharmacodynamics of most drugs are altered in severe renal disease because of decreased renal excretion and alterations in volume of distribution and protein-binding. In addition, children with chronic renal disease may be severely underdeveloped and therefore have lower dose requirements for many agents. The newer muscle relaxants, atracurium and vecuronium, do not rely on renal excretion for their clearance and are probably the relaxants of choice in renal disease. Atracurium is cleared by Hoffman elimination and enzyme hydrolysis, and vecuronium is mainly excreted via the liver.

The induction dose of thiopentone is significantly reduced in uraemic patients because of reduced protein-binding and lowered albumin levels. Narcotic analgesics should also be used with caution in renal failure, since the intensity and duration of their effects, with the possible exception of fentanyl, can be greatly enhanced. Fentanyl in high doses reduces the stress response to surgery and may improve renal function. Ketamine is largely metabolized in the liver and appears to have little effect on renal function, but should be avoided in patients with hypertension.

Table 12.3. Drugs used in the treatment of acute hypertensive crises (modified from Dillon, 1982)

Drug	Dose	Action	Comment
Labetalol	1–3 mg/kg/h i.v. (total 0.5–5.0 mg/kg)	α-Blocker and β-blocker	Use alone; stop infusate when blood pressure is controlled; effective 4–6 h
Sodium nitroprusside	0.5–0.8 µg/kg/min i.v.	Direct vasodilator	Very short duration of action; effective only while being infused
Diazoxide	2–10 mg/kg i.v. bolus	Direct vasodilator	Can cause hyperglycaemia, hypotension, and salt and water retention
Hydralazine	0.1–0.2 mg/kg i.v. or i.m.	Direct vasodilator	Can cause tachycardia, headache and flushing
Minoxidil	0.1–0.2 mg/kg p.o.	Direct vasodilator	Rapidly effective even though orally administered
Frusemide	1–2 mg/kg i.v.	Diuretic	Avoid unless saline overload is obvious
Phentolamine	0.1–0.2 mg/kg i.v.	α-Blocker	Hypertensive crisis of phaeochromocytomas

PLASTIC SURGERY

General principles

Plastic surgery in children covers a wide range of operations, from the removal of the most minor lesion to major reconstructive surgery. It is also performed in children of all ages, from the neonatal period to adolescence. There are, however, some general principles which apply to the majority of these operations.

Although plastic surgeons are sometimes involved in the treatment of emergency cases, particularly burns, most of the operations are elective, and relatively few are life-saving or urgent, so that it is essential that the child is as fit as possible before anaesthesia. There is evidence to suggest that there is a higher incidence of respiratory complications in children who have a history of upper respiratory tract infection in the 2 weeks prior to surgery (Tait et al, 1983), so that elective surgery should be delayed for at least 2 weeks after such an infection whenever possible. Following lower respiratory tract infection, surgery should probably be postponed for at least 4 weeks (Berry, 1986). On the other hand, some children suffer from almost continuously runny noses, and this is usually a sign of allergic disease. There is no evidence that there is an increased risk of anaesthesia in these children, and it is clearly impracticable to postpone surgery in all of them. If an assurance can be obtained from the parents that the child is as well as usual, and in the absence of pyrexia or clinical signs of respiratory infection, anaesthesia can safely proceed. There will inevitably be borderline cases where clinical judgement must be made after discussion with the parents.

Children requiring major reconstructive surgery often need repeated anaesthetics over many years, and careful preoperative preparation is necessary to minimize the psychological sequelae of frequent hospitalization. Effective premedication helps to relieve the anxiety of the immediate preoperative and induction periods, but may be difficult to achieve when surgery is performed on a day-stay basis.

Most plastic surgery involves the superficial tissues, and is therefore fairly stimulating, requiring effective analgesia throughout the operation. Movement during the operation or restlessness in the immediate postoperative period can increase bleeding and even prejudice the result of surgery. General anaesthesia in children is being increasingly augmented by regional blocks, which not only allow the anaesthetic to be conducted at a lighter plane, but help to provide a smooth recovery and also give good postoperative pain relief. These blocks are described in detail in Chapter 9.

Local infiltration with adrenaline is favoured by most plastic surgeons to reduce bleeding, and this may produce arrhythmias, especially if the heart has been sensitized by the use of halothane. Enflurane produces the least myocardial sensitization of the currently used inhalational agents, though halothane can be used safely with 1:200 000 adrenaline if ECG is monitored.

Surgery around the head

Cleft lip and palate

Congenital cleft lip is caused by failure of fusion of the medial and lateral nasal swellings which normally occurs by 35 days of intrauterine life. This may impair the subsequent closure of the palatine shelves, normally complete by the eighth to ninth week, so that cleft palate is frequently associated with cleft lip. Other secondary anomalies include defects in development of the teeth and incomplete growth of the ala nasi on the side of the cleft. The defect varies from a small notch in the upper lip to complete bilateral clefts of the lip and palate (Figure 12.2). Cleft lip occurs as part of a number of syndromes, all extremely rare.

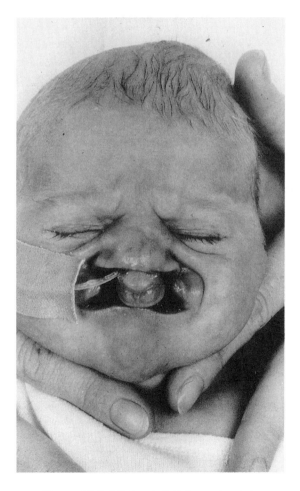

Figure 12.2. Bilateral cleft lip and palate.

Isolated cleft palate, without cleft lip, has a much higher incidence of associated congenital anomalies. Some of these form distinct syndromes (Table 12.4), but in any child with a cleft palate the possibility of other congenital anomalies should be remembered, particularly limb and ear deformities, umbilical hernia, congenital heart disease and cervical spine abnormalities. Many of these syndromes are associated with difficulty in intubation.

Table 12.4. Syndromes associated with cleft palate with anaesthetic implications (modified from Smith, 1982)

Syndrome	Other significant anomalies
Cerebrocostomandibular	Micrognathia
	Small thorax
	Tracheal and vertebral anomalies
Dubowitz	Microcephaly
	Micrognathia
	Hypertelorism
Femoral hypoplasia— unusual facies	Short lower limbs
	Micrognathia
Goldenhar	Micrognathia
	Malar and maxillary hypoplasia, usually unilateral
	Vertebral and cardiac anomalies
Hay–Wells	Maxillary hypoplasia
Klippel–Feil (see Figure 12.3)	Short, immobile neck
	Fused cervical vertebrae
	Neurological defects
	Cardiac defects
Mekel–Gruber	Encephalocoele, microcephaly
	Micrognathia
	Polycystic kidneys
Partial trisomy 10q	Microcephaly
	Ptosis
	Cardiac and renal anomalies
Pierre Robin	Micrognathia
	Glossoptosis
	Cardiac anomalies
Shprintzen	Deafness
	Micrognathia
	Cardiac anomalies
Stickler	Deafness
	Micrognathia
	Hypotonia
	Scoliosis
Treacher Collins	Micrognathia
	Malar and maxillary hypoplasia
	Ear deformities

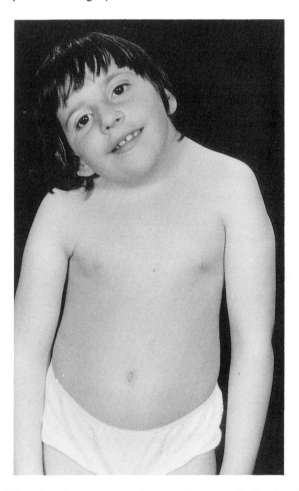

Figure 12.3. Klippel–Feil syndrome, showing fixed cervical spine deformity.

Pierre Robin syndrome (Figure 12.4)

The small mouth and large tongue in this condition cause severe airway problems in the supine position from birth. Traditionally, these babies have been nursed prone, but even then the mortality is high. Tracheal intubation can be very difficult, especially in the first few months of life. Various methods of surgical fixation of the tongue have been attempted, and more recently nasopharyngeal intubation has been advocated (Heaf et al, 1982). This method allows more normal development of the child than the prone position, but still requires skilled nursing care. In the worst cases tracheostomy may provide the only safe method of management.

Airway management becomes less difficult as the child grows older, though acute airway problems can arise in the postoperative period after closure of the cleft palate.

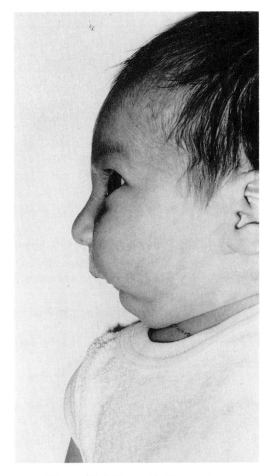

Figure 12.4. Pierre Robin syndrome.

Treacher Collins syndrome (Figure 12.5)

The main classical features of this condition are the antimongoloid slanting palpebral fissures, hypoplasia of the facial bones, ear deformities and cleft palate. Unilateral forms are more commonly referred to as Goldenhar syndrome or hemifacial microsomia.

Tracheal intubation can be exceedingly difficult in these cases, especially where there is asymmetry between the two sides of the face. In contrast to the Pierre Robin syndrome, intubation tends to become more difficult as the child gets older.

Anaesthetic management.   Examination of the child at the pre-operative visit should give the anaesthetist advance warning of possible difficulties in intubation in most cases. Micrognathia is usually obvious if

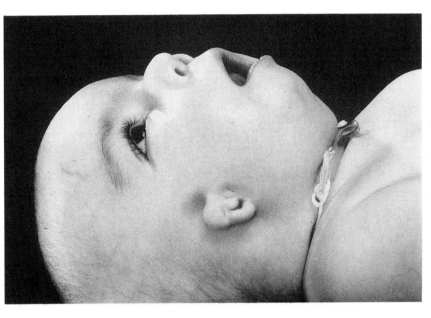

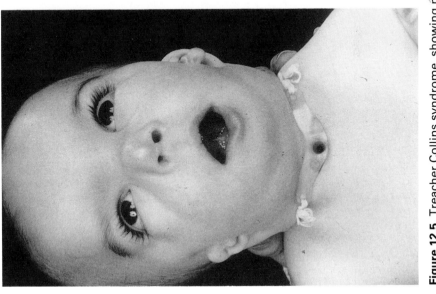

Figure 12.5. Treacher Collins syndrome, showing micrognathia, antimongoloid slanting of lower eyelids with absent eyelashes and deformity of the pinna of the ear.

looked for, but careful examination should also include an assessment of the degree of mobility of the neck and the amount of mouth opening. The presence of an anteriorly placed premaxilla in cases of cleft lip (Figure 12.6) may make insertion of the laryngoscope awkward, and the blade may slip into the cleft. When difficulty in intubation is suspected, however, it is not always easy to assess whether it will be mild, moderate or severe, and it is usually wise to assume the worst. Previous anaesthetic history; if available, can be extremely valuable. Mallampati (1983) described a simple method of assessment based on the view obtained when the patient's tongue is fully extruded. A more complex method of assessment has been described by Delegue et al (1980) based on measurement of the maxillo–pharyngeal angle on lateral X-ray. The normal angle is greater than 100°, and angles less than 90° suggest that it will be impossible to visualize the larynx with a laryngoscope. Between 90 and 100° it is likely that only the posterior commissure will be visible.

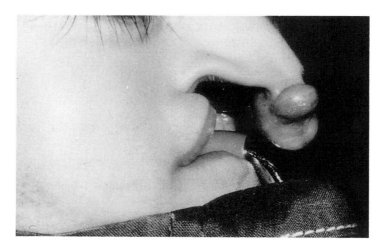

Figure 12.6. Bilateral cleft lip with anteriorly placed premaxilla.

It is wise to avoid sedative or narcotic premedication in children with severe upper airway problems, because of the risk of precipitating complete obstruction. Induction of anaesthesia is probably most safely performed with inhalational anaesthesia using halothane, and muscle relaxants should not be used unless the anaesthetist is sure that the lungs can be ventilated easily. This judgement can either be made from previous anaesthetic history, or by gentle inflation of the lungs after induction with spontaneous ventilation. Neither of these pointers are entirely reliable, however. The use of moderate amounts of continuous positive airway pressure with a tight-fitting mask during the early stage of induction can be very helpful, and will usually allow anaesthesia to be deepened to a stage where a pharyngeal airway can be inserted. Should this fail it is wise to discontinue the anaesthetic and consider the establishment of a tracheostomy under local analgesia. This should seldom be necessary in experienced hands, however.

A number of techniques are available to facilitate intubation when the larynx cannot be visualized. External compression over the larynx by an assistant is probably the most commonly used, and the passage of a malleable stilette through the tube to give it a more anterior curvature is also helpful. A variety of straight and curved bladed laryngoscopes should be available, together with a range of tubes of different sizes. In more difficult cases the stilette can be passed into the trachea first and the tube threaded over it. Blind nasal intubation may be possible, though decreasing numbers of anaesthetists are familiar with this technique. Fibreoptic laryngoscopes are now available in sizes small enough to accommodate at 4.5 mm tube, but practice is required in the use of this instrument in children with normal airways before attempting to use it in the difficult intubation problem. Retrograde intubation has been used successfully in infants (Cooper and Murray-Wilson, 1987) but requires careful advance preparation and is potentially dangerous. Tracheostomy is always a possibility, but is not easy to perform on unintubated infants, and is more appropriate when long-term airway management is required.

Many types of tracheal tube have been used for cleft lip and palate repair. Whichever tube is used, care should be taken to ensure that it cannot kink in the back of the pharynx—a common complication when the breathing system is directed downwards towards the chest. The most recently introduced tubes for this type of surgery are the preformed RAE tubes (Ring et al, 1975). These are usually satisfactory, though they can be compressed when the mouth gag is inserted, or even become wedged in the tongue plate if a split gag is used. A pharyngeal pack should be used for surgery on the lip, but most surgeons prefer to insert their own pack for palate repair.

An intravenous line should always be established, and ECG, blood pressure and temperature should be monitored. A precordial stethoscope is also extremely valuable to monitor breath sounds whenever there is a chance that the surgeon may interfere with the tracheal tube. Pulse oximetry is becoming routinely used in many centres. Maintenance of anaesthesia can be with spontaneous or controlled ventilation, the latter probably being preferable for primary lip repair because of the inefficiency of spontaneous ventilation in the first few months of life. The newer muscle relaxants, atracurium and vecuronium, have the advantage of rapid reversibility, and in operations of indeterminate length can be used by infusion, with response monitored by peripheral nerve stimulation. Nitrous oxide can be supplemented with either an inhalational agent or intravenous narcotic, though the latter should be used with caution in infants and in the presence of upper airway problems because of the risk of postoperative respiratory depression.

Where there has been difficulty in intubation or preoperative airway problems, extubation should not be performed until the child is fully awake and breathing well. The insertion of a tongue stitch before extubation to allow the tongue to be pulled forward is a wise precaution in the most difficult cases.

There has been some interest among plastic surgeons in recent years in the repair of cleft lip in the neonatal period. For this approach to be safe the anaesthetist must be fully aware of the specific problems of neonatal anaesthesia, and the operation should be performed in a centre where medical and nursing staff are handling surgical neonates on a regular basis. Early repair of cleft palate is likely to require more frequent blood transfusion. Time alone will tell whether improved results justify this new approach.

Major craniofacial reconstruction (see Chapter 16)

For several years there has been increasing interest in major craniofacial reconstruction for the craniofacial dysostoses, such as Crouzon's and Apert's syndromes (Tessier, 1971). The surgery is often approached as a joint procedure involving plastic, neuro- and faciomaxillary surgeons, and the procedure is usually a lengthy one. The problems facing the anaesthetist are those of major blood loss, hypothermia and prolonged anaesthesia, though intubation is occasionally difficult. Arterial and central venous pressure are usually measured, though internal jugular cannulation is not satisfactory for major head and neck surgery. Subclavian or femoral vein cannulation are recommended alternatives. The siting of the tracheal tube is frequently difficult, since nasal tubes are less liable to dislodgement, and are the only alternative to tracheostomy for postoperative care if the jaws are wired, but may interfere with the surgical field. The change from an oral to a nasal tube during surgery may be the only reasonable compromise, but if the intial intubation is at all difficult elective tracheostomy should be considered despite the increased risk of nosocomal infection.

Other head and neck surgery

Other commonly performed plastic surgical operations involve the head and neck. These include the correction of protruding ears, secondary corrections to nasal deformities related to cleft lip, excision of preauricular skin tags in children who may well have other congenital anomalies and the removal of unsightly lesions and scars around the face. Most of these operations pose little difficulty for the anaesthetist, though movement of the head during the operation may stimulate the patient to cough, so the application of topical lignocaine to the cords in a dose of up to 3 mg/kg is advisable.

Burns

The overall management of acute burns is described in detail elsewhere in this book (see Chapter 18). Children with severe burns may however need repeated anaesthesia for many years, first for changes of dressings and skin grafting and later for reconstructive plastic surgery. Burns around the head and neck may lead to severe contracture formation (Figure 12.7) causing serious intubation problems. In the worst cases division of the contracture under local anaesthesia must precede induction. It is essential that the anaesthetist understands not only the technical challenges which have to be faced, but also the serious psychological problems which are almost certain to arise (Szyfelbein et al, 1986).

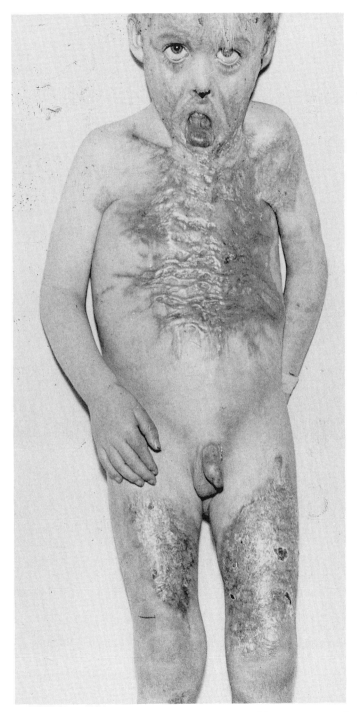

Figure 12.7. Severe burns to face, neck and chest with contracture formation (courtesy of Dr GH Bush).

Peripheral operations

Operations on the limbs, such as correction of syndactyly or other congenital anomalies, do not pose serious problems for the anaesthetist, though peripheral nerve blocks are being increasingly performed in these cases as an adjunct to anaesthesia and to provide postoperative pain relief. The pain of repeated injections into tissue expanders can be reduced by the topical application of a eutectic mixture of lignocaine and prilocaine cream (Emla).

The excision of large haemangiomata can not only cause massive blood loss, but also air embolism. Postoperative thrombosis may consume large quantities of platelets and other clotting factors and lead to a bleeding diathesis. Large arteriovenous fistulae may form, and become a cause of heart failure. Finally, it should be remembered that a coexisting subglottic haemangioma may be present, especially if the external lesion is situated around the face or neck (Figure 12.8).

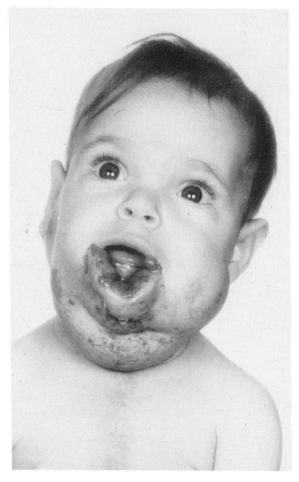

Figure 12.8. Large cutaneous haemangioma (associated with subglottic haemangioma).

REFERENCES

Barratt TM & Baillod RA (1982) Chronic renal failure and regular dialysis. In Williams DI & Johnston JH (eds) *Paediatric Urology*, pp 37–47. London: Butterworths.

Berry FA (1983) Anesthesia for genitourinary surgery. In Gregory GA (ed) *Pediatric Anesthesia*, pp 727–771. New York: Churchill Livingstone.

Berry FA (1986) The child with the runny nose. In Berry FA (ed) *Anesthetic Management of Difficult and Routine Pediatric Patients*, pp 349–367. New York: Churchill Livingstone.

Bonsu AK, Viby-Mogensen J, Fernando PUE, Muchhal K, Tamilarasan A & Lambourne A (1987) Relationship of post-tetanic count and train-of-four response during intense neuromuscular blockade caused by atracurium. *British Journal of Anaesthesia* **59**: 1089–1092.

Cooper CMS & Murray-Wilson A (1987) Retrograde intubation—management of a 4.8 kg, 5-month infant. *Anaesthesia* **42**: 1197–1200.

Cramolini GM (1987) Diseases of the renal system. In Katz J & Steward DJ (eds) *Anesthesia and Uncommon Pediatric Diseases*, pp 155–221. Philadelphia: Saunders.

Dear G de L, Hammerton M, Hatch DJ & Taylor D (1987) Anaesthesia and intraocular pressure in young children. A study of three different techniques of anaesthesia. *Anaesthesia* **42**: 259–265.

Delegue L, Rosenberg-Reiner S, Ghnassia M-D et al (1980) L'intubation trachéale chez les enfants atteints de dysmorphie cranio-faciales congenitales. *Anesthesia Analgesia Réanimation* **37**: 133–138.

Dillon MJ (1982) Hypertension. In Williams DI & Johnston JH (eds) *Paediatric Urology*, pp 57–72. London: Butterworths.

Fernando ON (1982) Renal transplantation in children. In Williams DI & Johnston JH (eds) *Paediatric Urology*, pp 49–56. London: Butterworths.

France NK (1983) Anesthesia for pediatric ophthalmic surgery. In Gregory GA (ed) *Pediatric Anesthesia*, pp 773–801. New York: Churchill Livingstone.

Heaf DP, Helms PJ, Dinwiddie R & Matthew DJ (1982) Nasopharyngeal airways in Pierre Robin syndrome. *Journal of Pediatrics* **100**: 698–700.

Henderson AM, Vallis CJ & Sumner E (1987) Anaesthesia in the prune-belly syndrome: a review of 36 cases. *Anaesthesia* **42**: 54–60.

Hull CJ (1986) Phaeochromocytoma—diagnosis, preoperative preparation and anaesthetic management. *British Journal of Anaesthesia* **58**: 1453–1468.

Johnston JH (1982a) The exstrophic anomalies. In Williams DI & Johnston JH (eds) *Paediatric Urology*, pp 239–250. London: Butterworths.

Johnston JH (1982b) Neuroblastoma, teratoma and other retroperitoneal tumours. In Williams DI & Johnston JH (eds) *Paediatric Urology*, pp 401–409. London: Butterworths.

Johnston RR, Eger EI II & Wilson C (1976) A comparative interaction of epinephrine with enflurane, isoflurane and halothane in man. *Anesthesia and Analgesia* **55**: 709–712.

Kaufman BH, Telander RL, van Heerden JA et al (1983) Phaeochromocytoma in the pediatric age group; current status. *Journal of Pediatric Surgery* **18**: 879–884.

Landers JWM, Sluiter HE, Thein TH et al (1985) Treatment of a phaeochromocytoma of the urinary bladder with nifedipine. *British Medical Journal* **290**: 1624–1625.

Lerman J, Eustis S & Smith DR (1986) Effect of Droperidol pretreatment on post-anaesthetic vomiting in children undergoing strabismus surgery. *Anesthesiology* **65**: 322–325.

Mallampati SR (1983) Clinical sign to predict difficult tracheal intubation (hypotensis). *Canadian Anaesthetists' Society Journal* **30**: 316–317.

Meyers EF, Krupin T, Johnson M & Zink H (1978) Failure of non-depolarising neuromuscular blockers to inhibit succinylcholine-induced increased intra-ocular pressure. A controlled study. *Anesthesiology* **48:** 149–151.

Nakayama DK, Harrison MR, Chinn DH & de Lorimer A (1984) The pathogenesis of prune belly. *American Journal of Diseases of Childhood* **138:** 834–836.

Pagon RA, Smith DW & Shepard TH (1979) Urethral obstruction malformation complex: a cause of abdominal muscle deficiency and the 'prune belly'. *Journal of Pediatrics* **94:** 900–906.

Potter D, Feduska N, Melzer J et al (1986) Twenty years of renal transplantation in children. *Pediatrics* **77:** 465–470.

Ridley SA & Hatch DJ (1988) Post-tetanic count and profound neuromuscular blockade with atracurium infusion in paediatric patients. *British Journal of Anaesthesia* **60:** 31–35.

Ring WH, Adair JC & Elwyn RA (1975) A new pediatric endotracheal tube. *Anesthesia and Analgesia (Cleveland)* **54:** 273–274.

Serfas D, Shoback DM & Lorell BH (1983) Phaeochromocytoma and hypertrophic cardiomyopathy: apparent suppression of symptoms and noradrenaline secretion by calcium channel blockade. *Lancet* **2:** 711–713.

Smith DW (1982) *Recognizable Patterns of Human Malformation.* Philadelphia: Saunders.

Solares G, Ramos F, Martin-Duran R et al (1986) Amiodarone, phaeochromocytoma and cardiomyopathy. *Anaesthesia* **41:** 186–190.

Szyfelbein SK, Martyn JAJ & Cote CJ (1986) Burns. In Ryan JF, Todres ID, Cote CJ et al (eds) *A Practice of Anaesthesia for Infants and Children,* pp 229–241. Orlando: Grune & Stratton.

Tait AR, Ketcham TR, Klein MJ et al (1983) Perioperative respiratory complications in patients with upper respiratory tract infections. *Anesthesiology* **59:** A433.

Tessier P (1971) The definitive plastic surgical treatment of the severe facial deformities of craniosynostosis: Crouzon's and Apert's diseases. *Plastic and Reconstructive Surgery* **48:** 419–442.

Anaesthesia for patients with cardiac disease

Anaesthesia for infants with cardiac disease, whether for palliative or corrective cardiac surgery or for associated or intercurrent disease, requires a full
knowledge of the pathophysiological background of the particular disease.
The anaesthetist is an invaluable member of the team involved in the
treatment of the patient from hospital admission to recovery.

In children, cardiothoracic surgery is mainly undertaken for congenital heart
disease which has a fairly constant worldwide incidence of 8 per 1000 live births.
Approximately 3500 children are operated on annually in the UK for heart
disease in nine supraregional centres. No specific causes are found in most cases,
but congenital rubella infection and fetal alcohol syndrome are well documented
causes of congenital heart disease. Some 30–40% of children with trisomy 21
(Down's syndrome) have heart disease and very many chromosomal abnormalities are associated with different cardiac lesions (Lenz, 1980). See p. 507 for
autosomal dominant and recessive syndromes which include cardiac malformations. More than 20% of infants die from cardiac disease in the first year of life
if left untreated, one-half within the first month (Esscher et al, 1975; Table 13.1).

Modern antenatal ultrasonography is identifying many forms of congenital heart disease with increasing accuracy allowing earlier identification
and treatment of affected babies. The incidence of other associated congenital abnormalities is very high, particularly midline defects such as cleft lip
and palate or gut atresias. Failure to thrive is a common sequel to untreated
congenital heart disease in the first weeks of life.

FUNCTIONAL GROUPING OF LESIONS

Four basic functional groups of patients can be identified, each of which
poses distinct anaesthetic problems.

1. Patients with increased pulmonary blood flow, including patent ductus
   arteriosus (PDA), septal defects, aorto-pulmonary (A-P) windows,
   truncus arteriosus and total anomalous pulmonary venous drainage
   (TAPVD). Inhalational induction is normal, but respiratory failure may
   occur because of reduced pulmonary compliance and increased work of
   breathing. Untreated cases die early in cardiac failure or develop pulmonary vascular disease and eventually Eisenmenger's syndrome
   (reversal of shunt). A fall in systemic vascular resistance may cause reversal of the shunt, severe cyanosis and even death.

Table 13.1. Incidence of congenital heart disease

Disease	Incidence	Treatment
Patent ductus arteriosus (PDA)	10–15%	Newborn—trial of indomethacin ligation or clipping Older—ligation
Ventricular septal defect (VSD)	10–20%	Closure on bypass
Atrial septal defect (ASD) (secundum)	5–15%	Closure on bypass
Atrial septal defect (ASD) (primum)	1–3%	Closure on bypass
Atrioventricular septal defect (AVSD)		Closure on bypass
Total anomalous pulmonary venous drainage (TAPVD)	1–2%	Immediate repair on bypass
Pulmonary stenosis (PS) (valvular)	5–10%	Newborn—valvotomy; inflow occlusion Older—valvotomy on bypass
Coarctation of aorta	2–5%	Subclavian angioplasty or resection
Aortic arch anomalies	0.5–1%	
Persistent truncus arteriosus	1–2%	Correction with conduit right ventricle to pulmonary artery (RV–PA)
Aortic stenosis (all types)	3–5%	Newborn—valvotomy; inflow occlusion Older—Konno on bypass
Tetralogy of Fallot	5–10%	Correction on bypass Blalock shunt; correction later
Pulmonary atresia + VSD	1%	Blalock shunt
Tricuspid atresia (TA)	1–3%	Blalock shunt; Fontan later
Transposition of great arteries (TGA)	5–15%	Rashkind septostomy Arterial switch on bypass Older—Senning on bypass
Corrected TGA (CTGA)	below 1%	
Univentricular heart (UVH)	1–2%	Banding of pulmonary artery
Ebstein's anomaly	below 1%	Tricuspid valve replacement ASD closure on bypass
Hypoplastic left heart syndrome	1–2%	Norwood on bypass

2. Patients with reduced pulmonary blood flow with often severe cyanosis and polycythaemia include Fallot's tetralogy, pulmonary stenosis or atresia and tricuspid atresia. Inhalational induction is very slow. Systemic hypotension causes increased right-to-left shunting and infundibular spasm causes catastrophic hypoxia and subsequent acidosis. Severe lesions of this type are dependent on patency of the ductus arteriosus and benefit from preoperative prostaglandin therapy.

3. Transposition of the great vessels which may be complicated by PDA and ventricular septal defect (VSD) has a combination of cyanosis and increased pulmonary blood flow. An arterial 'switch' operation is performed in the early days of life for 'simple' transposition before the pulmonary vascular resistance falls and the left ventricle can no longer support the systemic vascular resistance. With VSD or PDA the operation can be delayed, but not so long that pulmonary vascular disease develops. The alternative is to perform an atrial direction of flow during the first year of life (Senning or Mustard operation; Stark and de Leval, 1983). A Rashkind's balloon septostomy is always required soon after diagnosis to increase mixing at atrial level but even with good mixing at atrial level by 2 years of age the mortality without correction approaches 50%. Severe hypoxia and acidosis may develop during surgical manipulation before bypass.

4. Left ventricular outflow obstruction causing low cardiac output, myocardial ischaemia and eventually myocardial fibrosis occurs with aortic stenosis, subvalvular or valvular, aortic arch problems such as coarctation. Patients presenting with symptoms early in life often have very poor cardiac function and may require considerable preoperative support—mechanical ventilation, prostaglandins, inotropes, vasodilators, renal dialysis, etc.; however, surgery should not be delayed too long.

PATHOPHYSIOLOGY

Fetal and transitional circulation

The fetal channels, ductus arteriosus (DA) and foramen ovale are important in considerations of abnormal haemodynamics. In fetal life the DA is large so it allows equal pressures in the aorta and pulmonary artery. The blood flow to the lungs therefore depends on the relative resistances of the lungs and placenta. As the lungs are not expanded and have a high pulmonary vascular resistance (PVR) they take only 10% of the cardiac output. The vascular bed of the placenta has a low resistance and takes at least 50% of the total cardiac output. In all, 60% of the oxygenated blood from the placenta crosses from right to left through the foramen ovale to the aorta, coronaries and developing brain. The rest of the blood passes via the ductus venosus through the liver to the short inferior vena cava and is ejected by the right ventricle to the pulmonary artery, DA and hence to the lower part of the body. Fetal PaO_2 in the upper part of the body is approximately 4 kPa (60% saturated) and in the lower part 3 kPa (38% saturated).

After the first breath and clamping of the umbilical cord, cessation of umbilical blood flow causes a fall in right atrial pressure. Increasing pulmonary blood flow allows the left atrial pressure to rise and when this is at a sustained level—greater than right atrial pressure—the foramen ovale closes. Although it is potentially patent in 30% of normal adults, it may only be held closed by the difference in pressure between the two atria. Pulmonary vascular resistance falls further under the influence of increasing

PaO_2 and rising pH (falling $PaCO_2$), together with release of bradykinin from inactive precursors triggered by a fall in temperature and pH of umbilical venous blood at birth.

The media of the ductus contains spirally arranged dense smooth muscle which begins to contract from the pulmonary artery end under the influence of increasing PaO_2. Physiological closure is completed within 24 h but permanent closure, requiring fibrosis, takes at least 3 weeks. Isolated ductal tissue of the fetal lamb is relaxed by prostaglandins E_1 and E_2 which are the agents assumed to maintain patency during fetal life. The increased PaO_2 in the newborn period inhibits prostaglandin E_2 synthesis which, when coupled with the activation of cytochrome P-450 metabolism in mitochondria of periductal tissue, causes contraction of the smooth muscle of the ductus (Coceani, 1986). Persistent patency beyond the age of 4 months may be caused by a defect in the media of the PDA. Prostaglandins are not stored but are synthesized from arachidonic acid and released in response to stimuli such as hypoxia. Synthesis is blocked by prostaglandin synthetase inhibitors such as corticosteroids, aspirin or indomethacin (Greeley et al, 1987).

The premature ductus is less sensitive to the factors which cause closure, so many more remain open in this age group. This is caused partly by exposure to low PaO_2 and also by factors such as fluid overload at a time when the oxygen mechanism for closure of the ductus is not fully developed. If the PVR is less than systemic there will be a left-to-right shunt through a PDA causing heart failure, pulmonary oedema and increased work of breathing so that the duct may require urgent medical or surgical attention. The presence of a PDA in a baby dependent on mechanical ventilation may contribute to the appearance of bronchopulmonary dysplasia and thus be an indication to close the ductus.

It is possible to monitor the effects of a closing ductus using echocardiography because the size of the left atrium decreases with the reduction in the left-to-right shunt. Indomethacin is given orally for three 6-hourly doses of 0.2 mg/kg, but PVR is increased, an effect intensified by hypoxia and more marked in the preterm than the mature baby. This rise in PVR may outweigh the advantage of the 'medical' closure of the ductus.

Prostaglandin E_1 or E_2 are used therapeutically in doses of 0.05–0.1 µg/kg/min by intravenous infusions to maintain ductal patency in babies with severe cyanotic congenital heart disease with very low pulmonary blood flow. Such duct-dependent lesions include severe Fallot's tetralogy and pulmonary atresia with intact septum. Opening of the duct increases pulmonary blood flow and oxygenation, allowing stabilization of the infant and subsequent surgery in more favourable circumstances. Prostaglandin E_1 is also useful in patients with reduced systemic blood flow, such as in coarctation of the aorta. Prostaglandin therapy has undoubtedly made a major contribution to the reduction in mortality and morbidity in these lesions. High doses of prostaglandin E_1 cause apnoea and facilities for respiratory support should always be readily available.

Pulmonary vasculature

Changes in PVR are of the greatest importance in congenital heart disease as they may affect the successful outcome of any corrective surgery. Normally, PVR is low, falling from systemic levels to adult levels within the first few weeks of life. At birth the media of the peripheral pulmonary arterioles have abundant smooth muscle which regresses gradually, during which time the pulmonary vascular bed is very reactive. Vasoconstrictive reaction to hypoxia, hypercarbia and acidosis by an adrenergic mechanism may cause fetal channels to re-open with a right-to-left shunt and critical hypoxaemia. Transmembrane influx of Ca^{2+} may be involved in pulmonary vasoconstriction and intravenous $CaCl_2$ bolus injection almost always increases PVR.

Irreversible fixed pulmonary vascular disease is often the limiting factor in operability of congenital heart disease. Abnormalities such as ventricular septal defect, PDA, atrioventricular septal defects, transposition of great arteries and truncus arteriosus cause a high pulmonary artery pressure and an initially high pulmonary blood flow with subsequent development of pulmonary vascular disease. Initially the small vessels become muscularized very rapidly, possibly within days of birth, first on the arterial and then the venous side, and subsequently the intra-acinar vessels which normally develop during late fetal life and form mainly after birth, fail to do so (Haworth and Hall, 1986). This causes both a fixed increase in PVR as well as the potential for a reversible component by constriction of the abundant smooth muscle, at least in the earlier stages of pulmonary vascular disease.

Dependent shunts occur when ventricular pressures are equal and flow is determined by the relative resistances but an *obligatory* shunt occurs from a high pressure chamber to a lower (Rudolph, 1974) e.g. with atrioventricular septal defect blood shunts from left ventricle to right atrium, causing a continuous shunt. Most infants with large left-to-right shunts have a low PVR and high flow with hyperaemic lungs and tachypnoea. Pulmonary vascular disease is a serious risk if the pulmonary artery (PA) pressure is greater than half systemic pressure with a pulmonary:systemic flow ratio greater than 3:1. Resistance usually rises after the first year of life, but the Eisenmenger syndrome does not appear until after the age of 10–20 years. Cyanosis, causing pulmonary vasoconstriction and polycythaemia, which increases resistance to blood flow, complicates pulmonary vascular disease and greatly accelerates its course. Down's syndrome children develop pulmonary vascular disease earlier than other children with similar cardiac lesions.

Preoperative assessment of pulmonary vascular resistance is made using cardiac catheter data to obtain the ratio of pulmonary to systemic resistance ($R_p:R_s$), which is normally 0.2. The use of ratios has the advantage that assumptions used for the calculation of both resistances cancel each other out, as absolute values of pulmonary blood flow (Q_p) are difficult to obtain (Table 13.2).

With difficult or advanced cases a lung biopsy is taken and the progressive series of obliterative structural changes in the peripheral pulmonary arteries are classified into six grades (Haworth, 1986), from medial hypertrophy to acute arterial necrosis. Grades IV or more are irreversible, but grades III and IV increase the risk of correcting the abnormality—death from low cardiac output and right ventricular failure or the persistence of pulmonary hypertension. Even those in whom the PA pressure falls to normal postoperatively may show an abnormal increase in PA pressure on exercise, indicating a permanent reduction in the overall capacity of the pulmonary vascular bed.

Table 13.2. Calculation of pulmonary vascular resistance

$$Q_p = \frac{\text{oxygen uptake}}{\text{pulmonary A-V } O_2 \text{ difference}} \qquad Q_s = \frac{\text{oxygen uptake}}{\text{systemic A-V } O_2 \text{ difference}}$$

$$\therefore \frac{Q_p}{Q_s} = \frac{\text{systemic A-V } O_2 \text{ difference}}{\text{pulmonary A-V } O_2 \text{ difference}} \text{ because } R_p = \frac{P_p}{Q_p} \text{ and } R_s = \frac{P_s}{Q_s}$$

$$R_p/R_s = \frac{P_p}{P_s} \times \frac{Q_s}{Q_p} = \frac{P_p}{P_s} \times \frac{\text{pulmonary A-V } O_2 \text{ difference}}{\text{systemic A-V } O_2 \text{ difference}}$$

Q_p = pulmonary blood flow; Q_s = aortic blood flow; R_p = pulmonary resistance; R_s = systemic resistance; P_p = pressure drop across pulmonary vascular bed; P_s = systemic pressure difference.

Fall in peripheral resistance is not well tolerated when PVR is severe and sudden shunt reversal may occur. Prolonged diuretic therapy may make this situation more likely as circulating blood volume may be depleted and hypotension easily occurs, especially with induction of anaesthesia.

Low pulmonary blood flow

A *dependent* right-to-left shunt occurs when venous and systemic circulations communicate and the resistance of the right ventricular outflow is variable, e.g. in Fallot's tetralogy. An *obligatory* right-to-left shunt occurs when the normal pulmonary pathway is obstructed and blood shunts to the left side at a more proximal level, e.g. in pulmonary stenosis or atresia. In transposition of great arteries the obligatory shunt is of systemic venous blood to systemic arterial circulation and pulmonary to pulmonary.

Cyanotic patients make a number of adaptations to compensate for reduced oxygen delivery to the tissues. The oxygen dissociation curve is shifted to the right to allow improved unloading of oxygen to the tissues, a shift caused by a mild persistent metabolic acidosis and a rise in level of 2,3 diphosphoglycerate in red cells. There is enlargement of the systemic venous bed, doubling of blood volume with collateral formation (clubbing) and the oxygen-carrying capacity of the blood is increased by a rising haemoglobin which sometimes exceeds 20 g/dl. Progress of the disease, e.g. pulmonary atresia, is easily monitored from haemoglobin levels and a rising level may be an indication for further palliative surgery or even total correction. As the haematocrit rises there is an increase in blood viscosity, impairing perfusion of vital organs such as the kidneys. At levels above 70% there is sludging of cells in peripheral vessels and a danger of thromboembolism, especially in the cerebral circulation, particularly if the child becomes dehydrated. Preoperative starvation, diuretic therapy or sudden diarrhoea are all common contributory factors to such a catastrophe. Exchange transfusion with plasma may be necessary to reduce the haematocrit. A further compensatory mechanism is a coagulopathy with reduced prothrombin and poor platelet function which often causes bleeding problems after bypass surgery. Blood products such as platelet-rich plasma, fresh frozen plasma and cryoprecipitate should be available.

Cyanotic attacks, which are sometimes very severe (hypercyanotic) occur in Fallot's tetralogy if systemic resistance is reduced or right ventricular outflow tract resistance rises. They can occur during crying or feeding but commonly are associated with cardiac catheterization or during the pre-bypass phase of surgery, particularly induction of anaesthesia. The squatting which is so characteristic of the Fallot is an attempt to minimize right-to-left shunting by increasing peripheral resistance. Attacks can be controlled with β-blockade (e.g. propranolol) which is usually discontinued before surgery because of its myocardial depressant effect after bypass. Hypercyanotic attacks require urgent treatment, including sedation with morphine (0.2 mg/kg), oxygen, sodium bicarbonate (1 mmol/kg), propranolol (0.2 mg/kg) and an infusion of noradrenaline. Noradrenaline (dose range 0.01–0.5 μg/kg/min, 30 μg/kg in 50 ml 5% dextrose at 5 ml/h i.v. = 0.05 μg/kg/min), is the drug of first choice for attacks occurring during surgery. Surgery becomes more urgent as the combination of systemic hypotension, hypoxaemia and acidosis may be rapidly fatal. Mechanical ventilation may further decrease pulmonary blood flow especially if more than minimal distending pressure is used.

Congestive cardiac failure

Heart failure is associated with large left-to-right shunt, mitral or aortic valve disease, TAPVD or valve atresias and may be precipitated by respiratory infection or anaemia. Signs include hepatomegaly since the liver is so distensible in infancy, tachycardia with a gallop rhythm and tachypnoea, but peripheral oedema is a very late occurrence. Wheezing heard by auscultation of the chest in infancy is a sign of increased interstitial lung water, not asthma as there is no bronchial musculature in infants. Digoxin and diuretics (frusemide up to 1 mg/kg 8-hourly) with potassium supplements (1 mmol/kg b.d.) are standard treatment. Prolonged therapy with diuretics often leads to hypovolaemia in infancy as well as reduction in total body potassium, manifest by a metabolic alkalosis. Digoxin therapy is usually stopped preoperatively because of toxicity post-bypass and stronger inotropic agents such as dopamine used if necessary at that stage (Table 13.3).

Myocardial function

Differences in cardiovascular function in the infant are discussed elsewhere (p. 258), but animal work does show that fetal myocardium develops much less active tension during isometric contraction than the adult and is much more sensitive to the depressant effect of inhalational anaesthetic agents. Newborn myocardium contains only 30% contractile mass whereas the adult has 60%, causing the stroke volume of the infant to be relatively fixed. Increases in cardiac output can only come from increases in cardiac rate and bradycardia causes a severe fall in cardiac output. Infants have a lower blood pressure than that found later in life—average systolic blood pressure is 80 mmHg.

Table 13.3. Dose regimen for digitalization of children

	Total digitalizing dose in 24 h		Maintenance dose in 24 h	
Age	Oral (mg/kg)	Parenteral (mg/kg)	Oral (mg/kg)	Parenteral (mg/kg)
Neonates and infants (less than 3.0 kg)	0.04	0.03	0.015	0.010
Infants (over 1 month) and children to 2 years	0.06	0.04	0.025	0.015
Children 2–10 years	0.04	0.03	0.015	0.010
	Half the total dose is usually given at once, a quarter after 8 h and the remaining quarter 8 h later		Usually given as a divided dose twice and occasionally three times daily	

CARDIAC INVESTIGATION

A good history and proper physical examination remain the basis of diagnosis in paediatric cardiology, but in addition, chest X-ray, ECG, echocardiography and cardiac catheterization are often necessary.

From the *chest X-ray* an evaluation of cardiac size, shape, position and pulmonary vascularity can be made as well as lung fields generally. Cardiothoracic ratio is 0.6 in infancy and the thymus may mimic cardiac enlargement. Classically transposition of great arteries has an egg-shaped heart and Fallot's a boot shape, but a normal configuration does not necessarily rule out a specific defect. Pulmonary hyperaemia and underperfusion are easily seen, as are all stages of pulmonary oedema.

ECG has specific changes in the very young, with dominance of the right ventricle and right axis deviation, so that a left axis configuration is always abnormal. The adult pattern is seen by 3 years of age. Information on enlargement of chambers, cardiac malpositioning and rhythm abnormalities is also provided.

Modern *echocardiography* has revolutionized cardiac diagnosis and frequently information gained from this non-invasive technique is of superior quality (Macartney, 1986). M-mode echo records motion of the heart from which it is possible to measure the thickness of the chamber walls and left ventricular function. If the ECG is recorded at the same time, measurement of systolic time intervals can be made. Left ventricular function is assessed from the shortening fraction (above 0.3 in infants) and left ventricular systolic time intervals. The time between onset of the ECG Q wave and aortic valve opening is the pre-ejection period (PEP) and the ejection time

(ET) is the time the aortic valve is open. The PEP:ET ratio should be less than 0.3. The echo shows the velocity of fibre shortening (less than 1 circumference/s) of the walls and septum (Feigenbaum et al, 1982). Serial echo investigations are of great importance postoperatively to assess ventricular function and are particularly important after the arterial switch operation for transposition of great arteries, where the coronary arteries are reimplanted and after the Senning operation for atrial correction of transposition of great arteries, where the systemic right ventricular function may not be optimal. Two-dimensional echocardiography allows an accurate diagnosis of connections of all chambers and great vessels. Pericardial effusions are easily seen and the dimensions of septal defects can be estimated and shunts seen using bubble injections into the venous circulation. Doppler echocardiography detects changes in the velocity of blood flow so that shunts and obstructions as well as cardiac output can be measured (Sullivan, 1986).

Cardiac catheterization is required less often, but is necessary to obtain pressures, quantitative flows and for the calculation of systemic and pulmonary resistances (Table 13.4).

An increasing number of therapeutic manoeuvres are now performed— balloon atrial septostomy; transluminal angioplasty of aortic coarctation; balloon valvuloplasty of aortic and pulmonary valves; angioplasty of stenotic pulmonary arteries and occlusion of collaterals. Angiography with its contrast load may be poorly tolerated in sick infants as the circulation has to cope with a biphasic insult—first from a load of hyperosmolar solution followed by an osmotic diuresis. Protection against hypothermia is necessary.

At the Hospital for Sick Children in London most cardiac catheterizations are performed using sedation and local anaesthesia (lignocaine up to 3 mg/kg) and this has been the practice for more than 12 years (Table 13.5). In other centres, all children are anaesthetized but overall in the UK, 50% of older children and infants are anaesthetized; for newborns, one-third have no sedation or anaesthesia; one-third have sedation, and one-third general anaesthesia (O'Higgins, 1988).

In addition diazepam 0.2 mg/kg may be given via the catheter as necessary. Full monitoring includes ECG, blood pressure and pulse oximetry; blood up to 10 ml/kg is replaced by dextrose and serial haematocrits, blood sugar (BM sticks) and blood gas estimations are made.

Anaesthesia is rarely required but is used for very sick patients with severe lesions, such as pulmonary vascular disease, severe rhythm problems, severe heart failure due to obstructive lesions and the growing number of patients undergoing therapeutic catheterization.

Anaesthesia always involves a relaxant technique with controlled ventilation and a fixed inspired oxygen concentration, usually 30% to simplify the calculation of shunts. The anaesthetist must be prepared to deal with periods of low cardiac output and dysrhythmia so monitoring of arterial pressure is usually direct, though access to the central venous circulation is via the catheter. Patients with increased pulmonary vascular resistance are given a period of 100% oxygen to determine whether there is a reversible component. Tolazoline 0.5–1 mg/kg may also be given. A hypercyanotic attack in Fallot's tetralogy is common during cardiac catheterization.

Table 13.4. Normal cardiovascular values for children

	% Saturated O_2	Systolic	Diastolic	Mean
		Pressure (mmHg)		
Superior vena cava	65–75			2–6
Inferior vena cava	75–80			2–6
Coronary sinus	30–40			2–6
Right atrium	75	a = 5–10	v = 4–10	2–6
Right ventricle	75	15–30	0–5	
Neonate		65–80	0–5	
Pulmonary artery	75	15–30	5–10	10–20
Neonate		65–80	35–50	40–70
Pulmonary artery wedge	96	a = 3–7	v = 5–15	5–12
Pulmonary vein	96–100	a = 6–12	v = 8–15	5–10
Left atrium	96–100	a = 6–12	v = 8–15	5–10
Left ventricle	96–100	80–130	0–10	
Aorta	96–100	80–130	60–90	70–80

	Age		
	< 2 years	> 2 years	Adult
LV end-diastolic volume (ml/m²)	42 ± 10	73 ± 10	70 ± 20
LV end-systolic volume (ml/m²)	13.4	27 ± 7	24
LV stroke volume (ml/m²)	28.6	44 ± 5	45 ± 13
LV ejection fraction	0.68 ± 0.05	0.63 ± 0.05	0.67 ± 0.08
LV mass (g/m²)	92 ± 16	86 ± 11	96 ± 11
RV end-diastolic volume (ml/m²)	53 ± 3	75 ± 2	
Left atrial maximum volume (ml/m²)	26 ± 5	38 ± 8	34 ± 10

Cardiac index	3–5 l/min/m²
Systemic arteriolar resistance	10–15 Wood units (mmHg/l/min/m²)
Pulmonary arteriolar resistance	8–10 Wood units (neonate) and 1–3 units after 6–8 weeks (mmHg/l/min/m²)
Normal aortic valve area	2 cm²/m² (adult, 3–4 cm²)
Normal pulmonary valve area	2 cm²/m² (adult, 2–4 cm²)
Adult mitral valve	5 cm²
Adult tricuspid valve	10 cm²

ANAESTHETIC MANAGEMENT

The general principles of anaesthesia for cardiac surgery in children do not greatly differ from those in adults, but there are specific differences related to immaturity of all organ systems, and smaller blood volumes mean that sudden major haemorrhage is more likely to be catastrophic. Adequate depth of anaesthesia with analgesia is necessary to obtund a major stress response, which increases the chance of serious dysrhythmias, peripheral vasoconstriction, common anyway in infants and right ventricular outflow

Table 13.5. Sedation for children undergoing cardiac catheterization

---

These investigations are performed under *basal sedation* supplemented if required by i.v. diazepam (0.1–0.2 mg/kg).

No atropine
1. Trichloral syrup: 30 mg/kg orally nocte then Vallergan 3 mg/kg orally 3 h pre-catheter
2. Premedication: (all given i.m. *30 min pre-catheter*)
   (a) Newborns—1 month of age: may have pethidine injection compound up to 0.05 ml/kg
       No Vallergan
   (b) 1 month of age—15 kg: pethidine injection compound 0.1 ml/kg preceded by Vallergan in infants over 5 kg body weight. Maximum dose pethidine compound 1.5 ml. Smaller babies in poor condition should have a reduced dose
   (c) Over 15 kg: papaveretum and hyoscine preceded by chloral/Vallergan:

   Papaveretum   0.4–0.5 mg/kg
   Hyoscine   0.008–0.1 mg/kg
   (maximum dose papaveretum 15 mg)

Fallot's tetralogy patients may be more stable if given 0.2 mg/kg morphine rather than pethidine injection compound.
Children over 2½ years of age who are just under 15 kg body weight are usually better sedated if given papaveretum and hyoscine rather than pethidine injection compound. Most children require the full dose of sedation. The timing is important because of the patient preparation time and the duration of the investigation.

---

tract spasm in Fallot's tetralogy. Systemic embolism in children with right-to-left shunts such as transposition of great arteries and atrial septal defect is a potential danger. Great care must be taken to avoid injection of air or particulate matter and cerebral, coronary and renal arteries are at particular risk from embolization. Stopcocks are an important source of air so the line should be aspirated with the syringe before injection and the last millilitre from the syringe should not be used—injection with a needle into a rubber bung is an alternative.

Antibiotics (Table 13.6)

The prevention of bacterial endocarditis is a major concern in children; antibiotic prophylaxis is routine to cover all heart surgery because transient bacteraemia associated with intubation and vascular access is common. Routine cover is gentamicin 2 mg/kg and flucloxacillin 25 mg/kg i.v. at induction of anaesthesia, and again after bypass; then gentamicin 2 mg/kg 8-hourly i.v. and flucloxacillin 12.5 mg i.v. 6-hourly for 24 h postoperatively. For those allergic to penicillins vancomycin 20 mg/kg is substituted—this requires infusion over 1 h.

Assessment and premedication

Heart surgery is a tremendously anxious time for parents and patients and

Table 13.6(a). Antibiotic prophylaxis (Shanson, 1987)

Cardiac conditions	Surgical procedures
Prosthetic cardiac valves (including biosynthetic valves)	All dental procedures likely to induce gingival bleeding (not simple orthodontics or shedding of deciduous teeth)
Most congenital cardiac malformations	
Surgically constructed systemic pulmonary shunts	Tonsillectomy and/or adenoidectomy
	Surgical procedures or biopsy involving respiratory mucosa
Rheumatic and other acquired valvular dysfunction	Bronchoscopy, especially with a rigid bronchoscope
Idiopathic hypertrophic subaortic stenosis	Incision and drainage of infected tissue
Previous history of bacterial endocarditis	Genitourinary and gastrointestinal procedures
Mitral valve prolapse with insufficiency	
Endocarditis prophylaxis not needed for:	
Isolated secundum atrial septal defect	
Secundum atrial septal defect repaired without a patch 6 or more months earlier	
Patent ductus arteriosus ligated and divided 6 or more months earlier	

all aspects of anaesthesia and surgery including risks should be discussed fully, frankly and with courtesy. The patients have often been in hospital on previous occasions and anxiety may be intense. The preoperative visit also allows the anaesthetist to define the lesion and what the surgeon intends to do and to assess the clinical condition, degree of cyanosis, exercise tolerance, ability to feed etc. The presence of other congenital abnormalities should be noted. It is usual for the parents to be shown the postoperative intensive care unit on the day prior to surgery so that the shock of seeing their own child postoperatively should be lessened. Some small sick babies will already be receiving full intensive care and indeed a period of mechanical ventilation, fully monitored with prostaglandin and inotropic agents may be beneficial as myocardial glycogen stores may be replenished and poor renal function improved.

A checklist for preoperative investigations with the results is useful and should include haemoglobin, haematocrit, electrolytes, clotting studies and platelet count, a recent chest X-ray and the current status of drug therapy such as digoxin, diuretics or β-blockers. Any dental infection should be treated preoperatively together with the appropriate antibiotic cover. Children are given a dextrose drink 4 h preoperatively, but for small babies having 2–4-hourly feeds the last feed is omitted.

Establishment of a rapport with the child is beneficial but most children with cardiac disease tolerate full opiate premedication very well and indeed the use of morphine at this stage augments anaesthesia with much less disturbance to cardiovascular function than the same drugs given intravenously during the surgery (Table 13.7).

Table 13.6(b). Antibiotic dose regimens

Recommended antibiotic regimens for dental/respiratory tract procedures	
Standard regimen	
For dental procedures that cause gingival bleeding, and oral respiratory tract surgery	Penicillin V, 1–2 g orally 1 h before, then 0.50–1 g 6 h later, for patients unable to take oral medications, 1–2 million u aqueous penicillin G i.v. or i.m. 30–60 min before a procedure, and 0.5–1 million u 6 h later may be substituted
Special regimens	
Parenteral regimen for use when maximal protection desired, e.g. for patients with prosthetic valves	Ampicillin, 50 mg/kg i.m. or i.v. plus gentamicin, 2 mg/kg i.m. or i.v. 30 min before procedure followed by 0.5–1 g oral penicillin V 6 h later; alternatively, parenteral regimen may be repeated once 8 h later
Oral regimen for penicillin-allergic patients	Erythromycin, 20 mg/kg orally 1 h before, then 10 mg/kg 6 h later
Parenteral regimen for penicillin-allergic patients	Vancomycin, 20 mg/kg i.v. slowly over 1 h, starting 1 h before; no repeat dose is necessary
Recommended regimens for gastrointestinal/genitourinary procedures	
Standard regimen	
For genitourinary/gastrointestinal tract procedures	Ampicillin, 50 mg/kg i.m. or i.v. plus gentamicin 2 mg/kg i.m. or i.v. given 30 min before procedure; 1 follow-up dose may be given 8 h later
Special regimens	
Oral regimens for minor or repetitive procedures in low-risk patients	Amoxicillin, 1–3 g, orally 1 h before procedure and 0.75–1.5 g 6 h later
Penicillin-allergic patients	Vancomycin, 20 mg/kg i.v. slowly over 1 h, plus gentamicin 2 mg/kg i.m. or i.v. given 1 h before procedure; may be repeated once 8–12 h later

It is the author's practice to give sedative premedication to even the smallest baby as all require some respiratory support postoperatively.

Anaesthetic agents

There is no anaesthetic agent in common use which does not affect cardiovascular function and if the myocardium is poor the effects may be profound, particularly if the patient is hypoxic. All opioids cause hypotension,

Table 13.7. Anaesthetic premedication for cardiac patients

Intramuscular premedication: drug doses

Given 45–60 min preoperatively
1. Atropine
   Newborn 0.04 mg/kg (minimum 0.15 mg)
   Over 5 kg 0.02 mg/kg (maximum 0.5 mg)
2. Inj. pethidine compound (Toronto mixture)
   Used 1–18 months of age
   0.06–0.08 ml/kg (maximum 1 ml)
   This contains pethidine   25 mg ⎫
                  promethazine   6.25 mg ⎬ in 1 ml
                  chlorpromazine 6.25 mg ⎭
   (pethidine dose 1.5–2 mg/kg)
3. Papaveretum and hyoscine hydrobromide (combined ampoule contains papaveretum 20 mg, hyoscine hydrobromide 0.4 mg in 1 ml)
   Used over 2 years of age
   Papaveretum   0.4 mg/kg (maximum 15 mg)
   Hyoscine hydrobromide 0.08 mg/kg
4. Morphine and atropine sulphate
   Morphine   0.2 mg/kg (maximum 10 mg)
   Atropine sulphate 0.02 mg/kg

Oral sedation: drug doses

Used as pre-premedication or night sedation. May be given 3–6 h preoperatively. Not used routinely and not used under 18 months of age

1. Chloral hydrate syrup 20–30 mg/kg
2. Diazepam   0.4 mg/kg
3. Promethazine   0.5 mg/kg
4. Trimeprazine   1.5–2.0 mg/kg

and though fentanyl does preserve cardiac stability large doses should only be given after an initial test-dose. Myocardial depression with halothane may be severe; it is contraindicated except in minute doses in patients with obstructive lesions and not at all until full monitoring has been established. Hensley et al (1987) found that induction with halothane, nitrous oxide and oxygen actually increased oxygen saturation in children with cyanotic congenital heart disease, particularly in those with the potential for variable pulmonary outflow tract obstruction. Isoflurane is claimed to have a less depressive cardiac effect than halothane but it decreases systemic resistance, which is unwise in patients with balanced shunts. However it has been shown by Murray et al (1987) in children that halothane and isoflurane both decrease mean blood pressure from an awake level; both decrease cardiac index at 1.25 MAC (minimum alveolar concentration) with a significant decrease in ejection fractions. After a fluid load the ejection fraction decreased significantly with halothane but increased with isoflurane. This response to fluid may show that a greater cardiovascular reserve exists during isoflurane anaesthesia than with halothane. Isoflurane is a small vessel coronary dilator and this type of vasodilator may cause myocardial ischaemia by diverting flow from areas of borderline perfusion toward areas that are already well perfused. This so-called 'coronary steal' may be deleterious in paediatric patients whose coronary flow is already prejudiced (Becker, 1987). Ketamine causes tachycardia and increases cardiac output from catecholamine release, which may be undesirable in obstructive lesions, but is otherwise satisfactory (Morray et al, 1984).

Induction and monitoring—open heart surgery

Before induction of anaesthesia it is wise to have prepared clearly labelled syringes of 8.4% sodium bicarbonate, 1:10 000 adrenaline and 10 or 20% $CaCl_2$.

Whichever agents are preferred for induction minimal quantities to provide a smooth induction should be used and respiratory obstruction or depression avoided. The airway should be rapidly secured and mechanical ventilation commenced. At the Children's Hospital in London rapid induction of anaesthesia is achieved by either cyclopropane (50:50 with oxygen for 30–40 s) which has no cardiovascular effects over this brief period or thiopentone 2 mg/kg i.v. slowly. Thiopentone should be used with great care in patients with a fixed cardiac output, for example with aortic stenosis or constrictive pericarditis. Ketamine 2 mg/kg i.v. is a satisfactory alternative. Suxamethonium 1–2 mg/kg is used for rapid tracheal intubation and anaesthesia continued with oxygen/nitrous oxide and a long-acting muscle relaxant such as pancuronium (0.1 mg/kg). Pancuronium occasionally causes a troublesome tachycardia and tubocurarine or alcuronium are alternatives. The hypotension seen with tubocurarine in adults does not occur in children. Most infants undergoing cardiac surgery require some postoperative respiratory support so a firm nasal fixation of the tracheal tube is preferred. The tube should be of a sufficient size to allow a small air leak through the cricoid at 25 cm H_2O inflation pressure and at least 3 cm of tube should lie in the trachea. The author uses fixation with a Tunstall connector (Penlon Ltd.) which has proved very satisfactory over many years (Figure 13.1).

Monitoring during induction, a time of potential instability, should consist of a precordial stethoscope, ECG, automatic blood pressure device and a pulse oximeter. Most small children do not come to the induction room with venous access already established as this may prove to be rather upsetting; however, as soon as intubation has been achieved venous access should be established—a vein on the back of the hand using a 20 or 22 G cannula is satisfactory and this can be connected to an infusion line incorporating a warming coil for crystalloid, blood or plasma. Two 20 G or 18 G 50 mm cannulas are placed in the right internal jugular vein by direct puncture, one for monitoring and the other for continuous infusion of drugs. Alternatively a double-lumen catheter (e.g. Arrow Ltd.) can be placed using the Seldinger technique, but these are rather expensive and are not routinely used. Older children require 16 G × 80 mm cannulas. Other sites for central vein catheterization are less satisfactory, though the left internal jugular vein should be used if there is a persistent left superior vena cava or if a Glenn procedure is planned. It is often impossible to pass the cannula or catheter from the left

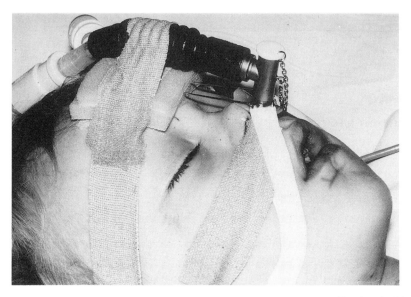

Figure 13.1. Fixation of the nasal tube using Tunstall connector (Penlon Ltd.).

into the right atrium even using a Seldinger wire. If a peripheral vein has been difficult to establish a third neck line can be placed. Three such cannulas are a basic requirement for open cardiac surgery. Great care should be taken not to introduce air into the circulation. Central venous pressure readings in infancy may not be reliable because the venous system has a great capacity as the liver is so distensible. Considerable volumes of fluid may be given with no rise in central venous pressure at all, though the liver has enlarged enormously. Right atrial pressure does not necessarily correspond with severity of congestive cardiac failure in small infants.

Direct monitoring of arterial pressure is via a 22 G Teflon cannula inserted percutaneously into a radial artery. Alternative sites include the ulnar axillary, femoral or temporal artery. Risks of air embolus and skin necrosis using this latter site have been described. In infants the technique of transfixation is likely to be more successful than a direct puncture technique. The cannula is connected to a short extension with a three-way stopcock to allow frequent sampling and is continuously flushed with heparinized saline (1 u/ml) using an 'intraflow' type of device (3 ml/h) except in very small babies when a syringe pump set to 1 ml/h is used.

This stage of anaesthesia should not take too long—10–20 min should be sufficient or the child will become vasoconstricted and acidotic. In addition a nasogastric tube (postoperative ileus), a silastic urinary catheter, peripheral temperature, nasopharyngeal temperature (reflecting cerebral temperature) and oesophageal temperature probes (reflecting cardiac temperature) are inserted. In patients at risk from postoperative pulmonary hypertensive crisis a 20 or 22 G catheter is coiled up in the right atrium via the right internal jugular vein to be passed on into the pulmonary artery by the surgeon before completing the operation. A Swan-Ganz catheter is rarely used. Other monitoring includes end-tidal CO_2, which is higher than $PaCO_2$ with reduced pulmonary blood flow, and pulse oximetry, which provides an index of tissue perfusion. The cerebral function monitor does not provide any useful information, though the new cerebral function analyser (CFAM) may do so (Prior and Maynard, 1986).

Maintenance of anaesthesia

The patient is transferred to the operating table on a heated mattress, which is at this stage switched off, and connected to a mechanical ventilator. A small bridge is used to lift the chest forward for median sternotomy. The chest movement is checked and ventilator adjustments made after blood gas analysis to give a $PaCO_2$ of 5 kPa. It should be remembered that patients with left-to-right shunts have non-compliant lungs whilst those with right-to-left shunts have compliant lungs; overventilation of these will further reduce pulmonary blood flow. When monitoring lines have been connected, anaesthesia is supplemented with fentanyl—first a test-dose (1 µg/kg) followed by up to 30 µg/kg i.v., repeated, together with a full dose of relaxant, just before bypass. These fentanyl dosages provide unique cardiovascular stability (Yasker, 1987). Diazepam (0.4 mg/kg) when used together with pancuronium can also be given to reduce the risk of awareness. Inspired oxygen concentration is adjusted to give a reasonable PaO_2, depending on the lesion, but 100% should be used if cardiac output falls— the balance is best made up with nitrous oxide. During opening of the chest, particularly by sternotomy, low doses of inhalational agents such as halothane or isoflurane will control the hypertension and may actually be beneficial to the myocardium (Murray et al, 1987); a systolic pressure of 90–100 mmHg is satisfactory. Serial blood gas analyses should be made as a tendency to an increase in acidosis is common and should be corrected if the base excess is greater than 5 mmol/l (weight/5 × ½ base deficit = ml 8.4% HCO_3).

Metabolic alkalosis is associated with a low total body potassium and increments of 0.5–1 mmol K^+ diluted are given slowly to keep serum levels over 4 mmol/l.

Rapid transfusion may be necessary at any time, e.g. during aortic cannulation, so equipment to pressurize the infusion should be available. Bleeding from sternotomy in older children with cyanotic disease may be enormous and in repeat operations there is a danger that one of the cardiac chambers is entered inadvertently. Surgical manipulation always interferes with cardiac output, especially when putting in venous pursestrings and 'snuggers' for the venous tourniquets. It is now usual to begin bypass with only the superior vena cava cannula and to put the second in as soon as bypass is established. A bolus injection of $CaCl_2$ is a powerful inotropic stimulus but it should be remembered that severe bradycardia and even asystole may occur if K^+ is low or if myocardial oxygenation is very borderline. A very small dose of 1 in 100 000 adrenaline may be better to improve cardiac output if the systemic blood pressure does not return to a reasonable level after surgical manipulations have stopped.

A control level of activated clotting time (ACT) is measured prior to heparinization and should be in the region of 90–140 s (Hemochron R automatic ACT device; Verska, 1977). Heparin 300 u/kg is given i.v. before aortic cannulation and ACT should be greater than 400 s before and during bypass. Further heparin would be necessary if the ACT fell below that level, but in practice with heparin given to the bypass prime and hypothermic conditions, further heparin is seldom needed. However, ACT continues to be used because a few patients have a decreased response (Gravlee et al, 1987) and inadequate anticoagulation may result in damaging low-grade fibrinolysis.

Cardiopulmonary bypass

A further full dose of relaxant and analgesic is given a few minutes before bypass to allow time for the drugs to fix at the end-plate and to achieve complete muscular paralysis. It is a disaster if respiratory movements start during deep hypothermic circulatory arrest; if air is sucked into the heart with an atrial septal defect air embolism is a very real possibility. There is no agreement on how to manage the lungs during bypass, but ventilation continues until there is full flow from the bypass and the venous drainage blood looks well oxygenated, after which the lungs may be left to collapse or maintained with 3–5 cm H_2O distending pressure with oxygen or oxygen and air. Lung damage is more likely to occur from the vascular side and blood from the left side must be vented continuously. Left-to-right shunts through a PDA or Blalock shunt must be immediately controlled.

A high perfusion pressure at the start of bypass should be assumed to be due to light anaesthesia causing peripheral vasoconstriction, until proved otherwise (e.g. 4 mg/kg thiopentone). Pressures between 30–70 mmHg are considered suitable at full flow (2.4 l/m²/min). Vasoconstrictors are not used, but the long-acting blocking agent phenoxybenzamine 1 mg/kg is given to those patients at risk from pulmonary hypertensive crisis—this may be given prior to bypass without serious cardiovascular effects, though the systemic pressure tends gradually to fall over a 10-min period. Sodium nitroprusside 5–20 μg/kg/min may also be necessary, and is used routinely anyway during the rewarming period (see below). At low temperatures cerebral metabolism and oxygen consumption are greatly reduced; at 20°C they are only 17% of basal requirements. Periods of circulatory arrest of up to 70 min may be used at this temperature. Deep hypothermic circulatory arrest is used routinely for periods of time in open heart surgery for very small babies with gradually improving results and allows the most complex of repairs to be performed. The venous cannulas are removed after circulatory arrest and replaced prior to recommencement of bypass. Catecholamine levels are enormously elevated after deep hypothermic circulatory arrest, contributing to extreme vasoconstriction; surface cooling (see below) causes even higher levels (Wood et al, 1980; Firmin et al, 1985). Lactate and pyruvate levels are surprisingly low even after long periods of arrest and myocardial protection is maximized by preventing the heart being rewarmed by surrounding tissues. Alternatively low flow can be maintained where possible (venus cannulas left in situ) at flow levels as low as 0.5 l/m^2/ min. Uniform cooling before arrest is very important and requires *all* temperatures to read 17–18°C with *at least* 12 min of bypass. Methylprednisolone 30 mg/kg to stabilize membranes is given before arrest and moderate haemodilution to a haematocrit of 20 is used to promote peripheral blood flow. Newborns who have difficulty in excreting a large fluid load may require ultrafiltration towards the end of bypass or peritoneal dialysis in the early postoperative period. Stow et al (1987) show decreases in cerebral perfusion pressure during cooling and rewarming on bypass after deep hypothermic circulatory arrest.

Surface cooling

The technique of surface cooling before beginning surgery has largely been abandoned in favour of a very short pre-bypass period and core cooling on bypass. It was claimed that the technique produced more even cooling, particularly of the peripheral muscular bed to prevent readjustment of temperatures and possible rewarming after arrest. A measure of cerebral protection would be achieved if cardiac output fell or cardiac arrest occurred during sternotomy (Barratt-Boyes et al, 1971). No metabolic differences have been found between surface cooling and core cooling. Icebags are packed around the baby over the major arteries after anaesthesia, but care is taken to avoid the precordium, kidneys or limb extremities. Peripheral vasodilatation is promoted by adequate anaesthesia (isoflurane) and as the temperature falls, CO_2 production is diminished so 2.5–5% CO_2 is added to the inspired gases to maintain $PaCO_2$ over 6 kPa. This improves cerebral perfusion. Very frequent blood gas (corrected for temperature) and K^+ analysis are essential and severe acidosis is corrected. Cardiac stability is easily achieved during cooling if K^+ supplements are given (0.5–1 mmol) as K^+ levels fall with movement into the cells. Crystalloid 10–20 ml/kg i.v. helps to maintain peripheral blood flow. Active cooling is discontinued when the nasopharyngeal temperature is 26°C. A 2°C afterdrop is to be expected and surgery then proceeds.

Cardioplegia

It is commonplace to infuse cold cardioplegic solution into the root of the aorta after aortic cross-clamping to cause asystole and cool the myocardium (Buckberg, 1979). The cardioplegic solution (e.g. Ringer's solution containing KCl 1.193 g, procaine 272.8 mg and magnesium chloride 3.253 g/l) is infused at 150 mmHg pressure at a dose of 20–30 ml/kg bodyweight to preserve myocardial function. A half-dose is repeated at intervals of 30 min of aortic cross-clamping to prevent electrical activity. As the aorta is clamped the solution is aspirated by the discard suction from the right atrium and none goes into the perfusate. There is some anecdotal evidence that the presence of procaine may increase the incidence of atrioventricular block in the immediate post-bypass period, but this does not appear to be of any clinical significance.

Extracorporeal circulation

Extracorporeal circulation is now safe and routine with flow rates at normothermia of 2.2–2.5 l/min/m^2 providing a margin of safety (Kirklin et al, 1985). Although pulsatile flow from the pump may help organ perfusion, particularly the kidneys, it is not routinely used (Finlayson, 1987) as there seems to be no proven clinical advantage. The peripheral circulation should be maximal at any temperature and this is related to oxygen consumption (Figure 13.2). The temperature gradient between perfusate and the patient should never exceed 15°C on rewarming, but it is commonplace to begin bypass with a perfusate cooled to 10°C to achieve very rapid cardiac and cerebral cooling. Systemic venous pressure should always be low (less than 10 mmHg) or cerebral oedema will occur, so the largest possible venous cannulas should be used.

The following is the formula for calculating haematocrit of the prime for cardiopulmonary bypass:

$$Htpm = \frac{(kg\ body\ weight \times f \times 1000)\ (Htp)}{(kg\ body\ weight \times f \times 1000) + machine\ B.V.}$$

Htpm is the desired total haematocrit (25–30), Htp is the Ht of the patient and f is 0.08 in infants and young children.

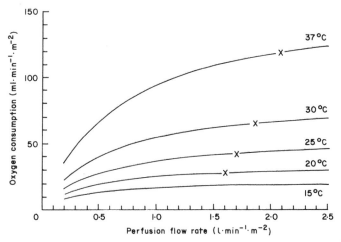

Figure 13.2. Normogram of the relation between oxygen consumption ($\dot{V}O_2$) and perfusion flow rate ($\dot{Q}$) at various temperatures from Kirklin et al, 1985, with permission.

Stored blood should ideally be less than 5 days old and requires 3000 units of heparin, 10 ml 8.4% $NaHCO_3$ and 5 ml 10% $CaCl_2$ to be added to each 500 ml of blood. Hartmann's solution is used for dilution. Blood sugar levels are always well maintained on bypass (Ratcliffe et al, 1985) but will require close monitoring afterwards. Many centres currently use the Terumo Capiox range of membrane oxygenators with low priming volumes; PaO_2 levels are held between 15 and 25 kPa, but $PaCO_2$ is more controversial. At the Hospital for Sick Children in London we add CO_2 to the gas mixture, but at the risk of having a high $PaCO_2$ after temperature correction.

Other constituents of the prime include 100 ml 20% albumin to increase the oncotic pressure and 0.5 g/kg mannitol to promote osmotic diuresis. Approximately 0.5–1 mmol/kg of potassium is required during bypass and this can be given incrementally after aortic cross-clamping to maintain a serum K^+ of at least 4.5 mmol/l.

Occasionally in infancy cardiopulmonary bypass may produce lung and tissue damage, including severe extravasation of plasma and greatly increased interstitial fluid plus a coagulopathy. Complement activation is assumed to play an important role in the lung damage, possibly with sequestration of polymorphs in the lungs (Kirklin et al, 1983; Chenoweth et al, 1981).

Rewarming

Just before the aortic clamp is released, rewarming starts with a temperature gradient of no more than 15°C between patient and perfusate or perfusate and heat exchange. During rewarming heat is provided mainly by the heat exchanger, but in addition to this, heat also comes from the heating mattress which is now turned on and from heated humidified inspired gases. At this stage it is routine to infuse sodium nitroprusside to overcome the intense vasoconstriction which hypothermia induces and to allow rapid and even rewarming. Higher doses than those used postoperatively are required at this stage and a mean perfusion pressure of 35–45 mmHg is satisfactory. The infusion is stopped at 36°C. Suction is attached to the aortic needle vent as the cross-clamp is removed. Removal of every trace of air is crucial to avoid cerebral air embolism. The cardiac action should be vigorous and the lungs inflated to drive air out of the pulmonary veins; venous pressure is increased and the heart, especially the left atrial appendage is massaged. The heart begins to eject at this point and mechanical ventilation is recommended. It is also usual to position the patient in the head-down position so any ejected air bubbles do not go to the brain.

Intracardiac lines are placed into pulmonary artery or left atrium at this stage. Monitoring of the left atrial pressure is necessary whenever left ventricular or mitral valve function requires close monitoring and is particularly important in the Fontan operation. Intracardiac lines, if placed with meticulous care, have a very low morbidity. Gold et al (1986) report a complication rate of 0.59% with left atrium (LA) lines (catheter retention and bleeding) and 1.07% with PA lines. It is wise to leave the chest drains in situ and to have a unit of blood cross-matched before these lines are removed in the postoperative period.

Post-bypass

Partial bypass is established after deaeration so that the heart can eject and bypass is slowly withdrawn by constriction in the venous drainage line. After venous drainage is stopped the patient is transfused via the aortic cannula to an arterial pressure of 80 mmHg and superior vena cava of 10–12 mmHg with LA no more than 15 mmHg. If arterial pressure remains low with high filling pressures then inotropic support is necessary, as it is essential that the heart is not left with poor myocardial perfusion pressures and poor myocardial oxygen delivery, causing increasing hypoxia and acidosis. It is acceptable to provide an initial inotropic 'kick' to the myocardium with a small bolus of 1 in 100 000 adrenaline or 10% $CaCl_2$ and in many cases this is all that will be necessary. Other patients will require dopamine 5–10 μg/kg/min, which is the author's first choice, or dobutamine in a similar starting dose for those patients judged to have a labile pulmonary vascular resistance, but these may be less effective than adrenaline at the time of coming off bypass (Steen et al, 1978). It is logical to use both dopamine and dobutamine, the former in a low renal vasodilating dose and the latter in higher dosage for inotropic action without vasoconstriction (Table 13.8).

Table 13.8. Cardiac drugs with dosages

Dopamine 6 mg/kg in 100 ml 5% dextrose	1 ml/hr = 1 μg/kg/min dose, 5–10 μg/kg/min
Dobutamine 6 mg/kg in 100 ml 5% dextrose	1 ml/hr = 1 μg/kg/min dose, 5–10 μg/kg/min
Adrenaline 60 μg/kg in 100 ml 5% dextrose	1 ml/hr = 0.01 μg/kg/min dose, 0.01–0.5 μg/kg/min
Isoprenaline 60 μg/kg in 100 ml 5% dextrose	1 ml/hr = 0.01 μg/kg/min dose, 0.01–0.5 μg/kg/min
Noradrenaline 60 μg/kg in 100 ml 5% dextrose	1 ml/hr = 0.01 μg/kg/min dose, 0.01–0.5 μg/kg/min
Dextrose/insulin 2 g dextrose:1 unit insulin	dose, 0.5 g/kg
Calcium chloride	10–20 mg/kg
Sodium nitroprusside 6 mg/kg in 100 ml 5% dextrose	1 ml/hr = 1 μg/kg/min dose, 0.5–5 μg/kg/min

It should be remembered that the venous system is very compliant and it is dangerously easy to overload a small patient with colloid without any change in central venous pressure. Small babies have a rate-dependent cardiac output so chronotropic drugs such as isoprenaline may be required. This can be infused separately or added to the dopamine. Once all the cardiac cannulas have been removed, colloid is tranfused to keep filling pressures within normal limits, using whole blood if the haematocrit is below 40, or fresh frozen plasma if the haematocrit is high. Initially, ventilation is with 100% oxygen to ensure complete oxygenation before the first blood gas analysis (pulse oximetry should give saturated O_2 100%) rather than avoiding nitrous oxide for the theoretical reason it may expand any air bubbles remaining in the circulation.

Protamine is given to reverse heparin in doses up to 6 mg/kg with ACT control though very small patients may require greater doses. Heparin levels in the patient coming off bypass are often in excess of those before going on as a result of heparin added to the prime; although ACT is not specific for heparinization, it is useful to know whether the level has returned to the baseline. Protamine causes a degree of hypotension in most patients and this is occasionally profound, possibly coming from the release of histamine or other vasoactive substances by the heparin–protamine moiety (Colman, 1987). Vascular effects of protamine can be minimized by very slow infusion, possibly after a small test-dose, into a peripheral rather than central vein or even into the left side of the heart via the LA line, although this should be done with meticulous care to avoid air embolism. Fresh frozen plasma, cryoprecipitate and platelet-rich plasma may all be necessary before haemostasis is finally achieved and the ACT has returned to the baseline level.

Towards the end of bypass and afterwards, urine flow should be at least 1 ml/kg/h. Urine output before bypass and during periods of low flow and hypothermia is of no interest. The incidence of acute renal failure associated with open heart surgery in the very young is high (Rigden et al, 1982) and mannitol in the prime, low renal vasodilating doses of dopamine (3–4 µg/kg/min) and small doses of frusemide (0.25 mg/kg) may help to minimize this. Where renal failure existed preoperatively in patients with major lesions, e.g. truncus arteriosus, it is wise to insert a peritoneal dialysis catheter before returning to the intensive care unit. Failure to respond to diuretics is a further indication for early dialysis.

The insertion of temporary pacemaker wires is routine; these can be for direct ventricular pacing or atrioventricular sequential pacing. Rhythm problems in children are not particularly common, but troublesome dysrhythmias do occur—supraventricular tachycardias, junctional rhythm and atrioventricular block with a fall in cardiac output when the myocardium is under stress or with electrolyte and blood gas abnormalities. Slow dysrhythmias are often easily corrected by small doses of isoprenaline. Fast dysrhythmias with an acute fall in cardiac output may be treated by DC shock or adenosine. If the change in rhythm is less catastrophic it can be treated by digoxin, β-adrenergic blockade or amiodarone 5 mg/kg by slow i.v. infusion (Deanfield, 1987).

When the haemodynamics are stable, pressures in all the cardiac chambers are measured by direct needle puncture and of particular interest is the right ventricular pressure, e.g. after repair of VSD or tetralogy of Fallot or gradients across repaired valves. Measurement of cardiac output is not routinely performed as it has many limitations in the infant patient (Nadeau and Noble, 1986). Many patients benefit from reduction in the left ventricular afterload, particularly in infants where vasoconstrictive compensatory mechanisms are very active. Sodium nitroprusside 1–2 µg/kg/min is the first choice, but nitroglycerine, which in low doses may specifically dilate venous capacitance vessels, is particularly indicated in mitral valve regurgitation and coronary artery dysfunction (e.g. after the arterial switch operation for transposition of great arteries).

Respiratory and cardiac support is continued into the postoperative period where indicated. Patients with simple lesions are weaned from the ventilator and extubated after a very short time, but others may require a prolonged weaning period. It is usually beneficial to continue inotropic support until the patient is weaned from the ventilator. Analgesia is with a continuous morphine infusion 0.5 mg/kg in 50 ml at 2 ml/h (= 20 µg/kg/h), which continues until after the chest drains have been removed, usually on the first postoperative day.

Pulmonary hypertensive crisis

In conditions of left-to-right shunt and TAPVD the smooth muscle of the media of the pulmonary arterioles does not regress at birth as normally happens. In fact there is an overgrowth of muscle so that these small vessels in the lung peripheries become unusually contractile and allow the PVR to be extremely labile. The vessels constrict with the stimuli of hypoxia and acidosis, probably via an adrenergic mechanism. If the fetal channels PDA and patent foramen ovale (PFO) are open the increase in PVR causes the reversion to a transitional circulation and critical hypoxaemia, but if these channels are closed as they are after surgery, then severe right heart failure is followed by left heart failure since in infancy both ventricles fail in parallel.

The patients at risk from postoperative pulmonary hypertensive crisis are those with a previously high pulmonary blood flow from left-to-right shunt; unrestrictive VSD; atrioventricular canal defect, especially Down's syndrome; truncus; transposition of great arteries and VSD; and TAPVD, and all these patients now have monitoring of PA or right ventricular pressure. Previously the PA catheter was directly introduced by the surgeon via the RA, but this has disadvantages of bleeding after removal and the need to leave a chest drain in place until after removal of the catheter. Now a 20 or 22 G catheter is put in using the Seldinger technique in the anaesthetic room via the right internal jugular vein and allowed to coil in the RA until the surgical repair is complete, when the surgeon threads it into the PA. This has the advantage of lasting for several days postoperatively if necessary. Only by monitoring PA pressure in relation to the systemic pressure can the effects of restlessness, tracheal suctioning, or weaning from intermittent positive pressure ventilation be seen, so for these at-risk patients we routinely monitor systemic, superior vena caval, PA pressure and transcutaneous oxygen tension ($P_{tc}O_2$).

Rises in PA pressure can be categorized into minor events if PA pressure acutely exceeds 80% of systemic, but without a fall in systemic pressure, and a major crisis if PA pressure exceeds systemic, with a fall in systemic pressure and reduction in $TcPO_2$ and cardiac output (peripheral temperature falls). Experience with the management of transitional circulation in the newborn shows that achieving and then maintaining cardiorespiratory stability is of the utmost importance. Phenoxybenzamine (1 mg/kg) used during surgery in high-risk cases may prevent some crises, but is of no help once a crisis has developed. This α-adrenergic blocking agent is continued for 48 h postoperatively (1 mg/kg 12-hourly). The patient remains on full mechanical ventilation with mild hyperventilation and PaO_2 over 14 kPa; paralysis with pancuronium or vecuronium is an advantage. Morphine infusions which are routinely used for postoperative analgesia in other patients may cause pulmonary vasoconstriction and hypotension, whereas fentanyl has no effect on the pulmonary vasculature. A fentanyl infusion of 4–10 μg/kg/h plus boluses of up to 25 μg/kg blunts stress responses associated with tracheal suctioning (Hickey et al, 1985).

If the pulmonary artery pressure rises to the level of systemic pressure or above, immediate steps must be taken to reverse the pulmonary vascular resistance; as the patient becomes hypoxic, pulmonary vasoconstriction gets worse and may be very difficult to reverse at this stage. Sedation and hyperventilation by hand with 100% oxygen may be effective and is the first-line approach, but if the PA pressure remains high, an infusion of the pulmonary vasodilating drug tolazoline (1 mg/kg/h) or prostacyclin (4–20 ng/kg/min) may be necessary for sustained pulmonary hypertension (PHT), multiple minor events or a crisis. Low doses of both agents may be more effective and are associated with fewer side-effects, e.g. gastric erosions. Approximately one-third of at-risk patients develop multiple minor or major crises and those with major crises have a significant mortality in spite of treatment. It is necessary to maintain tolazoline during weaning from mechanical ventilation. Tolazoline is a histamine agonist and will cause gastric erosions and haematemesis unless an H_2-blocker, such as ranitidine, is also administered. Aluminium hydroxide 5 ml should be put down the nasogastric tube 2-hourly.

REOPERATIONS

Many patients whose cardiac surgery has involved the use of a conduit (truncus arteriosus, pulmonary atresia, Rastelli operation) will eventually require this to be replaced either because it is non-functional with increasing calcification, or because the conduit put in in infancy has become inadequate with growth of the child. The conduit usually lies just beneath the sternum and may even be attached to it. The greatest care is required for the opening of the sternum and usually the iliac artery is prepared for bypass should one of the cardiac chambers be opened inadvertently. An external defibrillator plate is placed beneath the chest before surgery starts. It is advisable to secure extra venous access for these cases, to have blood and colloid in readiness, together with pressure infusion devices in case urgent transfusion should become necessary. The second operation is always well tolerated and is not necessarily a lengthy procedure.

CLOSED CARDIAC AND PALLIATIVE SURGERY

In any unit which receives the whole range of paediatric cardiac anomalies, approximately half the surgical procedures are performed without bypass, often via a thoracotomy. The patients may be in end-stage disease where palliation is all that can be offered, occasionally leading to a future heart or heart–lung transplant. Sick patients may require pre- and postoperative intensive care with respiratory and cardiac support. Direct monitoring of arterial pressure is usual and this also gives access for frequent blood gas analysis. If inotropic or cardiac resuscitation drugs are required at least one central venous line is also necessary. Other monitoring includes ECG, oximetry and central and peripheral temperatures. Small babies are hand-ventilated using a T-piece, though mechanical ventilation is used for older children. A nasogastric tube is inserted as ileus is very common after thoracotomy. For patients expected to be extubated at the end of the procedure fentanyl dose should not exceed 5–10 µg/kg and anaesthesia can be supplemented with small doses of an inhalational agent such as isoflurane or halothane. However, a great number of patients are extremely sick and inhalational agents are contraindicated, so that full doses of opioids may be given and postoperative respiratory support via a nasotracheal tube is undertaken.

Patent ductus arteriosus

Any premature baby is at risk from PDA because the mechanisms which cause the duct to close are also immature; fluid overload in the neonatal period may also cause the ductus to remain open. PDA is also associated with many forms of congenital heart disease, but may be a single chance finding. It is estimated that 25% of babies weighing below 1500 g and recovering from hyaline membrane disease have a PDA. The greatly increased pulmonary blood flow will contribute to the development of bronchopulmonary dysplasia and any small baby who is ventilator-dependent should have a PDA ligated. There may be no murmur so echocardiographic investigation should be routine. These small patients may be fragile, already ventilated and will require very careful monitoring, with the operation sometimes even being performed in the intensive care unit. A relaxant technique with oxygen, nitrous oxide or air and oxygen mixtures with fentanyl 10 µg/kg is an excellent technique for a small baby not expected to breathe spontaneously in the early postoperative period (Robinson and Gregory, 1981; Anand et al, 1987). Oxygen saturation should remain between 90 and 92% to minimize the risk of retinopathy of prematurity and the ventilation is best controlled by hand. The surgical approach is via a left thoracotomy and the ductus is either doubly ligated or clipped. Sudden ligation of the ductus may cause a surge in arterial pressure and increase the possibility of intraventricular cerebral haemorrhage in this vulnerable age group (Marshall et al, 1982). Before the PDA is finally ligated, a trial clamping takes place to demonstrate any serious cardiovascular consequences and there should be two suckers, vascular clamps and blood ready to transfuse in the unlikely event that the ductus is torn during ligation. Transfusion of blood is otherwise rarely necessary.

Older patients do not require direct arterial monitoring and are usually extubated at the end of the operation. During the ligation of a very large and tense ductus a reduction in systemic blood pressure, for example with isoflurane or a small dose of sodium nitroprusside, makes the surgery safer. As for any thoracotomy, intercostal nerve blockade by the surgeon into the open chest with bupivacaine 0.5–1 ml 0.25% per space will provide analgesia well into the postoperative period.

Coarctation of the aorta

Neonatal

These babies are often in terminal left ventricular failure with a tight preductal stenosis or a hypoplastic aortic arch and little, if any, collateral flow. Clinical diagnosis is confirmed by echocardiography. Preoperative care should include mechanical ventilation, prostaglandin and dopamine therapy and all vascular access should have been achieved in the intensive care unit before surgery is undertaken. The arterial line must be in the right arm or a temporal artery, as the left subclavian artery is often incorporated in the surgical repair which takes place via a left thoracotomy. The anaesthetic technique which provides the greatest stability for these very sick patients is relaxant, oxygen and fentanyl (10–25 µg/kg); inhalation agents such as halothane are contraindicated. Total body potassium is frequently very low and contributes to cardiac instability. The time of greatest risk is at unclamping of the aorta when hypotension reduces myocardial perfusion. The aorta can be repeatedly clamped to increase coronary perfusion pressure and with transfusion of 10–20% blood volume, the clamp can eventually be completely removed. The peripheral vasculature is often reactive so an infusion of sodium nitroprusside may be necessary later to maintain the blood pressure between 80 and 100 mmHg in the postoperative period. Respiratory support should continue for 48 h postoperatively, though recovery is usually rapid if the repair is satisfactory and other lesions, e.g. VSD, are not present.

Older child

The patients are not usually unfit, but may be hypertensive with large collateral flow through the intercostal arteries. Without mild induced hypotension the thoracotomy may bleed profusely. Mild hypotension without tachycardia is easily achieved with a combination of 0.5–1 mg/kg labetalol i.v. and isoflurane. Severe hypertension after application of the aortic clamps, indicating poor collateral circulation, is an indication for further induced hypotension, e.g. with sodium nitroprusside. Satisfactory cerebral, renal and spinal cord perfusion during the repair is ensured if the distal aortic pressure is kept above a mean of 45–50 mmHg. The clamping time should never exceed 20–25 min without the use of a temporary heparinized bypass. Sodium nitroprusside infusion is usually required postoperatively to maintain the blood pressure between 90 and 100 mmHg and although the patients are extubated before returning to the unit they do require full analgesia and sedation.

Blalock shunts

Palliative anastomosis of a subclavian artery to the pulmonary artery of the same side to improve pulmonary blood flow is frequently required in patients with pulmonary or tricuspid atresia or severe Fallot's tetralogy if the diameter of the main pulmonary arteries is less than 30% of the aorta. At the Hospital for Sick Children in London tetralogy patients below 8 kg are not corrected at this stage, but have a Blalock shunt as palliation if required. The shunt not only increases peripheral oxygen saturation and prevents damaging hypercyanotic attacks but the increased flow into the pulmonary artery will stimulate its growth to a degree, hopefully allowing patients with pulmonary atresia to be fully corrected at a later stage. The shunt most commonly performed is the modified Blalock using 4–6 mm Gore-Tex tube, usually on the side opposite the aortic arch. Direct anastomosis from aorta to pulmonary artery (Waterston's shunt) is not now performed because of the difficulty in judging its size and the increased risk of pulmonary vascular disease which would make subsequent corrective surgery, e.g. Fontan procedure for tricuspid atresia, impossible.

The patients are always cyanotic, often with a very high haematocrit, and excessive ventilation will further reduce pulmonary blood flow. Arterial monitoring should be from the side opposit to the thoracotomy and one or two lines are inserted into an internal jugular vein. Great care must be taken not to damage the subclavian artery on the side of the shunt during the insertion of these neck lines. Transfusion during the procedure is with plasma to replace blood loss. An anaesthetic technique with relaxant, oxygen, nitrous oxide or oxygen, air and fentanyl is satisfactory and hand ventilation helps the surgeon during the delicate anastomoses in the mediastinum. Heparin 1 mg/kg i.v. is given after the Gore-Tex has been sutured to the subclavian artery, before it is joined to the pulmonary artery. Increasing acidosis is a common finding and 1 mmol/kg sodium bicarbonate is invariably necessary during the procedure. After the shunt is completed peripheral oxygenation and graft patency depend on a normal perfusion pressure and an infusion of, for example, dopamine 6 µg/kg/min may be necessary to achieve this. A short period of intubation postoperatively is invariably beneficial, particularly if the shunt is large and pulmonary compliance falls. If large aortopulmonary collaterals have developed these may need to be ligated to optimize flow into the main pulmonary artery.

Closed valvotomy

In the small infant aortic and pulmonary valvotomy may be performed without bypass, using a very short period of inflow occlusion and circulatory arrest. This is simple, avoiding the use of cardiopulmonary bypass and is the technique of choice for sick newborns. The approach is a median sternotomy and monitoring is as for a bypass with reliable venous access for the rapid transfusion of warmed blood. For aortic valvotomy, the patient is ventilated with 100% oxygen for a few minutes and 1 mmol/kg HCO_3 is given before the cavae are snared. The aorta is clamped and opened and the valvotomy performed under direct vision, during which time 10–15% of the blood volume is transfused, so that the heart rapidly fills after the cavae have been unsnared, and ejects to remove air which escapes through the aortic suture line. Cross-clamping time should not exceed 3 min. Syringes containing 1:10 000 adrenaline, 10% calcium chloride and 8.4% sodium bicarbonate are drawn up ready for use. Postoperative respiratory support may be required for several days if ventricular function is poor.

Pulmonary artery banding

Banding the main pulmonary artery in patients with a large left-to-right shunt not amenable to early corrective surgery causes equalization of pressures in both ventricles, reducing the volume of the shunt. Pulmonary engorgement is diminished, compliance improves and the work of the left ventricle is reduced, as is the risk of permanent pulmonary vascular disease. Full arterial and venous monitoring is used and respiratory support is invariably required postoperatively as the patients have failed to thrive with unremitting cardiac failure. The surgical approach is a left thoracotomy and the band is tightened around the PA until the distal PA pressure is at least half the systemic. Systemic pressure usually rises as PA pressure falls. If the band is too tight the shunt becomes right-to-left with profound desaturation, bradycardia and a fall in cardiac output. Pulse oximetry is most useful in warning of over-banding (Casthely et al, 1987) and the final PaO_2 should be at least 7 kPa (80% saturation).

Blalock–Hanlon septectomy

This operation, performed via a right thoracotomy, is designed to remove a section of atrial septum to equalize the two atrial pressures. In the past the procedure allowed greater mixing of atrial blood in patients with transposition of great arteries to increase peripheral oxygen saturation, but nowadays is required only for complicated transposition of great arteries, where the Rashkind has failed, or other complex conditions not amenable to corrective surgery where decompression of the left atrium gives considerable palliation, e.g. mitral atresia. Problems include the potential for severe haemorrhage and periods of very low cardiac output after the pulmonary veins have been snared. Full monitoring and postoperative ventilation are required.

Vascular ring

The vascular ring around the trachea and oesophagus is commonly based on a double aortic arch with many variations, less frequently by a pulmonary artery sling, with the left PA arising from the right. The patients often present with stridor and the diagnosis is confirmed by a barium swallow which shows indentation of the oesophagus. The effect on the trachea is variable, ranging from mild tracheomalacia to severe tracheal stenosis. Vascular ring is a cause of respiratory arrest and sudden infant death. The operation via a left thoracotomy divides the PDA and one limb of the double aortic arch, freeing the oesophagus and trachea. Anaesthesia is little more complicated than for a simple PDA, but care should be taken with intubation to have the tip of the tracheal tube at least in the mid-trachea and hand ventilation allows early warning of tracheal obstruction during the dissection. Most patients may be extubated at the end of the procedure and nursed in a humidified headbox.

Pre-existing stridor may be intensified because of tracheal oedema and this may respond to dexamethasone 0.25 mg/kg i.v. A small group of patients with severe stridor and secretion retention may require nasotracheal intubation and continuous positive air pressure for several days. Tracheomalacia responds to the distending pressure, which may be continued in the infant with one nasal prong after extubation.

Phrenic nerve palsy

Infants rely solely on function of the diaphragm to breathe. The phrenic nerves are vulnerable during cardiac surgery and are frequently damaged by diathermy, cold injury or traction. A phrenic palsy should be suspected if a small baby fails to wean from the ventilator when cardiac output and pulmonary compliance are normal. The plain chest X-ray may show an elevated hemidiaphragm—two vertebral spaces above the contralateral side are diagnostic, but the diagnosis should also be confirmed by fluoroscopy; occasionally both sides are affected. Often, recovery can be expected between 3 and 6 weeks from the injury; however, the period of respiratory support will be greatly reduced if surgical plication of the diaphragm is undertaken to prevent the damaging respiratory effects of paradoxical movement. Plication will not prejudice normal diaphragmatic function if the nerve regenerates at a future time (Stone et al, 1987).

FLUID BALANCE

Accurate control of fluid balance is crucial to the success of cardiac surgery. In the pre-bypass period maintenance fluids of 5–10 ml/kg/h may be given as 5% dextrose, 4% dextrose/0.18% saline or lactated Ringer's solution. These fluids are not strictly necessary in small babies where sufficient volume of crystalloid is maintained by flushing and diluted drugs, but are of greater importance in patients with a high haematocrit or if surface cooling is used. Blood loss is replaced by colloid.

In the postoperative period, severe fluid restriction is used and post-bypass patients should be administered with 20 ml/m^2/h 5 or 10% dextrose for the day of surgery (day 1); 30 ml/m^2/h on day 2, and 40 ml/m^2/h on day 3; 1 g KCl (13 mmol) can be put into 500 ml of 5% dextrose to maintain serum K$^+$ around 4 mmol/l.

Nasogastric feeds usually begin on day 2 or 3, starting with half-strength milk, but the total fluid intake should not be exceeded. Blood sugar is never low during surgery, but is checked 2–4-hourly postoperatively and if low, boluses of 25% dextrose are given. Closed cases are given 3 ml/kg/h 5 or 10% dextrose on day 1; 4 ml/kg/h on day 2, and 5 ml/kg/h on day 3.

The infusion of colloid matches losses from the chest drains, though extra volumes are often required to maintain reasonable cardiac filling pressures and warm peripheries. Crystalloid input matches urine output, though on days 1 and 2 urine output should always exceed input and regular doses of diuretics may be necessary to achieve this. Continuous infusions of inotropes such as dopamine may require increased concentrations if fluid restriction is to be maintained—the dilutions are in multiples of 6 ml/kg in 100 ml 5% dextrose for ease of calculation.

NON-CARDIAC SURGERY

Increasing numbers of patients with cardiac disease which has been corrected, palliated or uncorrected, require surgery for non-cardiac reasons (Moore, 1981). Patients with corrected cardiac disease may have residual lesions or may never be able to respond to stress with a full cardiac output, e.g. after Mustard or Senning operation for transposition of great arteries the active atrial component of ventricular filling may be lost. Patients after the Fontan operation whose success depends on normal pulmonary vascular resistance may poorly tolerate intermittent positive pressure ventilation and anaesthesia, and many patients have a relatively fixed cardiac output. It is wise preoperatively to seek the opinion of a cardiology colleague to assess the current clinical status of the patient. It may even be necessary to perform the cardiac surgery before any general surgery is undertaken. Conditions such as corrected transposition and Ebstein's anomaly have a high incidence of dysrhythmias, such as supraventricular tachycardia and atrioventricular block.

Assessment must include the general condition of the patient, including associated pulmonary, renal and hepatic abnormalities. Exercise tolerance is the best guide to tolerance of anaesthesia, assessable in infants by the ability to feed and suck without breathlessness and whether growth and development has been normal. Cyanosis and its degree is noted, as well as which cardiac drugs are used, e.g. β-adrenergic blockers cause a relatively fixed cardiac output.

All patients having dental or general surgery require antibiotic prophylaxis (see p. 317) and anaesthetic considerations should include:

1. Full and careful monitoring—direct arterial monitoring is required for major surgery for continuous monitoring of pressure and vascular access for multiple blood samples. The use of a pulmonary artery catheter may be indicated for patients with raised PVR undergoing major surgery.
2. Cardiac output is maintained by a choice of suitable technique, which usually involves controlled ventilation with relaxants, since inhalational agents may be too hypotensive. Peripheral vasodilatation or vasoconstriction should not be excessive, particularly with balanced right-to-left and left-to-right shunts.

3. Blood volume should be well maintained with normal intraoperative fluids as well as colloid to cover blood and plasma losses.
4. Heart rate should be stable at a normal or slightly increased rate and judicial use of atropine intravenously may be necessary to achieve this. Pancuronium may cause undesirable tachycardia so atracurium or vecuronium by bolus or infusion may be more logical.
5. A high inspired oxygen concentration gives a margin of safety for periods of reduced cardiac output or pulmonary congestion and increased right-to-left intrapulmonary shunting.
6. Postoperative monitoring in a high dependence or intensive care unit may be required, as is an increased inspired oxygen concentration, delivered by facemask, nasal cannula or headbox.

REFERENCES

Anand KJS, Sippell WG & Aynsley-Green A (1987) Randomised trial of fentanyl anaesthesia in preterm babies undergoing surgery: effect on the stress response. *Lancet* **i**: 243–248.

Barratt-Boyes BG, Simpson M & Neutze JM (1971) Intracardiac surgery in neonates and infants using deep hypothermia with surface cooling and limited cardiopulmonary bypass. *Circulation* **43 (suppl. 1)**: 1–25.

Becker LC (1987) Is isoflurane dangerous for the patient with coronary artery disease? *Anesthesiology* **66**: 259–261.

Buckberg GD (1979) A proposed solution to the cardioplegic controversy. *Journal of Thoracic and Cardiovascular Surgery* **77**: 803–815.

Casthely PA, Redko V, Dluzneski J et al (1987) Pulse oximetry during pulmonary artery banding. *Journal of Cardiothoracic Anesthesia* **1**: 297–299.

Chenoweth DE, Cooper SW, Hugli TE et al (1981) Complement activation during cardiopulmonary bypass: evidence for generation of C3a and C5a anaphylatoxins. *New England Journal of Medicine* **304**: 497–503.

Coceani F (1986) Effects of eicosanoids on the ductus arteriosus. Proceedings of the Southeastern Symposium on Pulmonary and Cardiovascular effects of Eicosanoids (abstract).

Colman RW (1987) Humoral mediators of catastrophic reactions associated with protamine neutralisation. *Anesthesiology* **66**: 595–596.

Deanfield J (1987) Arrhythmias: paediatrics. *Current Opinions in Cardiology* **2**: 109–111.

Esscher E, Michaelsson B & Smedby B (1975) Cardiovascular malformation in infant deaths: 10 year clinical and epidemiological study. *British Heart Journal* **37**: 824–829.

Feigenbaum H, Henry WL & Popp RL (1982) Echocardiographic evaluation of ventricular function: an overview. *American Journal of Cardiology* **49**: 1311–1318.

Finlayson DC (1987) Nonpulsatile flow is preferable to pulsatile flow during cardiopulmonary bypass. *Journal of Cardiothoracic Anesthesia* **1**: 169–170.

Firmin RK, Bouloux P, Allen P et al (1985) Sympathoadrenal function during cardiac operations in infants with the technique of surface cooling, limited cardiopulmonary bypass and circulatory arrest. *Journal of Cardiovascular Surgery* **90**: 729–735.

Gold JP, Jonas RA, Lang P et al (1986) Transthoracic intracardiac monitoring lines in pediatric surgical patients: a 10-year experience. *Annals of Thoracic Surgery* **42**: 185–191.

Gravlee GP, Brauer SD, Roy RC et al (1987) Predicting the pharmacodynamics of heparin: a clinical evaluation. *Journal of Cardiothoracic Anesthesia* **1**: 379–387.

Greeley WJ, Leslie JB & Reves JG (1987) Prostaglandins and the cardiovascular system: a review and update. *Journal of Cardiothoracic Anaesthesia* **1**: 331–349.

Haworth SG (1986) Lung biopsies in congenital heart disease: computer assisted correlations between structural and hemodynamic abnormalities. In Doyle EF, Engle MA, Gersony WM, Rashkind WJ & Talner NS (eds) *Pediatric Cardiology*, pp 942–945. New York: Springer-Verlag.

Haworth SG & Hall SM (1986) Occlusion of intra-acinar pulmonary arteries in pulmonary hypertensive congenital heart disease. *International Journal of Cardiology* **13**: 207–217.

Hensley FA, Larach DR, Martin DE, Stauffer R & Waldhausen JA (1987) The effect of halothane/nitrous oxide/oxygen mask induction on arterial hemoglobin saturation in cyanotic heart disease. *Journal of Cardiothoracic Anaesthesia* **1**: 289–296.

Hickey PR, Hansen DD, Wessel DL et al (1985) Blunting of stress responses in the pulmonary circulation of infants by fentanyl. *Anesthesia and Analgesia* **64**: 1137–1142.

Kirklin JK, Westaby S, Blackstone EH et al (1983) Complement and the damaging effects of cardiopulmonary bypass. *Journal of Cardiovascular Surgery* **86**: 845–857.

Kirklin JK, Kirklin JW & Pacifico AD (1985) Cardiopulmonary bypass. In Arciniegas E (ed) *Pediatric Cardiac Surgery*, pp 67–77. Chicago: Year Book Medical Publishers.

Lenz W (1980) Aetiology, incidence and genetics of congenital heart disease. In Graham G & Rossi E (eds) *Heart Disease in Infants and Children*, pp 27–35. London: Arnold.

Macartney FJ (1986) Echocardiography versus catheterisation. In Marcelletti C, Anderson RH, Becker AE, Corno A, di Carlo D & Mazzera E (eds) *Paediatric Cardiology*, vol 6, pp 172–185. Edinburgh: Churchill Livingstone.

Marshall TA, Marshall F & Reddy PP (1982) Physiology changes associated with ligation of the PDA in preterm infants. *Journal of Pediatrics* **101**: 749–753.

Moore RA (1981) Anesthesia for the pediatric heart patient for noncardiac surgery. *Anesthesiology Reviews* **8**: 23.

Morray JP, Lynn A, Stamm SJ, Herndon P, Kawabori I & Stevenson J (1984) The hemodynamic effects of ketamine in children with congenital heart disease. *Anesthesia and Analgesia* **63**: 895–899.

Murray D, Vadewalker G, Matherne P & Mahoney L (1987) Pulsed Doppler and two-dimensional echocardiography: comparision of halothane and isoflurane on cardiac function in infants and small children. *Anesthesiology* **67**: 211–217.

Nadeau S & Noble WH (1986) Limitations of cardiac output measurement by thermodilution. *Canadian Anaesthetists' Society Journal* **33**: 780–784.

O'Higgins JW (1988) The anaesthetist and paediatric cardiac catheterization. *British Journal of Hospital Medicine* **40**: 58–63.

Prior PF & Maynard DE (1986) *Monitoring Cerebral Function*. Amsterdam: Elsevier.

Ratcliffe J, Elliott MJ, Wyse RKH et al (1985) Metabolic consequences of three different crystalloid pump priming fluids in children less than 15 kilos undergoing open-heart surgery. *Journal of Cardiovascular Surgery* **26(suppl)**: 86–91.

Rigden S, Barratt TM, Dillon MJ et al (1982) Acute renal failure complicating cardiopulmonary bypass surgery in children. *Archives of Disease in Childhood* **57**: 425.

Robinson S & Gregory GA (1981) Fentanyl-air-oxygen anesthesia for ligation of patent ductus arteriosus in preterm infants. *Anesthesia and Analgesia* **60**: 331–334.

Rudolph AM (1974) *Congenital Diseases of the Heart: Clinical–Physiologic Considerations in Diagnosis and Management*. Chicago: Year Book Publishers.

Shanson DC (1987) Antibiotic prophylaxis of infective endocarditis in the United Kingdom and Europe. *Journal of Antimicrobial Chemotherapy* **20 (suppl A)**: 119–131.

Stark J & de Leval MR (1983) *Surgery for Congenital Heart Defects*. London: Grune & Stratton.

Steen PA, Tinker JH, Pluth JR et al (1978) Efficacy of dopamine, dobutamine and epinephrine during emergence from cardiopulmonary bypass in man. *Circulation* **57**: 378–384.

Stone KS, Brown JW, Canal DF et al (1987) Long-term fate of the diaphragm surgically plicated during infancy and early childhood. *Annals of Thoracic Surgery* **44:** 62–65.

Stow PJ, Burrows FA, McLeod ME et al (1987) The effects of cardiopulmonary bypass and profound hypothermic circulatory arrest on anterior fontanel pressure in infants. *Canadian Anaesthetists' Society Journal* **34:** 450–454.

Sullivan ID (1986) Doppler echocardiography. *Current Opinion in Cardiology* **1:** 102–106.

Verska JJ (1977) Control of heparinisation by activated clotting time during bypass with improved postoperative hemostasis. *Annals of Thoracic Surgery* **24:** 170–175.

Wood M, Shand DG & Wood AJJ (1980) The sympathetic response to profound hypothermia and circulatory arrest in infants. *Canadian Anaesthetists' Society Journal* **27:** 125–131.

Yaster M (1987) The dose response of fentanyl in neonatal anaesthesia. *Anesthesiology* **66:** 433–435.

Anaesthesia for paediatric liver transplantation

Pioneering work in hepatic transplantation began under Starzl and Calne in the 1960s, but for many years results remained unimpressive. Since the early 1980s, however, survival figures have steadily improved. A number of factors have contributed, including greater public awareness of the need for organ donation, improved immunosuppression, advances in anaesthetic and postoperative management, and the support of a widening group of non-surgical hospital specialities. One-year paediatric survival rates in excess of 80% are now reported and longer-term results are also encouraging (Otte et al, 1987; Starzl et al, 1987). The value of transplantation in the management of children with end-stage liver disease is now widely recognized, and the number of centres offering the procedure is increasing rapidly (Bismuth et al, 1987).

The perioperative care of these patients presents a formidable challenge. Children with the severe physiological derangements of advanced liver disease are subjected to a lengthy surgical procedure in which profound cardiovascular, biochemical and haematological disturbances are commonplace. Major blood loss, myocardial depression, metabolic acidosis and electrolyte imbalance are routinely encountered, while transection of the inferior vena cava, renal hypoperfusion and a marked fall in body temperature are unavoidable. Successful anaesthetic management depends on good organization, full technical support, careful monitoring and timely manipulation of a number of critical physiological variables.

INDICATIONS AND RESULTS

A large number of acute and chronic liver disorders have been managed by transplantation (Figure 14.1). Some 50% of patients have congenital obstructive disorders, mainly extrahepatic biliary atresia, while 20% have metabolic disease, including α_1-antitrypsin deficiency and tyrosinosis. A further 20% suffer from primary parenchymal liver diseases including infectious and drug-related hepatitides, Wilson's disease and sclerosing cholangitis, while the remaining 10% have vascular disorders and tumours. Oxalosis, haemophilia and congenital protein C deficiency, conditions with normal hepatic function, have also been treated successfully by transplantation (Lewis and Bontempo, 1985; Watts et al, 1987; Casella et al, 1988).

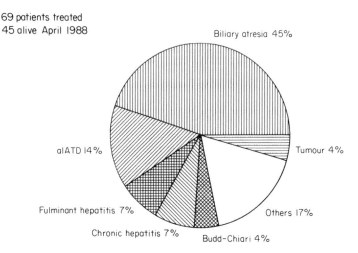

69 patients treated
45 alive April 1988

Biliary atresia 45%

Tumour 4%

aIATD 14%

Fulminant hepatitis 7%

Chronic hepatitis 7%

Budd-Chiari 4%

Others 17%

Figure 14.1. Indications for liver transplantation in 69 paediatric patients in the Cambridge/King's Series from January 1984 to April 1988.

Results in cases of hepatic malignancy have been poor, and these patients are now infrequently accepted into transplant programmes. Outcome otherwise appears to vary little between these diagnostic groups, although age at operation is of some importance. Infants (<1 year) present major technical difficulties and have a poorer prognosis: 1 year survival is approximately 50% (Starzl et al, 1987). Teenagers tend to do well, with 90% survival at 1 year and little subsequent attrition (Barnes, personal communication). Patients with very advanced disease and severe nutritional problems have poorer prospects than those who are relatively well at the time of transplantation (Van Thiel et al, 1984; Tizard et al, 1987), and early surgery is increasingly favoured. If all patients are included, current 1 year survival is in the range of 65 to 85%. Mortality beyond 1 year post-transplant is small and the quality of life of survivors appears to be excellent (Zitelli et al, 1987).

Transplantation is indicated when liver disease progresses to the point of major functional impairment and is likely to lead to death within 1 year (Neuberger, 1987). Deciding on the timing of operation may be difficult. In chronic conditions, poorer results associated with advanced disease must be weighed against the possible loss of months of relatively good health should complications follow an early operation. In fulminant cases recovery without transplantation may occur, yet delay can result in preventable death or permanent brain injury. As yet there are little published data to assist the clinician in these important decisions, although in practice the timing of surgery is often determined by the availability of a donor organ. As this must in all but the most desperate circumstances be ABO-compatible and of suitable size, a prospective recipient may wait weeks or even months once the decision to transplant has been taken, and some die before an organ is found.

PREOPERATIVE ASSESSMENT AND PREPARATION

Chronic liver disease in children is manifest by malnutrition, portal hypertension with ascites, and impaired hepatic synthetic function. Nutritional reserve is diminished by anorexia, malabsorption and impaired protein synthesis (Hehir et al, 1985), and is further depleted at the time of operation by the catabolic response to injury. This is likely to influence resistance to infection (Fredell et al, 1987), respiratory muscle function and wound healing. Preoperative dietary supplementation, bearing in mind the need for low sodium intake when ascites is present and protein restriction in patients with encephalopathy (Johnson et al, 1987), is to be encouraged for these reasons. Parenteral nutrition may be required in rare cases when portal hypertension is associated with near-complete malabsorption. Vitamins, iron and trace elements may also be beneficial and are routinely prescribed.

Portal hypertension may be associated with massive ascites, reduced lung volumes and limited exercise tolerance. Ascites is often easily reduced with diuretic therapy and infusion of albumin, which improves pulmonary function and makes most patients feel better. Oesophageal varices may be a source of significant bleeding preoperatively and portosystemic venous collaterals greatly increase blood loss during operation. Sclerotherapy is of value not only in the prevention of preoperative variceal bleeding but in reducing the risk of haemorrhage postoperatively, in the event of portal obstruction due to rejection or other pathological processes.

Impaired synthetic function is mainly reflected in reduced plasma concentrations of albumin and coagulation factors. Hypoalbuminaemia aggravates ascites and peripheral oedema, and may be corrected by infusion of 20% (salt-poor) human albumin solution. Coagulopathy is associated with gross intraoperative haemorrhage, particularly in the presence of extensive venous collaterals and abdominal adhesions related to previous surgery or peritonitis. Most coagulation factors, with the notable exception of factor VIII, are synthesized only in the liver and will be depressed in advanced liver failure even with adequate provision of vitamin K. Platelet numbers are also frequently reduced, usually due to hypersplenism. Correction of clotting defects by the administration of appropriate blood products immediately preoperatively is essential. This is discussed in detail below.

Preoperative laboratory investigations will often reveal further abnormalities. Haemoglobin values are depressed in a substantial minority of patients. This may be related to malnutrition, gastrointestinal bleeding or hypersplenism. Most patients have normal plasma electrolytes, although diuretic therapy, secondary hyperaldosteronism and other, poorly understood renal abnormalities may induce hyponatraemia and hypokalaemia. Preoperative correction of these is rarely necessary; considerable amounts of sodium and potassium are inevitably introduced into the circulation by blood transfusion at operation. Impaired metabolism of vitamin D may lead to osteomalacia and susceptibility to fractures. However even in these cases plasma concentrations of calcium, phosphorus and magnesium are usually normal. Hypoglycaemia is rarely observed in chronic hepatic failure, although in fulminant cases intravenous dextrose solutions may be needed.

Renal function is well preserved in the majority of patients, although renal insufficiency may be seen in children with acute hepatic failure or severe sepsis. Alterations in renal handling of sodium and water are recognized in liver disease but the mechanisms involved remain largely unexplained

(Epstein, 1986). Uncommon renal disorders include tyrosinosis, characterized by aminoaciduria and type 2 renal tubular acidosis, and oxalosis, which presents as chronic renal failure requiring simultaneous hepatic and renal transplantation (Watts et al, 1987). Renal microcirculatory changes may reduce the threshold for renal damage in many forms of chronic liver disease; however, evidence for this or any other specific causative mechanism in the 'hepatorenal syndrome' remains insubstantial (Wilkinson, 1987). Impairment of renal function, it should be noted, appears to be a strong predictor of postoperative sepsis and mortality (Cuervas-Mons et al, 1986), and measures to protect renal function during surgery should be part of routine practice. These are described in detail below.

Cardiovascular status is similarly well maintained in all but the most advanced cases of hepatic decompensation. Studies in adults (Bihari et al, 1985) have shown that liver failure is characterized by a disturbance of microcirculatory function causing arteriovenous shunting, increased cardiac output and flow-dependent oxygen consumption. There is little doubt that this also occurs in children and that its degree depends on the severity of the underlying hepatic disease. Myocardial reserve in most cases, however, is such that increased demand is not associated with left ventricular dilatation or pulmonary venous hypertension. An exaggerated basal flow murmur is a common clinical finding, and echocardiography should be done when this or other features raise the possibility of a structural abnormality. Children with biliary atresia in particular have a high incidence of associated congenital abnormalities (Miyomoto and Kajimoto, 1983), although these are usually confined to the abdomen. Alagille's syndrome (biliary hypoplasia, butterfly vertebrae and tetralogy of Fallot) presents a particular challenge. In the absence of a total correction of the tetralogy. pulmonary blood flow depends on the state of the palliative shunt; both systemic oxygen delivery and myocardial reserve may be poor. Successful transplantation has nonetheless been achieved in this condition.

Respiratory impairment is most often due to abdominal distension from ascites or hepatosplenomegaly, manifest by reduced lung volumes and tachypnoea. Ventilation/perfusion imbalance related to upward displacement of the diaphragm is likely to be the cause of the modest hypoxaemia often seen in these patients, although pulmonary arteriovenous shunting has also been demonstrated (Martin, 1986). Normocarbia or a mild respiratory alkalosis is the usual associated finding. Pulmonary oedema, often observed in the early postoperative period, is an unusual preoperative finding in ambulatory patients, although seen more often in patients with fulminant hepatic failure. It can be controlled by diuretic therapy and by cautious correction of hypoalbuminaemia. Aspiration and pulmonary infection are less frequent causes of preoperative lung dysfunction. Obstructive airways disease in children with α_1-antitrypsin deficiency has not been described.

SURGICAL TECHNIQUE

The abdomen is opened via bilateral subcostal incisions with a midline extension to the xiphoid. The structures of the free edge of the lesser sac and porta hepatis are dissected out and the liver freed of its supporting ligamentous attachments. The retrohepatic portion of the inferior vena cava is also mobilized and its branches ligated. Venous collaterals in the abdominal wall and mesentery may be extensive and will bleed heavily during this stage unless meticulous attention is paid to surgical haemostasis. This initial dissection phase of the procedure varies greatly in duration (about 1–6 h) and difficulty. Venous collaterals apart, post-inflammatory mesenteric scarring and adhesions from previous abdominal surgery cause major technical problems and substantially increase blood loss. Previous porto-enterostomy in biliary atresia (Kasai procedure) is a common source of difficulty.

Following dissection the bile duct, hepatic artery, portal vein and infrahepatic inferior vena cava are divided and a clamp placed across the suprahepatic cava at the level of the diaphragm. This too is then divided and the diseased liver removed along with the hepatic veins and the retrohepatic length of the inferior vena cava, beginning the 'anhepatic' phase. The donor liver is then removed from iced saline and placed in the hepatic fossa. Anastomosis of the suprahepatic cava and portal vein is performed and the infrahepatic caval anastomosis commenced. When the latter is nearly complete the new liver is perfused, via a cannula in the portal vein, with a crystalloid or colloid solution. This is meant to wash out storage perfusate and air, which escape via the incomplete lower caval anastomosis. The portal and suprahepatic caval clamps are then released, restoring circulation to the donor liver and beginning the final or 'reperfusion' phase of the operation. The infrahepatic caval anastomosis is rapidly completed and the cava is then unclamped. Hepatic artery and biliary anastomoses follow. Biliary drainage may be accomplished by a donor–recipient end-to-end anastomosis, by use of the donor gallbladder as a conduit between donor and recipient bile ducts, or by a Roux-en-Y cholecystojejunostomy, depending on the recipient's biliary anatomy (Figure 14.2).

Details of surgical technique vary between centres. In particular, unclamping of the three major anastomoses—portal vein, suprahepatic and infrahepatic cava—is done simultaneously in some centres, while in others release of the lower caval clamp is delayed several minutes to allow the cardiovascular changes associated with liver reperfusion to settle. Duration of surgery also varies widely, from 3 to more than 12 h depending on the patient and surgical team. A major recent departure from conventional technique has been the transplantation of livers reduced in size by excision of the right lobe. This may be undertaken when size discrepancy would otherwise prevent transplantation in young children, from whom the availability of donor organs of appropriate size is a major problem, and substantial success has been reported (de Hemptinne et al, 1987).

ANAESTHESIA

Preoperative preparation

An initial anaesthetic assessment should be performed when a patient is first referred to the transplant centre. This allows additional investigations

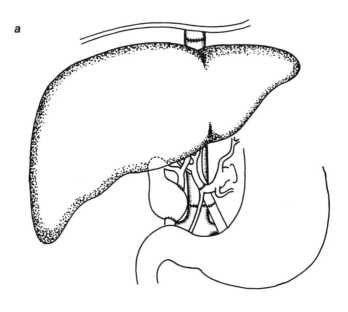

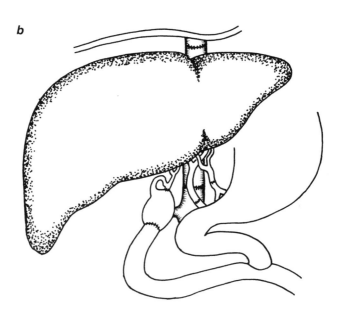

Figure 14.2. Orthotopic liver transplantation: diagram of operation; (a) with gall bladder conduit for biliary drainage; (b) Roux-en-Y cholecystojejunostomy. Note suprahepatic and infrahepatic anastomoses of inferior vena cava.

and preoperative preparation of the patient to be carried out well before surgery. Discussion with the patient's parents, particularly regarding the need for postoperative intensive care, is important and should be supported by a visit from an experienced member of the paediatric intensive care nursing team. If appropriate, the child should also be reassured about his or her comfort during the early postoperative period and about the free access of parents throughout this time.

Many seriously ill patients will stay on the ward until a donor is available and hence there will be adequate time for further assessment by the duty anaesthetic team when a transplant is scheduled. If a child is transferred from another centre without prior anaesthetic evaluation time may be short, since once a donor liver is removed it should be transplanted within 6–8 h. In practice, however, blood cross-matching will take 2 h and a basic clinical and laboratory assessment can be completed within this time. New organ preservation techniques will probably minimize such constraints in the near future (Kalayoglu et al, 1988).

Preoperative pathophysiological changes have been discussed above. Coagulopathy becomes the dominant consideration immediately prior to surgery and should be corrected. In consultation with the duty haematologist, fresh frozen plasma, cryoprecipitate and/or platelet concentrate are given as indicated. Fresh frozen plasma in a dose of 10–30 ml/kg over 30–60 min is given if the prothrombin time is more than 4 s prolonged. Cryoprecipitate should be added if the preoperative fibrinogen concentration is below 0.8 g/dl: 1 unit per 5 kg raises the plasma fibrinogen level approximately 0.075 g/dl (Gordon et al, 1987). Platelet concentrate should be given if the platelet count is less than $50\,000/mm^3$. A bag containing 4 units may be given: 1 unit per 10 kg may be expected to raise the platelet count by about 30 000 (Editorial, 1987).

The transplant anaesthesia team

A consultant experienced in paediatric anaesthesia directs and takes responsibility for all members of the anaesthesia team. In difficult cases two consultants will be needed. A senior registrar or experienced registrar provides assistance. Two highly trained theatre technicians prepare the theatre and assist in induction and monitoring procedures. They also run infusion pumps, blood administration apparatus and cell-saving equipment, and maintain detailed records of infusions and losses. A clinical measurement technician sets up and maintains monitoring equipment and performs routine measurements and blood sampling. Rapid access to biochemical and haematological laboratory facilities is essential. The results of routine studies, particularly arterial blood gases, haematocrit, serum sodium, potassium and ionized calcium, must be available within minutes. The importance of well organized and competent technical support cannot be overemphasized.

Anaesthetic technique

Premedication is important in children old enough to understand the scale of the procedure, particularly teenagers. Since intramuscular injections are best avoided in those with prolonged coagulation values, a short-acting oral benzodiazepine is the usual choice in children over 15–20 kg. Younger children often manage well without premedication. Indeed, given the unpredictable effects of orally administered agents and the risks of respiratory depression in patients who have marked abdominal distension, encephalopathy or impaired drug metabolism, premedication may be better avoided. Venous access tends to be easy, because of the low systemic vascular resistance and increased cardiac output which characterize advanced hepatic disease, and intravenous induction is therefore the method of choice. There is evidence of impaired gastric emptying in these children and, while aspiration has not been reported, a rapid sequence technique is recommended. Preoperative antacid therapy may also be indicated.

Intravenous atropine may be followed by any suitable induction agent, usually thiopentone, and suxamethonium. Clinical experience suggests that the effects of suxamethonium are little altered by deficiency of cholinesterase. Oral intubation may be followed by placement of a nasal tube if clotting is near normal, bearing in mind the likelihood of 24–48 h of postoperative mechanical ventilation. A nasogastric tube is required, since gastric distension may interfere with surgical access and since postoperative ileus, occasionally with marked gastric dilatation, occurs in all cases. These considerations outweigh the risks of traumatic bleeding from unidentified or untreated varices in patients with portal hypertension, although due care must be taken.

The choice of agents for maintenance of anaesthesia is determined chiefly by the need to preserve good myocardial function. Both preload and contractility may be dramatically altered during surgery and myocardial depression due to anaesthetic agents must be minimized. A well proven technique incorporates fentanyl 5–20 µg/kg, atracurium and air–oxygen–isoflurane. Nitrous oxide, though often used, has some disadvantages. Bowel distension may interfere with abdominal closure, particularly when the transplanted liver is relatively large. Prolonged exposure may affect DNA synthesis and bone marrow function by oxidation of vitamin B_{12} and interference with folate metabolism (Banks et al, 1968; Amess et al, 1978; Perry et al, 1979; Deacon et al, 1980). Although nitrous oxide is known to produce myocardial depression in cardiac patients given morphine (Lappas et al, 1975) and fentanyl (Lunn et al, 1979), this has not been seen in studies of healthy volunteers given nitrous oxide–oxygen–isoflurane (Stevens et al, 1971; Dolan et al, 1974), and effects in patients with hepatic disease are unknown. Animal work suggests that hepatic blood flow may be significantly reduced by nitrous oxide (Seyde et al, 1986), consistent with evidence that it causes sympathetically mediated vasoconstriction (Smith et al, 1970; Eisele and Smith, 1972). While of no consequence during the dissection phase this is likely to be undesirable once the new liver is reperfused. The possibility of air embolism, a recognized hazard in liver transplantation (Mazzoni et al, 1979; Borland et al, 1985) and probably more dangerous in the presence of nitrous oxide (Butler et al, 1987), may further contraindicate its use.

Cardiovascular stability favours the use of isoflurane over halothane or enflurane. Although isoflurane may reduce hepatic blood flow, data from animal studies suggest that this is likely to be much less than occurs with halothane (Hursh et al, 1987). Patients who are gravely ill and hypotensive may be anaesthetized with air–oxygen–trichloroethylene. This agent, while little studied, has a long record of safety in states of cardiovascular decompensation (Bethune et al, 1980) and in hepatic transplantation (Lindop and Farman, 1987). Techniques relying solely on high-dose opiates have not been described in paediatric liver transplantation. Variable hepatic function following grafting and the possibility of a washout effect related to massive blood replacement are theoretical disadvantages. Complete suppression of stress-related cardiovascular responses may not in any case be advantageous in this clinical context.

The choice of muscle relaxant presents less scope for controversy. Pancuronium has been used successfully for many years and its partial dependence on hepatic elimination has not proved clinically relevant. Atracurium lacks significant cardiovascular effects when given in appropriate dosage, and in contrast to other agents its half-life is not prolonged in patients with liver disease (Ward and Neill, 1983). An increase in infusion dose requirements related to increases in volume of distribution and plasma clearance, and to rapid turnover of blood volume with operative haemorrhage, may be observed. However the mean requirement reported in a group of adolescent and adult liver transplant patients of 0.38 mg/kg/h (Farman et al, 1986) suggests that these effects are not clinically important. The need for a period of postoperative mechanical ventilation, during which relaxants are rarely given, further diminishes the significance of relaxant kinetics.

Vascular access

Large-bore intravenous access is vital. Placement of cannulas is facilitated by the high cardiac output of advanced liver disease and it is usually possible to insert 16 G cannulas peripherally even in small children. These must be placed in the upper extremities since caval clamping renders femoral and saphenous routes useless during the anhepatic phase. Two lines dedicated to transfusion and a third available for infusion of other blood products and kept in reserve in case of failure of one of the transfusion lines is the minimum required. A wire-guided double- or triple-lumen polyurethane catheter, preferably placed via the internal jugular route, is also essential. This is used to monitor central venous pressure and for the infusion of drugs. A second central catheter, easily placed alongside the first, may act as a reserve volume infusion line. The subclavian route is associated with a higher risk of complications and is best avoided, particularly when clotting is abnormal.

Monitoring

Maintenance of cardiovascular stability during liver transplantation requires continuous direct monitoring of arterial and central venous pressure. Although experience in small children is limited, a pulmonary artery flotation catheter (5 FG placed through a 6 FG introducer) may assist intraoperative and postoperative cardiovascular management in some patients (Damen and Wever, 1987). Zeroing must be accurate, particularly in relation to cardiac filling pressures as these must be maintained within a narrow range during rapid changes in circulating volume. Monitoring catheters must be securely fixed and easily accessible in the event of technical difficulties.

ECG and temperature monitoring are also essential. Pulse oximetry provides beat-to-beat monitoring of peripheral oxygen delivery. Capnography allows a continuous assessment of alveolar ventilation, although changes in cardiac output and the administration of sodium bicarbonate may influence end-tidal carbon dioxide levels. Accurate monitoring of urine flow is also required, as is the efficient tallying of shed blood.

Measurement of arterial blood gases, sodium, potassium, glucose, ionized calcium and haematocrit should be performed at frequent intervals, at least hourly during the initial and closing phases of the operation and more often during the period in which caval clamping and hepatic reperfusion are carried out. All are subject to rapid changes, particularly in small children; these changes will be discussed in detail below. Accurate measurement of ionized calcium stands out as a significant recent advance in intraoperative monitoring, as this cannot be predicted from total calcium values. Citrate toxicity occurs readily in liver transplantation due to heavy transfusion requirements and impaired hepatic metabolism of citrate. Cardiovascular stability is greatly enhanced by the rapid identification and treatment of ionic hypocalcaemia.

The value of coagulation monitoring is also widely accepted, although practices vary (Bontempo, 1987). Rapid non-specific assessment of clotting is provided by the activated clotting time (Haemochron; Schriever et al, 1973). Thromboelastography, a more sensitive bedside technique quantifying the rate and quality of fibrin formation, is also advocated (Kang et al, 1985; Owen et al, 1987). Regular coagulation screening tests, now obtainable by rapid automated methods, are routine in many centres, as are measurements of clotting factors and tests of fibrinolysis, although the volumes of blood required limit the application of these to older patients. No method of coagulation monitoring, however, has been shown to be superior in terms of reduction of blood loss, and there is considerable scope for further investigation in this area.

Blood replacement and fluid management

Major operative haemorrhage is usual during hepatic transplantation. The magnitude of blood loss varies greatly, depending on the underlying disease, state of the portal circulation, presence of postsurgical or inflammatory adhesions, and surgical technique. An early paediatric series reported an average loss of 3.95 blood volumes (range 370 ml to 30 l; Borland et al, 1985). A total of 87 consecutive paediatric cases in the Cambridge/King's programme from June 1968 to March 1988 had a mean measured loss of 2.6 blood volumes (160 ml to 26.6 l).

Measurement of blood loss is difficult and may be complicated by the inclusion of ascites. Measured totals will lag far behind actual losses when bleeding is brisk, and volume replacement must always be guided by clinical judgement and cardiac filling pressure. This should be maintained at the upper end of the normal range, allowing a margin of safety in case very rapid blood loss should occur and reducing the risk of air embolism. A pressurized rapid infusion system for each of the two large-bore infusion lines is essential. A volumetric infusion pump incorporating a bypass limb for rapid infusion allows better control of the rate of infusion in small children (Smith et al, 1987). Microfiltration of blood is advisable (Derrington, 1985). Filters of 20 µ depth have been advocated for maximum clearance of microaggregates but are prone to obstruction; 40 µ screen filters are a more practical alternative.

Autotransfusion techniques have developed rapidly in recent years and may now reduce the use of bank blood by as much as 40% (Smith et al, 1987). In the Haemonetics system red cells are salvaged through heparinized suction lines, then washed and centrifuged before reconstitution in a heparin-free saline suspension with a haematocrit of about 55%. In practice blood loss exceeding 1 l is needed before processing can begin and the rate of processing limits reinfusion to a maximum rate of 100–125 ml/min, which is achieved through the use of a modified reinfusion bag system (Smith et al, 1987). Reinfused cells must be diluted if high haematocrits are to be avoided, and plasma proteins must be replenished from other sources. Cell-saving techniques are contraindicated in hepatic malignancy and in cases where bacterial soiling of the peritoneum has occurred.

Repeated measurement of haematocrit guides the choice of replacement products. It is normal practice for whole blood to be given in preference to concentrated red cells, since the use of large volumes of fresh frozen plasma, human albumin solution, synthetic colloid or crystalloid solutions all have significant disadvantages. A packed cell volume of 30–35% is considered desirable once the new liver is reperfused, as this is likely to allow optimum oxygen transport. A tendency to exceed this range is observed in spite of liberal administration of clear fluids, and occasionally phlebotomy is required.

Citrate given in transfused blood and plasma depresses plasma ionized calcium, which must be maintained near normal levels if myocardial depression is to be avoided. Calcium chloride is usually administered. Dose requirements depend on the volume of blood products given and on the liver's ability to metabolize citrate. The latter depends in turn on body temperature, hepatic perfusion and the severity of the underlying disease. Paediatric patients in the Cambridge/King's series have received a mean dose of 4.0 ml (4.0 mmol) of 13.4% calcium chloride per litre of citrated products (range 0.37–16.7 ml). Repeated bolus administration of 1–2 mmol per 10 kg is well tolerated.

The use of blood products to correct pre-existing coagulopathy and the intraoperative monitoring of coagulation have been discussed above. Intraoperative replacement therapy is guided in the first instance by clinical observation, and is indicated when efforts at surgical haemostasis remain unsuccessful and clot formation in the wound is poor. If not performed at regular intervals, laboratory assessment of coagulation, including prothrombin time, partial thromboplastin time, fibrinogen concentration, platelet count and fibrin degradation products should be obtained when such bleeding occurs. Fresh frozen plasma and platelets given preoperatively and early in the course of surgery to most patients usually forestalls the need for further therapy until hepatic reperfusion. However, an increased bleeding tendency is commonly observed at this stage (Bontempo, 1987; Kratzer et al, 1988; Luddington, 1988), characterized by further reduction of clotting factors and in some cases signs of fibrinolysis. Dilutional changes account for this in part, and may be managed by further infusion of fresh frozen plasma and platelets. However severe bleeding is usually associated with pathological fibrinolysis, and the best approach to this remains to be established. Cryoprecipitate is generally administered if fibrinogen levels are depressed and antifibrinolytics have been used. However in most cases gradual recovery is observed and treatment remains empirical.

Volumes of fresh frozen plasma given vary widely, depending on the severity of the coagulopathy and the haematocrit at the time of infusion. Aliquots of 20–30 ml/kg are usual. Platelets are supplied in bags containing 4–6 units, at 25–50 ml per unit. Patients generally receive these by the bag, the rate being titrated against filling pressures and haematocrit.

Losses of fluid other than blood must also be taken into account. Respiratory evaporative losses can be minimized through humidification of inspired gases or the use of a heat and moisture exchanging device, but urinary and nasogastric losses may be substantial. Probably more significant are evaporative and interstitial losses related to prolonged exposure and extensive traumatization of peritoneum. Sodium and protein losses are adequately replaced in the course of blood and colloid infusion, but water losses must be replaced by other means if hypernatraemia is to be avoided (Dyer et al, 1987). The infusion of 4–6 ml/kg/h of 0.18% sodium chloride in 4% dextrose throughout the procedure appears to accomplish this; to this must be added a further 2–4 ml/h of the same solution infused as flush solution in monitoring lines.

Electrolyte and acid–base changes

The infusion of large volumes of blood products and reperfusion of the donor liver may induce marked changes in plasma chemistry. Blood glucose is normal preoperatively in most patients but rises inexorably during the procedure due to the administration acid–citrate–dextrose blood and stress-related insulin resistance. Hypoglycaemia, occasionally observed preoperatively in very young children and in those with fulminant hepatic failure, has not been seen intraoperatively even when normal hepatic glucose release is interrupted during the anhepatic and early reperfusion phases. A decline in blood glucose levels once the new liver begins to function has been described (Borland et al, 1985) but appears to depend in part on the use of insulin and of dextrose-free maintenance fluids. When insulin is not given glucose levels in excess of 15–20 mmol/l are common, but no harm appears to result and control is readily achieved in the early postoperative period.

Serum sodium also tends to rise and may, with glucose, contribute to moderate hyperosmolarity at the end of the procedure (Dyer et al, 1987). Sodium citrate in blood products, sodium bicarbonate administration and evaporative water loss may be implicated. The use of a low sodium maintenance crystalloid solution appears to prevent hypernatraemia and is advocated (Berridge and Klinck, 1988). Serum potassium, low or normal initially, peaks dramatically on reperfusion as blood from the obstructed portal system acquires extracellular potassium from the ischaemic donor liver and rejoins the main circulation. Arterial plasma levels as high as 8 mmol/l may be measured, and characteristic electrocardiographic changes are seen. However redistribution follows within seconds, and a progressive fall is observed subsequently. Intraoperative potassium supplementation is sometimes necessary late in the procedure since reuptake by the grafted liver may result in dangerous hypokalaemia.

Metabolic acidosis, usually absent or minimal at first, tends to deepen during the operation and is the dominant acid–base disturbance. The cause is likely to be multifactorial. Transfused blood introduces a substantial quantity of exogenous acid, and lactate metabolism and renal function are impaired, especially during the anhepatic phase. Acid metabolites associated with venous stasis in the portal and lower body circulations, as well as those which accumulate in the new liver during transport and storage, are released into the general circulation on reperfusion, causing a further rise in hydrogen ion concentration. Thereafter acidosis gradually subsides, as normal cardiac output and renal function are restored. Treatment includes modest hyperventilation, support of the circulation if required and sodium bicarbonate. The value of bicarbonate administration has, however, been questioned and its use appears to be declining. Evidence that circulatory function is impaired by moderate metabolic acidosis is slight, while detrimental effects on oxygen delivery and intracellular pH associated with bicarbonate therapy have been described (Mattar et al, 1974; Bishop and Weisfeldt, 1976; Arieff et al, 1982; Bersin et al, 1986; Graf and Arieff, 1986). The common tendency to metabolic alkalosis postoperatively further discourages its use. Alternative buffers may be of value but remain to be assessed in controlled clinical trials.

Changes in ionized calcium may be marked and of great haemodynamic significance; these have been discussed above. Hypomagnesaemia has also been described in liver transplant patients (Martin, 1986; Burrows, personal communication) but the clinical relevance of this remains undefined.

Cardiovascular changes

Hypovolaemia due to haemorrhage presents the greatest threat, and the ability to replace blood rapidly has already been emphasized. Cardiac function may be impaired during the dissection phase by sudden obstruction of venous return during surgical manipulation of the liver, or by direct compression of the diaphragmatic surface of the heart. Clamping of the inferior vena cava for hepatectomy produces a marked fall in venous pressure and cardiac output (Carmichael et al, 1985; Marquez and Martin, 1986), although this may be attenuated in the presence of portosystemic venous collaterals. Systemic vascular resistance increases, but a moderate fall in blood pressure is expected. Provided cardiac filling pressures and contractility are maintained, however, frank hypotension is unusual. Lower filling pressures are accepted during the anhepatic phase as long as the lowest (presystolic) central venous pressures remains positive and arterial blood pressure remains satisfactory. Overtransfusion at this stage may result in dangerously high filling pressures following unclamping, with adverse effects on gas exchange and hepatic and renal blood flow.

Excessive bleeding and renal hypoperfusion related to the marked increase in portal and renal venous pressures when clamps are applied at the beginning of the anhepatic phase have encouraged the use of bypass techniques in adult patients. A venovenous system incorporating portal, femoral and axillary cannulas, heparin-bonded tubing and an atraumatic centrifugal pump is now used routinely during the anhepatic period in some centres, and a venoarterial (femorofemoral) system has also been employed (Calne et al, 1984). Venous decompression and support of cardiac output and renal blood flow are achieved, allowing prolongation of the anhepatic time and a reduction in bleeding from portal collaterals. However, the technique is time-consuming, technically complicated and of unproven benefit. It also exposes the patient to the risk of embolization of air or clot. Most would consider its use in children unnecessary and inappropriate.

Reperfusion of the transplanted liver is usually associated with significant changes in heart rate, contractility and peripheral vascular tone (Carmichael et al, 1985; Marquez and Martin, 1986). Portal unclamping alone, prior to release of the caval clamps, induces a transient fall in blood pressure, presumably related to a sudden drainage from dilated splanchnic veins and reduced resistance in the splanchnic arteriolar bed. Caval unclamping allows acidic, desaturated blood from the obstructed portal circulation, rendered cold, more acidic and potassium-rich by passage through the new liver, to perfuse the heart. Sinus slowing is observed, as are electrocardiographic signs of acute hyperkalaemia. These changes are typically mild and short-lived, but asystole and tachydysrhythmias, including ventricular fibrillation, have been seen (Borland et al, 1985). Blood pressure falls in almost all cases. This is due to myocardial depression and systemic vasodilatation, possibly related to inflammatory mediators from the ischaemic liver or to peptides released during splanchnic stasis. Treatment just prior to revascularization with calcium chloride and atropine may modify these effects (Martin et al, 1984). In most cases blood pressure and cardiac output are restored to preclamping values within minutes, although patients with very advanced hepatic failure may require inotropic support. Those undergoing urgent retransplantation for hepatic infarction may have preoperative circulatory failure; hypotension and acidosis following unclamping may be progressive and irreversible in this setting.

Cardiovascular instability resulting from air embolism has been described (Mazzoni et al, 1979; Borland et al, 1985), and maintenance of a positive venous pressure is recommended. In one published report high-frequency ventilation was associated with cerebral air embolization, raising the possibility of air entry via the pulmonary route, possibly through abnormal arteriovenous channels. The use of positive end expiratory pressure, while theoretically desirable for prevention of venous air embolism, must therefore be considered with caution.

Renal function

Significant changes in renal function during liver transplantation are related to alterations in cardiac output and renal blood flow. Urine flow is diminished during the period of caval clamping as cardiac output is reduced and renal venous pressure acutely raised. This improves to a variable degree following unclamping, but pre-existing renal disease, prolonged hypotension and high transfusion volumes are associated with a high risk of postoperative renal failure. Measures to prevent intraoperative renal damage include the use of a low-dose dopamine infusion (2 μg/kg/min), mannitol (0.5 g/kg over 30 min, followed by 0.1 g/kg/h), and intermittent frusemide (0.1–0.5 mg/kg). Oliguria associated with hypotension during or following the anhepatic phase may respond to dobutamine (5–15 μg/kg/min). Dopamine and mannitol prophylaxis is recommended for all cases (Polson et al, 1987; Salem et al, 1988).

Maintenance of body temperature

Core temperature invariably falls during liver transplantation. Factors contributing to this include the poor nutritional state of most patients, the exposure of body surfaces during preparation for surgery, substantial evaporative heat loss from the large area of peritoneum exposed during the operation, the infusion of large volumes of fluids, and the placement in the abdomen of a donor liver stored at 2–4°C. Hypothermia impairs coagulation, drug metabolism, renal function and myocardial contractility, and may alter the myocardial response to inotropes. Appropriate protective measures include the use of a warm water mattress, humidification and warming of inspired gases, and warming of all infused fluids. Further reduction of heat loss is achieved by wrapping exposed areas in polyethylene or reflective sheeting, particularly important during the period following induction when monitoring and infusion catheters are inserted. Increasing the operating room temperature and the use of a radiant warmer are also of value during the preparation period.

With these measures core temperature can usually be kept above 35°C until reperfusion of the donor liver, when a fall to 32–34°C is almost always observed. A gradual recovery then occurs as the operation is completed, although a subnormal core temperature or marked core–peripheral temperature gradient may persist for several hours postoperatively.

POSTOPERATIVE INTENSIVE CARE

A period of 1–3 days of postoperative ventilation is usual, although relatively fit older children and adolescents may be extubated 6–12 h postoperatively if temperature, circulation and gas exchange are satisfactory and bleeding is minimal. Potential respiratory problems include pulmonary oedema and pleural effusion, related to fluid overload, increased vascular permeability and transdiaphragmatic leakage of abdominal fluid; lobar atelectasis, most commonly the right upper lobe; and diaphragmatic restriction, often due to the use of a relatively large donor liver. Donor body weights up to three times the recipient's have been associated with a successful outcome, although weaning from artificial ventilation may be delayed due to high intra-abdominal pressures. Abdominal distension due to ileus, aerophagia or retained clot may also interfere with spontaneous ventilation. Aspiration is a rare complication, avoidable through frequent gastric aspiration and the use of 4–5 cm of positive end expiratory pressure. Right phrenic paresis, probably related to injury caused by application of the suprahepatic caval clamp, may also be seen.

Control of pain is achieved through the use of intravenous opiates, possibly by infusion. Intercostal blocks have proved useful in some patients, particularly for weaning (Shelly and Park, 1987), although a small dose of opiate or ketamine is needed for the procedure.

Maintenance of fluid and electrolyte balance in the early postoperative period may be complicated by continuing blood loss and rapid reuptake of potassium by the transplanted liver. Administration of calcium and potassium salts is required. A tendency to oliguria, in spite of normal or high cardiac filling pressures and the use of low-dose dopamine infusion, is common. This is managed empirically with intermittent administration of frusemide, since overfilling of the circulation leads readily to pulmonary oedema. Intraoperative metabolic acidosis gives way to postoperative metabolic alkalosis, probably related to metabolism of citrate (Driscoll et al, 1987), diuretic administration and hypokalaemia.

Cardiovascular stability depends mainly on maintenance of an adequate intravascular volume. Hypertension and bradycardia, however, are common features, particularly in young children. The cause is unknown; although cyclosporin A has recognized vasoconstrictive and nephrotoxic effects, elevated blood pressure is also seen in children not given this drug. Since myocardial infarction, encephalopathy and cerebral haemorrhage have occurred in hypertensive children following liver transplantation (Thompson, 1986), treatment with vasodilators is appropriate.

Surgical complications include uncontrolled bleeding, leakage or obstruction of biliary or bowel anastomoses, bowel perforation and formation of abdominal collections. Prompt reoperation may be necessary, so a dedicated operating theatre should be reserved.

The most serious problems arising early (<10 days) after transplantation, however, are related to failure of graft function or complications of immunosuppression. Hepatic infarction, which may be partial or complete and may occur with or without thrombosis of one or both afferent vessels, is a catastrophic complication seen most frequently in children under 5 years of age. Urgent retransplantation is required. Acute rejection and fulminant sepsis may be associated with hepatic infarction or may occur independently. Differentiation of these from infarction and from each other on clinical grounds may be difficult, and biopsy is usually required. Rejection in most cases can be controlled by increased immunosuppression. Sepsis, on the other hand, though often characterized by similar biochemical evidence of graft injury, requires reduction of immunosuppressive agents and aggressive antibiotic treatment if the patient is to survive. It is usually caused by Gram-negative enteric organisms; opportunistic infections of viral, protozoal and fungal origin tend to arise later and present less acutely. Shock, coagulopathy and haemorrhage, non-cardiogenic pulmonary oedema, renal failure and progressive cerebral oedema may all occur in association with fulminant graft failure after an uneventful initial postoperative course. Effective management requires competent intensive care nursing, full laboratory support, and close collaboration between the surgical, anaesthetic and paediatric members of the transplant team.

CONCLUSIONS

Liver transplantation has now secured a recognized place in the management of children with end-stage hepatic disease. The perioperative care of these patients demands a sound understanding of the pathophysiology of severe hepatice failure, of the major stages and potential pitfalls of the surgical procedure, and of the cardiovascular, biochemical and haematological changes which commonly occur. Successful anaesthetic management presents a technical and logistic challenge which should not be underestimated. It depends on careful and comprehensive monitoring, good communication with surgical colleagues, and a thoroughly organized team approach. The effort is rewarded by an increasing number of long-term healthy survivors, and ultimately by the prospect of better understanding and more able management of problems encountered in a much broader group of critically ill children.

REFERENCES

Amess JAL, Burman JF, Rees GM, Nancekievill DG & Mollin DL (1978) Megaloblastic haemopoiesis in patients receiving nitrous oxide. *Lancet* **ii:** 339–342.
Arieff AI, Park R, Leach W & Lazarowitz VC (1982) Systemic effects of $NaHCO_3$ in experimental lactic acidosis in dogs. *American Journal of Physiology* **242:** 586.
Banks RGS, Henderson RJ & Pratt JM (1968) Reaction of gases in solution. Part III. Some reactions of nitrous oxide with transition-metal complexes. *Journal of the Chemical Society (A):* 2886–2889.
Berridge JC & Klinck JR (1988) Paediatric liver transplantation: biochemical changes during surgery. Proceedings of the Liver Care Group of Europe Inaugural Meeting, 25–26 March 1988 (unpublished data).
Bersin R, Chatterjee K & Arieff AI (1986). Metabolic and systemic effects of bicarbonate in hypoxic patients with heart failure. *Kidney International* **29:** 180.
Bethune DW, Collis JM, Hardy I & Latimer R (1980) Anaesthesia for coronary artery surgery. In Longmore DB (ed) *Towards Safer Cardiac Surgery*, pp 267–279. Lancaster: MTP Press.
Bihari D, Gimson AES, Waterson M & Williams R (1985) Tissue hypoxia during fulminant hepatic failure. *Critical Care Medicine* **13:** 1034–1039.
Bishop RL & Weisfeldt ML (1976) Sodium bicarbonate administration during cardiac arrest. Effect on arterial pH, pCO_2, and osmolality. *Journal of the American Medical Association* **235:** 506.
Bismuth H, Castaing D, Ericzon BG et al (1987) Hepatic transplantation in Europe. *Lancet* ii: 674–676.

Bontempo FA (1987) Monitoring of coagulation during liver transplantation—how much is enough? *Mayo Clinic Proceedings* **62:** 848–849.

Borland LM, Roule M & Cook DR (1985) Anaesthesia for paediatric orthoptic liver transplantation. *Anaesthesia and Analgesia* **64:** 117–124.

Butler BD, Leiman BC & Katz J (1987) Arterial air embolism of venous origin in dogs: effect of nitrous oxide in combination with halothane and pentobarbitone. *Canadian Journal of Anaesthesia* **34:** 570–575.

Calne RY, Rolles K, Farman JV, Kneeshaw JD, Smith DP & Wheeldon DR (1984) Veno-arterial bypass in orthotopic liver grafting. *Lancet* **ii:** 1269.

Carmichael FJ, Lindop MJ & Farman JV (1985) Anaesthesia for hepatic transplantation: cardiovascular and metabolic alterations and their management. *Anesthesia and Analgesia* **64:** 108–116.

Casella JF, Lewis JH, Bontempo FA, Zitelli BJ, Markel H & Starzl TE (1988) Successful treatment of homozygous protein C deficiency by hepatic transplantation. Lancet **i:** 435–437.

Cuervas-Mons VE, Millan I, Gaveler J, Starzle TE & Van Thiel DH (1986) Prognostic value of pre-operatively obtained clinical and laboratory data in predicting survival following orthotopic liver transplantation. *Hepatology* **6:** 922–927.

Damen J & Wever JE (1987) The use of balloon tipped pulmonary artery catheters in children undergoing cardiac surgery. *Intensive Care Medicine* **13:** 266–272.

Deacon R, Chanarin I, Perry J & Lumb M (1980) Marrow cells from patients with untreated pernicious anaemia cannot use tetrahydrofolate normally. *British Journal of Haematology* **46:** 523–528.

de Hemptinne B, de Ville de Goyet J, Kestens PJ & Otte JB (1987) Volume reduction of the liver graft before orthotopic transplantation: report of a clinical experience in 11 cases. *Transplantation Proceedings* **XIX:** 3317–3322.

Derrington MC (1985) The current status of blood filtration. *Anaesthesia* **40:** 334–337.

Dolan WM, Stevens WC, Eger E II et al (1974) The cardiovascular and respiratory effects of isoflurane–nitrous oxide anaesthesia. *Canadian Anaesthetists' Society Journal* **21:** 557–568.

Driscoll DF, Bistrian BR, Jenkins RL et al (1987) Development of metabolic alkalosis after massive transfusion during orthotopic liver transplantation. *Critical Care Medicine* **15:** 905–908.

Dyer PM, Blanloeil YG & Farman JV (1987) Liver transplantation in children. Blood transfusion and metabolic disorders. *Annales Françaises d'Anésthésie et Réanimation* **6:** 163–168.

Editoral (1987) Platelet transfusion therapy. *Lancet* **ii:** 490–491.

Eisele JH & Smith NTY (1972) Cardiovascular effects of 40% nitrous oxide in man. *Anesthesia and Analgesia* **51:** 956–961.

Epstein M (1986) The sodium retention of cirrhossis: a reappraisal. *Hepatology* **6:** 312–315.

Farman JV, Turner JM & Blanloeil Y (1986) Atracurium infusion in liver transplantation. *British Journal of Anaesthesia* **58:** 96S–102S.

Fredell J, Takyi Y, Gwenigale W et al (1987) Fibronectin as possible adjunct in treatment of severe malnutrition. *Lancet* **ii:** 962.

Gordon JB, Bernstein ML, Oski FA & Rogers MC (1987) Hematologic disorders in the pediatric intensive care unit. In Rogers MC (ed.) *Textbook of Pediatric Intensive Care*, pp 1181–1221. Baltimore: Williams & Wilkins.

Graf H & Arieff AI (1986) Sodium bicarbonate in the therapy of organic acidosis. *Intensive Care Medicine* **12:** 285–288.

Hehir DJ, Jenkins RL, Bistrian BR & Blackburn GL (1985) Nutrition in patients undergoing orthotopic liver transplant. *Journal of Parenteral and Enteral Nutrition* **9:** 695–704.

Hursh D, Gelman S & Bradley ELJ (1987) Hepatic oxygen supply during halothane or isoflurane anaesthesia in guinea pigs. *Anesthesiology* **67:** 701–706.

Johnson PJ, O'Grady J, Calvey H & Williams R (1987) Nutritional management and assessment. In Calne RY (ed.) *Liver Transplantation*, pp 103–117. London: Grune & Stratton.

Kalayoglu M, Sollinger HW, Stratta RJ et al (1988) Extended preservation of the liver for clinical transplantation. *Lancet* i: 617–619.

Kang YG, Martin DJ, Marquez J et al (1985) Intraoperative changes in blood coagulation and thromboelastographic monitoring in liver transplantation. *Anaesthesia and Analgesia* 64: 888–896.

Kratzer MAA, Dieterich HJ & Knedel M (1988) Intraoperative monitoring of coagulation and specific treatment with blood products during liver transplantation. Proceedings of the Liver Care Group of Europe Inaugural Meeting, 25–26 March 1988 (unpublished data).

Lappas DG, Buckley MJ, Laver MB, Daggett WM & Lowenstein E (1975) Left ventricular performance and pulmonary circulation following addition of nitrous oxide to morphine during coronary artery surgery. *Anesthesiology* 43: 61–69.

Lewis HA & Bontempo FA (1985) Orthotopic liver transplantation in patients with haemophilia. *New England Journal of Medicine* 312: 1189–1190.

Lindop MJ & Farman JV (1987) Anaesthesia: assessment and intraoperative management. In Calne RY (ed.) *Liver Transplantation*, pp 157–177. London: Grune & Stratton.

Luddington RJ (1988) Changes in haemostatic factors associated with liver transplantation. In Proceedings of the Liver Care Group of Europe Inaugural Meeting, 25–26 March 1988 (unpublished data).

Lunn JK, Stanley TH, Eisele J, Webster L & Woodward A (1979) High dose fentanyl anaesthesia for coronary artery surgery: plasma fentanyl concentrations and influence of nitrous oxide on cardiovascular responses. *Anesthesia and Analgesia* 58: 390–395.

Marquez JM Jr & Martin D (1986) Anaesthesia for liver transplantation. In Winter PW & Kang YD (eds) *Hepatic Transplantation*, pp 44–57. New York: Praeger.

Martin D (1986) Hemodynamic monitoring during liver transplantation. In Winter PW & Kang YG (eds) *Hepatic Transplantation*, pp 95–102. New York: Praeger.

Martin DJ, Marquez JM, Kang YG et al (1984) Liver transplantation: hemodynamic and electrolyte changes seen immediately following revascularisation. *Anesthesia and Analgesia* 63: 246(S).

Mattar JA, Weil MH, Shubin H & Stein L (1974) Cardiac arrest in the critically ill. II: Hyperosmolal states following cardiac arrest. *American Journal of Medicine* 56: 162.

Mazzoni G, Koep L & Starzl TE (1979) Air embolus in liver transplantation. *Transplant Proceedings* 11: 267–268.

Miyamoto M & Kajimoto T (1983) Associated anomalies in biliary atresia patients. In Kasai M (ed) *Biliary Atresia and its Related Disorders*, pp 13–19. Amsterdam: Excerpta Medica, ics 627.

Neuberger J (1987) When should patients be referred for liver transplantation? *British Medical Journal* 295: 565–566.

Otte JB, de Ville de Goyet J, De Hemptinne B et al (1987) Liver transplantation in children: report of 2½ years' experience at the university of Louvain medical school in Brussels. *Transplantation Proceedings* XIX: 3289–3302.

Owen CA, Rettke SR, Bowie EJW et al (1987) Hemostatic evaluation of patients undergoing liver transplantation. *Mayo Clinic Proceedings* 62: 761–772.

Perry J, Chanarin I, Deacon R & Lumb M (1979) The substrate for polyglutamate biosynthesis in the vitamin B_{12} inactivated rat. *Biochemistry and Biophysics Research Communications* 91: 678–684.

Polson RJ, Park GR, Lindop MJ, Farman JV, Calne RY & Williams R (1987) The prevention of renal impairment in patients undergoing orthotopic liver grafting by infusion of low dose dopamine. *Anaesthesia* 42: 15–19.

Salem MG, Crooke JW, McLoughlin GA et al (1988) The effect of dopamine on renal function during aortic cross clamping. *Annals of the Royal College of Surgeons of England* **70:** 9–12.

Schriever HG, Epstein SE & Mintz MD (1973) Statistical correlation and heparin sensitivity of activated partial thromboplastin time, whole blood coagulation time and an automated coagulation time. *American Journal of Clinical Pathology* **60:** 323–329.

Seyde WC, Ellis JE & Longnecker DE (1986) The addition of nitrous oxide to halothane decreases renal and splanchnic flow and increases cerebral blood flow in rats. *British Journal of Anaesthesia* **58:** 63–68.

Shelly MP & Park GR (1987) Intercostal nerve blockade for children. *Anaesthesia* **42:** 541–544.

Smith MF, Thomas DG & Hesford JW (1987). Perioperative support, monitoring and autotransfusion. In Calne RY (ed) *Liver Transplantation*, pp 179–196. London: Grune & Stratton.

Smith NT, Eger E II, Stoelting RK, Whayne TF, Cullen D & Kadis LB (1970) The cardiovascular and sympathomimetic responses to the addition of nitrous oxide to halothane in man. *Anesthesiology* **32:** 410–421.

Starzl TE, Esquivel C, Gordon R & Todo S (1987) Pediatric liver transplantation. *Transplantation Proceedings* **XIX:** 3230–3235.

Stevens WC, Cromwell TH, Halsey MJ et al (1971) The cardiovascular effects of a new inhalational anesthetic, Forane, in human volunteers at constant carbon dioxide tension. *Anesthesiology* **35:** 8–16.

Thompson AE (1986) Aspects of pediatric intensive care following liver transplantation. In Proceedings of the Second Symposium on Liver Transplantation, 14–16 September, 1986. University of Pittsburgh, Pittsburgh (unpublished data).

Tizard EJ, Pett S, Pelham AM, Mowat AP & Barnes ND (1987) Selection and assessment of children for liver transplantation. In Calne RY (ed) *Liver Transplantation*, pp 119–129. London: Grune & Stratton.

Van Thiel DH, Schade RR, Gavaler JS, Shaw BW, Iwatsuki S & Starzl TE (1984) Medical aspects of orthotopic liver transplantation. *Hepatology* **4** (suppl 1): 79S–83S.

Ward S & Neill EAM (1983) Pharmokinetics of atracurium in acute hepatic failure (with acute renal failure). *British Journal of Anaesthesia* **55:** 1169–1172.

Watts RWE, Calne RY, Rolles K et al (1987) Successful treatment of primary hyperoxaluria type I by combined hepatic and renal transplantation. *Lancet* **ii:** 474–475.

Wilkinson SP (1987) The hepatorenal syndrome revisited. *Intensive Care Medicine* **13:** 145–147.

Zitelli BJ, Gartner JC Jr, Malatack JJ et al (1987) Pediatric liver transplantation: patient evaluation and selection, infectious complications, and life-style after transplantation. *Transplantation Proceedings* **XIX:** 3309–3316.

Heart and heart–lung transplantation in children

HISTORY

The results of John Hunter's successful transplant experiments on animals performed over 200 years ago can be seen at the Royal College of Surgeons, London. However, it was not until 1960 when Sir Peter Medawar received the Nobel Prize for his pioneering work on acquired immunological tolerance that the golden age of immunology began. Medawar's work was stimulated by the desperate need for skin grafting to help airmen burnt during the war.

In 1967, Barnard performed the first orthotopic human heart transplant, and later in the same year, Kantrowitz introduced cardiac transplantation in neonates when his group transplanted a heart from an anencephalic neonate to a 3-week-old infant with tricuspid atresia. The child only survived a few hours. With the introduction of cyclosporin in 1980, and the continued improvement in results, heart and heart–lung transplantation have evolved from being experimental procedures to being the accepted treatment in selected patients with end-stage heart and lung disease.

According to the register of the International Society for Heart Transplantation (1987 report) over 4000 heart and heart–lung transplants have now been performed worldwide. Only 2.7% of these were performed in children under 15 years (Kaye, 1987). The combined experience of Papworth and Harefield Hospitals accounts for over 60 of these children.

PROCUREMENT OF DONOR ORGANS

The success of any transplant programme ultimately depends on the viability of the procured organs. As a result good medical management of the cadaveric donor before and during the period of organ procurement has become an essential part of the transplant programme.

Criteria for the selection of heart–lung donors

Screening for hepatitis antigen and human immunodeficiency virus infection must be negative. The donor's cytomegalovirus (CMV) status and the

ABO blood grouping should also be known. It is now the practice to match donors and recipients for CMV status. This is because CMV infection is a significant problem in heart and lung transplantation. There is some evidence to suggest that clinical illness, usually CMV pneumonitis, is common in those recipients who seroconvert from negative to positive CMV status following transplantation (Dummer et al, 1985; Burke et al, 1986; Griffith et al, 1987).

The period of mechanical ventilation should be short, preferably less than 48 h, as beyond this period the incidence of microbial contamination of the bronchial tree increases (Johnson et al, 1969, 1972; Cross and Roup, 1981; Ruiz-Santana et al, 1987). The donor should be afebrile and have no evidence of systemic infection. Blood culture and sputum sample should be taken for routine screening.

Size

In order to match the donor with the recipient for organ size, measurement of the donor's weight and height should be made. From these measurements, the total lung capacity can be calculated and compared with the recipient (Cotes, 1979). It is usual to select as far as possible donor organs slightly smaller than the recipient's thoracic capacity as the reverse leads to difficulties in closing the chest wall and postoperative pulmonary collapse.

Lung function

Formal lung function testing is not necessary. However, what is required is that the most recent chest X-ray should be free of any evidence of pulmonary oedema or atelectasis. The airway pressure generated by a tidal volume of 10 ml/kg body weight should be less than 30 cm H_2O. Similarly, the gas transfer properties of the lung should be such that on an inspired oxygen of 40% the arterial oxygen tension (PaO_2) will be greater than 20 kPa. Positive end expiratory pressure (5 cm) is usually added to the ventilatory settings to keep the lungs slightly distended.

Heart

A 12-lead ECG should be normal. If on dopamine, the dose necessary to maintain a normal arterial pressure should be less than 10 μg/kg/min.

Congenital heart disease can largely be excluded by reviewing the clinical, electrocardiographic and radiographic data. It is possible to evaluate the quality of the donor heart and its protection during transport by taking a biopsy of the left ventricle just before the heart is removed. Two further biopsies are taken, just before and after implantation. These biopsies are examined by the birefringence method for an assessment of myocardial contractility (Darracott-Cankovic et al, 1987). The contractility data however are not available prior to implantation. It is hoped that research in this area will allow such information to be obtained prior to the excision of the donor's heart.

Darracott-Cankovic et al (1987) have reported very interesting findings based on 78 consecutive donor heart biopsies obtained at the time of excision through to the time of implantation. They discovered that about one-third of the donor hearts were poorly functioning at the time of excision and remained so during transportation and implantation. Another third were normally functioning at the time of excision but deteriorated during transportation and were poorly functioning subsequently. The last third were normally functioning from the onset and remained so subsequently. This grading by birefringence into three groups was also reflected in the immediate performance of the transplanted hearts and subsequent recipient morbidity. This report highlights the need for a more reliable method for donor selection and the fact that the ideal method for myocardial protection during storage and transport is yet to be found.

Potential donors often do not match these selection criteria, as shown by the experience of the Stanford group, that only 10–16% of heart donors can be used as heart and lung donors (Harjula et al, 1987). Nevertheless, it is important for the referring donor hospital to establish the suitability of their patient for heart and lung donation by discussing the case with the transplant centre.

Management of the donor operation

Initially the donor was moved to the hospital where the recipient operation was to be performed. This had obvious logistic and emotional disadvantages. With improvement in organ preservation, distant procurement is now normally practised.

As indicated above, the management of the donor is crucial to the subsequent function of the harvested organs. Good medical management of the donor organs is owed not only to the memory of the deceased benefactor but also to the recipient. The anaesthetist, by virtue of his or her training in the care of the critically ill, is perhaps the most suitable clinician to assume the responsibility for protecting the donor organs from ischaemic injury both before and during harvesting. There is some evidence that newborn hearts are more vulnerable to global ischaemic injury than adult hearts (Chu-Jeng Chiu and Bindon, 1987).

Periods of hypotension or dysrhythmias leading to cardiac dilatation will affect graft function postoperatively. Accordingly, at Papworth, a senior anaesthetist is part of the procurement team for harvesting organs for combined heart and lung transplantation.

Ideally the donor management should begin as soon as brain stem death has been confirmed by two independent suitably qualified clinicians and consent for organ removal has been obtained from the relatives. The primary diagnosis of the majority of the donors is irreversible brain injury secondary to a road traffic accident or sudden intracranial haemorrhage. The standard supportive management of these patients includes reduction of intracranial pressure using mannitol and fluid restriction. The net result of this treatment is a reduction of central circulatory volume.

Consequently these donors often arrive in the operating theatre for the donor operation with a very low or negative central venous pressure. If there is an associated cranial diabetes insipidus, this problem may be exacerbated. A number of these donors will also require inotropic support to maintain their blood pressure. At this stage, the severe dehydration must be corrected. However, what should be used and how much remains controversial. The special needs of the lungs, heart and kidneys may conflict.

There is a need to keep the lungs dry in order to achieve optimum graft function postoperatively. This means that transfused fluids should remain in circulation and not diffuse out into interstitial spaces. In addition, the volume of fluid transfused should perhaps be less than optimal in order to reduce the risk of pulmonary oedema.

To support the heart, a proportion of these donors will be receiving inotropic drugs to maintain arterial pressure in the normal range. The need for the inotropic support arises from the fact that the circulatory volume has been significantly reduced and not because the heart is actually failing. In a brain-dead patient there is a vasomotor paralysis leading to a total inhibition of sympathetic reflexes. This results in the reduction of the effectiveness of the heart as a pump to about 80% of normal (Guyton, 1976), without losing its heterometric response.

It is a clinical axiom not to use inotropic agents on an empty heart for fear of inducing an ischaemic injury. In addition, there is some evidence to suggest that acute head injury itself may produce myocardial damage in some patients (McLeod et al, 1982). When an adequate circulatory volume has been achieved, using the central venous pressure as a guide, in most cases the inotropic support can be safely reduced or discontinued.

There is also the need to maintain the urinary output in the physiological range in order to preserve the renal function and minimize the risk of pulmonary oedema. Large volumes of synthetic plasma volume expanders may cause renal tubular damage.

Newton and Wesenhagen (1986) have suggested that in most situations the use of pure albumin preparations and blood would be the most appropriate. However, because of the problems of availability of albumin preparations and the fact that a significant proportion of donors have a raised haematocrit, the above suggestion may not be practical. It is our experience since the start of the heart and lung transplant programme in 1984 that a combination of albumin, plasma, gelatin volume expanders and blood adequately fulfils the requirements.

Work from animal models has shown that very shortly after brain death there is a rapid loss of several plasma hormones, especially tri-iodothyronine (T3) and thyroxine (T4); (Novitzky et al, 1984). This has been confirmed in human brain-dead patients (Robert et al, 1986). The fall in T3 and T4 levels is associated with a shift from aerobic to anaerobic metabolism leading to reduced myocardial energy stores. However, at present, it is uncertain whether the hormonal abnormalities should be restored by exogenous T3, cortisol or insulin. It is hoped that current work will provide some insight into this phenomenon.

It is essential that the donor is closely monitored. On arrival in the operating theatre, an ECG, a reliable peripheral venous line, a right internal jugular line and a left radial artery line are established. The right internal jugular vein and the left radial artery are preferred because the innominate vein and the right subclavian artery are ligated very early during the dissection of the heart.

The heart–lung donor operation often involves the harvesting of liver, kidneys and other organs, frequently necessitating the involvement of several surgical teams. As a result the harvesting process may take up to 6 h. Fluid losses incurred during this procedure are similar to any major thoracoabdominal operation and must be replaced in order to maintain adequate organ perfusion. Because blood transfusion is sometimes necessary, 4 units of blood should be cross-matched for every adult donor operation and proportionately less for smaller donors. The total amount of fluids transfused during the whole procedure may be as much as 8 l.

By definition, anaesthesia is not necessary for the operation. However, certain haemodynamic changes occur in response to surgical stimuli, reminiscent of living patients. These responses occur in only a proportion of the donors and take the form of hypertension sometimes with tachycardia but unassociated with diaphoresis. These responses are usually of short duration but if they persist, they should be treated in the same way as any hypertensive episode during anaesthesia. Wetzel et al (1985) have reported similar observations.

Although the underlying mechanisms of these responses are not fully understood, they do not invalidate the brain death criteria as set out by the Conference of the Medical Royal Colleges (1976). Spinal reflex arcs between pain afferents and sympathetically mediated efferents (Johnson et al, 1975) and humoral responses involving the stimulation of the adrenal medulla have been invoked to explain the haemodynamic changes (Naftchi et al, 1974; Guyton, 1981). The lungs are ventilated with an air and oxygen mixture or nitrous oxide in oxygen if medical air is not available. Muscle relaxation is sometimes necessary to aid surgical access.

No attempt is made to describe the surgical technique in detail but the salient features which affect organ perfusion will be mentioned. During multiorgan harvesting, the surgical teams take turns in dissecting for the various organs. The dissection for the liver and the kidneys invariably starts first and may take up to 3 h. There is usually no haemodynamic instability during this period provided fluid losses are replaced and obstruction of the inferior vena cava (IVC) is avoided. These organs are however left in situ until after cardioplegia solution has been given to the heart.

After median sternotomy, the lungs should be inspected to confirm the absence of any gross abnormality and that there is full expansion of all lobes, especially the left lower lobe. The heart is also examined. The superior vena cava (SVC) is next palpated to ensure that the central venous catheter tip is superior to the site to be ligated. The trachea is also checked for the position of the tracheal tube.

Prior to cannulating the pulmonary artery (PA), 3 mg/kg heparin is given. The cannula has a side arm through which the PA is perfused with prostacyclin. Prostacyclin is a potent vasodilator and in order to prevent any ensuing hypotension, the central venous pressure has to be maintained. The infusion of prostacyclin starts about 15 min before the aorta is cross-clamped at a dose of 2 ng/kg/min progressively going up to 20 ng/kg/min.

The SVC and IVC are later ligated. This effectively excludes any venous return to the heart, hence the need to maintain the filling pressure prior to this point in order to minimize any hypotensive episodes. Immediately after the caval ligation, the aorta is cross-clamped and 10 ml/kg of cold crystalloid cardioplegia solution is infused via the aortic cannula to stop the heart in diastole. Infusion of pulmoplegia solution at 4°C via the PA cannula starts at the same time as the cardioplegia. It is infused at a pressure of 60 cm H_2O through a heat-exchanger into the PA (Figure 15.1). A vent in the left atrial appendage allows excess pulmoplegia solution to drain out.

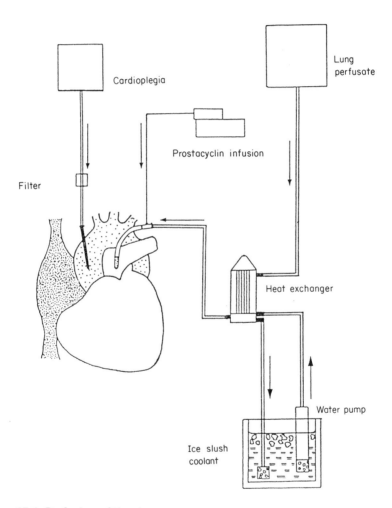

Figure 15.1. Perfusion of the donor organs.

When the delivery of pulmoplegia solution is complete, the lungs are held inflated with room air and the trachea clamped a few centimetres above the carina. In order to reduce the incidence of postoperative atelectasis, all the lobes of the lung must be seen to be fully inflated before the trachea is clamped. Room air is used to inflate the lungs in order to reduce the risk of absorptive atelectasis. The heart and lungs are removed en bloc, kept cold with cold cardioplegia solution and prepared for transportation back to the transplant centre.

The need to procure organs from distant hospitals has led to the various transplant centres evolving different methods for organ preservation when the organs have been harvested. The current technique at Papworth Hospital has been found to preserve the organs for up to 4 h. The technique is called the single pulmonary flush method. It is unique to the Papworth group. Other groups have used more complex methods. The Pittsburgh group uses a warm, beating, autoperfusing, ventilated heart–lung preparation.

The Harefield team cools the donor on cardiopulmonary bypass prior to harvesting the organs. The constituents of the Papworth pulmoplegia solution are as set out in Table 15.1. The volumes given are scaled down proportionately for smaller donors.

Table 15.1. Pulmoplegia solution

Constituents
400 ml of the donor blood
200 ml of 20% albumin
100 ml of 10% mannitol
10 000 units of heparin
700 ml of Ringer's solution
63 ml of citrate phosphate dextrose (CPD)

The organs are transported in a special box containing a pneumatic cushion which protects the organs from mechanical injury during transport and also acts as a thermal insulator. The box can maintain the organs at 4°C for a period of 20–40 h depending on the ambient temperature (Figure 15.2).

Because the donor operation is often timed to suit both the donor and the receiving hospitals, the majority of transplant operations are performed at night. In order to reduce the cold ischaemic time of the donor organs to the minimum, frequent communication from the procurement team to update the base hospital is essential. This has been facilitated with the recent development of portable telephone systems.

MANAGEMENT OF THE RECIPIENT

Assessment

Children referred to a transplant unit for assessment often undergo further investigation, for example cardiac catheterization, and myocardial or lung biopsy (Bricker and Frazier, 1987). Most children under the age of 10 will need general anaesthesia, and the hazards of the procedure itself, such as

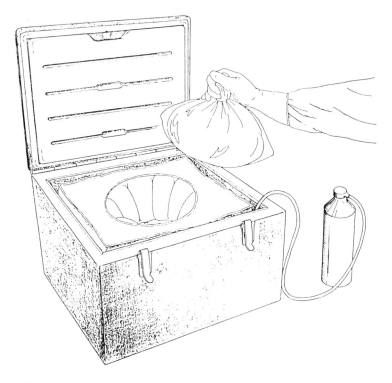

Figure 15.2. Equipment for transport of the donor organs (see text).

the adverse cardiovascular effects of radiopaque dye, may exacerbate their already serious condition. As much care must be taken with these children undergoing investigations as is taken with their definitive procedure. As well as confirming the diagnosis in complex abnormalities, it is vital to measure the pulmonary vascular resistance (PVR). It has long been recognized in adult heart transplantation that undetected high PVR in the recipient due to chronic left ventricular failure imposes an often intolerable load on the normal right ventricle of the donor heart. Sadly, small children with heart disease develop a high PVR early, necessitating heart–lung rather than heart transplantation. Uncorrected congenital defects with an increased pulmonary blood flow, such as ventricular septal defect, lead to pulmonary hypertension. If pulmonary pressures exceed systemic arterial pressures, then reversal of the shunt occurs (acquired Eisenmenger's syndrome). It is essential to avoid systemic hypotension in these patients (see p. 309). There is no absolute level of pulmonary hypertension above which a normal heart fails. As world experience grows, the limits will be defined more clearly. At present, few surgeons would accept a patient with an irreversible PVR of more than 6 mmHg/l/min or a pulmonary vascular resistance index (PVR$_1$) of more than 10 mmHg/l/min/m^2 for cardiac transplantation. If the disease has been of short duration, for example viral cardiomyopathy, then although the child is in severe failure, the PVR may still be low, and heart transplantation alone is needed. The shortage of suitable donors means that many of these acutely ill children are unlikely to survive long enough to receive a transplant.

Hypoperfusion of the lungs due to pulmonary atresia may also be treated by heart–lung transplantation if conventional surgery is not feasible. Table 15.2 shows the diseases for which children have received heart and heart–lung transplants.

Table 15.2(a). Possible indications for heart transplantation

Cardiomyopathy
Idiopathic
Familial
Viral
Fibroelastosis
Adriamycin toxicity
Storage disease
Impaired development
Hypoplastic left heart syndrome
Congenital heart disease (without pulmonary vascular disease)
Coronary artery abnormalities with damaged ventricles

Table 15.2(b). Possible indications for heart and lung transplantation

Parenchymal lung disease
Cystic fibrosis
Fibrosing alveolitis
Primary or idiopathic pulmonary hypertension
Congenital heart disease (with pulmonary vascular disease)
Eisenmenger's syndrome
Complex pulmonary atresia

Having been assessed, most children are discharged home, or to their referring hospital. Only the most gravely ill are kept at the transplant centre awaiting surgery, as the availability of small donor organs is limited. Several patients with pulmonary hypertension receive prostacyclin at home via a tunnelled central line while waiting (Jones et al, 1987).

Immunosuppression

Immunosuppression regimes vary from unit to unit; the current immuno-suppression regime at Papworth is shown in Table 15.3. Preoperative cyclosporin is now omitted because of its nephrotoxicity and the majority of patients have poor renal function preoperatively. Antithymocyte globulin gave rise to severe hypotension when given at induction, and is now given after bypass has been established without adverse effect. Once the cardio-vascular status of the patients is improved by surgery, they can easily tolerate antithymocyte globulin. Postoperative steroids are only given in heart–lung transplantation to treat rejection, as their use prevents healing of the tracheal anastomosis.

Table 15.3. Immunosuppression regimen currently in use at Papworth Hospital

Drug	Preoperative	Postoperative
Azathioprine	3 mg/kg i.v.	1.5–2 mg/kg o.d.
Methylprednisolone	1.5 mg/kg i.v.	For heart transplant only 1 mg/kg o.d. reducing to 0.3 mg/kg/day at 3 weeks
Cyclosporin (therapeutic blood levels: for whole blood 800–1000 μg/l; for plasma 150–200 μg/l)	—	Induction dose of 100–150 mg Maintenance dose of 50 mg/day
Antithymocyte globulin	10 mg/kg i.v. on bypass	1st–2nd postoperative days. Dose depends on % of T- cells

Premedication

When a suitable donor is found for a child, the time available in which to admit that child and prepare him or her for surgery may vary from as little as 2 to 3 h up to several days. The calm preoperative assessment of the child with the family, adequate fasting and premedication are rarely achieved, largely due to the current organization of organ harvesting in this country. If there is time, and if the child is cardiovascularly stable, then trimeprazine 2 mg/kg is given orally 2 h preoperatively followed by papaveretum 0.3 mg/kg and hyoscine 0.006 mg/kg i.m. 1 h preoperatively. Trimeprazine is omitted if time is short. Children under 1 year and extremely sick children are unpremedicated, or given atropine 0.02 mg/kg i.m. 1 h preoperatively.

Preparation of the anaesthetic room

All invasive procedures must be done aseptically, and scrupulous attention to cleanliness is maintained when managing these children.

Anaesthetic drugs are ready drawn up in labelled syringes, and infusions of isoprenaline and antithymocyte globulin are prepared.

A variety of different sized tracheal tubes should be available, as these children are often small for their age. The authors use nasotracheal intubation with an uncuffed Portex tube and a Tunstall frame fixation for small children (see p. 320), and oral cuffed tubes for the larger children. For heart–lung transplantation the tubes must be 1 cm or so shorter than usual, in order to avoid the tracheal anastomosis, which is about 2 cm above the carina.

Induction of anaesthesia

The greatest problems encountered at induction of anaesthesia are in children with primary cardiac pathology. Children undergoing heart–lung transplantation with parenchymal lung disease do not usually present great difficulty. It cannot be over-emphasized how unpredictably children with heart disease may respond to anaesthesia, and how rapidly their condition may deteriorate. Patients with pulmonary hypertension and poor right ventricular function may rapidly enter a downward spiral of increasing hypoxia and cardiac decompensation, leading to cardiac arrest.

The position of the haemodynamically unstable patient is critical. Some children are just compensated when semi-recumbent, and if made to lie flat will rapidly deteriorate as blood 'transfused' into the central circulation from the periphery increases the already high ventricular filling pressures. Anaesthesia should be induced in the slightly head-up position in these children.

At Harefield there is no standard regime, and the choice of technique depends on the anaesthetist's assessment of the clinical situation. A review of the records of 22 children under the age of 10 years undergoing heart or heart–lung transplantation showed that 50% received either a narcotic or a narcotic–benzodiazepine induction (sometimes with incremental etomidate); 36% had an inhalational induction with nitrous oxide, oxygen and halothane; and 14% received ketamine. At Papworth, because the average age of the paediatric transplant patient is 13 years (range 6–16 years) the same technique is used as for any high-risk cardiac patient: incremental papaveretum or midazolam is given for sedation, and anaesthesia is induced with nitrous oxide, oxygen and trichloroethylene, which gives a quick, pleasant and stable induction. Halothane is used for rapid induction of anaesthesia in the younger patient.

Halothane is a potent cardiac depressant, but it is also used to induce light anaesthesia in order to gain peripheral venous access. Once this is done, a narcotic and a relaxant are given. Intramuscular ketamine (3–4 mg/kg) may be used for the same purpose.

Drugs are given in low doses which are carefully titrated against their effect. Low cardiac output will prolong the circulation time, and response may be slow.

Fentanyl is usually the opiate of choice, but papaveretum or phenoperidine are also used. Intubation is facilitated with suxamethonium if the stomach is full. Otherwise, pancuronium (which has a useful chronotropic effect) or vecuronium is used.

A small-bore nasogastric tube is passed in the younger children to allow feeding and cyclosporin to start as soon as there is enteral absorption postoperatively.

Monitoring

Ideally, direct arterial pressure should be monitored during induction of anaesthesia. Pre-induction intra-arterial cannulation under local anaesthesia is possible only in a few children, who are either especially co-operative or particularly ill, and who have easily palpable arteries.

An automatic non-invasive blood pressure machine, set to measure every minute, electrocardiogram and pulse oximeter give adequate monitoring during induction, and are usually well tolerated.

After induction central and peripheral venous and arterial cannulas are inserted. Superficial veins are often sparse, and neck or femoral veins are used. The largest possible cannula is inserted. Two internal jugular cannulas (or a double-lumen catheter) are the minimum requirement for measurement of central venous pressure and administration of drugs and inotropes. If heavy blood loss is anticipated, the external jugular vein is a useful vessel. At Harefield, the left side of the neck is used whenever possible, leaving the right side untouched for future endomyocardial biopsies. At Papworth, the right side of the neck is used because it is anatomically more favourable for line insertion, and there have been no complaints from those taking subsequent biopsies.

A urinary catheter is inserted to monitor urine output and temperature is monitored with a nasopharyngeal probe.

Maintenance of anaesthesia

Maintenance of anaesthesia is by a nitrous oxide–narcotic–relaxant sequence, supplemented by a low concentration of a volatile agent or a benzodiazepine or etomidate. At Papworth 0.5% trichloroethylene is used, as it gives excellent cardiovascular stability and postoperative analgesia (Bethune et al, 1988). A Pall Ultipor BB50T heat-and-moisture exchanger is incorporated in the breathing circuit at the catheter mount, which also acts as a bacterial and viral filter (Shelley et al, 1986).

Just as position may adversely affect the awake patient, so may positioning on the operating table. Venesection, the use of 5–10° of head-up tilt, and nitroprusside to reduce afterload prevent an increase in ventricular filling pressures. Nitrous oxide is discontinued after heparinization to reduce the third gas effect, and to minimize the size of any microbubbles (Bethune, 1976). This is especially important in children with a right-to-left shunt.

Cardiopulmonary bypass (see p. 322)

For children under 10 kg the pump prime contains fresh whole blood. If the child is polycythaemic, fresh frozen plasma replaces some of the blood in order to reduce the haematocrit towards the normal. The haematocrit is kept above 30% in small children. Hypothermia is induced on bypass, to 25°C at Harefield, and to 30°C at Papworth (Wheeldon et al, 1986). Haemofiltration is performed on bypass to remove fluid from those children who are in cardiac failure with peripheral oedema. Some children who have impaired renal function can be haemodialysed on bypass (Hakim et al, 1985).

Papworth and Harefield differ in their practice of potassium replacement during cardiopulmonary bypass. Unusual sensitivity of the transplanted heart to potassium has been reported from Harefield (Grebenik and Robinson, 1985). This is not the experience at Papworth, where potassium supplements are given to maintain serum potassium above 4.5 mmol/l: normokalaemia appears to reduce the incidence of junctional and ventricular arrhythmias.

On two occasions the authors have encountered difficulty in coming off bypass because of high pulmonary arterial pressures. This is in spite of trying to identify patients with pulmonary hypertension preoperatively, as described above. As a last resort, we have infused prostacyclin into the pulmonary artery, which reduced the PVR and relieved the strain on the right ventricle. The antiplatelet properties of prostacyclin made haemostasis more difficult.

When coming off bypass, isoprenaline is used for its positive chronotropic and pulmonary vasodilator effects. Most patients are successfully taken off bypass on isoprenaline alone, but occasionally dopamine may be necessary in addition. Pacing may also be useful at a rate of 110 beats/min, in order to prevent the ventricular distension associated with the bradycardia inherent in the denervated heart.

We have also had difficulty weaning a patient from bypass who was refractory to β-agonists. The use of enoximone, a phcsphodiesterase inhibitor, produced a rapid improvement and the patient did well (Crawford, 1987).

Perioperative problems

Acid–base status

The trend of acid–base balance is assessed by frequent blood gas analysis. These children often have a profound metabolic acidosis due to poor tissue perfusion, and this should be corrected. However, a metabolic acidosis developing towards the end of the bypass period should not be corrected so vigorously, as a postoperative metabolic alkalosis may ensue.

Haemorrhage

Peri- and postoperative haemorrhage is a major problem, particularly in heart–lung transplantation. Liver dysfunction and preoperative anticoagulation predispose to bleeding, as do the rich bronchial blood supply, collateral vessels, pleural adhesions and previous chest surgery. It is crucial to achieve haemostasis in the posterior mediastinum after removal of the recipient's heart and lungs, as this area is inaccessible when the donor organs are transplanted. Time is often limited at this stage, as the total ischaemic time for the donor heart and lungs should be as short as possible.

Fresh whole blood, fresh frozen plasma and platelets are routinely ordered in generous amounts for heart–lung transplantation. Perioperatively the tracheal tube should be gently suctioned in order to prevent bleeding from the tracheal anastomosis forming clots in the lower airways. Postoperative haemorrhage is frequent; at Papworth 3 of 5 paediatric heart–lung transplant patients were re-explored for bleeding.

Urine output

A renal dose of dopamine may be useful to optimize renal function, which is often impaired, and may be exacerbated postoperatively by cyclosporin.

Gas exchange

Although preoperative gas exchange may be poor, oxygenation and removal of carbon dioxide are rarely difficult to achieve when the child is intubated and ventilated. It is possible that transplanted lungs may be particularly sensitive to damage by oxygen-free radicals, so the inspired oxygen concentration should be limited to that which produces PaO_2 of 12–15 kPa.

When the donor organs are transplanted, there is an increase in physiological dead space. The minute volumes needed to maintain a normal PCO_2 may initially be higher than expected.

Damage to nerves and thoracic duct

During the removal of the heart and lungs from the recipient, care is taken to ensure preservation of the phrenic, vagus and recurrent laryngeal nerves. The ability to cough after a recurrent laryngeal nerve palsy can be improved by Teflon paste injection of the vocal cords (Bodenham et al, 1987). One patient had a chylous leak causing a pleural effusion which persisted for several weeks.

Postoperative management

The major postoperative problems are haemorrhage, infection and rejection.

Children are ventilated routinely after heart and heart–lung transplant until they are awake, warm and haemodynamically stable. Early extubation reduces the likelihood of colonization of the bronchial tree. Sedation and analgesia are provided by intermittent boluses of intravenous papaveretum, and diazepam or midazolam. If there has been retention of carbon dioxide before heart–lung transplant, then there will be insensitivity to CO_2 in the immediate postoperative period, and narcotics must be used with particular caution. The authors avoid using neuromuscular relaxants unless there is cardiovascular instability or extreme restlessness.

Vigorous physiotherapy, including postural drainage, is needed after heart–lung transplantation as the lungs are denervated, and there will be no stimulus to clear secretions below the tracheal anastomosis. Occasionally, an enlarged pulmonary artery may damage the recurrent laryngeal nerve, and clearance of secretions is impaired even more.

Positive end expiratory pressure of 5 cm H_2O helps to prevent atelectasis after heart–lung transplant. Fluid overloading is carefully avoided in heart–lung transplant children, as lymphatic drainage from the lungs is interrupted. Humidification prevents inspissation of secretions.

Neurological complications are more common after paediatric than after adult heart transplantation. A patent foramen ovale in the donor heart allows paradoxical embolization, and hypertensive convulsions may be associated with cyclosporin. Fever and metabolic disturbances in children may also be a cause of convulsions.

Renal function deteriorates further in the postoperative period, and cyclosporin therapy may have to be withheld.

Infection

There is a high incidence of chest infection after heart and heart–lung transplantation. The source of the infection is often endogenous or from the transplanted organs or donor blood. While on the ventilator the inspiratory gases are filtered with a bacterial and viral filter. The child is barrier-nursed for at least the first 3 postoperative days.

CMV infection was one cause of the early high mortality after heart–lung transplantation. Since 1986, the Papworth team has screened all donor organs for CMV, in order to prevent transplanting a CMV-positive organ into a negative recipient. False negatives may occur, and double-checking is necessary (Gray et al, 1987). CMV infection commonly causes a pneumonitis, and is diagnosed serologically by viral culture and by histological demonstration of inclusion bodies. In a suspected case, hyperimmune globulin is started immediately and the antiviral agent Ganciclovir has been used successfully (Hutter et al, 1988b).

Pneumonia may be due to common organisms, such as *Streptococcus pneumoniae*, *Staphylococcus aureus*, *Pseudomonas*, and *Haemophilus influenzae*. In the immunosuppressed patient opportunist organisms, such as *Aspergillus*, *Pneumocystis* and tubercle, as well as dissemination of latent herpes simplex or varicella, may be troublesome.

Rejection

One of the greatest challenges facing the transplant teams early in the programme was the search for a reliable and sensitive means of diagnosing rejection. Clinical features include failure to thrive, cardiovascular instability, dyspnoea and oedema in heart transplant patients, and wheezing with alveolar shadowing on X-ray in heart–lung transplant. A technique of transbronchial biopsy in heart–lung transplantation has been developed at Papworth (Higenbottam et al, 1987; Hutter et al, 1988a; Stewart et al, 1988). It is well tolerated under light sedation, for example using propofol, and allows early diagnosis of lung rejection. From the biopsy material, CMV may be detected. Early diagnosis and treatment of lung rejection in heart–lung transplant has reduced the incidence of obliterative bronchiolitis, and cardiac rejection is now almost unknown. Because timely diagnosis of lung

rejection prevents cardiac rejection, endomyocardial biopsy is now only performed routinely in children who are too small to allow flexible bronchoscopy.

GENERAL SURGICAL PROBLEMS

Following successful transplantation, the patients are restored to a normal
life and may present with surgical problems unrelated to their transplanted
organs (Steed et al, 1985). A wide variety of general and regional anaesthetic
techniques have been used in patients who have had heart and heart–lung
transplants with little evidence of superiority of a particular technique
(Grebenik and Robinson, 1986). There are theoretical advantages in the use
of regional techniques whenever possible. They avoid any problems with
intubation and possible infection by the tracheal route, and in the heart–
lung transplants ensure that the patient can be given chest physiotherapy
immediately following the operation. Preoperative assessment should include contact with the patient's transplant centre to determine the results of
the most recent follow-up assessment. This is important for several reasons,
but the main interest will be in the possibility of graft atherosclerosis having
been detected at follow-up coronary arteriography, as these patients cannot
suffer the pain of angina with their denervated hearts. The possibility of
active rejection should be considered if the patient appears unwell.

CONCLUSIONS

Organ transplantation in children raises a number of ethical issues which
are not easily resolved (Moskop, 1987). Children are unable to understand
the implications of terminal disease, transplantation or immunosuppression. The natural desire of the parents for life at all costs may not
always be in the true interests of the child (English, 1983). On the other
hand, the mother of a child who died after transplantation stated that the
only thing worse than her child's death was if the child were to have 'died
without being given the chance with the transplant' (Gold et al, 1985).
Transplantation offers hope in desperate situations: children presenting for
transplant surgery have only weeks or months to live. The authors feel that
the hope of transplantation must improve the quality of life in the final
phase of otherwise terminal illness.

The 1-year survival rate for heart–lung transplantation in children at Papworth is 60%, compared with 75% for adults. For heart transplantation,
the figures are 75 and 90% respectively. Clearly, surgery carries a greater
risk for children than for adults, but those children who do survive have
full and active lives. More experience with paediatric transplantation will
improve survival further. The rapid advances in this field make anaesthesia for paediatric heart and heart–lung transplant surgery particularly
rewarding.

REFERENCES

Bethune DW (1976) Organ damage after open heart surgery. *Lancet* **ii:** 1410.

Bethune DW, Hardy I, Kneeshaw J, Latimer RD & Oduro A (1988) Anaesthesia and cardiopulmonary bypass for cardiac transplantation. In Wallwork J (ed.) *Heart and Heart Lung Transplantation*, vol. 8, pp 131–139. Orlando: Grune & Stratton.

Bodenham A, Latimer RD & Bethune DW (1987) Respiratory obstruction following vocal cord injection. A complication on induction of anaesthesia. *Anaesthesia* **42:** 289.

Bricker JT & Frazier OH (1987) Preoperative evaluation of the paediatric heart transplant candidate. *Clinical Transplantation* **1:** 164–168.

Burke CM, Glanville AR, Macoviak JA et al (1986) The spectrum of cytomegalovirus infection following human heart–lung transplantation. *Journal of Heart Transplantation* **5:** 267–272.

Chu-Jeng Chiu R & Bindon W (1987) Why are newborn hearts vulnerable to global ischemia? *Circulation* **767 (suppl V):** V146–V149.

Conference of the Medical Royal Colleges and their Faculties (1976) Statement issued by the honorary secretary. *British Medical Journal* **ii:** 1187–1188.

Cotes JE (1979) *Lung Function—Assessment and Applications in Medicine*, 4th edn, pp 369–370. Oxford: Blackwell Scientific Publications.

Crawford MH (1987) Intravenous use of Enoximone. *American Journal of Cardiology* **60:** 42c–45c.

Cross AS & Roup B (1981) Role of respiratory assistance devices in endemic nosocomial pneumonia. *American Journal of Medicine* **70:** 681–685.

Darracott-Cankovic S, Wheeldon D, Cory-Pearce R et al (1987) Biopsy assessment of 50 hearts during transplantation. *Journal of Thoracic and Cardiovascular Surgery* **93:** 95–102.

Dummer JS, White LT, Ho M et al (1985) Morbidity of cytomegalovirus infection in recipients of heart or heart–lung transplants who received cyclosporin. *Journal of Infectious Diseases* **152:** 1182–1191.

English TAH (1983) Is cardiac transplantation suitable for children? *Pediatric Cardiology* **4:** 57–58.

Gold LM, Kirkpatrick BS, Fricker FJ & Zitelli BJ (1986) Psychosocial issues in pediatric organ transplantation: the parents' perspective. *Pediatrics* **77:** 738–744.

Gray JJ, Alvey B, Smith DJ & Wrightt TG (1987) Evaluation of a commercial latex agglutination test for detecting antibodies to cytomegalovirus in organ donors and transplant recipients. *Journal of Virological Methods* **16:** 13–19.

Grebenik CR & Robinson PN (1985) Cardiac transplantation at Harefield. *Anaesthesia* **40:** 131–140.

Grebenik CR & Robinson PN (1986) Anaesthesia for surgery in a patient with a transplanted heart. *British Journal of Anaesthesia* **58:** 1199–1200.

Griffith BP, Hardesty RL, Trento A et al (1987) Heart–lung transplantation: lessons learned and future hopes. *Annals of Thoracic Surgery* **43:** 6–16.

Guyton AC (1976) *Textbook of Medical Physiology*, p 306. Philadelphia: WB Saunders.

Guyton AC (1981) *The Autonomic Nervous System. Textbook of Medical Physiology*, pp 710–721. Philadelphia: WB Saunders.

Hakim M, Wheeldon D, Bethune DW et al (1985) Haemodialysis and haemofiltration on cardiopulmonary bypass. *Thorax* **40:** 101–106.

Harjula A, Baldwin JC, Starnes VA et al (1987) Proper donor selection for heart–lung transplantation. *Journal of Thoracic and Cardiovascular Surgery* **94:** 874–880.

Higenbottam T, Stewart S, Penketh A & Wallwork J (1987) The diagnosis of lung rejection and opportunistic infection by transbronchial biopsy. *Transplant Proceedings* **19:** 3777–3778.

Hutter JA, Higenbottam T, Stewart S & Wallwork J (1988a) Routine endomyocardial biopsy is redundant in heart–lung recipients. *Journal of Heart Transplantation* (in press).

Hutter JA, Despins P, Higenbottam T, Stewart S & Wallwork J (1988b) Heart lung transplantation: better use of resources. *American Journal of Medicine* **85**: 4–11.

Johnson WG, Pierce AK & Sanaford JP (1969) Changing pharyngeal bacterial flora of hospitalized patients. *New England Journal of Medicine* **281**: 1137–1140.

Johnson WG, Pierce AK, Sandford JP et al (1972) Nosocomial respiratory infections with Gram negative bacilli. *Annals of Internal Medicine* **77**: 701–706.

Johnson B, Thomson R, Palleares U & Sadive MS (1975) Autonomic hyperreflexia. A review. *Military Medicine* **140**: 345–359.

Jones PK, Higenbottam T & Wallwork J (1987) Treatment of primary pulmonary hypertension with intravenous Epoprostenol (prostacyclin). *British Heart Journal* **57**: 270–279.

Kaye MP (1987) The registry of the International Society for Heart Transplantation. *Journal of Heart Transplantation* **6**: 63–67.

McLeod AA, Neil-Dwyer G, Meyer CHA et al (1982) Cardiac sequelae of acute head injury. *British Heart Journal* **47**: 221–226.

Moskop JDC (1987) Organ transplantation in children: ethical issues. *Journal of Pediatrics* **110**: 175–180.

Naftchi NE, Wooten GF, Lowman EW & Axelrod J (1974) Relationship between serum dopamine–β-hydroxylase activity, catecholamine metabolism and haemodynamic changes during paroxysmal hypertension in quadriplegia. *Circulation Research* **35**: 850–861.

Newton DEF & Wesenhagen H (1986) The role of the anaesthetist in transplantation. VII European Congress of Anaesthesiology Proceedings.

Novitzky D, Wicomb WN, Cooper DKC et al (1984) Electrocardiographic, haemodynamic and endocrine changes occurring during experimental brain death in the Chacma baboon. *Journal of Heart Transplantation* **4**: 63–69.

Robert RM, Gifford MD, Weaver AS et al (1986) Thyroid hormone levels in heart and kidney cadaver donors. *Journal of Heart Transplantation* **5**: 249–253.

Ruiz-Santana S, Jimenz AG, Esteban A et al (1987) ICU pneumonias: a multi-institutional study. *Critical Care Medicine* **15**: 930–932.

Shelley MP, Bethune DW & Latimer RD (1986) A comparison of five heat and moisture exchangers. *Anaesthesia* **41**: 527–532.

Steed DL, Brown B, Reilly JJ et al (1985) General surgical complications in heart and heart–lung transplantation. *Surgery* **98**: 739–745.

Stewart S, Higenbottam T, Hutter JA, Penkath ARL, Zebro TJ & Wallwork J (1988) Histopathology of transbronchial biopsies in heart–lung transplantation. *Transplant Proceedings* **20**: 764–766.

Wetzel RC, Setzer N, Stiff JL & Rodgers MC (1985) Haemodynamic responses in brain dead organ donor patients. *Anaesthesia and Analgesia* **64**: 125–128.

Wheeldon DR, Bethune DW & Gill RD (1986) Perfusion for cardiac transplantation. *Perfusion* **1**: 57–61.

Anaesthesia for neurosurgery in paediatrics

Anaesthesia for neurosurgery in children requires an intimate knowledge not only of the pathophysiology and control of raised intracranial pressure (ICP), but also of neonatal and infant physiology and an acute awareness of the problems which can so readily arise during major surgery in small children.

The nervous system develops in both size and complexity, like the other systems of the body from the early stages of fetal life, but unlike the other systems which only increase in size after birth, the nervous system not only grows but becomes massively more complex.

The very early phase of development begins early in intrauterine life; cerebrospinal fluid production commences between 6 and 8 weeks of gestational age. Between 10 and 18 weeks the brain growth is mainly neuronal resulting from neuroblast multiplication. This explains the extreme sensitivity of the central nervous system to external noxious effects, such as viral infection, drugs, toxins and X-rays, during this stage of fetal development. At birth the number of neurones is almost complete so that postpartum growth is mainly glial, dendritic arborization with synaptic formation and myelination. At birth only about a quarter of the number of all cells are present, reaching two-thirds by 6 months and growth is completed during the second year of life. Differential growth rates occur in different areas: the cerebellum is less developed at birth but completes its development during the first year of life, prior to the cortex and brain stem.

Nutrition is important both prenatally and postnatally in achieving full cerebral development; malnourished infants have evidence of reduced cell numbers, dendritic connections and also cerebral lipid and protein content.

CONTROL OF INTRACRANIAL PRESSURE (ICP)

Children with intracranial pathology have certain differences from adults which may be advantageous. The fontanelles and non-fused sutures, which may separate even into early adolescence, provide protection from gradual changes in intracranial volume which results in an increase in head size prior to a rise in pressure. Acute changes are not absorbed in this way, because of the rigidity of the fibrous tissue bridging the fontanelles and sutures. Secondly, children of all ages are fortunate in having healthy blood vessels devoid of atheroma, and therefore all areas of the brain should be equally perfused during treatment for raised ICP.

Despite a lack of definitive studies on cerebral blood flow regulation in children, the same mechanisms are thought to apply as in adults. Cerebral blood flow in *normal* children over 3 years has been studied and is almost double that of adults: the oxygen consumption is increased by approximately one-third (Kennedy and Sokoloff, 1957). Clinical experience suggests that the effects of hypo- and hypercarbia and hypoxia are the same in children as in adults. The lower limits of autoregulation are not known in children, but are assumed to be related to their normal systemic pressure. However, sick newborn infants with respiratory distress syndrome or birth asphyxia have been shown to have impaired autoregulation with cerebral blood flow following systemic blood pressure, which may explain the susceptibility of these patients to the development of intraventricular haemorrhage (Lou and Friis-Hansen, 1979).

Good operative conditions for neurosurgery are produced by controlling the ICP, that is the cellular pressure, extracellular fluid, cerebrospinal fluid and cerebral blood volume affected by cerebral blood flow and venous drainage. Raised ICP from obstructive hydrocephalus or tumours associated with large cysts is little affected by the anaesthetist's skills and will only be markedly improved by removal of the encysted fluid. Marked reduction of the pressure or volume of the surrounding normal brain may result in creation of space for further fluid expansion, and should not be performed routinely in these cases, except where there has been a critical rise in ICP.

Steroids have been shown to provide dramatic improvement in the amount of oedema present and the clinical picture in patients with cerebral oedema secondary to tumours. Dexamethasone 0.25 mg/kg initially, with subsequent doses of 0.1 mg/kg every 6 h is a typical dosage regimen. An advantage from steroids in head injury and routine neurosurgery has not been proven but most units employ a short course of steroids perioperatively, rapidly reducing the dosage over 1 week.

Cerebral dehydration, with reduction in both intracellular and extracellular fluid volume, is achieved with diuretics. Mannitol 20% solution, apart from its use in the treatment of acute rises in ICP, is best reserved for specific surgical situations where access to deep structures is difficult. Because of the excellent renal function expected in children and the small circulating blood volume, mannitol should be used with caution and a maximum dose of 1 g/kg administered. Urine output must be carefully monitored and an indwelling catheter is essential. If urine in excess of the infused volume plus 10% of blood volume is produced, increased intravenous fluid replacement will be required. It has been suggested that if a marked reduction in intracranial volume is produced prior to surgery, the dural veins may rupture, producing a haematoma. Cerebral dehydration can also be produced using intravenous frusemide 0.5 mg/kg, which, despite the advantages of not providing an osmotic load to the circulation, has not replaced mannitol as agent of first choice in most units.

Good positioning is essential in the production of a low venous pressure, and is much harder to achieve in children due to the relatively short necks and larger heads which may result in venous obstruction if the head is rotated. A slightly head-up position is employed routinely, but this may be associated with air embolism, especially if hypovolaemia is present.

Positive end expiratory pressure is also avoided during ventilation of neurosurgical patients except in situations of poor respiratory function, where the risks of hypoxia are greater than the increased venous pressure transmitted via the great veins. Manual ventilation via the Jackson Rees modification of the T-piece, the standard technique for infants having general surgical procedures, is avoided in neurosurgery because of the difficulty in ventilating manually without applying positive end expiratory pressure. Manual ventilation is reserved for those infants with decreased pulmonary compliance where further changes may be critical. Ventilators of the T-piece occluder pattern are popular in paediatric practice, but hyperventilation may be difficult to achieve, as increasing the minute volume by increasing the rate results in rebreathing unless very high fresh gas flows are used (Nightingale et al, 1965). If the tidal volume is increased expiration time may also need to be lengthened to prevent rebreathing. Children over 20 kg and those with abnormal lungs below this weight should be mechanically ventilated using an alternative system, preferably a non-rebreathing type. Adequate oxygenation is also essential for good neurosurgical conditions. Some neurointensive care units suggest hyperoxia (PaO_2 greater than 20 kPa) may have a beneficial effect in patients with gross cerebral oedema, from the greater tissue gradients (Swedlow, 1983). During anaesthesia this level is usually maintained. The combination of routine monitoring of inspiratory and end-tidal CO_2 using an infrared capnometer together with pulse oximetry now means that a breath-to-breath check of adequate ventilation is constantly available.

Induced arterial hypotension must be associated with deep anaesthesia and adequate muscle relaxation, good oxygenation and moderate hyperventilation, normovolaemia and normothermia. Hypotensive agents should not be given to children without direct arterial monitoring especially in a situation where sudden or heavy blood loss may be expected. Good operative conditions in paediatric practice are best achieved by a relatively slow heart rate for the particular size of patient. In a neonate a heart rate of 110 beats/min is considered slow, whereas in an 8-year-old it would be considered abnormally fast. If the rate is fast, initial measures should include deepening anaesthesia and increasing the rate of transfusion, with a check of arterial gases to ensure normal values, prior to embarking on active measures. Beta-blockers either alone (propranolol, incrementally to a maximum dose of 0.05 mg/kg) or in combination with an alpha-blocker (labetalol, incrementally to a maximum dose of 1 mg/kg) are suitable for heart rate reduction with an associated fall in arterial pressure. If the heart rate is already slow or a more profound fall in pressure is required, such as for vascular malformations, either sodium nitroprusside 0.5 mg/kg/min (maximum dose 1 mg/kg/24 h) or trimetaphan (0.2% solution) may be used. Hypotensive techniques should only be employed in paediatric practice where the surgical conditions are inadequate and not solely to achieve a blood pressure thought to be desirable. In general children are more resistant to hypotensive agents than adults.

PREOPERATIVE ASSESSMENT AND PREMEDICATION

As in all neurosurgical patients an accurate assessment of the neurological status must be made, including evidence of raised ICP, alteration in conscious level, and any focal findings, in particular cranial nerve palsies. Bulbar palsies from brain stem pathology may be associated with reduction in cough reflex and silent aspiration resulting in pulmonary collapse, consolidation and hypoxaemia.

Raised ICP in children commonly presents with vomiting and may cause dehydration and hypovolaemia, making the child liable to hypotension following induction of anaesthesia. Urea and electrolytes should be checked routinely and corrected if necessary. Routine haemoglobin measurement is carried out and *all* patients are cross-matched. Children with chronically infected shunt systems may have toxic depression of the bone marrow and may be very anaemic and require preoperative transfusion. Lesser degrees of anaemia can be corrected perioperatively. In the presence of dehydration from vomiting, the initial haemoglobin level may be falsely raised by 1–2 g/dl. Pathology of other systems is extremely rare in most patients with central nervous system neoplasia; however in certain patients multisystem disease is likely and requires careful assessment. Such patients are ex-premature infants with hydrocephalus secondary to intraventricular haemorrhage, patients with cerebral abscess from cyanotic congenital heart disease and patients with various syndromes having craniofacial surgery.

Sedative premedication should be avoided in all infants and children having intracranial surgery. Children with raised ICP, especially those with blocked shunt systems, may appear well apart from complaining of headaches and vomiting. However, many of these children will have markedly raised ICP and minor triggers such as sedation may cause a spiralling effect with massive rises in pressure.

Atropine 0.02 mg/kg (minimum dose 0.15 mg) is administered intramuscularly 30 min prior to surgery, for all small children and older children having surgery sitting, prone or in any other position where salivation may result in dislodgement of the tracheal tube.

Discussion in simple terms should take place with those children able to understand about the nature of the anaesthetic induction technique and postoperative monitoring and equipment, without frightening them with details about which they will not be aware. Alleviation of parental anxiety, as far as possible, will be helpful in preventing its transmission to their child, especially in the younger child unable to communicate with language. Children not having intracranial surgery, for example spinal surgery, may have a standard sedative premedication (see Appendix).

ANAESTHETIC TECHNIQUE

It is well known that anaesthetic gases and volatile agents increase ICP, though isoflurane and low concentrations of halothane in the presence of moderate hyperventilation have an insignificant effect. A smooth induction is the aim and therefore in paediatric practice, a non-traumatic gaseous induction may have a less deleterious effect on the ICP than an intravenous induction resulting in crying and breath-holding in an already cerebrally irritable child.

Isoflurane, because of its reduced effect on cerebral blood flow, appears to be an ideal agent, but the longer induction time and high incidence of breath-holding and coughing especially in unsedated children detracts from its routine use as an induction agent in paediatric neuroanaesthesia.

Light inhalational anaesthesia may be induced prior to administration of thiopentone 4 mg/kg and suxamethonium 1–2 mg/kg, to facilitate intubation. Suxamethonium rarely causes fasciculation in small children and rapid intubation and securing of the airway outweigh the theoretical advantages of using a non-depolarizing muscle relaxant routinely in paediatric neurosurgery. The longer periods of ventilation with a facemask needed when intubating with a non-depolarizing muscle relaxant may not produce hyperventilation, because of the difficulty producing a seal with the facemask and also because air always enters the stomach and this may cause splinting of the diaphragm and decreased compliance.

The airway is secured using an uncuffed tracheal tube of correct size (age/4 + 4.0 mm), which has a small leak at the cricoid level; too great a leak may result in hypoventilation. Armoured tubes are always used in neurosurgery to enable the head to be moved freely without risk of kinking the tube. Latex armoured tubes are very thick-walled and therefore have a much smaller lumen for a given size of tube and consequently greater resistance. The Magill pattern, red rubber reinforced tubes are no longer manufactured but plastic or silastic armoured disposable tubes are as satisfactory. The disadvantage of the plastic tube is that the external surface is extremely smooth and fixation can be very difficult especially if lubricant inadvertently covers the external surface. The silastic tubes are much less slippery for fixation but because of the nature of the material, writing on the tube is very difficult and the manufacturers have only marked 4 cm spaces, which makes positioning of the tube tip in the trachea difficult. After intubation it is essential to check with a stethoscope for bilateral lung ventilation with the head both in a neutral position and in its final operative position, and again after fixation of the tube, as only 1 cm may be the difference between a good position and bronchial intubation.

Maintenance anaesthesia is with a standard technique of moderate hyperventilation with nitrous oxide 66% and oxygen with an opiate and muscle relaxant administered at the first signs of returning muscle tone. D-tubocurarine 0.4–0.5 mg/kg is the muscle relaxant of choice in paediatric neuroanaesthesia as significant falls in blood pressure are rarely seen, whereas pancuronium may be associated with marked tachycardia and hypertension and therefore prevents the production of good operative conditions. For short procedures or those in high-risk patients atracurium 0.4–0.5 mg/kg or vecuronium 0.08–0.1 mg/kg may be used. Vecuronium provides excellent cardiovascular stability, whereas atracurium seems an ideal agent in very high-risk preterm infants with multisystem disease or immaturity where the hydrolysis of the drug ensures its short duration of action, and minimizes the need for mechanical postoperative ventilation. Severe bronchospasm has been reported with atracurium in children (Woods et al, 1985).

Analgesia is provided with fentanyl (up to 5 µg/kg) with incremental doses of 1 µg/kg/h. A maximum dose of 6 µg/kg is usually sufficient unless surgery is prolonged (greater than 3–4 h). Higher doses are used where postoperative ventilation is planned. Supplementary anaesthesia is with isoflurane 0.5–1%, though halothane 0.5% was previously used.

At the end of surgery residual muscle relaxation is always reversed using atropine 0.025 mg/kg and neostigmine 0.05 mg/kg unless postoperative ventilation is planned. Extubation is performed only when the child is breathing well and awake.

MONITORING

Routine monitoring for all paediatric neurosurgery should include a precordial or oesophageal stethoscope, ECG, and a blood pressure cuff of suitable size attached to an automatic blood pressure machine or oscillotonometer. In general for small children the largest cuff which fits easily on the upper arm is the correct size, making allowance for increased axillary and forearm subcutaneous fat.

All major cases should have direct arterial pressure measurement via radial artery cannulation. Adequate ventilation is monitored using an infrared capnometer with either the paediatric or adult cuvette. The Hewlett Packard machine is particularly good in paediatrics as no gas samples are taken and the small size of the cuvettes does not result in a significant increase in dead space. Combined with pulse oximetry adequate ventilation can be checked breath by breath. Venous access should consist of at least two free-flowing venous cannulas, except for simple shunt procedures, as major blood loss can occur in any neurosurgical procedure in children, despite optimal conditions. Central venous catheterization is not routinely used in the author's unit as the most reliable route with least complications in children is via the internal jugular vein, which might result in obstruction to the venous drainage of the head especially if associated with a marked degree of head flexion to produce optimal surgical positioning. The antecubital fossa is not a reliable route in small children; the veins are rarely adequate for percutaneous central catheterization before the age of 5 years. A long catheter via the femoral vein is an alternative route. Central venous pressure monitoring is reserved for cases where either massive blood loss is expected or those such as craniopharyngiomas where fluid balance due to diabetes insipidus may be a problem. Routine blood and fluid replacement is given on a basis of heart rate and general cardiovascular parameters.

Rectal temperature is monitored routinely in all patients. Urinary catheters are only required where large volumes of urine may cause fluid balance problems, either after diuretics or in patients who have or are expected to develop diabetes insipidus.

Temperature control

The surface area of a normal child's head represents 18% of the total body surface area, double that of an adult. In general children have much larger surface area to weight ratio than adults, and also have much less subcutaneous fat. General heat losses by conduction, convection and radiation, and once the head is open by the latent heat of vaporization, must be minimized and active measures must be available for rewarming as required

(Nightingale and Meakin, 1987). The introduction of the hot air mattress (Howarth Air Engineering Company) has enabled the anaesthetist to have a much better control of patient's temperature, not only preventing excessive heat loss but also being able to rewarm the patient if necessary. Passive measures to prevent heat loss include wrapping the child in aluminium foil and covering with gamgee. If rapid transfusions of blood are required— greater than 20% blood volume per hour—a blood warmer should be used. It is essential to monitor body temperature closely, preferably with a rectal thermistor, as hypothermia with peripheral circulatory shutdown and metabolic acidosis may be very difficult to reverse even with increased transfusion rates. Hyperthermia should also be avoided because of the increased cerebral metabolism with increased body temperature. Ideally a temperature between 36 and 36.5°C should be maintained. However, where there are surgical difficulties, a lower temperature may have a cerebral protective action by reducing cerebral metabolism, enabling surgery to be completed while the cerebral circulation is somewhat compromised. Temperatures over 34.5°C may provide cerebral protection without putting the child in jeopardy from cardiac arrhythmias and metabolic changes (Berntman et al, 1981). This can usually be achieved by discontinuing active heating and heat-conserving measures, and does not require active cooling. Postoperative hyperpyrexia is associated with some forms of neurosurgery and if not treated vigorously has a poor prognosis, especially if the temperature exceeds 40.5°C. Active cooling methods include increased transfusion of room temperature fluids and fanning. If these measures are not successful peripheral vasodilatation may be achieved using small doses of chlorpromazine 0.1–0.2 mg/kg intravenously, or other vasodilator drugs of choice, while closely monitoring and correcting any fall in blood pressure. If the temperature still fails to respond and remains over 40°C other steps which can be taken are the use of ice bags over the great vessels and liver, and rectal, bladder or gastric washouts with ice-cold saline. Frequent blood gas analysis will also be required to ensure adequate oxygenation and ventilation during a period of increased metabolism. Electrolyte imbalance also requires correction, because of both cellular dysfunction and rapid transfusion. Hyperpyrexia is more likely after craniopharyngioma resection and hypothalamic, pontine and mid-brain manipulation.

Fluid balance

As mentioned previously, the head of a child is proportionately twice as big as that of an adult and therefore neurosurgery in a paediatric population is associated with proportionately greater blood losses. In children under 25 kg blood transfusion is almost invariably required for a craniotomy, except when performed in the sitting position, where in the author's experience only about 50%, including those under 10 kg, require transfusion. Blood loss is extremely difficult to measure during neurosurgery because of the high percentage which contaminates the drapes rather than being collected on swabs which can be weighed, or in the suction bottle. Also the blood will be mixed with both cerebrospinal fluid and saline used during bone work. The use of ultrasonic suction devices which have a constant spray of saline is another cause for difficulty in assessing blood loss. Heart rate remains an extremely sensitive monitor of normovolaemia, especially in conjunction with other cardiovascular parameters, pressure, capillary filling and core–peripheral temperature difference, enabling the practised paediatric anaesthetist to maintain normovolaemia. Heavy losses of 10–20% of blood volume can be expected during skin closure of a large craniotomy wound. Further bleeding will occur postoperatively and allowance must be made for this.

Exchange transfusions will often be required during neurosurgical procedures on small children despite provision of optimal operative conditions. Fresh frozen plasma or cryoprecipitate should be administered at approximately 10% of the blood volume per exchange transfusion to ensure adequate clotting factors, once 1–2 blood volumes have been transfused. Calcium supplements will usually only be required with rapid transfusion—greater than 40% of the blood volume per hour (Abbott, 1983). In these circumstances arterial gases should be checked and any base deficit corrected if greater than −5. Correction of base deficits causes excessive alkalosis postoperatively with citrate metabolism.

Routine maintenance fluids are also administered, care being taken to avoid overtransfusion with crystalloid as this may contribute to postoperative cerebral oedema. Very small preterm infants may require intravenous fluids preoperatively to avoid hypoglycaemia because of their poor energy reserves in the liver and as body fat.

Postoperative fluids are given as 4% glucose in 0.18% saline or similar solution, again to avoid hypoglycaemia, on a basis of 2.5–3 ml/kg/h, reducing to 2 ml/kg/h by 15–20 kg, and further reducing to 1–1.25 ml/kg as adult size is approached. If nasogastric losses are excessive, normal saline and potassium replacement will be required.

Hyperglycaemia occurring in patients with head injuries has been shown to be associated with a less favourable outcome and this may be the explanation for lack of benefit from steroid administration in these cases. However, in small children hypoglycaemia is a more likely occurrence perioperatively, especially if there has been a long period of reduced fluid and food intake prior to surgery, or because of vomiting and drowsiness, and if large volumes of blood have been required during the operation. Where the metabolic response to stress may be unable to compensate fully the blood sugar will remain low.

POSTOPERATIVE CARE

Routine postoperative ventilation is usually reserved for children who either have had very long operations or where there is a particular neurosurgical or airway indication. All patients who have had craniotomies have continuous direct arterial pressure and ECG monitoring until the next day. Careful evaluation of the neurological status and cardiorespiratory function is carried out regularly, along with fluid balance.

Analgesia can be provided by codeine phosphate 1 mg/kg intramuscularly, which provides good pain relief without altering consciousness and pupil size. Later oral paracetamol 10–15 mg/kg with a maximum dose of 60 mg/kg/day can be substituted. Antiemetics are not routinely prescribed in children under 5 years unless vomiting is troublesome, when prochlorperazine 0.15–0.2 mg/kg or metoclopramide 0.1–0.15 mg/kg may be used.

Children having craniotomies will be given prophylactic antiepileptic drugs, but children having less major procedures, especially very small babies having shunt insertions or revisions, benefit from phenobarbitone 1–1.5 mg/kg for a short while postoperatively. This reduces the cerebral irritation caused by blood in the ventricles. Phenobarbitone in these circumstances has a more beneficial effect than analgesics.

Children who receive postoperative ventilation will require sedation and analgesia postoperatively. For those patients in whom the risks of intracerebral complications are slight, a morphine infusion provides excellent sedation. However, where for example mid-brain function requires to be assessed during ventilation, intermittent administration of diazepam seems preferable and analgesia is provided by intramuscular codeine. Codeine phosphate should never be administered intravenously as there is a high incidence of cardiovascular collapse (Shanahan et al, 1983).

NEURORADIOLOGY

The rapid advances in radiology which have occurred in the last decade with the general availability of computerized tomography (CT) scanning and ultrasound and the introduction of magnetic resonance imaging (MRI) have transformed the work of the anaesthetist in the X-ray department.

The indications for general anaesthesia in children are for investigations which are either painful or prolonged or require a degree of co-operation and immobility with which the child is unable to comply. See Appendix for CT and MRI scan sedation requirements.

At the Hospital for Sick Children, London, major investigations such as cardiac catheters are performed under sedation, with less than 10% of the 2500 CT scans performed annually requiring general anaesthesia. Many of these will either have acutely raised ICP or be grossly subnormal or hyperactive children. Small babies can be fed and swaddled and allowed to sleep naturally during the scan, or may be given chloral hydrate 30 mg/kg 1 h in advance. Babies over 3-months without signs of raised ICP may be sedated as suggested in Appendix. Occasional top-ups with a maximum dose of 0.3 mg/kg of diazepam i.v. are required, especially if contrast is used.

MRI provides more challenges for the paediatric anaesthetist, but most are employing a technique using either ketamine or sedation, provided ICP is normal. When planning MRI facilities, monitoring for small children must be considered, so that the equipment, such as pulse meters, ECG and automatic blood pressure devices, can be suitably insulated from the magnetic field at the time of installation. At present pulse oximeters cannot be satisfactorily screened for use during MRI.

Angiography and myelography are routinely performed under general anaesthesia, though children of normal intelligence over the age of 10–12 years may accept myelography under premedication and local anaesthesia. Myelography is usually carried out under a standard paediatric anaesthetic technique of intubation and spontaneous respiration of nitrous oxide, oxygen and halothane or other volatile agent of choice. Angiography requires paralysis and moderate hyperventilation to produce clearer demarcation of the vasculature. Care must be taken to avoid hypoxia during the apnoea required for subtraction films, especially in small children. A careful note of the blood loss and volume of hypertonic contrast medium injected during prolonged investigations is also required in children with small blood volumes.

Embolization techniques have recently become part of the neuroradiologist's skills, providing not only a major challenge to the radiologist, but frequently also to the anaesthetist. Vein of Galen aneurysms present in neonates as high-output cardiac failure and in older children with either increasing head size or neurological features from an intracranial bleed. Embolization of these aneurysms may be very hazardous but results compare favourably with those of surgery for this condition. Infants will require invasive monitoring. The other problems for the anaesthetist are those of prolonged anaesthesia, fluid balance and temperature control. The disconnection of the balloon or other embolus may be associated with major cardiovascular disturbances, especially if the catheter is in the basilar artery. Arteriovenous malformations may be embolized relatively easily with injections of small particles or acrylic glue to block the vessels of the malformation.

ANAESTHESIA FOR SOME SPECIFIC NEUROSURGICAL PROCEDURES

Neonatal neurosurgery

Neurosurgery in the neonatal period is usually for the repair of meningomyelocoeles or encephalocoeles, which are usually occipital but may be frontal or nasal, the latter being repaired via a bifrontal craniotomy and usually delayed until the child is older. Early surgery is indicated to close the defects where there is a flimsy dural sac which can easily become damaged or infected, leading to meningitis. Following the introduction of shunt procedures for hydrocephalus in 1952 and new antibiotics to treat meningitis, a policy of early surgery for all patients, irrespective of their neurological function, was carried out until the early 1970s. This resulted in large numbers of grossly damaged children of low intelligence unable to lead an independent existence, wheelchair-bound, with gross kyphoscoliosis and eventual respiratory failure, renal failure from the complications of a neuropathic bladder, and skin problems from pressure on anaesthetic areas, with chronic infection leading to repeated shunt infections and blockages. Nowadays a selective policy is usual in many units, where neonatal repair is reserved for those with good leg function with or without anal tone. Routine antenatal screening of α-fetoprotein and subsequent therapeutic abortion has resulted in a marked decrease in the number of babies with open neural tube defects reaching term. Suspicion of a neural tube defect may also arise from antenatal ultrasound scanning showing a widened spinal canal or increased head size from the associated hydrocephalus, present in 80% of patients with meningomyelocoele.

However, the early antenatal diagnosis does not explain totally the reduction in numbers of patients with neural tube defects (Sellar, 1987). There is also marked regional variation with the highest incidence in Northern Ireland; Europe has a higher incidence than Asia or Africa (Leck, 1974).

Following atropine 0.15–0.2 mg and vitamine K 1 mg, a standard neonatal anaesthetic technique should be used, with preoxygenation and intubation with a reinforced tube. Positioning the baby with the sac of the meningocoele or occipital encephalocoele in a 'doughnut' head ring and with the remainder of the baby supported on a folded towel provides a neutral supine position for intubation, without damaging the flimsy dural sac (Figure 16.1). Alternatively, the lateral position may be used but this makes intubation more difficult. A relaxant, nitrous oxide, oxygen technique is used supplemented intermittently as required with low dose halothane or isoflurane, ventilating manually so that pulmonary compliance can be constantly assessed.

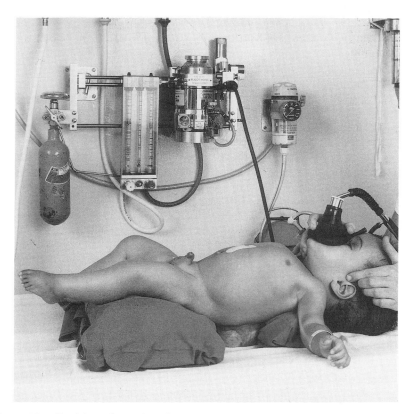

Figure 16.1. Position of a patient for induction of anaesthesia and intubation with meningomyelocoele.

The operations are carried out prone, except for frontal encephalocoeles, and great care must be taken with positioning not only to produce a free abdomen for easy ventilation but also to reduce blood loss by avoiding inferior vena cava compression and increased paraspinal venous pressure. Many of these neural tube defects have an associated haemangioma in the skin and underlying tissues and this may result in increased bleeding. In general, transfusion is only required for lesions with a base in excess of 3–4 cm. Large lesions may need rotation skin flaps, again with increased blood loss. Tissue expanders have now been used in some cases, with inflation over a 10–14-day period prior to closure of the defect.

Other neonatal neurosurgical procedures include elevation of depressed fractures, usually caused by difficult forceps delivery or for drainage of subdural or extradural haematomas secondary to birth trauma.

Hydrocephalus

Treatment for hydrocephalus is the commonest procedure in paediatric neuroanaesthesia. The hydrocephalus is produced by a blockage of the cerebrospinal fluid drainage and may be primary or secondary to intraventricular haemorrhage, meningitis or the Arnold–Chiari malformation associated with spina bifida. There is some evidence that primary, i.e. antenatal, hydrocephalus is due to intrauterine infection or haemorrhage. Prenatal diagnosis is now common, and antenatal surgery has been carried out successfully in a few centres. To reduce obstetric problems from the large head and to minimize permanent brain damage many of these infants are electively delivered around 32 weeks. The advantages of earlier treatment of the congenital defects must always be weighed up against the risks of prematurity and subsequent complications which may result in a poorer prognosis than allowing the baby with hydrocephalus to go to term.

While there has been a reduction in the number of infants with meningo-myelocoele being born, the numbers of very small babies surviving neonatal intensive care and suffering from intraventricular haemorrhage which results in hydrocephalus have risen rapidly over the last 10–15 years. It should be noted that provided the hydrocephalus is adequately treated, the long-term outcome need not necessarily be different from those without this complication. The presenting feature of secondary hydrocephalus is increasing head circumference, crossing the standard growth chart lines. The clinical picture of a baby with a massively enlarged head, bulging fontanelles, engorged head veins and sunsetting eyes is rarely seen nowadays.

All newborn babies have a high cerebrospinal fluid protein and cell count and after intraventricular haemorrhage the cerebrospinal fluid remains viscous for some time. Until the protein and cell counts approach normal infant levels the patients are not suitable for ventricular shunt insertion as the low flow rate and high viscosity will cause an unacceptably high valve blockage rate and subsequent infection. Initial treatment in these cases is either by intermittent ventricular tapping via the anterior fontanelle or by insertion of a percutaneous drain. Occasionally a ventricular catheter and Rickman cap are inserted to make intermittent tapping easier.

Ventriculo-peritoneal shunting is considered when all other factors are suitable. While there is no absolute minimum size suitable for surgery, after a trial period of operating on babies under 1 kg in the author's unit, the surgical complication rate was unacceptably high and now very few infants weigh less than 1.5 kg and most are nearer 2 kg when the valve system is inserted. These infants, who have usually survived long and stormy periods of intensive care, may still be less than 40 weeks postconceptual age, despite being 3 months old. Preterm infants, as is now well recognized, are more prone to postoperative complications even after minor surgery (Steward, 1982).

Preoperative assessment takes account not only of the neurological features of hydrocephalus but also the general condition. The high-risk preterm infant will have poor central and peripheral, respiratory control with frequent apnoeic spells leading to cyanosis and bradycardia, and may be oxygen-dependent due to bronchopulmonary dysplasia following prolonged ventilation for respiratory distress syndrome of the newborn. Nutritional status may be poor due to poor feeding from hypotonia and possibly vomiting from raised ICP. Preterm infants may have had a period of peripheral parenteral nutrition resulting in difficult venous access. Temperature control will be very poor both from central immaturity and lack of body fat. Liver function may be abnormal due to immaturity and under-nutrition, with abnormal clotting factors and increased sensitivity to drugs because of reduced plasma proteins.

Ventriculo-peritoneal shunting is the operation of choice, but if there are coexisting inguinal hernias, so common in preterm infants, these should be repaired at the same time or cerebrospinal fluid may accumulate in the hernia sacs. Contraindications to peritoneal drainage are any form of intraperitoneal pathology which may require surgery in the future, especially unresolved necrotizing entercolitis. Atrial shunts are not routinely performed nowadays because of the rare but disastrous complications of infection, causing bacterial endocarditis and pulmonary emboli leading to pulmonary hypertension. The insertion of an atrial shunt is associated with a greater blood loss, transfusion being common in infants, and there is also potential for air embolism. The pleural route is occasionally used but is usually reserved for drainage of cysts or subdural haematomas where a negative pressure effect may be advantageous. If large amounts of cerebrospinal fluid drain into the pleural cavity respiratory embarrassment can occur.

As is well recognized, preterm infants are very sensitive to anaesthetic agents and a technique of minimal anaesthesia should be used, such as atracurium with nitrous oxide and oxygen, supplemented with small doses of isoflurane, particularly during subcutaneous tunnelling. For all other children a standard technique is used. Airway control with a mask and intubation may be difficult due to occipital enlargement of the head unless the body is raised on a folded towel, bringing the head and neck into a neutral position. Heat losses are minimized by placing the baby, complete with diathermy pad and monitoring, in aluminium foil and exposing the burr hole site and a strip 3–4 cm wide across the thorax to the upper abdomen for surgical access.

When inserting peritoneal shunts blood transfusion is rare even in the smallest infants, as careful surgeons usually spill less than 10 ml; however, blood must be cross-matched in case the enlarged dural veins are damaged during the burr hole as control of the bleeding can sometimes be very difficult with limited access.

Postoperatively the preterm infants will require very close monitoring as the change in ICP often affects the central control of respiration, leading to apnoeic spells frequently associated with a fall in cardiac output. All babies under 46 weeks' postconceptual age must be monitored with an apnoea alarm and are likely to require increased inspired oxygen (FiO_2 0.3) to prevent bradycardia secondary to hypoxia. At the same time the risks of hyperoxaemia contributing to retinopathy of prematurity should be remembered. Transcutaneous oxygen monitors should be used in high-risk patients.

Opiates, including codein phosphate, are only given during surgery and postoperatively to babies over 5 kg because of the problems of respiratory depression. Phenobarbitone 1–1.5 mg/kg is very effective in treating the symptoms of cerebral irritation frequently seen in these patients.

Tumours

Malignancy is the second most common cause of death in children after accidents, and central nervous system tumours are second only to the leukaemias in the paediatric population, but despite this they are still relatively rare with less than 200 new cases each year in the whole of the UK. They arise at all ages with equal frequency.

Despite no major breakthrough in chemotherapy, the improvements in general care of the very ill child and neuroradiological advances leading to earlier diagnosis now result in approximately 50% of patients with medulloblastomas having a 5-year survival.

Posterior fossa tumours

The majority of brain tumours in children are in the posterior fossa and are usually midline, so the sitting position is the position of choice, producing excellent conditions, with less than 50% of all patients, including those under 15 kg, requiring blood transfusion, and of these the majority require 20% of blood volume or less.

Postural hypotension is rare in children unless they are clinically dehydrated, when they rapidly respond to 5 ml/kg glucose–saline infusion. Despite this stability the sitting position should be achieved slowly over a period of 3–4 min.

Careful positioning is very important both for maintaining venous pressure and preventing venous air embolism, and to ensure a free airway, as extremes of head flexion may cause the tube to bevel against the tracheal wall. The sitting position can be used in all ages but is more difficult to achieve before the development of a secondary lumbar curve, i.e. in those who do not yet sit independently (Figures 16.2, 16.3).

Venous air embolism is the major disadvantage of the sitting position. Most units in Britain rely on end-tidal CO_2 for the diagnosis, as the Doppler tends to be oversensitive and also has to be disconnected during the periods of highest risk because of diathermy interference. Evidence from the USA and Japan (Cucchiara et al, 1984; Furuya and Okumura, 1984) suggests that transoesophageal echocardiography may be of help in early detection of air emboli and especially of paradoxical embolus. Provided the surgeon and anaesthetist respond immediately the end-tital CO_2 begins to fall, the effects of the air embolus are minimized, and further entry is prevented. The surgeon fills the wound with a saline soaked pad, while the anaesthetist, using 100% O_2, hand ventilates with a small amount of positive end expiratory pressure and applies digital jugular vein compression. Once conditions are confirmed as stable the surgeon isolates the open vein, now bleeding because of the increased venous pressure, and coagulates it before continuing. Nitrous oxide should only be reintroduced when the end-tidal and arterial CO_2 values are approximately the same.

Significant air emboli are thought to be caused by boluses in excess of 0.5 ml/kg/min and therefore children, especially smaller ones, would be expected to have a higher incidence of significant emboli. This is not seen in practice, either at Great Ormond Street or at the Mayo Clinic (Cucchiara and Bowen, 1982).

Most units now use relaxants and intermittent positive pressure ventilation during posterior fossa surgery, therefore alterations in heart rate and blood pressure are the first signs of surgical interference with vital areas to which the surgeon must be alerted. Bradycardia is the commonest dysrhythmia, occasionally associated with hypertension. Cardiovascular instability is usually associated with tumours of the floor of the fourth ventricle, especially medulloblastomas and ependymomas, and is an indication for elective postoperative ventilation. Children with bulbar problems may require prolonged intubation for airway protection.

Craniopharyngioma

This is a rare tumour in childhood, but may cause complications because of diabetes insipidus which in small children causes major fluid balance problems. Synthetic vasopressin (DDAVP) may be required to control urine output postoperatively and can be administered i.m., i.v. or intranasally. Central venous pressure monitoring and a urinary catheter are essential aids to fluid balance in these patients, who are also prone to postoperative hyperpyrexia, which must be treated vigorously as described earlier, and will also complicate fluid balance.

Other tumours in infants may be extremely vascular, especially choroid plexus papillomas and some primitive tumours. Despite paying meticulous detail to providing optimal conditions, most centres still have a small but significant mortality from blood loss in these patients. Morbidity from massive blood loss is low in children during anaesthesia provided that there is good oxygenation before and during periods of reduced cardiac output. There is frequently evidence of air entering the circulation at the same time as the massive blood loss is occurring, but again this does not appear to cause long-term sequelae. Multiple rapid exchange transfusions are compatible with a good outcome provided massive brain swelling does not occur.

Craniofacial surgery

Rapid advancements have taken place in craniofacial surgery during the last two decades following the pioneering work of Tessier et al (1967), who showed that cranial and facial bones could be completely mobilized and

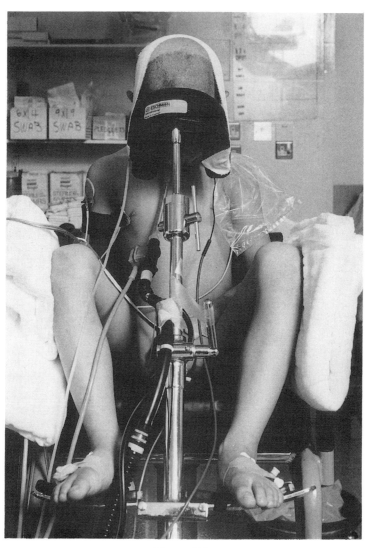

Figure 16.2.

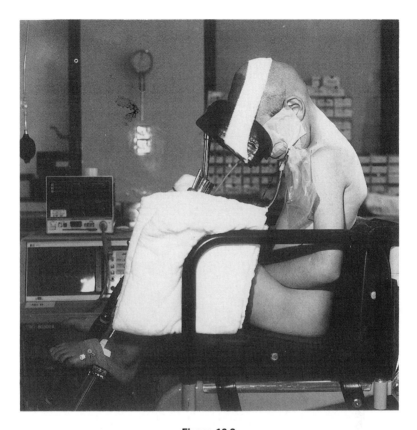

Figure 16.3.

Figures 16.2 and 16.3. The sitting position for posterior fossa exploration.

rearranged with good survival, and also that despite gross external abnormalities of the orbits the optic foramina are always normally situated and therefore orbital reconstruction does not affect vision.

Craniosynostosis covers a range of deformities, from the relatively simple sagittal fusion resulting in scaphocephaly, through unilateral and bilateral coronal fusion causing plagiocephaly and brachycephaly, to complex total synostosis usually associated with facial abnormalities, especially maxillary hypoplasia. The latter are usually part of a syndrome such as Crouzon's, Apert's, or Pfeiffer's, characterized by the associated abnormalities usually of the hands and feet, frequently syndactyly.

Early surgery is now considered to optimize brain growth; the rapidly growing brain of the infant is utilized to mould the repositioned bone flaps. Despite a lack of definite signs of raised ICP or slow development preoperatively, many of these children show accelerated development postoperatively. The optimal time for surgery is between 3 and 6 months, preferably when the infant weighs over 5 kg.

The development of the craniofacial team, consisting of plastic surgeons and neurosurgeons with ophthalmic, ear, nose and throat surgeons and specialist neuroradiologists, and for older children, psychologists, maxillary surgeons or orthodontists, speech therapists, etc. helps to optimize the timing and the nature of the surgery. It is essential to have a specialist anaesthetist familiar with both paediatric and neuroanaesthesia and intensive care, and a backing of skilled paediatric nurses.

The type of surgery planned will depend on which sutures are fused. Sagittal synostosis is treated by a simple craniectomy removing the fused suture—a relatively quick procedure associated with heavy blood loss despite good surgical conditions, with most patients receiving transfusions of the order of 30% of their blood volume, making allowance for postoperative losses. Some surgeons use silastic strips attached to the bone edges to prevent further fusion when regrowth takes place. This prolongs the operation and therefore adds to the total blood loss while not having marked long-term benefit.

Coronal or complex total synostosis is usually treated by a 'floating forehead' procedure (Marchac and Renier, 1979), involving frontal and orbital ridge advancement including the root of the nose and extending laterally to the level of the zygoma.

More major surgery involving maxillary mobilization is usually performed on older children either as a second stage or as a combined procedure in those who have not had early cranial surgery. Originally these procedures were performed on adolescents or pre-adolescents whose final facial growth had commenced, but now this type of surgery is often carried out on preschool children. The tracheal tube is extremely vulnerable in maxillary surgery, and many people employ nasal fixation or intradental fixation of an oral tube. It is sometimes necessary to change from oral to nasal tube before the maxilla is fixed, though this should not be done if intubation is difficult. Occasionally tracheostomy is necessary, especially if mandibular surgery is also planned as a single-stage operation. Sometimes in these complex craniofacial procedures ribs are taken for grafting and the anaesthetist must be alert to the possibility of a pneumothorax.

Preoperative assessment must be meticulous, especially with respect to intercurrent infection, as wound breakdown in these cases would be disastrous. Ease of feeding gives a good assessment of the nasal airway in a baby. Many infants with syndromes will have failed to thrive from general causes as well as from poor nasal breathing. Some may have required intermittent nasogastric tube feeding. Other associated abnormalities are noted. Premedication is with atropine 0.15–0.2 mg in infants. Older children may have a sedative premedication after careful assessment of neurological and airway status. Dexamethasone and prophylactic anticonvulsive therapy is started 24 h preoperatively, and antibiotics are also used routinely. A further dose of dexamethasone is given intravenously on induction. In infants a gaseous induction is safer, to ensure an adequate airway at all times, as airway obstruction will have a more deleterious effect on ICP. Producing a good seal with a facemask may also be difficult where there is gross proptosis.

As soon as inflation with the facemask has been shown to be possible the infant may be paralysed and intubated. If the facial abnormality is such that intubation difficulties are expected, laryngoscopy is performed under spontaneous ventilation and deep anaesthesia. Where maxillary surgery is also involved a throat pack is inserted and then removed immediately before tightening of the intradental fixation.

Venous access consisting of at least two free-flowing cannulas is essential and central venous catheterization may be required if massive blood loss is expected. The presence of syndactyly or other hand abnormalities may make radial artery cannulation difficult due to an abnormal position of the artery and an inability to extend the wrist. Posterior tibial artery puncture may be a suitable alternative.

As a moderate head-up position is employed, venous air embolism is a possibility, especially if blood replacement is lagging behind the loss. In patients with very abnormally shaped heads, such as clover leaf skulls, the surgeon requires radiological help to locate the major venous sinuses.

Routine urinary catheterization is not employed as light abdominal pressure will cause voiding if spontaneous micturition does not occur. The urine can be collected into an adhesive bag and output measured. In older children having prolonged surgery catheterization is advisable. Other monitoring and the anaesthetic technique are those used routinely for all neurosurgical procedures. Production of a relatively slow heart rate and blood pressure slightly below normal is ideal. Induced hypotension is not employed routinely, except during maxillary dissection, because of the duration of surgery. Sudden reflex hypotension or arrhythmias may occur during surgical dissection of the bony orbit or from traction on the skin transmitted via the tarsorraphies (Flandin-Bléty, 1982), an extreme variant of the occulocardiac reflex. The author now uses glycopyrrolate 2 µg/kg/h once the full effect of premedication is waning in an attempt to block this reflex.

Intraoperative blood loss will be proportional to the duration of surgery, but in most 'floating forehead' procedures it will be 300–400 ml, though it may be much greater if there is chronically raised ICP preoperatively with a copper-beaten skull making dissection more difficult. Infiltration of the skin with adrenaline 1:400 000 reduces blood loss by approximately 100 ml, and is now employed routinely. Blood loss continues into the postoperative period either as drainage or tissue swelling, and allowance must be made for these losses. Suction drains should be avoided because of the large bony defect resulting in the vacuum being directly transmitted to the brain, causing cardiovascular disturbance. The skin becomes very closely applied to the new bone shape and may cause pressure erosion if under tension.

Postoperatively all infants, and older children with hazardous airways, remain intubated for 24–48 h depending on the degree of swelling. At the end of the operation, if the nasal airway is suitable, the infants are reintubated nasally, otherwise orally, with a plain plastic tube. Fixation of the tube has to be carried out very carefully because the usual fixation to the forehead is not suitable, as this is now mobile. Moderate hyperventilation will keep swelling to a minimum. Continuous analgesia and sedation are provided while the infant is fully ventilated with a morphine infusion 0.5 mg/kg in 50 ml 5% dextrose at 3–4 ml/h. Spontaneous ventilation is usually established the following morning and extubation is performed when there is no residual sedation and swelling has subsided.

Spinal surgery

Congenital abnormalities of the lumbar spine are relatively common, frequently with cutaneous manifestations such as a hair tuft, capillary naevus, pigmented naevus or dermal pit as the only obvious feature.

All patients are investigated by myelography prior to surgery, which is usually carried out before the child starts walking. Blood loss, provided positioning of the patient is satisfactory, is usually of the order of 30–50 ml and therefore children over 6–7 kg are unlikely to require blood transfusion, where the lesion is limited to either lumbar or sacral segments.

Children with either primary or secondary spinal tumours are very different, with high blood losses despite good positioning, optimal anaesthesia and induced hypotension. Direct arterial monitoring should be employed for tumours and cervical spinal explorations. It must be remembered that surgical manipulation of the spinal cord is a very potent stimulus and may be associated with arrhythmias and falls in cardiac output.

SCOLIOSIS

Scoliosis, curvature of the spine, is classified by aetiology (Goldstein and Waugh, 1973; Table 16.1). The commonest cause, approximately 70% of all cases, is described as idiopathic or genetic and this diagnosis is made by exclusion. Idiopathic scoliosis is subdivided by age at onset into infantile (0–4 years), juvenile (4–9 years) and adolescent (10 years to the onset of bony maturity). A survey of 11 000 Edinburgh school children by Wynne-Davis (1968) gave an overall incidence of scoliosis diagnosed clinically and confirmed radiologically of 1.8 per 1000, subdivided into incidence in girls of 3.9 per 1000 and in boys of 0.3 per 1000. The sex difference is mainly due to the increased incidence of adolescent idiopathic curves in females, the commonest form of scoliosis. In the USA an incidence of 4 per 1000 was found purely radiographically by Strands and Esberg (1955).

There are two types of infantile scoliosis—resolving and progressive. The former rarely develops beyond 30° and requires no treatment. The progressive variety is more common in males, is usually left-sided, associated with severe deformity and has a poor prognosis.

Juvenile scoliosis is much rarer, and though recognized by the Scoliosis Research Society there is debate about its classification.

Adolescent idiopathic scoliosis is usually a right-sided thoracic curve involving 7–10 vertebral levels. If untreated, only 30% of patients will have curves less than 70° at the end of growth. It used to be thought that with the cessation of growth the curve did not deteriorate. A 25-year follow-up by Collis and Ponseti (1969) showed progression by an average of 30° but little cardiorespiratory effect. However, a 50-year follow-up by Freyschuss et al (1968) showed increased mortality with an average age at death of 46.6 years, mainly from respiratory or right heart failure. Of the survivors, with an average age of 62 years, almost half were cardiorespiratory cripples.

Congenital scoliosis is frequently associated with other major abnormalities, especially cyanotic congenital heart disease or as part of VATER syndrome with vertebral, anal, tracheo-oesophageal fistula, renal, radial

Table 16.1. Classification of scoliosis

Idiopathic (genetic)
Infantile 0–4 years
Juvenile 4–9 years
Adolescent over 10 years
Congenital
No neurological deficit, e.g. hemivertibrae, fused ribs
With neurological deficit (closed), e.g. diastematomyelia
With neurological deficit (open),
e.g. meningomyelocoele
Neuropathic
Upper motor neurone, e.g. cerebral palsy
Lower motor neurone, e.g. poliomyelitis
Myopathic
Static, e.g. amyotonia congenita
Progressive, e.g. muscular dystrophy
Neurofibromatosis
Mesenchymal disorders
Congenital, e.g. Marfan's; Morquio's; dwarfism
Acquired, e.g. Still's disease
Traumatic
Vertebral, e.g. fracture, surgery
Extravertebral, e.g. burns, thoracic surgery

and cardiac abnormalities. Children with spina bifida who have severe scoliosis usually have a major neurological deficit.

Many neuromuscular disorders may be associated with scoliosis but following the almost universal uptake of poliomyelitis vaccination this infection is no longer a major cause of scoliosis in developed countries. Compared with idiopathic scoliosis, paralytic scoliosis, both neuro- and myopathic, has a worse prognosis and there is progressive deterioration after cessation of growth. The prognosis will also be affected by coexisting cardiac disease. Obesity is another poor prognostic factor.

Preoperative preparation

Preoperative assessment includes detailed examination of the respiratory, cardiovascular, neuromuscular and renal systems because of the high incidence of associated abnormalities.

If a 'wake-up' test is to be performed a full explanation must be given to the patient, though in a series of 150 patients studied by Hall et al (1978) only 12 recalled the test. Children likely to require postoperative ventilation should have this and the need for nasal intubation explained. This should not be discussed too far in advance as it may provoke anxiety.

Respiratory assessment

Two major factors which affect pulmonary function are the degree of curvature and neuromuscular dysfunction.

Patients with idiopathic scoliosis rarely develop significant respiratory impairment unless the curve is greater than 65°. There is a restrictive pattern with the greatest reduction occurring in vital capacity with smaller changes in total lung capacity and functional residual capacity (Kafer, 1980). Ventilation–perfusion mismatch and alveolar hypoventilation result in early hypoxaemia while carbon dioxide levels remain normal until late in the disease process and are an ominous prognostic feature.

Restriction of the pulmonary vascular bed and hypoxaemia cause pulmonary hypertension and subsequently right heart failure. ECG changes of right heart strain are a late feature. Coexistence of either neuromuscular disease or cyanotic heart disease further compromises these patients. However, surgery is usually well tolerated in patients with marked reductions in vital capacity, though those with a vital capacity of less than 30% of predicted values usually require postoperative ventilatory support (Jenkins et al, 1982). Predicted values are calculated using span, as height is reduced by the spinal curve. Formal pulmonary function testing may be very difficult in young children and patients with severe cerebral palsy, due to an inability to comply with instructions.

Treatment

Non-operative treatment is with either plaster localizer casts with or without halo traction or with bracing. External fixation is the sole treatment for less severe degrees of scoliosis. In younger patients localizers are used as a stop-gap procedure to enable further growth to occur without deterioration in the curve prior to spinal fusion. Bracing is also used postoperatively to provide external stability while bony fusion occurs.

Spinal fusion was first performed in 1911 by Russell Hibbs but the introduction of the Harrington rod in 1962 and the Dwyer apparatus in 1968 have resulted in the massive increase in posterior and anterior spinal fusion seen today.

The anterior approach is used where there is marked fixation of the curve, especially in the lower thoracic and lumbar levels and usually is the first stage of a two-stage operation prior to posterior fusion. The anterior approach uses a thoracoabdominal incision involving removal of the diaphragm from its peripheral attachments. The intervertebral discs are removed at several levels and this results in a dramatic increase in spinal mobility. Anterior spinal fusion using transverse screws is usually performed, or alternatively a postoperative period of halotibial traction prior to posterior spinal fusion may give improved results in younger patients where growth is still in progress. The complications of the anterior approach result from the large thoracoabdominal wound and diaphragmatic disruption, causing severe postoperative pain and an increased incidence of postoperative ventilation. Another effect of extensive anterior dissection is unilateral and occasionally bilateral lumbar sympathectomy. A chest drain with underwater seal should be used routinely following anterior spinal fusion.

Posterior fusion is also an extensive procedure using a distraction rod applied to the concavity of the curve fixed at either end with hooks to the facet joints and usually stabilized with sublaminar wiring (Luqué). There is extensive decortication of the vertebrae and application of bone graft from the iliac crest.

Anaesthesia

Premedication with papaveretum and hyoscine provides an excellent basis for hypotensive anaesthesia, though many children may require considerably reduced doses because of poor respiratory function.

Specific problems which may cause technical difficulties for the anaesthetist are associated limb deformities, which may make venous access and arterial cannulation more difficult. Spina bifida patients with hydrocephalus may have or have had previous atrial shunts which may cause difficulty with internal jugular cannulation for central venous pressure measurement. Facial abnormalities, especially Goldenhar's syndrome which has a high incidence of scoliosis, may present difficulties with intubation, as may patients in spinal jackets, particularly those with halo attachments. In this case the plaster should either be bivalved or have the anterior part removed prior to induction of anaesthesia and tools should be available for removal of the halo traction rods if that should become urgently necessary.

In patients being placed prone a reinforced trachael tube should be used. For anterior surgery in the older adolescent a small double-lumen tube may improve ventilatory control.

An anaesthetic technique of nitrous oxide, oxygen and relaxant with fentanyl and supplemented with either halothane or isoflurane is recommended. Most patients with neuromuscular disease should not be given suxamethonium and non-depolarizing relaxants should be used with care. The response of patients with neuromuscular disorders to muscle relaxants has been reviewed by Azar (1984). Some patients will also be susceptible to malignant hyperpyrexia (see p. 528).

Because of the extensive nature of the surgery one of the major complications of posterior spinal fusion is massive blood loss. Many factors affect the volume of blood loss, the first being the duration of surgery because of the large raw bony surface, and secondly, venous pressure in the vertebral veins, which is controlled by good positioning in the vertebral veins, which is controlled by good positioning in the prone position ensuring a free abdomen with low intra-abdominal pressure and a lack of inferior vena caval compression. In some patients with fixed lordotic deformities it may be impossible to achieve good positioning and these cases are always associated with increased venous bleeding.

Moderate hyperventilation to $PaCO_2$ 3.75–4 kPa is also recommended but marked reductions should be avoided because vasoconstriction will cause reduced spinal cord blood flow, especially if arterial hypotension is also employed.

In several series without arterial hypotension the average blood loss for posterior spinal fusion in adolescent idiopathic scoliosis was 2.5 l and with induced hypotension this was reduced to 1.5 l (McNeill et al, 1974). These results have led to the widespread use of induced hypotension for these operations. However, some patients will always have increased blood losses despite control of arterial pressure, due to increased venous bleeding. These include severely lordotic patients, those with large meningomyelocoeles and those with myopathies.

Hypotension is induced using a standard technique, described on p. 379, in conjunction with adequate levels of anaesthesia, normal oxygenation and acid–base balance. Normovolaemia is also essential, especially in those patients with cardiac disease.

Spinal cord damage occurred in approximately 1% of patients reviewed by MacEwen et al in 1975, with a better prognosis for incomplete lesions and for those patients in whom the stabilizing metal work was removed within 3 h. Because of the potential risks of this type of surgery intraoperative 'wake-up' tests became popular but more recently have been replaced by spinal cord monitoring. Somatosensory-evoked potentials from stimulation of the peroneal nerves are recorded from epidural electrodes inserted percutaneously via a Tuohy needle during anterior procedures or directly above the operative site in posterior fusions. It has been demonstrated that adequate wave generation is recorded with 60% nitrous oxide and up to 1.0 MAC (minimum alveolar concentration) isoflurane or enflurane and 0.75 MAC halothane (Pathak et al, 1987). Recently motor function has also been studied (Boyd et al, 1986).

Postoperative pain relief is very important after major surgery but will need to be administered cautiously in those patients with poor respiratory function. Anterior fusion is a much more painful procedure but excellent analgesia can be provided with intercostal nerve blocks performed at the end of the operation. Subsequently and for patients having posterior fusion a morphine infusion will provide good pain relief.

Patients with spasticity, especially those with cerebral palsy, experience extreme pain following all orthopaedic procedures and have increased analgesic requirements. A background of diazepam or baclofen 5–15 mg 6-hourly administered regularly is useful in reducing the muscle spasm and also the analgesic requirements.

Results

After scoliosis surgery, despite marked improvement of the spinal curve, there is little demonstrable effect on lung volumes (Shneerson and Edgar, 1979) though Shannon et al in 1970 showed a decrease in physiological dead space and improvement in hypoxaemic patients. Whether long-term follow-up will demonstrate prevention of the late sequelae of untreated scoliosis has yet to be proved and studies into the next century will be needed to compare with the 50-year follow-up by Freyschuss et al (1968).

REFERENCES

Abbott TR (1983) Changes in serum calcium concentrations during massive blood transfusions and cardiopulmonary bypass. *British Journal of Anaesthesia* **55**: 753–760.

Azar I (1984) The response of patients with neuromuscular disorders to muscle relaxants: a review. *Anesthesiology* **61:** 173–187.

Berntman L, Welsh FA & Harp JR (1981) Cerebral protective effect of low-grade hypothermia. *Anesthesiology* **55:** 495–498.

Boyd SG, Rothwell JC, Cowan JMA et al (1986) A method of monitoring function in corticospinal pathways during scoliosis surgery with a note on motor conduction velocities. *Journal of Neurology, Neurosurgery and Psychiatry* **49:** 251–257.

Collis DK & Ponseti IV (1969) Long term follow up of patients with idiopathic scoliosis not treated surgically. *Journal of Bone and Joint Surgery* **51:** 425–445.

Cucchiara RF & Bowen B (1982) Air embolism in children undergoing suboccipital craniotomy. *Anesthesiology* **57:** 338–339.

Cucchiara RF, Nugent M, Seward JB et al (1984) Air embolism in upright neurosurgical patients: detection and localization by two-dimensional transesophageal echocardiography. *Anesthesiology* **60:** 353–355.

Flandin-Bléty C (1982) Anesthesia and intensive care for craniofacial surgery in children. In Marchac D & Renier D (eds) *Craniofacial Surgery for Craniosynostoses*, pp 39–45. Boston: Little Brown.

Freyschuss W, Nilsonne U & Lundgren KD (1968) Idiopathic scoliosis in old age. 1. Respiratory function. *Acta Medica Scandinavica* **184:** 365–372.

Furuya H & Okumura F (1984) Detection of paradoxical air embolism by transesophageal echocardiography. *Anesthesiology* **60:** 374–377.

Goldstein LA & Waugh TR (1973) Classification and terminology of scoliosis. *Clinical Orthopedics* **93:** 10–22.

Hall JE, Levine CR & Sudhir KG (1978) Intraoperative awakening to monitor spinal cord function during Harrington instrumentation and spinal fusion. *Journal of Bone and Joint Surgery* **60:** 533–536.

Jenkins JG, Bohn DJ, Edmonds JF et al (1982) Evaluation of pulmonary function in muscular dystrophy patients requiring spinal surgery. *Critical Care Medicine* **10:** 645–649.

Kafer ER (1980) Respiratory and cardiovascular functions in scoliosis and the principles of anesthetic management. *Anesthesiology* **52:** 339–351.

Kennedy C & Sokoloff L (1957) An adaption of the nitrous oxide method to the study of the cerebral circulation in children: normal values for cerebral blood flow and cerebral metabolic rate in childhood. *Journal of Clinical Investigation* **36:** 1130–1136.

Leck I (1974) Causation of neural tube defects: clues from epidemiology. *British Medical Bulletin* **30:** 158–163.

Lou HC & Friis-Hansen B (1979) Impaired autoregulation of cerebral blood flow in the distressed newborn infant. *Journal of Pediatrics* **94:** 118–121.

MacEwan GD, Bunnell WP & Sriram K (1975) Acute neurological complications in the treatment of scoliosis. A report of the Scoliosis Research Society. *Journal of Bone and Joint Surgery* **57:** 404–408.

Marchac D & Renier D (1979) Le front flottant, traitement précoce des faciocraniostenoses. *Annales de Chirurgie Plastique* **24:** 121–126.

McNeill TW, DeWala RL, Kuo KN et al (1974) Controlled hypotension anesthesia in scoliosis surgery. *Journal of Bone and Joint Surgery* **56A:** 1167–1172.

Nightingale P & Meakin G (1987) A new method for maintaining body temperature in children. *Anesthesiology* **65:** 447–448.

Nightingale DA, Richards CC & Glass A (1965) An evaluation of rebreathing in a modified T-piece during controlled ventilation of anaesthetised children. *British Journal of Anaesthesia* **37:** 762–771.

Pathak KS, Ammadro M, Kalamchi A et al (1987) Effects of halothane, enflurane and isoflurane on somatosensory evoked potentials during nitrous oxide anaesthesia. *Anesthesiology* **66:** 753–757.

Sellars MJ (1987) Unanswered questions on neural tube defects. *British Medical Journal* **294:** 1–2.

Shanahan EC, Marshall AG & Garrett CPO (1983) Adverse reactions to intravenous codeine phosphate in children. *Anaesthesia* **38:** 40–44.

Shannon DC, Riseborough EJ & Kazemi H (1970) Ventilation–perfusion relationships following correction of kyphoscoliosis. *Journal of the American Medical Association* **217:** 579–584.

Shneerson JM & Edgar MA (1979) Cardiac and respiratory function before and after spinal fusion in adolescent idiopathic scoliosis. *Thorax* **34:** 658–661.

Steward DJ (1982) Preterm infants are more prone to complications following minor surgery than are term infants. *Anesthesiology* **56:** 304–306.

Strands AR & Esberg HB (1955) The incidence of scoliosis in the state of Delaware. *Journal of Bone and Joint Surgery* **37:** 1243–1249.

Swedlow DB (1983) Anesthesia for neurosurgical procedures. In Gregory GA (ed) *Pediatric Anesthesia*, vol. 2, pp 679–706. New York: Churchill Livingstone.

Tessier P, Guigot G, Rougerie J, Delbet JP & Pastoriza J (1967) Osteotomies cranionasio-orbitales. Hypertelorisme. *Annales de Chirurgie Plastique* **12:** 103–118.

Woods I, Morris P & Meakin G (1985) Severe bronchospasm following the use of atracurium in children. *Anaesthesia* **40:** 207.

Wynne-Davies R (1968) Familial (idiopathic) scoliosis—a family survey. *Journal of Bone and Joint Surgery* **50:** 24–30.

Anaesthesia for ear, nose and throat surgery

GENERAL CONSIDERATIONS

Minor ear, nose and throat (ENT) procedures in children are commonplace and frequently take place in adult centres where little other paediatric surgery is performed. Many operations are short and simple; however, the potential for both anaesthetic and surgical complications is great, particularly in procedures where surgeon and anaesthetist share the airway. The dangers of allocating an inexperienced anaesthetist, unsupervised, to a 'tonsil' list, where the surgeon is also very junior must be realized.

Minor operations on the ear may not demand any great expertise; however, diagnostic procedures in infants and small babies with upper airways obstruction require considerable anaesthetic expertise and the importance of co-operation and understanding between surgeon and anaesthetist during these procedures cannot be over-emphasized.

This chapter outlines a few general principles and describes in more detail the management of specific procedures and conditions. The list is far from exhaustive and those procedures whose management differs little from adult practice have been omitted or only touched on briefly.

Preoperative considerations

Many minor ENT operations are performed on a day-stay basis; however as this is usually a surgical decision it is important for patients to arrive at the hospital early enough to allow time for full anaesthetic assessment preoperatively and premedication if appropriate (see Chapters 1 and 2).

Particularly common in ENT practice is the child with the 'snuffly' nose (Berry, 1986). This is often a feature of adenoidal hypertrophy and should not be a contraindication to surgery. It should be distinguished from an acute upper respiratory tract infection (URTI), as general anaesthesia in the presence of an URTI will result in an increased incidence of laryngeal spasm both on induction and emergence, and in postoperative lower respiratory tract infections.

Upper airways obstruction of varying degrees at nasal, pharyngeal or laryngeal level may be present in many patients, so it is particularly important for the anaesthetist to see all children to assess the degree of any respiratory obstruction. Anticipating a difficult airway problem and being suitably prepared in the anaesthetic room will go a long way to reducing anaesthetic complications.

The anaesthetist should also be alerted to any unusual conditions or syndromes known to be associated with airway and intubation difficulties. This includes the Pierre Robin syndrome, hemifacial microsomia (Goldenhar syndrome), Treacher Collins syndrome and the mucopolysaccharidoses.

As bleeding from the tonsillar fossa or vascular tissues in the nose can result in serious morbidity, history of a bleeding tendency either in the child or the family is important, as a bleeding disorder may as yet be undiagnosed in a small child. If there is any doubt at all, coagulation studies should be carried out preoperatively. Drug history should be carefully taken and due to its anticoagulant properties it is recommended that aspirin should be withheld for at least 1 week prior to tonsillectomy (Paradise, 1981); its use in children is not now advised because of risk of Reye's syndrome.

Direct questioning about loose teeth is wise, as these can be dislodged during anaesthesia and accidentally inhaled or swallowed. It may be advisable to remove a very loose tooth following induction to prevent such accidents.

Premedication

Although protocols for premedication depending on age and type of operation are helpful, each child should be assessed individually. There may be no real benefit from premedication in some older ambulant children having minor surgery, whereas in the 2–4-year age group preoperative sedation can be invaluable. Children in the 2–4-year age group are particularly likely to suffer emotionally from hospital admission and a preoperative visit to establish a good rapport with parents and child will help to minimize this.

The type and dose of premedication must be tailored to suit the preoperative status of the patient and the intended anaesthetic technique.

Children under the age of 6–7 years for minor ear procedures and adenotonsillectomy are better premedicated with a non-respiratory depressant such as oral trimeprazine and atropine, which provides moderate sedation combined with significant antiemetic effect. As trimeprazine is devoid of any analgesic action, it is best combined with 1 mg/kg codeine phosphate given intramuscularly just before extubation. Children over 6–7 years are premedicated with a reduced dose of papaveretum (0.2–0.3 mg/kg) and hyoscine. Patients with disturbed sleep patterns due to chronic upper airways obstruction and those with less severe obstruction due to preexisting maxillofacial deformities should have intramuscular atropine only. As most patients for endoscopy also have a degree of airways obstruction this group should also have atropine alone (Table 17.1).

Monitoring

Nowhere in paediatric anaesthetic practice is monitoring so important as in paediatric otolaryngology. Frequently the theatre lighting is dimmed during

Table 17.1. Premedication for ENT surgery

Adenotonsillectomy
1. Under 7 years of age: oral trimeprazine 3–4 mg/kg with atropine 0.05 mg/kg orally 2 h preoperatively
2. Over 7 years of age: papareveretum and hyoscine in dose 0.3 mg/kg
3. Postoperative sedation: codeine phosphate only, 1 mg/kg i.m. before leaving theatre

Endoscopy
Atropine only (children with tracheostomy may have sedation)

---

use of the microscope or headlight. The patient may be almost totally covered in drapes, and when the airway is being shared there is always the potential for hypoxia, whether due to inadequate ventilation, kinking of an endotracheal tube or accidental extubation.

Monitoring requires close, continuous clinical observation combined with a precordial stethoscope, ECG, blood pressure measurement and pulse oximetry. Though expensive, pulse oximetry today must have high priority in this field and should become essential monitoring for endoscopy as arterial oxygen saturation falls before there is clinical evidence of hypoxia.

Postoperative care

As many ENT operations involve the airway, nursing care during the recovery period must be of the highest standard, so that danger signals are recognized early and appropriate action taken before serious complications occur. When there may be blood in the pharynx (for example, after adeno-tonsillectomy and nasal operations) patients should be nursed not only on their side, but also with a pillow under the chest, so that any blood will run out of the mouth or nose and not into the larynx with the risk of laryngeal spasm or obstruction due to blood clot. No patient should be returned to the ward until full recovery has taken place.

Codeine phosphate 1 mg/kg i.m. provides adequate analgesia for most ENT operations; however, it should never be given intravenously to children as severe falls in cardiac output may occur (Shanahan et al, 1983).

Opiates should be avoided in all operations on or around the airway, but can be used following ear surgery provided an antiemetic is also prescribed.

Operations on the ear

Myringotomy and insertion of grommets

The treatment of recurrent otitis media and persistent effusion in the middle ear, with surgical myringotomy and insertion of ventilation tube, is a very common procedure today. Unless combined with adenoidectomy it is well suited to day-case surgery.

If no anaesthetic or surgical problems are anticipated maintenance of anaesthesia with a mask and airway is safe. Intubation may be required, however, if the airway is difficult to maintain, or the external auditory meatus is very narrow, making surgical access difficult.

Major ear surgery

Major ear surgery may involve two groups of operation—congenital defects of the ear, and myringoplasty, exploration of the middle ear and mastoidectomy.

Congenital defects of the ear.

Surgery for reconstruction of congenital defects of the ear includes formation of an external auditory meatus to enable a hearing aid to be fitted. These congenital defects are associated with two important syndromes—Treacher Collins and Goldenhar's syndrome (or hemifacial microsomia). Treacher Collins syndrome is an autosomal dominant mandibulofacial dysostosis which includes severe mandibular hypoplasia and malformation of the pinna and external auditory meatus. In Goldenhar's syndrome, in addition to unilateral hypoplasia of the malar, maxilla and mandible, there is deformity or absence of the pinna, external auditory meatus and middle ear, and congenital heart disease (usually a ventriculoseptal defect or tetralogy of Fallot).

As these children are often difficult to intubate, and have difficult airways to maintain both on induction and emergence, sedative premedication should be avoided. Inhalational induction with halothane is safest and spontaneous respiration must be maintained until mask ventilation has been shown to be possible (mask fit in Goldenhar's may be a problem, making mask ventilation inadequate even in the presence of a clear airway). Whether short-acting muscle relaxants are used or not, a wide range of tubes, laryngoscopes and bougies should be available. Visualization of the larynx is aided by firm backward pressure from the front of the neck, bringing an anteriorly placed larynx more into view. A semi-rigid bougie is helpful in directing the tube into the larynx.

These children often have staged surgical procedures, therefore careful anaesthetic records describing technique and degree of difficulty will often help for future anaesthetics.

Once intubation has been achieved anaesthesia is best maintained with muscle relaxant, intermittent positive pressure ventilation (IPPV) and minimal supplement (such as 0.5% halothane) so that there is rapid return to full consciousness at the end of the procedure allowing safe extubation.

Myringoplasty, exploration of the middle ear and mastoidectomy.

Myringoplasty and exploration of the middle ear may be required when infection has badly damaged the tympanic membrane. Exploration of the mastoid air cells for removal of infected tissue or cholesteatoma is rare today. There are three special concerns with this type of surgery—bleeding, graft displacement and preservation of the facial nerve:

1. *Bleeding*: The operating microscope is used for these procedures, making

even small amounts of blood troublesome. Venous bleeding due to raised venous pressure in the superior vena cava or internal jugular vein is usually the result of poor anaesthetic technique. Causes include partial airways obstruction during spontaneous respiration, raised mean airway pressure during IPPV, or abdominal compression. Arterial bleeding in children is related more to cardiac rate and cardiac output than directly to peak systolic pressure. A stormy induction with crying, coughing and straining will increase catecholamine secretion, producing an increase in pulse rate and cardiac output which may last for up to 30 min.

Meticulous attention to detail is therefore necessary if a bloodless field is to be obtained. Induction should be smooth, avoiding coughing and straining during or after intubation. The use of curare, IPPV and 0.5–1% halothane, followed by careful positioning of the patient on the table with a 15–20° head-up tilt, will give a systolic pressure of 80–90 mmHg and good conditions in the majority of cases.

Hypotensive agents may rarely be required to reduce pressure further, but they should not be used to compensate for bad anaesthetic technique.

Trimetaphan (Arfonad) (0.1% solution) causes autonomic ganglion blockage. It rapidly produces a compensatory tachycardia which may lead to poorer operating conditions than before its use; however, a small tiltrated dose of β-blocker will prevent this. As it is associated with histamine release it should never be used in asthmatic patients.

Sodium nitroprusside (Nipride) is a rapidly direct-acting peripheral vascular dilator producing profound hypotension. It is difficult to manage safely without the use of an indwelling arterial cannula and its use is not justified normally in this field.

Labetalol (Trandate) is the best agent available at present for this sort of surgery. It has both α and β effects, producng both peripheral vasodilatation and β-blockade so that compensatory tachycardia is not seen. It produces modest falls in blood pressure, so that direct intra-arterial monitoring is not as necessary as with other agents, provided a reliable automatic blood pressure monitor is available. It is given in a bolus starting with 0.2 mg/kg and repeated at 5-min intervals until the desired effect is achieved. Due to its β-blocking effect it should be avoided in asthmatics. Bradycardia, if excessive, responds to intravenous atropine.

2. *Graft displacement*: Nitrous oxide is three to four times as soluble as nitrogen, therefore in closed cavities it diffuses in much more rapidly than nitrogen can escape. If the cavity is distensible the volume will increase, but if non-distensible the pressure within the cavity will rise. This effect reaches a peak about 30 min after administration of the gas. During anaesthesia for myringoplasty, when nitrous oxide is discontinued, pressure in the middle ear will become negative once the cavity is closed, causing displacement of the tympanic membrane graft. To avoid this, nitrous oxide should be discontinued at least 20 min before closure of the middle ear space, and anaesthesia continued with oxygen or an oxygen/air mixture together with an increase in the concentration of volatile agent to prevent awareness.

3. *The facial nerve*: For mastoidectomy, myringoplasty and exploration of the middle ear a postauricular incision is used. In small children the mastoid process is not developed and the stylomastoid foramen with emerging

facial nerve is relatively superficial and more easily damaged with a postauricular incision. Some surgeons may wish to preserve neuro-muscular function until the facial nerve has been positively identified with a nerve stimulator.

Operations on the nose, nasopharynx and pharynx

Choanal atresia

Choanal atresia may be unilateral, bilateral, membranous or bony. Some 60% are associated with one or more congenital defects including the CHARGE association (Kaplan, 1985). Although every postnatal examin-ation should include passage of an 8 French gauge catheter through each nostril into the nasopharynx, unilateral atresia may not be diagnosed for months or years. In contrast, bilateral atresia causes acute respiratory dis-tress in the neonate and unless an oral airway is inserted the baby will become severely hypoxic and may die. The airway is taped to the baby's cheeks and orogastric tube-feeding is provided until surgery is undertaken at 1–2 days (Figure 17.1). Atropine premedication is given and following preoxygenation an orotracheal tube is inserted after induction of anaes-thesia or in the awake state. Puncture of the choanae is usually performed transnasally with dilators or a shielded dental drill, but if the transpalatal route is anticipated blood loss will be significant and blood must be cross-matched preoperatively. As there is no Doughty mouth gag small enough for neonates, a Boyle–Davis gag is used. This has no split in the tongue plate, so compression and obstruction of the tracheal tube can be a problem. A 3 mm preformed tube (e.g. Oxford) is satisfactory. Ventilation is controlled using a relaxant technique with all the precautions and monitoring neces-sary for neonatal surgery. Provided a mouth gag is used and the surgeon has a direct view of the pharynx a throat pack is unnecessary. After nasal puncture is complete, splints, made from a plastic tracheal tube, are passed into each nostril and fixed in position with a heavy nylon tie around the nasal septum. These provide a patent nasal airway and are removed after 6 weeks. At the end of the procedure extubation should be performed with the baby fully awake after careful suctioning of the pharynx.

Adenotonsillectomy

The Department of Health and Social Services (DHSS) statistics show that between 70 000 and 90 000 tonsillectomies and/or adenoidectomies were performed annually in England and Wales between 1979 and 1983 (DHSS 1978–1983). Although the numbers of tonsillectomies has diminished due to effective treatment of acute tonsillitis with antibiotics, adenotonsillectomy is still one of the commonest operations carried out in children. It should never be regarded as a minor operation as morbidity and mortality still occur (Richmond et al, 1987).

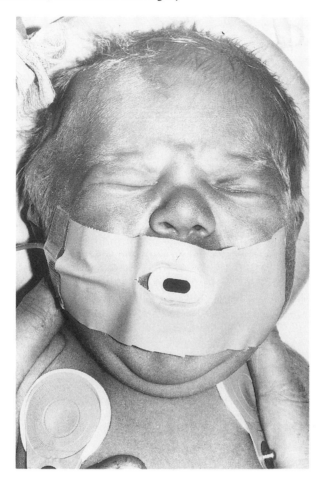

Figure 17.1. Neonate with bilateral choanal atresia showing oral airway taped in place.

Mortality has been estimated variously from 1 in 1000 to 1 in 27000 (Paradise, 1981). The commonest cause of death is postoperative haemorrhage, leading to hypovolaemia with or without respiratory obstruction due to aspiration of blood or clots. Equally important is the danger of respiratory depression from postoperative sedation. Common errors in management are: delay in effective treatment for haemorrhage, underestimation of blood loss due to swallowed blood, and postoperative sedation for restlessness due to hypoxia or bleeding (Tate, 1963).

Economic factors have seen a trend towards day-case surgery in some centres for adenotonsillectomy (Shott et al, 1987). However, in many centres it is felt unwise to discharge any patient following such surgery for at least 24 h, although longer may be unnecessary (Siodlak et al, 1985).

Adenoids are removed because they cause obstruction to the eustachian tubes and the nasopharyngeal airway. Tonsillectomy is usually performed for recurrent tonsillitis, but rarer indications include peritonsillar abscess and chronic upper airways obstruction. Occasionally chronic upper airways obstruction may lead to the sleep apnoea syndrome, where there is disordered central control of respiration and inco-ordination of oropharyngeal musculature (Guilleminault et al, 1976; Bradley and Phillipson, 1985; Thach, 1985). Hypoxia and hypercarbia may in turn result in pulmonary vasoconstriction with right ventricular hypertrophy and, rarely, right heart failure (Macartney et al, 1969). Adenotonsillectomy will cure many children with the sleep apnoea syndrome (Brouillette and Fernbach, 1982), but as hypoxaemia may continue into the postoperative period, these children must be closely monitored postoperatively and added oxygen and a nasopharyngeal airway used if indicated. Postoperative sedation must be avoided.

As already mentioned, premedication should be tailored to fit both the child and the anaesthetic technique used. Inhalational induction with cyclopropane or halothane is best suited to children sedated with trimeprazine. Despite the newer inhalational agents, enflurane and isoflurane, halothane remains superior for induction of anaesthesia. During induction, the airway of children with nasal or pharyngeal obstruction due to enlarged adenoids or tonsils can be difficult to maintain, though it is helped by maintaining a tight reservoir bag. Keeping the mouth slightly open under the mask will often help until an oral airway can be safely inserted. Although traditionally in the past insufflation techniques using ether and a Boyle–Davis gag have been used, the airway is best maintained with an orotracheal tube.

Suxamethonium may be used for intubation and there are advantages in using an extended metal connector (for example, Worcester) on the tracheal tube (Figure 17.2). This will prevent compression between the tongue plate and the teeth when the Doughty gag is opened. Newer preformed plastic RAE tubes can be used, but these soften once in situ, and particularly with the smaller sizes may become compressed if excessive opening of the gag is required. Inability to remove the gag without extubating the patient due to wedging of the tube in the split in the blade has also been reported (Wood, 1987).

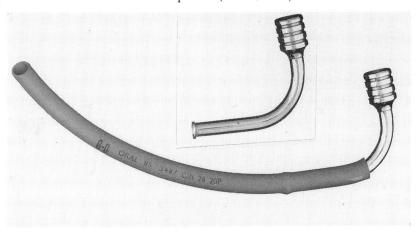

Figure 17.2. Worcester connector (inset) and tracheal tube for use in adenotonsillectomy. The long extension for the connector within the tube prevents its compression between the gag and the teeth.

Spontaneous respiration with nitrous oxide, oxygen and halothane is satisfactory in children premedicated with trimeprazine, but in older children who have had opiate premedication and intravenous induction, a spontaneously breathing technique is difficult to conduct. Irregular breathing and hypoventilation occur making adequate depth of anaesthesia difficult to achieve and these patients are more safely managed with a muscle relaxant and IPPV.

Monitoring should include precordial stethoscope, ECG, blood pressure measurement and pulse oximetry.

Blood volume should be calculated (75–80 ml/kg) and a careful watch should be kept on blood loss. It has been shown that 40% of children lose 10% or more of their blood volume during adenotonsillectomy, with an occasional patient losing up to 20% (Shalom, 1964). An intravenous cannula, therefore, should always be in situ and remain there until full recovery.

Intravenous fluids are not normally required in older children unless there is continuing bleeding, vomiting or excess insensible loss during hot weather, but patients under 12 kg should be maintained with intravenous fluids until oral intake is satisfactory.

At the end of the operation the pharynx should be carefully suctioned for blood and debris prior to extubation. In younger children who have had trimeprazine premedication and maintained breathing spontaneously with halothane, deep extubation is safe. These children recover consciousness quickly and the incidence of laryngeal spasm is low. In the older child who has had an opiate premedication and intravenous induction, recovery is slow, and the incidence of laryngeal spasm will be high if deep extubation is attempted. These children should be extubated awake; this is more readily achieved using a relaxant technique with minimal additional volatile anaesthetic. Children who have had trimeprazine premedication have a more peaceful recovery if a single dose of codeine phosphate 1 mg/kg i.m. is given prior to extubation. All patients should be nursed in the classic 'tonsillar' position, head-down and on their side until awake. Postoperative care must be of a high standard, and the child should be returned to the ward fully awake, with no bleeding and a good cough reflex.

The bleeding tonsil

The incidence of re-operation for bleeding following adenotonsillectomy has been estimated at 1–2%. Postoperative bleeding should never be underestimated and a decision to return the child to theatre should be made promptly, as waiting for several hours to see if the bleeding improves is a dangerous practice. Re-anaesthetizing children who have continued to bleed following adenotonsillectomy can be hazardous (Davies, 1964) and there are three main problems to consider:

1. *Full stomach*: Blood trickling or oozing from the operative site is usually swallowed, resulting in a stomach full of blood.
2. *Hypovolaemia*: Frequently, blood loss is seriously underestimated due to hidden losses in the stomach and lack of visible blood in the bed. There

may have been a significant loss at the initial operation and, combined with large quantities of swallowed blood, a very large deficit may be present.
3. *Residual narcosis*: As there may be residual narcosis from sedative or anaesthetic drugs given earlier in the day, no further sedation should be given preoperatively.

Blood should be cross-matched early and preoperative volume replacement undertaken with crystalloid, plasma or blood, depending on the condition of the patient. Signs of serious losses include restlessness, pallor, tachycardia and poor peripheral circulation.
The operating theatre should be prepared in the following way:

1. Two suckers should be available with wide-bore tubing to remove blood clots. The first sucker may become blocked just when it is most needed.
2. Two laryngoscopes are necessary as the bulb often becomes obscured with blood and the larynx cannot be visualized.
3. Several tracheal tubes of smaller sizes than the one used for the first operation should be prepared as postoperative oedema may have reduced the lumen of the larynx.
4. A competent assistant should be available.

There is little agreement on the safest anaesthetic technique for a bleeding tonsil; whether an intravenous or inhalational induction should be used; whether the patient should be supine or lateral and whether relaxants should be used. Probably the most important factor is that the anaesthetist should be aware of the problems and use a technique with which he or she is thoroughly familiar.
Following atropine premedication the patient is probably safest anaesthetized in the head-down, lateral position on the operating table, with the surgeon standing by. If the anaesthetist has never intubated a patient in the lateral position, the supine position may be justified.
Most anaesthetists advocate a rapid sequence i.v. induction with reduced dose of thiopentone and suxamethonium. Others prefer inhalational induction with 100% oxygen and halothane (cyclopropane should be avoided in this situation as it may cause vomiting and laryngeal spasm). Once the child is anaesthetized a laryngoscope blade can be gently introduced on to the tongue so that the bleeding may be assessed. Provided it is not excessive and the patient is well oxygenated with no signs of airways obstruction, the mask is re-applied to ensure full oxygenation, then intravenous suxamethonium is given and cricoid pressure applied until the trachea is intubated. Ventilation via a facemask should be avoided as it may precipitate massive regurgitation of blood clot from the stomach. Intubation under deep halothane without relaxants may be used, but in an already hypovolaemic patient high concentrations of halothane may cause critical hypotension. The minimum alveolar concentration (MAC) of halothane for tracheal intubation is 1.33% (Yakiatas et al, 1977) which is close to the level which causes severe cardiovascular depression. If intubation is attempted too soon laryngeal spasm may occur, resulting in dangerous hypoxia.
Once the child is intubated a large-bore gastric tube should be passed to

empty the stomach (not through the nose if adenoidectomy has been under-taken). During surgery the patient should be closely monitored and blood and fluids transfused as necessary. Extubation should be in the lateral, tonsillar position once the child is fully awake.

Endoscopy

Most infants referred for diagnostic laryngoscopy and bronchoscopy, and treatment if indicated, have mild to moderate airways obstruction. Stridor is usually the presenting sign and the type of stridor (see p. 483) together with a chest X-ray, lateral X-ray of the neck, and barium swallow, will give a clue to the cause and help to anticipate difficulties.

Close co-operation and understanding between operator and anaesthetist are vital and many endoscopists would be prepared to acknowledge that the ability to make an accurate diagnosis lies in the hands of the anaesthetist. Unless the surgical requirements are met, diagnosis is impossible. Require-ments for diagnostic laryngoscopy are a still, spontaneously breathing patient, who can be maintained almost awake and without laryngospasm, so that careful assessment of cord and cricoarytenoid movement can be made.

Anaesthetic requirements are as follows:

1. *Avoidance of hypoxia*: This is the single most important requirement. Not only should one be in a position to provide adequate oxygenation to the patient at all times, but the oxygen reserve should be as great as possible, precluding the use of nitrous oxide during endoscopy: 100% oxygen should always be used, even in premature babies, where the dangers of hypoxia far outweigh the risk of retinopathy of prematurity. Before the advent of the pulse oximeter the detection of hypoxia was often delayed. All too frequently bradycardia was the first indication of hypoxia and it cannot be over-emphasized that during laryngoscopy or bronchoscopy bradycardia must always be assumed to be due to hypoxia until proved otherwise.
2. *Control of secretions*: This is essential for endoscopy for three reasons: Firstly, unless an anticholinergic agent has been used, the incidence of coughing, breath-holding and laryngospasm on induction, emergence and during endoscopy will be greatly increased. Secondly, if there are copious secretions, repeated suctioning will be required with an increased risk of hypoxia and prolongation of the procedure. Thirdly, generous topical anaesthesia is essential for good operating conditions and if drying of secretions has not been achieved the local anaesthetic will be diluted, with diminished effect (Whittet et al, 1988).
3. *Protection of the airway from acid gastric contents*: The risk of regurgitation of acid gastric contents is much greater in the presence of upper airways obstruction where induction of anaesthesia may be prolonged and diffi-cult, making gastric distension more likely. Silent aspiration postopera-tively as a result of topical anaesthesia to the larynx also makes strict preoperative starvation mandatory.

4. *Avoidance of coughing, breath-holding, laryngospasm and bronchospasm*: It is impossible to assess any part of the airway accurately if coughing and breath-holding occur, and mistakes in diagnosis may be made unless the anaesthetist can produce adequate conditions for the operator. Good topical anaesthesia and adequate depth of anaesthesia are required, whatever technique is used, and despite the newer inhalational agents, halothane remains the agent of choice as it is least irritant to the airway.
5. *Adequate ventilation*: Whether spontaneous, assisted or controlled ventilation is used, it must be adequate to prevent hypoxia, hypercarbia and ensuing acidosis. In assessment of the larynx and subglottis much of the examination must be done without the safety of a tracheal tube, therefore a technique relying on spontaneous respiration is essential. Assisted or controlled ventilation may be required during bronchoscopy, but this can readily be achieved without relaxants in infants via the Storz ventilating bronchoscope. Again, halothane is the inhalational agent of choice, as it produces less respiratory depression than either isoflurane or enflurane.
6. *Rapid wakening*: Preoperative sedation should always be avoided as rapid wakening is important not only for protection of the airway in the presence of upper airway obstruction, but for the assessment of cord and cricoarytenoid movement.

PREOPERATIVE CONSIDERATIONS

Before embarking on an endoscopy on a baby with upper airways obstruction, the anaesthetist, operating theatre staff and equipment should be properly prepared. There should always be skilled anaesthetic assistance. A wide range of tracheal tubes should be available, down to the smallest, together with semi-rigid tube introducers. The anaesthetist must be familiar with the bronchoscopic equipment and its hazards and limitations. Finally, emergency resuscitation drugs should be at hand in the event of total obstruction and inability to secure an artificial airway, as should instruments and personnel for emergency cricothyroid puncture or tracheostomy.

GENERAL ANAESTHESIA

Premedication is with intramuscular atropine in a dose of 0.02 mg/kg. This not only dries secretions, but also produces a more rapid heart rate, which helps to maintain cardiac output in the presence of halothane. Sedation should be avoided. The importance of preoperative starvation has already been emphasized.

Inhalational induction is safest, using 100% oxygen and an increasing concentration of halothane. Once consciousness is lost, the use of a tight-fitting facemask and semi-occlusion of the T-piece reservoir bag achieves a raised airway pressure which will improve gas exchange. The functional stridor of laryngomalacia will often improve or completely disappear, whereas the fixed biphasic stridor or subglottic stenosis will only improve minimally.

It should be remembered that in the presence of significant obstruction, induction of anaesthesia will be prolonged, taking many minutes to achieve sufficient depth of anaesthesia for intubation. Assisted ventilation will help to speed up this process.

Whilst anaesthesia deepens, monitoring is applied, intravenous access obtained, and a decision made whether to intubate using deep anaesthesia or a short-acting muscle relaxant. If mask ventilation is difficult relaxants should not be used. If any doubt exists, a preliminary look at the larynx will indicate the safety of paralysis.

If a short-acting muscle relaxant is used the glottis is sprayed with lignocaine before intubation. In the presence of spontaneous respiration, however, the risk of laryngospasm is high, even in experienced hands, and it is definitely safer to spray the glottis after intubation. A metered-dose 10% lignocaine spray, up to a maximum of 4–5 mg/kg, is used (the commonly used proprietary preparation contains 10 mg per aliquot). Pelton et al (1970) reported safe levels of lignocaine with a dose of 3 mg/kg, which gives a blood level of about 3 mg/l. The toxic level is between 5 mg/l (Foldes et al, 1960) and 10 mg/l (Bromage and Robson, 1961) in unanaesthetized and anaesthetized patients respectively. It is known that general anaesthesia raises the toxicity threshold and with this in mind, the higher dose of 4–5 mg/kg has been used in many large series without complications (Eyers et al, 1978).

Microlaryngoscopy

The trachea is intubated with an appropriate sized plastic nasotracheal tube (oral intubation may be preferred initially). This gives a guide to subglottic size and allows anaesthesia to be continued with a secure airway for transfer from the anaesthetic room and setting up the suspension laryngoscope and microscope for preliminary assessment of the airway. Once this is completed the tracheal tube is withdrawn to the nasopharynx and anaesthesia is maintained by insufflation of oxygen and halothane. Unless bronchoscopy is indicated, the patient is then allowed to wake up with the tip of the laryngoscope in the vallecula to allow assessment of vocal cord and cricoarytenoid movement. This technique using spontaneous respiration is the most satisfactory in infants and babies. The use of an injector attached to the laryngoscope has been used (Borland and Reilly, 1987); however, under the age of 7–8 years the gas jet distorts the glottis, ventilation is often inadequate and any functional assessment is impossible. Bronchoscopy is performed, if indicated. However it should be avoided if significant subglottic stenosis is present, as it may precipitate postoperative subglottic oedema and critical obstruction.

Bronchoscopy

Indications for bronchoscopy are either diagnostic in association with microlaryngoscopy, upper and lower airway lesions, or therapeutic as for removal

of inhaled foreign body (see p. 500), and treatment of refractory atelectasis
in older children.

Anaesthetic technique depends to a great extent on the equipment available. There are two types of rigid bronchoscope—the Negus (Figure 17.3)
and the Storz (Figure 17.4). Both have their advantages and disadvantages
(Table 17.2).

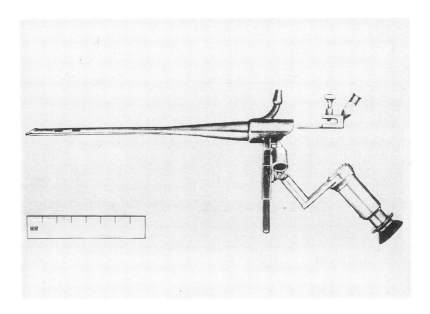

Figure 17.3. The Negus suckling bronchoscope with Venturi needle attachment
(right) and side arm for oxygen and anaesthetic gases (above). From Hatch and
Sumner (1986).

Table 17.2. Comparison of the Storz and Negus bronchoscopes

Characteristics	Storz	Negus
Intermittent positive pressure ventilation	Yes	No
Jet ventilation	No	Yes
Smallest size	2.5 mm (external diameter 4.0 mm)	Suckling (external diameter 5.0 mm)
Optics	Very good	Poor
Shape	Straight-sided	Tapered
Removal of foreign body	Difficult	Easier

Most paediatric centres use the Storz bronchoscope for its superior optical
characteristics and its side arm which allows attachment of an anaesthetic
T-piece for ventilation. With the Hopkins telescope in place it is a closed
system allowing controlled ventilation; however, there are two situations
where adequate ventilation may not be possible.

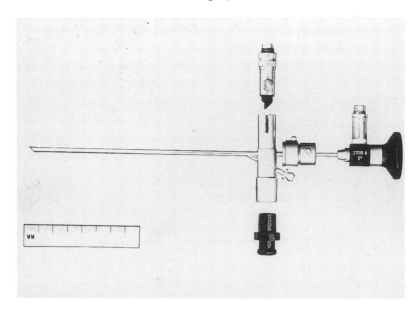

Figure 17.4. The Storz bronchoscope with light carrier (above) and attachment for anaesthetic T-piece (below). From Hatch and Sumner (1986).

Firstly, the bronchoscope has an anti-fog sheath, which if used in sizes smaller than the 5 mm (nominal size) produces unacceptable increase in resistance. The sheath should be replaced by a spacing block which prevents the telescope from projecting from the end of the bronchoscope.

Secondly, with the telescope in place, as the size of the bronchoscope decreases, the resistance to air flow increases. With the smallest 2.5 mm bronchoscope, the resistance is quite unacceptable (Table 17.3). Attempts to achieve ventilation result in prolonged expiration, air-trapping, the risk of pneumothorax and reduced venous return and cardiac output.

Table 17.3. Resistances in Storz paediatric bronchoscopes

	Gas flow resistance ($cmH_2O/l/s$)			
	Measured at 5 l flow		Measured at 10 l flow	
Bronchoscope size (mm)	Bronchoscope only	Bronchoscope and telescope	Bronchoscope only	Bronchoscope and telescope
2.5	42	1512	80	2700
3.0	21	40	30	65
3.5 (short)	12	16	15	26
3.5 (long)	12	34	19	39
4.0	8	20	15	25
5.0	6	12	12	18

From Battersby and Ridley (unpublished data).

Adequate gas exchange can very simply be achieved by frequent removal of the telescope to allow unimpeded ventilation through the bronchoscope.

The Negus bronchoscope is optically inferior to the modern bronchoscopes. The smallest (suckling) bronchoscope has an external diameter of 5 mm and is therefore rather large for small babies. Although it is not a ventilating brochoscope, its tapered shape, with wide proximal opening, allows the use of the Venturi injector for jet ventilation, and makes instrumentation easier for the removal of foreign bodies.

Although small fibreoptic bronchoscopes are now available (down to 2.7 mm external diameter) and have been used without general anaesthesia for evaluation of upper airways obstruction (Wood, 1984), their use with general anaesthesia is limited. They may have a place in difficult intubations as a guide for placement of a tracheal tube (Kleeman et al, 1987).

Premedication and induction of anaesthesia are as described for laryngoscopy, followed by full local anaesthesia of the respiratory tract.

Some anaesthetists intubate all children having bronchoscopy, although it is not strictly necessary. The child may have an abnormal airway (e.g. subglottic stenosis) and it is important that a bronchoscope of appropriate size is used (Table 17.4). It should be remembered that in a small baby 1 mm of oedema at subglottic level can reduce the airway by more than 60%. By intubating first, the surgeon can be advised of a safe size of bronchoscope to use and prevent too large a one being forced through the subglottis.

Table 17.4. Appropriate sizes of bronchoscopes and their external diameters

Size of bronchoscope (internal diameter) (mm)	External diameter (mm)	Age range
2.5	4.0	Premature to neonate
3.0	5.0	Neonate to 6 months
3.5	5.7	6–18 months
4.0	7.0	18 months to 3 years
5.0	7.8	3–8 years
6.0	8.2	> 8 years

When the surgeon is ready the tube is removed and the bronchoscope inserted. If the Storz instrument is being used the anaesthetic T-piece is connected to the side arm and anaesthesia is continued with oxygen and halothane. Assisted ventilation is usually required to maintain adequate gas exchange in infants, although paralysis is neither necessary nor advisable for diagnostic procedures where functional assessment is required.

If the Negus bronchoscope is being used, jet ventilation based on the Venturi principle is the safest way of achieving effective ventilation (Sanders, 1967). If the driving pressure is at standard pipeline pressure (413 kPa; 60 psi) it is necessary to reduce jet size to prevent barotrauma to the lungs in small children. Miyasaka et al (1980) confirmed the safety of a 19 G needle jet even in small babies. With the needle attachment at the proximal end of a tapered bronchoscope, such as the Negus, it is unlikely that the pressure reaching the lungs will be greater than 3 kPa, even with the 3 mm (suckling) bronchoscope.

Whichever bronchoscope is being used, constant communication with the operator is vital throughout the procedure, since altered position of the bronchoscope and prolonged suction may result in ineffective ventilation. Hypercarbia, hypoxia and too light or too deep anaesthesia may all cause cardiac arrhythmias such as nodal rhythm, ventricular ectopic beats, bigeminy, and bradycardia. Withdrawal of the bronchoscope into the trachea and manual hyperinflation of the lungs with 100% oxygen, adjusting the level of anaesthesia if necessary, will usually abolish any arrhythmia or bradycardia. Hypoventilation and hypoxia must be recognized early and prompt action taken to avoid serious consequences.

Monitoring for both laryngoscopy and bronchoscopy requires close constant clinical observation combined with precordial stethoscope, ECG and pulse oximetry to ensure adequate oxygenation at all times.

Postoperatively, the patient should be carefully watched until fully awake and nursed postoperatively in humidified air, or air and oxygen, in a tent or headbox. If stridor or other signs of laryngeal oedema develop racemic adrenaline or dexamethasone 0.25 mg/kg i.v. followed by three further doses of 0.1 mg/kg i.m. 6-hourly should be given. If signs of obstruction do not resolve tracheal intubation may become necessary. It is wise to give the patient nil by mouth for 3 h after the larynx has been sprayed with lignocaine.

Removal of inhaled foreign body

This is the commonest indication for bronchoscopy in children between the ages of 1 and 3 years. Although many objects and foods have been inhaled, peanuts are encountered most often in the UK. They are particularly dangerous as the oil in the nut produces mucosal irritation, oedema and often a severe pneumonitis distal to the obstruction. Typically there is a history of choking followed by coughing, stridor and occasionally dyspnoea or cyanotic attacks. Although the child may be brought to hospital straight away, in up to 30% of cases the foreign body may have been there for more than 1 week (Brown, 1973).

On examination there may be unilateral decreased air entry or wheezing. The foreign body may be visible on chest X-ray with pulmonary collapse beyond it, but if a ball-valve obstruction has occurred there will be hyperinflation on the affected side. This will be most obvious on a chest X-ray taken in expiration, if the child is old enough to co-operate (Figure 17.5).

The basic principles of anaesthesia are the same as for diagnostic bronchoscopy, although removal of a foreign body will usually take much longer. Anaesthetic technique should include atropine premedication, deep halothane anaesthesia maintaining spontaneous respiration, good local anaesthesia of the airway and avoidance of muscle relaxants. Unless the foreign body is in the trachea, intubation is useful prior to passage of the bronchoscope (see above). Air entry to both lungs should be monitored as the surgeon may dislodge the foreign body from one side to the other.

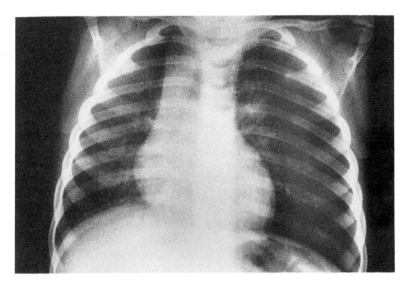

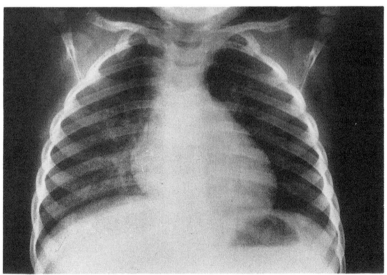

Figure 17.5. Chest X-ray of a child with an inhaled foreign body in the left main bronchus. Top: taken in expiration. Bottom: taken in inspiration. Note that on the film taken in expiration the hyperinflation of the left lung is more marked and there is mediastinal shift. From Hatch (1985), with permission.

The Storz bronchoscope is used to locate the foreign body, but often the Negus bronchoscope is used for its removal as instrumentation is easier through its larger lumen. Although there is a background of spontaneous respiration with 100% oxygen and halothane, assisted ventilation with the Storz bronchoscope or use of the Venturi injector on the Negus bronchoscope may be required to prevent hypoxia and hypercarbia.

The biggest danger occurs when the foreign body is withdrawn into the trachea and falls out of the forceps, lodging just below the cords and totally obstructing the airway. The use of a single dose of suxamethonium has been advocated just before the foreign body is pulled through the cords, but if anaesthesia is sufficiently deep, and with good local anaesthesia, this is not necessary and can be a hazardous practice. Spontaneous breathing is safer because the tracheal diameter increases during inspiration. If the foreign body does become lodged in the subglottis, rather than persevere with its removal and risk the child becoming severely hypoxic, it should be pushed back down far enough to allow adequate ventilation and a second attempt made at its removal.

The bronchoscope may have to be removed along with the foreign body, of which the external diameter often exceeds the internal diameter of the bronchoscope. The larynx may become traumatized as the bronchoscope often has to be removed and reinserted several times, making a 24-h regimen of dexamethasone, as already described on p. 419, advisable. Humidity with or without oxygen and regular physiotherapy are essential postoperatively. Antibiotics may be required if infection is present.

OPERATIVE PROCEDURES ON THE LARYNX AND TRACHEA

With the introduction of newer technology, such as the operating microscope and carbon dioxide laser, operative procedures on the larynx and trachea are being performed with increasing frequency. These procedures make specific demands on the anaesthetist for several reasons. Many of the children require repeated surgery at regular intervals over a prolonged period, and their preoperative preparation must be carefully managed. It is helpful where possible to ensure that the same anaesthetist is involved each time, so that he/she gets to know the children and parents well. Individual needs must be assessed, but most children appreciate the security of well defined preoperative rituals which do not change from week to week. The precarious nature of the airway may be a contraindication to sedative premedication, which reinforces the need for meticulous psychological preparation for surgery.

Inhalational induction with halothane is universally regarded as the safest technique in the child with the difficult airway, as it provides the smoothest induction with the lowest incidence of laryngospasm. This factor outweighs the slight risk of halothane hepatitis with repeated administration. The use of the pulse oximeter, with an audible signal which informs both the surgeon and anaesthetist of falling oxygen saturation, has significantly improved the safety of these shared airway procedures.

Microlaryngeal surgery

Many minor surgical procedures can be performed using the suspension laryngoscope without the need for tracheostomy. Various techniques for managing these cases have been used but none is ideal.

Endotracheal anaesthesia and insufflation

Spontaneous respiration with deep halothane anaesthesia is combined with topical anaesthesia as for bronchoscopy. As much surgery as is possible is performed with a small nasotracheal tube in place, which is then withdrawn to the pharynx for the remainder of the operation. In practice this technique is very satisfactory for short procedures and no special equipment is required.

Jet ventilation

This is a derivative of the Sanders bronchoscopic jet; however, as there is no tapered tube, there is little or no gas entrainment. Satisfactory blood gases can be maintained for a relatively long time using a normal ventilatory rate with the jet pressurized with oxygen at 207–413 kPa; 30–60 psi (Spoerel and Greenaway, 1973). Complete muscle paralysis must be maintained after initial deep anaesthesia and topical anaesthesia to the larynx. Intravenous supplements may be required to maintain anaesthesia. In addition to being sited on the laryngoscope blade the jet may be placed in the trachea, as described by Benjamin and Gronow (1979). The 'Ben jet' has four soft side flanges near the tip maintaining the jet in mid-trachea thus avoiding movement and damage to the tracheal mucosa as the jet is pressurized. The paediatric tube used is 16 gauge and therefore requires a driving pressure well below standard pipeline pressure, which can be achieved using the Komesaroff bronchoflator (Komesaroff and McKie, 1972). Jet ventilation is not without risk and unless the glottis is unobstructed at all times, serious barotrauma with bilateral pneumothorax may occur. The operative procedure must not obstruct the glottis at any time. Serious gastric distension and regurgitation may occur if there is poor alignment of the jet on the laryngoscope blade.

High-frequency positive pressure ventilation

High-frequency positive pressure ventilation has been used for laryngoscopy and bronchoscopy (Eriksson and Sjostrand, 1977) either via a transglottic catheter (Borg et al, 1980) or via a percutaneous transtracheal catheter (Klain and Smith, 1979). Again, muscle paralysis is essential to maintain an open glottis; however the risk of barotrauma is less as the peak inspiratory pressure is usually below that of conventional ventilation. This technique requires the use of a specially designed high-frequency jet ventilator, for example Sechrist, and as conventional chest movement is not present to assess ventilation, close monitoring including pulse oximetry is essential.

Microlaryngeal laser surgery

The carbon dioxide laser was first introduced into clinical practice in the early 1970s and is now firmly established for the treatment of obstructive lesions of the paediatric airway. It has been used in choanal atresia, nasal, nasopharyngeal and oral lesions, but its use is confined in most centres to microlaryngeal surgery, particularly for laryngeal papilloma, haemangioma and cystic hygromas extending to the base of the tongue.

For laryngeal surgery the CO_2 laser is coupled to an operating microscope and the invisible CO_2 laser beam is guided round the operating field with a visible helium neon laser. The beam can be very accurately aimed and the depth of tissue destruction precisely controlled, firstly by adjusting the power of the laser (maximum 40 W) and secondly by selecting exposure times from 0.1 to 1 s (continuous exposure is also possible). Tissue destruction is by cell vaporization and as the intracellular temperature never rises above 100°C and tissues are poor conductors of heat, there is minimal damage to contiguous areas. Healing is good and almost pain-free with minimal postoperative oedema and scarring (McGill et al, 1983). Tissue destruction is almost bloodless as vessels up to 0.5 mm in diameter are sealed by the laser.

All these advantages are especially valuable when dealing with the small dimensions of a child's airway. Laser surgery greatly reduces the incidence of postoperative difficulties and may obviate the need for a tracheostomy in some cases.

Anaesthesia for laser surgery has been reviewed by Wainwright (1987) and any anaesthetist involved in its use must be aware of the hazards involved (Carruth et al, 1980; Wainwright et al, 1981). The main problem is that all rubber and plastic tubes if ignited will burn in 100% oxygen and some in as little as 25% oxygen. Nitrous oxide supports combustion as effectively as oxygen, so its use does not reduce the problem. Gas mixtures themselves will not absorb a laser beam and therefore cannot be heated, ignited, decomposed or exploded unless some solid object first absorbs the beam. If the laser beam strikes metal (including aluminium foil) it will be deflected and the energy scattered.

The following safety precautions should be taken for all microlaryngeal surgery using a laser:

1. If a tracheal tube is used it should be a foil-wrapped red rubber tube (Figure 17.6; plastic is more inflammable than red rubber). Flexible metal tubes are available for adult use (Norton and DeVos, 1978) and these are being developed for small children.

   The tracheal tube should be wrapped with adhesive aluminium tape (3M no. 425 has been recommended). Reflective tapes are available that are non-metallic, but they present a serious fire hazard as they do not reflect CO_2 laser energy and should never be used. Application of the tape requires great care, winding it evenly with at least one half-width overlap on every turn. Wrapping from the tip and proceeding proximally prevents the laser beam from getting under the edge of the tape, and any rough edges will be less traumatic on extubation than intubation.

2. Some children will have a tracheostomy and a plastic tracheostomy tube should be changed for a silver one. The tube should not be of the fenestrated variety as this may allow the laser beam to travel down the trachea.

3. The patient's eyes and face must be protected with damp gauze and theatre personnel should wear protective goggles. The operator is protected by the optics of the microscope.

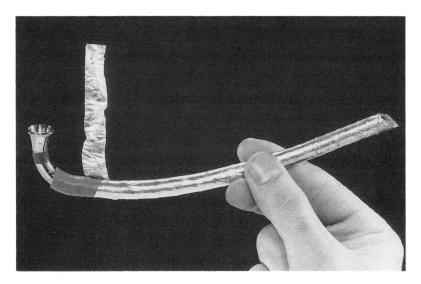

Figure 17.6. Foil-covered red rubber tracheal tube for use with laser.

4. All exposed areas in the mouth or larynx should be protected by moist
   gauze swabs (which will absorb laser energy).
5. Intravenous access is generally required.

Many workers claim that paralysis is mandatory for laser surgery (Simpson and Strong, 1983); however, at the Hospital for Sick Children, London,
we have not found that necessary. Over 500 anaesthetics have been administered using spontaneous respiration, without problems. Good topical
anaesthesia is combined with oxygen and halothane, administered via a
foil-wrapped tracheal tube to maintain deep anaesthesia. Spontaneous
respiration is retained throughout and the tube withdrawn to the pharynx
to allow areas previously obscured by it to be treated. The obvious disadvantage of this technique is the risk of ignition of the tube; however, there have
been no complications. The technique is simple, and having a tube in place
allows the surgeon to put a moist swab below the cords to protect the trachea
from the laser beam travelling beyond its target. Alternative techniques
using paralysis and supraglottic or intratracheal jet ventilation have been
described and have their advocates (Norton and DeVos, 1983; Simpson and
Strong, 1983; Scammen and McCabe, 1984); however, due to serious complications that can occur, using a tracheal tube with spontaneous respiration is
a simple and safe technique especially for babies and small children. There is
a theoretical risk that the tracheal tube may seed laryngeal papillomata
down the airway. Total intravenous techniques are unlikely to be as satisfactory in children as in adults, since the increased volume of distribution
delays recovery.

Whenever laser surgery is performed on the paediatric airway, it is safest
in the hands of an experienced team. Because of the specialized nature of the
work, and its hazards, it should not be undertaken lightly.

Supraglottic cysts

These are rare and are normally single, but may be multiple. They give rise to intermittent episodes of upper airways obstruction, but much of the time the patient may be symptom-free. A good quality lateral X-ray of the neck will usually confirm the diagnosis. Treatment is to deroof the cyst and marsupialize the base, using the suspension laryngoscope. The principles of anaesthesia are the same as for any child with upper airways obstruction. Muscle relaxants must be avoided prior to intubation as the cyst may 'ball-valve' over the glottic opening, making controlled ventilation impossible. If the larynx is unrecognizable it is useful to remember that its opening always lies behind the cyst, which is anteriorly placed arising from the vallecula. In extreme difficulty the cyst may be aspirated with a needle attached to a suction unit. Following surgery the patient should be awake before extubation, but as there is little tissue damage or oedema, recovery is usually trouble-free.

Laryngeal cleft

This is a condition that is often missed on direct laryngoscopy as the glottis appears normal superficially. A probe will reveal the deficiency posteriorly of interarytenoid tissue, which prevents competent glottic closure during swallowing. These children have episodes of aspiration and the longer the cleft the more severe the pulmonary results of aspiration. They usually require a low tracheostomy plus a feeding gastrostomy, and repair of the cleft is either achieved via an anterior laryngofissure or lateral pharyngotomy. Minor forms can be closed by direct suture using the suspension laryngoscope.

Laryngotracheoplasty

This is an operation for the relief of subglottic stenosis (Evans and Todd, 1974; Cotton and Evans, 1981). The patient will already have a low tracheostomy and the operation is performed through a collar incision immediately above the tracheostome. The cricoid ring is enlarged with a stepped incision, or if too abnormal or the first tracheal ring is stenosed, a costal cartilage graft is used. The cricoid and trachea may be closed over a roll of silastic sheet which remains sutured in place for at least 6 weeks. To allow good surgical access the head is extended and a suitable tracheostomy tube free of bulky connectors is used. A cuffed latex armoured tube, inserted into the tracheostome and taken through 180° to connect with the anaesthetic circuit over the chest, provides the most satisfactory airway. There are, however, problems attached to its use. It is important to make sure the entire cuff is within the airway or it is likely to extrude during the operation. With a low tracheostomy the distance between it and the carina is short, making accurate placement of the tube essential. Its tip must be clear of the carina to allow ventilation of both lungs, which can be achieved more readily by abolishing the bevel at the end of the tube.

The walls of these cuffed armoured tubes are very thick and occasionally it is impossible to pass even the smallest size. A shortened preformed plastic tube (e.g. Mallinckrodt, RAE tube) is an alternative, but does not have the advantages of a cuffed tube. The use of a cuffed tube prevents anaesthetic gases leaking into the operation site, and more important, blood trickling down into the trachea.

Anaesthesia consists of any technique using muscle paralysis and IPPV, having first induced anaesthesia via the tracheostome and sprayed the glottis with lignocaine. Further clearance of secretions should always be attempted using saline and suction prior to changing to the armoured tube.

The tube is inserted (using a semi-rigid tube introducer if necessary) and securely strapped in place after positioning the child for surgery with a sandbag under the shoulders and the neck extended (Figure 17.7). A suitable connector (e.g. Cardiff or Cobbs) should be used to allow easy access for further suction, if it becomes necessary. A nasogastric tube is inserted, as swallowing and drinking may be delayed postoperatively.

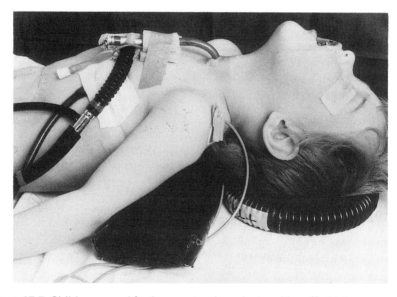

Figure 17.7. Child prepared for laryngotracheoplasty with cuffed latex armoured tube in place via tracheostome and neck hyperextended over a sandbag.

Extensive monitoring is essential and includes a precordial stethoscope, airway pressure gauge and disconnection alarm. ECG, automatic blood pressure monitor and pulse oximetry should also be routine.

Access to the patient once surgery has commenced is very limited, making close continuous monitoring of ventilation mandatory.

Intravenous fluids are administered as necessary and continued post-operatively, as the use of a silastic splint, if too long, may give rise to glottic incompetence, allowing aspiration to take place.

If a rib graft is taken a postoperative chest X-ray is essential to exclude pneumothorax.

All patients are nursed in humidified air, with added oxygen if necessary, and chest physiotherapy should not be forgotten, as there is often a temporary increase in secretions postoperatively.

Tracheostomy

Tracheostomy in infants and children still has a mortality of approximately 5%. This has not improved significantly since that estimated by Friedberg and Morrison (1974) at 3–10%. The operation is obviously safest when performed on a still, well oxygenated, anaesthetized patient. Tracheostomy should rarely be done as an emergency procedure in an unintubated, unanaesthetized patient.

With the advent of long-term nasotracheal intubation, the number of tracheostomies for respiratory support alone has been greatly reduced. Nowadays the main indications for tracheostomy relate to the many causes of congenital and acquired upper airways obstruction and the management of prolonged respiratory support.

Many patients come for tracheostomy already intubated, in which case sedative premedication may be appropriate, but unintubated patients with upper airways obstruction should have atropine alone. Inhalational induction is safest with 100% oxygen and a gradually increasing percentage of halothane. Relaxants should be avoided in the presence of upper airways obstruction and if subglottic stenosis is suspected a wide range of cut and uncut tracheal tubes should be available, down to the smallest sizes. Occasionally the stenosis is so severe that the smallest Portex tube (2.5 mm) in common usage will not pass. In this situation the smallest Cole neonatal resuscitation tube (8 French gauge) is useful; it has an external diameter of just over 2.5 mm (A 2.5 mm Portex tube has an external diameter of 3.4 mm). It must, however, be remembered that the internal diameter of an 8 French gauge Cole tube is only 1.5 mm, which poses an unacceptably high resistance to spontaneous respiration. Portex tubes of 2 mm have been manufactured, but they are so soft that it has proved impossible to pass them through a tight subglottic stenosis. The Cole tube is much more rigid, and impacted onto tight subglottic stenosis can provide a temporary airway in a difficult situation.

Local anaesthetic spray applied to the larynx and trachea prevents coughing or bucking when the trachea is being manipulated, if a spontaneous respiration technique is used. An intravenous line and full monitoring are essential.

The patient is carefully positioned with a sandbag under the shoulders and the head fully extended to bring the trachea into prominence. The surgical operation for tracheostomy in infants and children is a skilled procedure and two important rules must be observed. First, cartilage should never be excised because of the risk of tracheal collapse and stenosis, and second, the incision in the trachea should always be below the first tracheal ring, because of the risk of tracheal stenosis. A vertical incision is made in the second and third tracheal rings. If the incision is too low there is a risk of dislodgement of the tube and bronchial intubation. Two 'stay' sutures are inserted, one on each side of the tracheal incision, and these are taped to the chest wall at the end of the operation.

Before the tracheal incision is made 100% oxygen is administered and the tracheostomy tube and connectors checked. It is usual to select a tube one size larger than the anticipated tracheal tube size for the child's age. The Great Ormond Street (Aberdeen) non-cuffed plastic tracheostomy tubes prove generally satisfactory, although at the moment no British Standard connections are available for them (Figure 17.8). Portex and Shiley (silastic) are also satisfactory. When the tracheal wall is incised the tracheal tube is withdrawn into the upper trachea (it is safer not to remove it completely until the tracheostomy tube is taped in place). Once the tracheostomy tube is in place anaesthesia is continued via a sterile connector. Before the tube is tied in place the sandbag should be removed from behind the shoulders to allow the head to flex. Unless the head is flexed the ties will be too loose and the tube may fall out. It is notoriously difficult to replace a dislodged tracheostomy tube in the first few days before a tract has formed and it is for this reason that tracheal 'stay' sutures are inserted. Should the tube become accidentally dislodged, the tracheal opening is more easily re-entered by pulling the sutures apart.

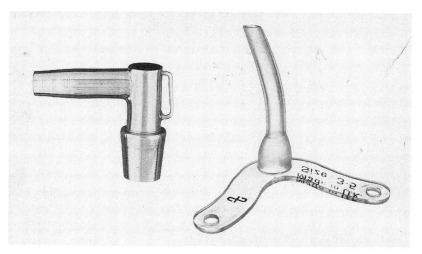

Figure 17.8. Great Ormond Street pattern tracheostomy tube with connector.

Postoperatively a chest X-ray is taken to confirm correct positioning of the tube and to exclude pneumothorax. The patient is nursed in humidified air, with added oxygen if necessary, via a tent or tracheostomy mask. Suction, following instillation of 0.5 ml normal saline, is performed at least half-hourly initially to prevent crusting of secretions and blockage of the tube. A spare tube, tapes and tracheal dilators should be at the bedside in addition to oxygen and suction, and for the first 4 h the child should never be left unattended. Babies are nursed more easily with a small roll behind the neck to prevent the chin obstructing the tracheostomy. Humidity can usually be discontinued after 2–3 weeks.

Complications of tracheostomy can be fatal; however, with careful management most should be avoidable. Tube dislodgement, obstruction of the tube with crusted secretions and bleeding usually occur in the first few days, whereas granuloma formation and vascular erosion are late complications.

REFERENCES

Benjamin B & Gronow D (1979) A new tube for microlaryngeal surgery. *Anaesthesia and Intensive Care* **7**: 258–263.

Berry FA (1986) The child with the runny nose. In Berry FA (ed) *Anaesthetic Management of Difficult and Routine Paediatric Patients*, pp 349–367. New York: Churchill Livingstone.

Borg U, Eriksson I & Sjostrand U (1980) High-frequency positive pressure ventilation (HFPPV). A review based on its use during bronchoscopy and for laryngoscopy and microlaryngeal surgery under general anaesthesia. *Anaesthesia and Analgesia* **59**: 594–603.

Borland L & Reilly J (1987) Jet ventilation for laryngeal surgery in children. Modification of the Saunders jet ventilation technique. *International Journal of Paediatric Otomicrolaryngology* **14**: 65–71.

Bradley TD & Phillipson EA (1985) Pathogenesis and pathophysiology of the obstructive sleep apnoea syndrome. *Medical Clinics of North America* **69**: 1169–1185.

Bromage PR & Robson JG (1961) Concentrations of lignocaine in the blood after intravenous, intramuscular, epidural and endotracheal administration. *Anaesthesia* **16**: 461–478.

Brouillette RT & Fernbach J (1982) Obstructive sleep apnoea in infants and children. *Journal of Pediatrics* **100**: 31–40.

Brown TCK (1973) Bronchoscopy for the removal of foreign bodies in children. *Anaesthesia and Intensive Care* **1**: 54.

Carruth JAS, McKenzie AL & Wainwright AC (1980) The carbon dioxide laser. Safety aspects. *Journal of Laryngology and Otology* **94**: 411.

Cotton R & Evans JNG (1981) Laryngeal reconstruction in children. *Annals of Otology, Rhinology and Laryngology* **90**: 516–520.

Davies DD (1964) Re-anaesthetising cases of tonsillectomy and adenoidectomy because of persistent postoperative haemorrhage. *British Journal of Anaesthesia* **36**: 244–249.

DHSS (1978–1983) *Hospital Inpatient Enquiry*. London: HMSO.

Eriksson I & Sjostrand U (1977) A clinical evaluation of high frequency positive pressure ventilation (HFPPV) in laryngoscopy under general anaesthesia. *Acta Anaesthesiologica Scandinavica* **64** (suppl): 101–110.

Evans JNG & Todd GB (1974) Laryngotracheoplasty. *Journal of Laryngology and Otology* **88**: 589–597.

Eyers RL, Kidd J, Oppenheim R & Brown TCK (1978) Local anaesthetic plasma levels in children. *Anaesthesia and Intensive Care* **6**: 243–247.

Foldes FF, Molloy R, McNall PG & Koukal LR (1960) Comparison of toxicity of intravenously given local anaesthetic agents in man. *Journal of the American Medical Association* **172**: 1493–1498.

Friedberg J & Morrison MD (1974) Paediatric tracheostomy. *Canadian Journal of Otolaryngology* **3**: 147.

Guilleminault C, Tilkian A & Dement WC (1976) The sleep apnoea syndromes. *Annual Review Medicine* **27**: 465–484.

Hatch DJ (1985) Acute upper airway obstruction in children. In Atkinson RS & Adams AP (eds) *Recent Advances in Anaesthesia and Analgesia*, vol. 15, pp 133–153. Edinburgh: Churchill Livingstone.

Hatch DJ & Sumner E (1986) *Neonatal Anaesthesia and Perioperative Care*, 2nd edn, pp 187–188. London: Edward Arnold.

Kaplan LC (1985) Choanal atresia and its associated anomalies. Further support for the CHARGE association. *International Journal of Paediatric Otorhinolaryngology* **8:** 237–242.

Klain M & Smith RB (1977) High frequency percutaneous transtracheal jet ventilation. *Critical Care Medicine* **5:** 280–287.

Kleeman PP, Jantzen JAH & Bonfils P (1987) The ultra-thin bronchoscope in management of the difficult paediatric airway. *Canadian Journal of Anaesthesia* **34:** 606–608.

Komesaroff D & McKie B (1972) The bronchoflator. A new technique for bronchoscopy under general anaesthesia. *British Journal of Anaesthesia* **44:** 1057–1068.

Macartney FJ, Panday J & Scott O (1969) Cor pulmonale as a result of chronic nasopharyngeal obstruction due to hypertrophied tonsils and adenoids. *Archives of Disease in Childhood* **44:** 585–592.

McGill T, Freidmann EM & Healy GB (1983) Laser surgery in the paediatric airway. *Otolaryngologic Clinics of North America* **16:** 865–870.

Miyasaka K, Sloan IA & Froese AB (1980) An evaluation of the jet injector (Sanders) technique for bronchoscopy in paediatric patients. *Canadian Anaesthetists' Society Journal* **27:** 117–124.

Norton ML & DeVos P (1978) New endotracheal tube for laser surgery of the larynx. *Annals of Rhinology and Laryngology* **87:** 554–557.

Paradise JL (1981) Tonsillectomy and adenoidectomy. *Pediatric Clinics of North America* **28:** 881.

Pelton DA, Daly M, Cooper PD & Conn AW (1970) Plasma lidocaine concentrations following topical aerosol application to the trachea and bronchi. *Canadian Anaesthetists' Society Journal* **17:** 250–255.

Richmond KH, Wetmore RF & Baranak CC (1987) Postoperative complications following tonsillectomy and adenoidectomy. *International Journal of Otorhinolaryngology* **13:** 117–124.

Sanders RD (1967) Two ventilating attachments for bronchoscopes. *Delaware Medical Journal* **39:** 170–175.

Scammen FL & McCabe BF (1984) Evaluation of supraglottic jet ventilation for laser surgery of the larynx. *Anesthesiology* **61:** A447.

Shalom AS (1964) Blood loss in ear nose and throat operations. *Journal of Laryngology and Otology* **78:** 734–756.

Shanahan EC, Marshall AG & Garrett CPO (1983) Adverse reactions to intravenous codeine phosphate. *Anaesthesia* **38:** 40–43.

Shott S, Myer CM & Cotton RT (1987) Efficacy of tonsillectomy and adenoidectomy as an outpatient procedure: a preliminary report. *International Journal of Paediatric Otorhinolaryngology* **13:** 157–163.

Simpson GT & Strong MS (1983) Recurrent respiratory papillomatosis. The role of the carbon dioxide laser. *Otolaryngologic Clinics of North America* **16:** 887–894.

Siodlak MZ, Gleeson MJ & Wengraf CL (1985) Post-tonsillectomy secondary haemorrhage. *Annals of the Royal College of Surgeons of England* **67:** 167–168.

Spoerel WE & Greenway RE (1973) Technique of ventilation during endolaryngeal surgery under general anaesthesia. *Canadian Anaesthetists' Society Journal* **20:** 369–377.

Tate N (1963) Deaths from tonsillectomy. *Lancet* **ii:** 1090–1091.

Thach BT (1985) Sleep apnoea in infancy and childhood. *Medical Clinics of North America* **69:** 1289–1315.

Wainwright AC (1987) Anaesthesia and laser surgery. In Kaufman L (ed) *Anaesthesia Review*, vol. 4, pp 159–165. London: Churchill Livingstone.

Wainwright AC, Moody RA & Carruth JAS (1981) Anaesthetic safety with the carbon dioxide laser. *Anaesthesia* **36:** 411.

Whittet HB, Hayward AW & Battersby E (1988) Plasma lignocaine levels during paediatric endoscopy of the upper respiratory tract. Relationship with mucosal moistness. *Anaesthesia* **43:** 439–442.

Wood P (1987) Difficulty in extubation. *Anaesthesia* **42:** 220.

Wood RE (1984) Spelunking in the pediatric airways: explorations with the flexible fiberoptic bronchoscope. *Pediatric Clinics of North America* **31:** 785.

Yakiatas RW, Blitt CD & Angiulo JP (1977) End-tidal halothane concentration for endotracheal intubation. *Anesthesiology* **47:** 386–388.

Yelderman M & New W (1983) Evaluation of pulse oximetry. *Anesthesiology* **59:** 349–352.

Emergencies in paediatric anaesthesia

INTRODUCTION

In spite of the major advances in all fields of medicine over the past two decades, there is still a significant incidence of morbidity and mortality associated with anaesthesia and surgery (Lunn et al, 1983). These advances are, paradoxically, contributing factors to the continuing mortality in that patients are coming to surgery who would previously have died or have been considered inoperable. Nowhere is this more true than in paediatrics where our better understanding of many pathophysiological processes, better perinatal and neonatal intensive care and improved transport mean that more sick infants are reaching centres where they can be operated on. One of the best examples of this is congenital diaphragmatic hernia where the continuing high mortality is largely due to the early survival of more severe cases.

Other causes of perioperative mortality are more difficult to identify precisely, although type of surgery, experience or otherwise of anaesthetist and surgeon, and age and preoperative status of the patient all play their part. One factor that is common to all studies however is that emergency surgery is associated with increased operative mortality and accounts for 50–60% of anaesthetic-related deaths (Harrison, 1978; Hovi-Viander, 1980; Lunn et al, 1983). Although the mortality totally attributable to anaesthesia is low, 83% of this is avoidable. For example, a recent confidential enquiry into perioperative deaths found that preoperative assessment and fluid replacement was inadequate in one-third of the cases, leading to untreated hypovolaemia and hypotension (Buck et al, 1987). This was often due to undue haste. Also prominent amongst the causes of death in these reports is regurgitation with pulmonary aspiration of gastric contents and the problems associated with anaesthesia and a full stomach will be discussed in some detail. The general problems associated with neonatal anaesthesia are described in Chapter 11, but specific problems of those congenital anomalies severe enough to require urgent treatment in the newborn period will be discussed in this chapter.

PREOPERATIVE ASSESSMENT

Special attention must be paid to the psychological aspects of a child undergoing emergency treatment who may be frightened, in pain and unable to comprehend his or her situation and surroundings. Children in the age group of 6 months to 5 years in particular have been shown to suffer the most severe emotional upset on hospitalization and a sympathetic approach is imperative, though not always rewarding. Although a thorough history and examination are not always possible it is essential that certain basic facts should be established. The importance of the degree of hydration and the state of the circulation have already been noted and are covered in more detail below. The respiratory system must also be thoroughly examined and any evidence of airway obstruction or embarrassment sought and treated; this is especially important in burned children who may have upper or lower respiratory tract involvement. Burned children also readily develop acute gastric distension which may impair diaphragmatic movement and thus respiratory efficiency. Gastric distension also increases the risk of regurgitation and may occur with other sick children, particularly if they are hypoxic or acidotic. In neurosurgical or trauma cases the level of consciousness must be established and any neurological deficit noted. Treatment of raised intracranial pressure with diuretics or artificial ventilation may have already been instituted. Other injuries must be identified and any medication given so far noted. The haemoglobin level should be checked, as should the serum electrolytes where there has been fluid loss. Where possible surgery should be delayed while these are corrected. Following major trauma, patients often develop secondary complications such as multiple organ failure, and frequently a coagulopathy. Measures to correct or at least to improve a coagulopathy, such as the administration of platelets or freshly thawed plasma, should be started prior to surgery, and haematological advice may be needed. In neonates calcium and glucose should also be checked as they are often low. Acid–base balance and blood gas status must be checked where there is any evidence of respiratory or cardiovascular impairment and appropriate support instituted. Finally, while it is important to establish how long it has been since the last oral intake, it should be remembered that a long period of starvation does not guarantee an empty stomach, particularly in the emergency situation.

Circulatory status (see Chapter 8)

The most frequent cause of circulatory insufficiency in infants and children is intravascular volume depletion and this may result from:

1. blood loss—external or internal;
2. plasma loss—burns, peritonitis or sepsis;
3. water and electrolyte loss—decreased intake, vomiting etc.

The active vasomotor tone of infants results in peripheral vasoconstriction as the blood volume contracts. This decreased peripheral perfusion in turn produces a metabolic acidosis and a core–periphery temperature gradient. Furthermore, decreasing pulmonary blood flow leads to hypoxia which may increase pulmonary vascular resistance, causing further hypoxia and restlessness. A full assessment of the state of hydration therefore depends on the evaluation of heart rate, blood pressure, peripheral perfusion and temperature, arterial blood gases and acid–base balance. This may be difficult and presents a challenge to all anaesthetists, particularly those not used to dealing with children. Table 18.1 illustrates some of the clinical signs that may help in this evaluation. It should be noted that these deficits relate to total body water, which in young infants represents 75–80% of body weight. An infant with a 10% deficit will therefore need approximately 80 ml/kg volume replacement, in addition to normal maintenance requirements. Total body water declines to the adult value of approximately 60% by about 1 year of age. Insensible water loss may be increased by over 100% in critically ill neonates nursed under radiant heaters, particularly if the infants weigh less than 1.5 kg (Wu and Hodgman, 1974) or if they are being ventilated (Baumgart et al, 1981), and this should be taken into account when assessing fluid replacement.

Table 18.1 Clinical signs of dehydration (from Graves, 1982)

5%	Clear sensorium
	Dry mucous membranes
	Skin turgor fair
10%	Clouded sensorium
	Dry mucous membranes
	Skin turgor poor
	Sunken fontanelle
	Raised pulse and respiratory rate
	Blood pressure may be decreased
	Urine output decreased
15%	Stuporous
	Dry, parched mouth
	Sunken fontanelle and eyes
	Rapid thready pulse
	Decreased blood pressure
	Respiratory distress
	Oliguria

Hypotension is readily caused by anaesthesia, particularly in the first 3–4 months, especially in the presence of hypovolaemia; wherever possible blood volume should be restored before surgery. The nature of the fluid replacement depends on the nature of the loss and what is available. Crystalloids are the most readily available fluids and are suitable in many cases, though expansion with plasma or 4.5% human albumin solution is longer-lasting and requires less volume. Plasma substitutes such as dextran 70 or Hespan (6% hetastarch in 0.9% sodium chloride) are as effective as plasma in restoring intravascular volume and are cheaper, though adverse reactions can occur rarely. They may however interfere with coagulation factors and should be limited to 7 ml/kg. Whole blood is the fluid of choice for major bleeding but with the trend towards blood component therapy this is increasingly difficult to obtain. In this situation packed red cells should be accompanied by recently thawed fresh frozen plasma, which contains coagulation factors. Where hypovolaemia is severe, 20 ml/kg or more may be needed and measurement of central venous pressure may be helpful. This is feasible by many routes. Right-sided filling pressures give a much better indication of the cardiac output in children than in adults and thus pulmonary artery catheters and indirect left atrial pressure measurements are rarely necessary in children without cardiac anomalies. The examination of the urine output and specific gravity (SG) are also helpful pointers. A urine output of less than 0.5 ml/kg/h suggests volume depletion, but needs to be assessed over several hours. Robinson and Gregory (1977) have shown urinary SG to be a valuable predictor of the state of hydration in the neonate. With an SG below 1009 there was no hypotension (defined as a 30% decrease in systolic blood pressure) with halothane anaesthesia, while a SG above 1009 was associated with a 75% incidence of hypotension. It should be emphasized that this is only a screening test.

REGURGITATION

It is important at the outset to distinguish between active vomiting and passive regurgitation. Vomiting is a series of co-ordinated movements involving the diaphragm, stomach, oesophagus, palate and glottis, in which there is usually sufficient preservation of laryngeal reflexes to prevent pulmonary aspiration. Regurgitation is not a co-ordinated act but the unimpeded movement of gastric contents into the oesophagus because of a pressure gradient. This has been shown to occur in up to 8% of general anaesthetics using contemporary techniques (Blitt et al, 1970) and is of far more concern to the anaesthetist because of its silent nature. In the normal conscious individual the main barrier to this flow is the lower oesophageal sphincter (LOS), a rather indistinct structure extending a few centimetres either side of the diaphragm which is affected by many drugs. It maintains a resting pressure greater than intragastric pressure, thought to be due to the spontaneous active tension developed in the circular muscle layer of the oesophagus. Any increase in intragastric pressure, such as may occur with a full stomach, or decrease in LOS pressure increases the risk of reflux. In healthy individuals, there is a reflex adaptive increase in LOS pressure to an increase in intra-abdominal pressure, thus preventing reflux (Figure 18.1; Lind et al, 1966).

It is now well established by manometric, radiological and pH studies that gastro-oesophageal reflux is exceedingly common in the first year of life. This has been attributed to the fact that the intra-abdominal segment of the oesophagus is virtually non-existent at this age so there is an abnormal LOS (Carre, 1984). The majority of infants with symptoms of reflux will improve spontaneously by 18 months of age, though up to 30% may continue to have symptoms up to the age of 4 years (Herbst, 1981). This reflux occurs readily when the stomach is distended and has been implicated as a cause of apnoea, asthma and recurrent pneumonia (Berquist et al, 1981). Aspiration during anaesthesia is three times more frequent in children than in adults (Olsson et al, 1986) and is of great importance in young infants requiring emergency anaesthesia.

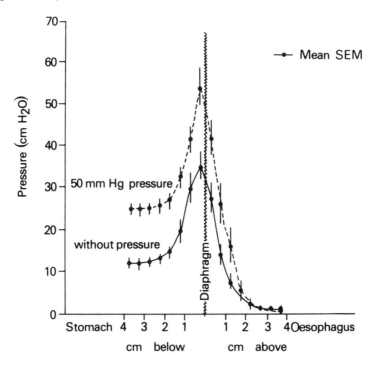

Figure 18.1. The lower oesophageal sphincter (LOS) in relationship to the dia-phragm. Also shown is the effect of increasing intra-abdominal pressure, which causes an increase in LOS pressure. From Lind et al (1966), with permission.

Death has been reported in up to 62% of adult patients following signifi-cant aspiration (Cameron et al, 1973) and may occur either by obstruction of airways or by a chemical pneumonitis, the severity of which depends on the nature and amount of the aspirate. Mendelson (1946) demonstrated that it was the acidity of gastric contents which caused the severe pulmonary damage and subsequent work has shown that a gastric pH of less than 2.5, together with a volume of more than 0.4 ml/kg, are important risk factors (Teabeaut, 1952; Roberts and Shirley, 1974). Recent work in the rat has confirmed and extended knowledge of this important interaction between gastric pH and volume in pulmonary aspiration (James et al, 1984). It is of great concern therefore that over 92% of children presenting for emergency surgery have a gastric pH of less than 2.5 and 63% also have a volume of more than 0.4 ml/kg. (Salem et al, 1976; Cote et al, 1982; Yildiz et al, 1984). This appears to be independent of the period of starvation. Olsson and Hallen (1982) found that gastric volume was directly related to severity of injury in children and there are numerous anecdotal reports that pain and anxiety delay gastric emptying. More recent studies however do not support this (Marsh et al, 1984), and Cote et al (1982) found no differences in gastric pH or volume between calm and anxious children. Since it is well recognized that prolonged fasting does not guarantee an empty stomach (Hester and Heath, 1977), all patients presenting for emergency surgery should be assumed to have a full stomach, even if starved for 6 h or more.

ANAESTHESIA IN THE PRESENCE OF A FULL STOMACH

Various methods have been suggested to minimize the risks of aspiration in these patients. Neither the use of emetics such as apomorphine nor the passage of a nasogastric tube guarantees emptying of the stomach (Holdsworth et al, 1974). Metoclopramide, by stimulating gastric emptying, has been shown to decrease significantly the volume of gastric contents in children with trauma (Olsson and Hallen, 1982) and is also known to increase LOS pressure, thereby reducing the risk of regurgitation. Unfortunately its effects on gastric emptying are completely abolished by narcotics (Nimmo et al, 1975) and its beneficial effects on the LOS are counteracted by atropine (Cotton and Smith, 1981a). Indeed all the anticholinergic agents, which are considered essential by most paediatric anaesthetists, have been shown to decrease LOS pressure significantly, if given intravenously, resulting in increased reflux as demonstrated by pH testing in the lower oesophagus (Brock-Utne et al, 1977; Cotton and Smith, 1981b). However atropine given intramuscularly produces little effect on LOS over 1 h and should not therefore increase the risk of regurgitation (Fell et al, 1983).

Another approach has been to reduce the pH of gastric contents by administering antacids. Although commonly used in obstetric anaesthesia they are only effective if properly mixed with gastric contents. They have the disadvantages of increasing gastric volume and delaying gastric emptying time. Furthermore there are numerous reports of severe lung damage and death following aspiration of antacid-containing gastric contents and the particulate antacids have been shown to produce an extensive pulmonary reaction in dogs (Gibbs et al, 1979). The non-particulate antacid 0.3 mol/l sodium citrate (0.4 ml/kg) is effective in raising gastric pH in children (Henderson et al, 1987) and would appear to be the best option. There may however be an increase in serum gastrin concentration and a subsequent acid rebound following a number of antacids (Feurle, 1975) leading to an increased postoperative risk. Much more effective are the two H_2 antagonists, cimetidine and ranitidine, both of which have shown marked inhibition of basal gastric acid secretion and that secreted in response to gastrin. Cimetidine given orally in a dose of 10 mg/kg is fully effective in children in raising gastric pH above 2.5 but is very time-dependent and must be given 2–3 h prior to induction (Yildiz et al, 1984). It has greatly decreased efficacy in children with burns however, probably due to rapid clearance, and much larger doses will be needed (Martyn, 1985). Neither agent has any effect on acid already present in the stomach and they have therefore limited usefulness in emergency anaesthesia, even if given intravenously. Results to date suggest that ranitidine is the superior agent since its longer duration of action may persist into the postoperative period but neither agent is used routinely. Adult studies suggest that a combination of cimetidine and metoclopramide is the most effective but no method is reliable.

It is apparent from the numerous articles on the subject that there is no ideal premedicant. Sedative agents should be avoided in neonates and in neurosurgical cases, and where there is any respiratory obstruction. The delaying effect of narcotics on gastric emptying should also be borne in mind. Although the use of anticholinergics in adults has been questioned it is accepted that infants and children are different, having brisk vagal reflexes and a predominantly parasympathetic innervation of the heart. Bradycardia is readily induced and unwanted secretions may easily block the small-diameter tracheal tubes used in infants. Most paediatric anaesthetists thus favour the use of anticholinergics, though many will omit them in the immediate newborn period where vagal reflexes are not so brisk and the drying effect may predispose to pulmonary complications. Although glycopyrronium (0.01 mg/kg) produces better gastric emptying (Salem et al, 1976), atropine (0.02 mg/kg) is the preferred drug because of its better vagal blocking action and its lesser drying effect. The dose should be reduced where mucociliary clearance is impaired, as in cystic fibrosis, and if the patient is febrile because sweat gland activity is also blocked. Many anaesthetists prefer to give the atropine intravenously at induction, but it should be remembered that this causes a significant fall in LOS pressure, whereas intramuscular atropine does not.

If gastric distension is present, a nasogastric tube should be passed and the stomach aspirated prior to induction. Since no single method can be relied upon to prevent regurgitation of acid gastric contents, various mechanical manoeuvres have been suggested to prevent soiling of the lungs. A head-down tilt during induction has been proposed in the hope that any contents which reflux will flow into the mouth where they can be removed by suction. However this posture inevitably increases intragastric pressure, thus increasing the likelihood of regurgitation. It may be combined with a left lateral position, though this can make intubation more difficult. Alternatively, a steep head-up (almost sitting) position during induction has been advocated on the grounds that intragastric pressure is then insufficient to lift gastric contents to the larynx. This manoeuvre is of little value in an infant because of the short length of its oesophagus. Should gastric contents reach the larynx they will amost certainly be aspirated. Furthermore, the sitting position increases the possibility of hypotension on induction, particularly if there is underlying hypovolaemia. Most anaesthetists have therefore not adopted either of these two approaches and induce their patients flat, with the facility to tip the trolley head-down should regurgitation occur. Suction apparatus should be immediately available and trained assistance is imperative. The most effective method of preventing aspiration is cricoid pressure, as described by Sellick (1961), provided that it is properly applied. It has been shown to be effective in infants even in the presence of a nasogastric tube (Salem et al, 1972).

The method of induction is a matter of personal preference and experience, the aim being to secure the airway quickly without allowing aspiration. The well established rapid induction–intubation sequence involves preoxygenation for 3–4 min followed by the intravenous administration of thiopentone 4–6 mg/kg and suxamethonium 1–2 mg/kg. Cricoid pressure should be applied by a skilled assistant as consciousness is lost and until the trachea has been intubated and its correct placement confirmed. To prevent gastric distension the lungs should not be inflated via a facemask.

It has long been taught that suxamethonium raises intragastric pressure, due to muscle fasciculation, thus increasing the risk of regurgitation. Precurarization with a small dose of non-depolarizing relaxant was thus advocated to prevent this. It has been shown however that whilst this rise in intragastric pressure does occur, suxamethonium produces a larger rise in LOS pressure (Figure 18.2; Smith et al, 1978). There is thus no increased risk of regurgitation and precurarization is unnecessary.

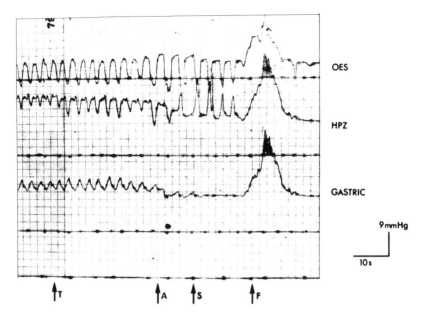

Figure 18.2. Pressure recordings following the administration of thiopentone (T) and suxamethonium (S). The patient was asleep at A, and F denotes the onset of fasciculations. HPZ is the high pressure zone, an alternative name for the lower oesophageal sphincter (LOS). Note that the increase in LOS pressure is greater than the increase in gastric pressure. From Smith et al (1978), with permission.

If it has not been possible to correct hypovolaemia and hypotension prior to induction and surgery can no longer be delayed, ketamine 2–3 mg/kg should be used as the induction agent. Where inadequacy of veins precludes an intravenous induction or where there is a major anatomical airway problem an inhalational induction may be used. Again the aim is to secure the airway as soon as possible and whichever inhalational agent is used, cricoid pressure should be applied as consciousness is lost. Intubation may then be carried out using suxamethonium intravenously or intramuscularly, or under deep inhalational anaesthesia, although the latter may not be advisable in the hypotensive patient. Maintenance of anaesthesia depends on the nature of the surgery being undertaken, and it should be remembered that the risks of regurgitation are as great at the end of the operation as at induction. Extubation should be carried out after airway reflexes have returned and with the patient on his or her side. Occasionally regional anaesthesia may be appropriate, although frightened children are often not the best subjects for this. Regional techniques are discussed in Chapter 9.

ABDOMINAL EMERGENCIES

Surgical procedures involving the gastrointestinal tract or abdominal wall account for a large proportion of emergencies in infants and children, and the principles of anaesthesia are essentially those outlined earlier, namely the restoration of circulating volume and the prevention of regurgitation. Several other conditions warrant further discussion.

Intestinal obstruction

In the newborn period, this is quite common with an incidence of 1 in 1500 births. One-third are due to the congenital atresias, of which the majority are ileal and duodenal. They are often associated with other anomalies, for example duodenal atresia with Down's syndrome and cardiac anomalies. Malrotation is the failure of the bowel to rotate and become fixed in its normal position. Obstruction may then occur either by a midgut volvulus, where the blood supply may also be compromised, by a peritoneal band, or more rarely by forming an intra-abdominal hernia. Meconium ileus occurs in 10% of infants with cystic fibrosis and is due to the impaction of thick viscous meconium in the lumen of the bowel. In some instances this is so thick that it is exceedingly difficult to express or aspirate this meconium, even from opened bowel.

The signs of obstruction depend primarily on its site but are classically those of vomiting, distension and failure to pass meconium or faeces. With a high obstruction vomiting is the predominant sign and there may be a history of maternal polyhydramnios. Dehydration and a hypochloraemic metabolic alkalosis occur, with disorders of plasma sodium and potassium, especially if the diagnosis and treatment are delayed. In duodenal atresia, a 'double bubble' on a plain abdominal X-ray may be seen, with gas in the stomach and proximal duodenum but nowhere else. Where the obstruction is low, distension is the cardinal sign and abdominal X-rays may reveal dilated loops of bowel.

In infants over 2 months of age intussusception is the commonest cause of obstruction, occuring mainly in the first year of life. This is the invagination of one section of the bowel into the next, usually at or near the ileocaecal valve. The majority of such cases are of unknown aetiology, though there is a definitive cause such as a polyp or inverted Meckel's diverticulum in 5%. As the invagination generally involves part of the mesentery there is usually venous obstruction, engorgement and eventually mucosal bleeding. The classic symptoms are of sudden paroxysms of pain of increasing frequency in a previously fit child. The pain may be severe enough to cause profuse sweating and pallor, but between paroxysms the infant may appear well. The blood and mucus that appears in the stools of over 60% of these patients has been likened to redcurrent jelly and there may be a sausage-shaped mass in the abdomen. This can occasionally be reduced by barium but will often require surgery. The affected portion of the bowel may become gangrenous and perforation and peritonitis may complicate the picture.

The general management of all these conditions is similar and surgery can usually be delayed while gastric decompression, rehydration and correction of electrolyte imbalance take place. In some situations however, such as intussusception or volvulus, there may be a compromised blood supply to the bowel and delay can increase the chances of and danger from ischaemia, necrosis, perforation and septic shock. Occasionally the metabolic acidosis that accompanies this chain of events cannot be properly corrected until the necrotic segment of bowel has been resected. It should be noted that fluid can be lost into the bowel readily, particularly in intussusception where volume depletion may be much greater than expected. These children presenting with hypotension and markedly reduced peripheral perfusion often need as much as 30–40 ml/kg of colloidal fluid. If this is given as plasma rather than blood, which is often the case in the acute situation, it is important to check the haematocrit prior to surgery. This is particularly necessary with intussusception where there may be considerable blood loss from the venous congestion that occurs from the invaginated bowel (see p. 204).

Congenital pyloric stenosis

This is a relatively common surgical problem in infancy with an incidence of 1 in 3000–4000 births, mainly males. The exact aetiology of the hypertrophy of the muscularis layer of the pylorus is unknown but the increasing obstruction it produces results in vomiting, usually presenting at 3–6 weeks. The usual clinical course is of progressive dehydration and electrolyte loss which, if not diagnosed early, may lead to gross metabolic changes. The loss of ions in the gastric fluid results in hypochloraemic alkalosis to which the kidney initially responds by excreting an alkaline urine. In an attempt to conserve sodium, chloride and extracellular volume, however, the kidney then excretes potassium and hydrogen ions in exchange for sodium, thereby exacerbating the alkalosis and producing hypokalaemia. A compensatory respiratory response to this alkalosis may result in hypoventilation and even apnoea. The concomitant fluid loss may lead to a fall in cardiac output and in urine output and subsequently to hypoxia and metabolic acidosis.

Rehydration with normal saline is urgent and the accompanying electrolyte loss must be replaced prior to surgery. This commonly takes 24–48 h but may take 3–4 days and surgery should not take place until this has been achieved. Once hydration and electrolyte status have been corrected these cases must be treated as for any high intestinal obstruction. These infants are generally too old and lusty for an awake intubation, and, as an i.v. line is always present, a rapid sequence intravenous induction with cricoid pressure should be performed (after the stomach has been aspirated.) It is the author's practice to paralyse and ventilate these patients and, depending on the speed of the surgeon, atracurium or vecuronium would appear ideal relaxants. Extubation is carried out when the infant is wide awake and able to maintain the airway. Postoperative respiratory depression is occasionally seen but this is probably related to incomplete preoperative electrolyte correction and cerebrospinal alkalosis.

Exomphalos and gastroschisis

Although these are embryologically unrelated their anaesthetic and surgical management are identical. Exomphalos is caused by an incomplete return of gut contents to the abdominal cavity during fetal life, resulting in a varying degree of intestinal herniation into the umbilical cord. This may include other organs, such as liver or spleen, and is covered with a thin transparent membrane, though this may be ruptured. These infants are often premature and there may be other major congenital anomalies, particularly cardiac ones. Gastroschisis is a herniation of intestinal contents through a defect in the lateral abdominal wall, usually on the right and is not covered by a membrane. Both anomalies require replacement of contents into the abdominal cavity and several problems may be expected. The large surface area of bowel exposed to air predisposes to infection and can result in large evaporative heat and water losses. Fluid requirements may be 100% higher than normal and there may be significant protein loss from the bowel.

There is often a poorly developed abdominal wall and it may be difficult to replace the abdominal contents entirely without causing respiratory embarrassment. However, primary closure can usually be achieved by stretching the abdominal wall and, as with all neonates, anaesthesia should include paralysis and controlled ventilation. Manual ventilation will allow the anaesthetist to warn the surgeon if the abdominal pressure produced by replacing the abdominal contents has too great an effect on lung compliance, especially as some cases are associated with a relatively small chest.

Respiratory embarrassment frequently occurs postoperatively and should be treated by ventilatory support until abdominal pressure and distension diminish. There is often impaired venous return and oedema of the lower body after primary closure and intravenous lines are better sited in the arms. There is also often a prolonged ileus postoperatively and parenteral nutrition may be required for several weeks.

Where it is impossible to replace the abdominal contents completely the extra-abdominal portion can be encased in a pouch of Prolene mesh. This can then be slowly reduced in size over a period of days until all the contents are back in the abdominal cavity and the defect fully closed. This technique has now become the procedure of choice for exomphalos in the author's unit as postoperative ventilatory support is rarely necessary and enteral feeding can be started earlier. Infection, which was a problem with the earlier Dacron pouches, does not appear to be a problem with the Prolene.

Necrotizing enterocolitis

This serious disease of newborns is seen particularly in premature infants and is characterized by varying degrees of ischaemia or necrosis of the intestinal wall. Its rising incidence probably reflects the improved survival of sick, low birthweight babies. The aetiology is still unknown but is associated with hypoperfusion of the bowel resulting in mucosal ischaemia and increased susceptibility to bacterial and hyperosmolar damage. Factors

implicated in this include prenatal asphyxia, umbilical artery catheterization, hyperosmolar feeds and exchange transfusion. A patent ductus
arteriosus is also seen quite commonly and it is postulated that this reduces
intestinal blood supply. Presenting signs generally include abdominal
distension, ileus and bloody stools, although peritonitis or septicaemia may
occur before the intestinal lesion is suspected and the infant may become
acidotic, shocked and develop a coagulopathy. There is generally a characteristic X-ray showing gas in the bowel wall (pneumatosis intestinalis).
Aggressive medical management, including the stopping of feeds, gastric
decompression, antibiotics, intravenous feeding and the removal of
potentially compromising umbilical lines etc. is often successful but surgery
is occasionally needed where the bowel has perforated or to resect any
necrotic bowel. Hypovolaemia and acidosis should be corrected if possible
and it may be necessary to ventilate these infants preoperatively. An arterial
line is helpful for monitoring pressure and acid–base balance and it is
important to have reliable venous access as bleeding can be excessive.

It has been recommended that nitrous oxide should be avoided for fear of
increasing the size of gas bubbles in the submucosa. However these infants
are often premature, with the risk that excessive oxygen may cause retinopathy of prematurity. If available, an air/oxygen mixture supplemented with
a narcotic such as fentanyl may be a sensible alternative as postoperative
ventilatory support may be needed for other problems associated with
prematurity, such as hyaline membrane disease or apnoeic episodes.

Diaphragmatic hernia

With an incidence of 1 in 4000–5000 births, this is a rare but serious cause of
respiratory distress and cyanosis at birth. Despite major improvements in its
clinical management the overall mortality remains high at 40–60% because
of the severe pulmonary hypoplasia and abnormal pulmonary vasculature,
together with associated anomalies, that accompanies this condition (David
and Illingworth, 1976). An intriguing theory that pulmonary hypoplasia is
the primary lesion in this disorder, resulting in failure of diaphragmatic
development, has been proposed by Iritani (1984). The primary defect
however is probably failure of closure of the diaphragm, allowing abdominal contents to herniate into the thoracic cavity. Some 80% of these hernias
occur through the posterolateral foramen of Bochdalek which is the last
portion of the diaphragm to close, and the slightly later closing on the left
explains the 5:1 predominance of this side. The presence of abdominal
contents in the thorax at this time leads to the disrupted development of the
ipsilateral (and to a lesser extent, contralateral) lung, usually at the 10–13-
week stage. There is therefore a severe reduction in the number of
generations of airways, particularly the distal ones, and a decreased number
of alveoli. The degree of this hypoplasia depends on the extent and exact
timing of this herniation but in severe cases the lung weight can be only
2–3 g, compared with the normal 35 g. There is also impaired development
of the pulmonary vasculature, with a reduced number and size of vessels,
and a failure of regression of the smooth muscle surrounding them. This

accentuates the normally labile tone of the neonatal pulmonary vasculature, predisposing these infants to a transitional circulation with pulmonary hypertension and right-to-left shunting. There may also be congenital cardiac anomalies, and because the normal rotation and fixation of the bowel has not occurred there is a high incidence of malrotation.

These infants generally present soon after birth with severe respiratory distress and cyanosis, a scaphoid abdomen and a characteristic chest X-ray. With large hernias the mediastinum may be displaced, compressing the contralateral lung. This condition used to be considered a true surgical emergency and these infants were operated upon immediately with little or no preoperative care. Operating on acidotic, hypoxic, hypothermic neonates is undesirable and often leads to worsening hypoxia and acidosis. Removing the abdominal contents from the thorax does not cure the underlying problem of pulmonary hypoplasia in the more severely affected infants and there is some evidence that respiratory mechanics deteriorate after surgery (Sakai et al, 1987). It is essential to improve the condition of these patients before surgery and this should include paralysis and mechanical ventilation via a tracheal tube. Ventilation by a facemask should be avoided as this will inflate the gut in the chest and increase the distress, and a nasograstric tube should be passed to decompress the stomach. These infants should ideally be ventilated to $PaCO_2$ around 5 kPa and a $PaCO_2$ around 11 kPa to avoid the acidosis and hypoxia that provoke pulmonary hypertension. Because of the pulmonary hypoplasia, however, compliance is low and there is a tendency to increase ventilator pressures to achieve this gas exchange. This should be avoided as far as possible because of the danger of causing a pneumothorax on either side. It is often better to increase rate rather than pressure and to accept a higher $PaCO_2$. The ability to achieve normocarbia without excessive ventilation is a good indicator of the degree of pulmonary hypoplasia and an accurate predictor of mortality (Bohn et al, 1984, 1987). During this period of stabilization an arterial line should be inserted for continuous pressure monitoring and blood gas sampling. Ideally this should be in the right arm so that preductal blood is sampled. A second postductal arterial line to assess ductal shunting is helpful but a transcutaneous oxygen electrode is usually sufficient.

Those patients with only mild hypoplasia can usually be stabilized and prepared for surgery within a few hours but this may take longer in infants with more hypoplastic lungs. Where there is severe pulmonary hypoplasia alternative methods of support, such as high-frequency ventilation or extracorporeal membrane oxygenation (ECMO) have been advocated (Hardesty et al, 1981). ECMO has major technical and staffing implications with significant morbidity of its own. It is unlikely that either of these approaches will help where there is insufficient lung to sustain life and the mortality in this group remains 100%. There is an intermediate group with moderate pulmonary hypoplasia who are potentially salvageable but in whom the abnormal pulmonary vasculature causes grave problems. These patients exhibit all the features of persistent pulmonary hypertension with progressive hypoxia and acidosis leading to right-to-left shunting at ductal and atrial level. The worsening hypoxia and acidosis themselves cause an increased pulmonary vascular resistance which exacerbates the situation, leading to an inexorable fall in cardiac output. Much attention has been directed at the pulmonary circulation in an attempt to prevent or break this vicious circle but as yet without universal success, though tolazoline has been effective in many cases (Sumner and Frank, 1981). This is given as a bolus of 1–2 mg/kg followed by an infusion of 1–2 mg/kg/h. As these vasodilators are not specific to the pulmonary circulation, systemic hypotension may also occur, requiring intravenous fluids and occasionally dopamine. Isoprenaline (0.05–1 µg/kg/min) may also be effective, combining inotropic and pulmonary vasodilating action.

Further work may reveal that vasoactive substances such as thromboxane are involved and that prostacyclin (4–20 ng/kg/min) may help, though none of these vasodilators can be effective where there is gross pulmonary hypoplasia.

The most effective treatment for a hypertensive crisis at present remains correction of hypoxia and acidosis by manual hyperventilation with 100% oxygen. Surgery to remove the abdominal contents from the chest and close the defect is carried out once the patient has been stable with acceptable blood gases for 24 h. This is usually through an abdominal approach and anaesthesia involves continuation of the paralysis and ventilation. High-dose fentanyl may prevent a pulmonary vasoconstrictive response to the stress of surgery and may also be useful in the pre- and postoperative management (Vacanti et al, 1984). Airway pressures must be carefully monitored and any sudden deterioration should alert the anaesthetist to the possibility of a pneumothorax. Similarly, the lungs should not be hyper-inflated in an attempt to expand the small lung at the end of surgery.

Postoperatively these infants should remain paralysed and ventilated with minimal handling for at least 48 hours as even slight disturbances can provoke a pulmonary hypertensive crisis. Attempts to prevent ductal shunting by ligating the duct have not proved successful and generally rapidly precipitate right ventricular failure. Advances in ultrasonography have made it possible to diagnose congenital diaphragmatic hernia prenatally and in-utero correction may be a solution. However the patients who will benefit from in-utero repair are those who go on to develop persistent pulmonary hypertension. Until it is possible to diagnose this high-mortality group reliably this approach is not practical (Puri and Gorman, 1987). Lung transplantation may be the only solution.

THORACIC SURGERY

In general, non-traumatic paediatric thoracic emergencies involve congenital anomalies that are severe enough to have presented during or shortly after the neonatal period. This includes tracheo-oesophageal fistula, congenital lobar emphysema, and some cardiac anomalies, discussed in Chapter 13. Problems to be anticipated include hypoxia due to intrapulmonary shunting caused by lung retraction, or contusion. The potential for major blood loss means that there should be wide-bore intravenous access. There may also be cardiovascular instability due to mediastinal manipulation and vagal traction, and the possibility of a pneumothorax must always be considered.

Double-lumen tracheal tubes, which are widely used in adults to isolate one lung, are not available in small paediatric sizes. Bronchial blockade can, however, be achieved using an embolectomy catheter passed with the help of a bronchoscope. One-lung anaesthesia can also be achieved with selective bronchial intubation although it must be remembered that the right upper lobe bronchus leaves the main bronchus just below, and occasionally at, the carina. However, neither of these manoeuvres is usually required except for fluid-filled cysts or lung abscesses.

Tracheo-oesophageal fistula and oesophageal atresia

This condition, which has an incidence of 1 in 3500, was universally fatal 50 years ago and represents one of the success stories of paediatric anaesthesia and surgery. In recent years survival in the term infant with no other anomalies has approached 100% (Spitz, 1987). Many infants are of low birthweight, approximately 30% being premature, and 20–25% have a major cardiac anomaly. In these infants, previously classified group C (Waterston et al, 1962) survival is not so good (approximately 90%). The majority have oesophageal atresia with a distal fistula, and the various types with their incidences are illustrated in Figure 18.3. The diagnosis may be suspected if there has been polyhydramnios if the midwife notes that the baby is 'mucusy' after birth, and diagnosis is usually made when a catheter cannot be passed into the stomach. Sometimes the diagnosis is not made until the child chokes or becomes cyanosed on feeding. Barium studies should never be used for confirmation as pulmonary aspiration may occur. A plain X-ray demonstrates a radiopaque catheter in the oesophageal pouch, and the presence of a gas bubble in the stomach confirms the lower pouch fistula. The main risks of this condition are aspiration of secretions or feeds, or of gastric contents via a fistula, with subsequent pulmonary infection. The oesophageal pouch should therefore be kept free of secretions, for example by using a double-lumen Replogle tube and continuous suction. If significant aspiration has already occurred chest physiotherapy and antibiotics may be required preoperatively. Anaesthetic management should include an awake intubation because of the high incidence of laryngeal abnormalities and the remote possibility of being unable to ventilate the baby after muscle relaxant.

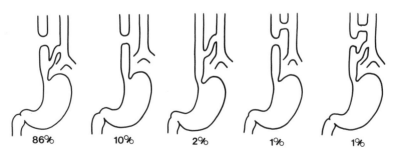

Figure 18.3. The various types of tracheo-oesophageal fistula/oesophageal atresia, with their approximate incidences.

The position of the tip of the tracheal tube is all-important in this condition with the fistula usually arising from the posterior tracheal wall, 1–2 cm above the carina. By listening over the chest and stomach, with gently assisted ventilation, it is usually possible to position the tube to achieve good lung expansion without significant gastric distension. Advancing or withdrawing the tube or rotating the bevel may be necessary to achieve this. Thereafter anaesthesia is maintained using a non-depolarizing muscle relaxant, controlled ventilation, nitrous oxide and oxygen and 0.25–0.5% halothane. Where postoperative ventilation is anticipated a short-acting narcotic may be used.

The fistula is isolated and ligated through a right thoracotomy, and the atresia repaired where possible. This is usually via an extrapleural approach unless there is an urgent need to control the fistula. There are other potential problems to be anticipated. Ventilation may be impaired by surgical retraction and secretions or blood may block the tracheal tube. Therefore manual ventilation is indicated so that any change in inflating pressure can be quickly and easily noticed. It is also important to remember that a third of these infants are premature and at risk of developing retrolental fibroplasia. If an arterial line is not available for blood gas analysis, a transcutaneous oxygen electrode or pulse oximeter may be useful.

In general these patients can be extubated at the end of surgery, but postoperative ventilation may be required if the infant is very small or has aspirated preoperatively. Ventilation may also be indicated when the primary oesophageal repair is under tension and in an attempt to limit neck movement and prevent breakdown of the repair it is the author's practice to keep these patients paralysed for 5 days. Where the gap between the upper and lower oesophageal pouches is too large for primary repair, cervical oesophagostomy and gastrostomy are performed.

Occasionally these infants have defective cartilage at the site of the fistula and develop tracheomalacia, requiring respiratory support for several days. Where this does not resolve, aortopexy may be indicated and this is frequently successful.

Congenital lobar emphysema

Although this may not cause problems for perhaps 6 months, it occasionally presents in the newborn period with severe respiratory distress. The emphysematous lobe, which is usually the right or left upper or right middle, may be due to intrinsic or extrinsic bronchial obstruction, though the aetiology is often unknown. The lobe may compress the unaffected ipsilateral or contralateral lung, and may produce marked mediastinal shift. The diagnosis is dependent on the chest X-ray where the radiolucent lobe must be distinguished from congenital lung cysts, diaphragmatic hernia, and pneumothorax. There are often associated cardiac defects such as a ventricular septal defect or a patent ductus arteriosus. These infants generally require lobectomy. Positive airway pressure and, theoretically, nitrous oxide may further distend the emphysematous lobe. Anaesthesia should therefore be induced using halothane in 100% oxygen, with gentle controlled ventilation. When the chest is opened, the lobe usually herniates out, relieving the intrathoracic compression, and bronchial intubation is unnecessary.

TRAUMA

Children are unfortunately prone to accidents, and trauma is the leading cause of death after the first year of life. The vast majority of these accidents are the result of blunt-impact trauma and half of these children suffer multiple organ injuries. It is especially important therefore that a systematic approach to assessment and resuscitation is carried out, particularly when anaesthesia appears necessary. During this assessment it should be remembered that 30–50% of children with extradural haematomas never lose consciousness and intracranial pathology must always be considered. The increased compliance of intracranial contents in children results in a greater ability to compensate for volume changes, and the normal signs of raised intracranial pressure may therefore be delayed. The discovery of a subdural haematoma in an infant under 1 year old is often due to child abuse and necessitates a thorough examination for other injuries, both old and new. Indeed, all those involved in the care of injured children should be alert to the possibility of non-accidental injury.

It appears to be neither the number of organ systems involved nor the initial blood loss that has the greatest bearing on mortality in paediatric trauma but whether or not there is an associated head injury (Colombani et al, 1985). In one series, three-quarters of the children dying during hospitalization for injuries had a significant brain injury (Mayer et al, 1981). Aggressive medical and surgical management of children with severe head injuries can reduce this mortality and morbidity and the anaesthetist has a vital role in this. Whilst the initial insult is beyond our control, further brain damage, due to cerebral ischaemia or oedema, may result from inappropriate management. Systemic hypotension, hypoxia and hypercarbia all compromise cerebral perfusion and must be treated early. Indeed 26% of head-injured patients have airway problems and 22% have hypotension (Rose et al, 1977). A secure airway must be established promptly to ensure adequate oxygenation and ventilation. This is particularly important where there are associated maxillofacial injuries, which themselves may compromise the airway and complicate intubation. Blood, debris or loose teeth may be found in the airway, and a fractured mandible can allow the tongue to fall backwards, causing obstruction.

When intubation is necessary the orotracheal route is most appropriate but a nasotracheal tube will be necessary if there are major intraoral injuries or where mandibular fixation is required. Nasotracheal intubation is inadvisable however where there is major nasopharyngeal damage or where there is concern about a basal skull fracture. The latter is often found in severe head injuries, and if accompanied by a meningeal tear allows leakage of cerebrospinal fluid from the nose or ear. This may lead to meningitis and must be covered by antibiotics.

The maintenance of a clear airway is of paramount importance however, and occasionally a tracheostomy may be necessary. Some 35% of patients with head injuries have extracranial injuries (Horton, 1976) and unless X-rays have excluded a cervical spine injury intubation should be performed with as little manipulation of the head and neck as possible.

Hypotension is rarely due to the head injury itself and if associated with tachycardia suggests hypovolaemia from bleeding elsewhere. If it is accompanied by bradycardia cervical spinal cord damage should be suspected and inotropic or chronotropic support may be necessary. Whether for airway support, radiological investigation such as computerized tomography, or surgical intervention, anaesthesia must be conducted without unduly raising intracranial pressure. Mannitol (0.25 g/kg) may be useful in reducing a critically raised intracranial pressure whilst awaiting surgery. Sedative agents may cause hypoventilation and should not be used as premedicants. As all the volatile anaesthetic agents and ketamine raise intracranial pressure, thiopentone is the induction agent of choice. Suxamethonium may cause a significant increase in intracranial pressure in patients with compromised intracranial compliance, possibly due to afferent input from muscle spindle receptors. This does not appear to be related to the degree of muscle fasciculation, although it can be prevented by pretreatment with a small 'defasciculating' dose of non-depolarizing relaxant (Stirt et al, 1987). Where there is the danger of a full stomach however, suxamethonium should still be used as part of the standard rapid induction–intubation sequence.

Acute rises in intracranial pressure during laryngoscopy and intubation are well documented, particularly where intracranial pressure is already raised, and numerous techniques have been proposed to prevent this. Most involve hypotensive agents or a second dose of thiopentone (Unni et al, 1984) which may not be advisable in the hypovolaemic patient undergoing a rapid induction–intubation sequence; therefore these techniques have not been widely adopted. After intubation adequate anaesthesia must be provided to prevent rises in intracranial pressure from surgical stimulation and a balanced technique with nitrous oxide, oxygen, muscle relaxants and a short-acting narcotic such as fentanyl (2–5 μg/kg) should be used.

Moderate hypocapnia lowers intracranial pressure and one should aim for a $PaCO_2$ of about 4 kPa. It appears that a low concentration of halothane in the presence of established hypocapnia is not associated with a rise of intracranial pressure (Adams et al, 1972). Isoflurane may be preferable as it is the least potent cerebral vasodilator. In low concentration (<1.0 MAC (minimum alveolar concentration)) it does not raise intracranial pressure, even with normocarbia (Eger, 1981) and maintains autoregulation. It may also confer some protection from cerebral hypoxia and ischaemia (Michenfelder at al, 1987).

The principles outlined above apply equally to the child undergoing surgery for non-neurosurgical injuries if there is any suspicion of head involvement and surgery cannot be delayed. Thoracic injuries occur in about 10% of blunt trauma cases but rarely require major operative intervention, though they may interfere with ventilation. Flail chest is uncommon due to the compliant chest wall and soft ribcage in children, although it can occur with separation of costochondral joints and posterior rib fractures. Lung contusion may be more common and will cause intrapulmonary shunting and increased oxygen requirements. Rupture of the diaphragm is more frequent in children than in adults and nitrous oxide should be avoided if there is significant bowel in the thorax. Chest drains with underwater seals should be inserted before surgery if pneumothorax or haemothorax are present. Tracheal or bronchial trauma should be suspected where there is bloody sputum, stridor, respiratory distress and subcutaneous emphysema of the upper chest or face. Bronchoscopy should be conducted using spontaneous ventilation. Bronchial intubation may be necessary to bypass the injury and high-frequency jet ventilation is effective where there is a major air leak. Haemopericardium may present with a large heart shadow, a high central venous pressure, tachycardia and a low cardiac output, and can be confirmed by echocardiography. If present, the pericardium must be drained under local anaesthesia before induction, otherwise anaesthesia and controlled ventilation are poorly tolerated. A widened mediastinal shadow on X-ray may also represent major vessel damage, though this is uncommon.

In recent years there have been encouraging results with non-operative management of renal, splenic and hepatic injuries in children (Wesson et al, 1981; Grisoni et al, 1984) and this has been helped by improvements in non-invasive imaging. Exploration is only carried out if the patient is unstable or there is continuing blood loss requiring replacement in excess of 40 ml/kg. In this situation good intravenous access is essential and should ideally be via a central line. Ketamine is often necessary in these situations to prevent a further fall in blood pressure on induction. Thereafter ventilation should be controlled using pancuronium (0.1 mg/kg). The same principles apply when surgery is required for intrathoracic bleeding.

Where there has been massive muscle damage, as in crush injury or electrical burns, hyperkalaemia may be present and suxamethonium should be used with caution. Myoglobinuria from the rhabdomyolysis can cause acute renal failure and measures to encourage urine output are necessary to prevent this. Other simple isolated injuries such as minor limb fractures or other soft tissue injuries do not present anaesthetic problems, provided standard 'full stomach' precautions are taken. Major fractures such as shaft of the femur do not cause major blood loss in children as they do in adults, so that if signs of shock exist then other sources of bleeding such as ruptured spleen should be sought (Fallis, 1987).

ANAESTHESIA FOR EMERGENCY EYE SURGERY

Penetrating eye injury may require removal of any foreign bodies and early wound closure and often cannot be delayed to ensure an empty stomach. This has become one of the most contentious areas of anaesthesia because of two conflicting arguments. On the one hand, the possibility of a full stomach demands rapid intubation for airway protection and this is best achieved by the rapid induction–intubation sequence using suxamethonium. On the other hand, there is the need to protect the eye from a rise in intraocular pressure since this may cause extrusion of ocular contents through even very small wounds, leading to total loss of vision in that eye. Suxamethonium causes a transient but definite rise in intraocular pressure, even in the absence of fasciculation (Feneck and Cook, 1983; Dear et al, 1987), which cannot be reliably prevented, and should not be used. Many authorities therefore recommend that intubation should be performed using a large dose of a non-depolarizing relaxant while cricoid pressure is maintained. Although pancuronium (0.2 mg/kg) has the advantage of raising LOS pressure, which has not been demonstrated with either vecuronium or atracurium (Hunt et al, 1984a, b), it was hoped that the latter drugs might act faster than pancuronium and be more suitable for a rapid intubation sequence. Although clinical impressions are favourable, studies to date have not entirely supported this (Gramstad et al, 1983), possibly because of difficulties in defining ideal intubating conditions (Bencini and Newton, 1984). The development of priming techniques to accelerate the onset of non-depolarizing blockade or its administration prior to the induction agent do not always provide good intubating conditions (Mallaiah et al, 1986). Premature attempts at intubation provoke coughing, which significantly raises intraocular pressure and should be avoided.

The balance of opinion has thus shifted in recent years and the use of suxamethonium to provide optimal intubation conditions in a rapid induction sequence is widely accepted. One of the causes of this controversy stems from the desire to establish a rigid protocol for the management of patients with a penetrating eye injury and this may not be in the best interests of the patients. A number of patients may already have lost most of the vitreous, or have sealed the wound with lens or iris tissue and in these patients a rise of intraocular pressure is of much less importance. Unfortunately, this cannot always be assessed until the eye has been examined under anaesthesia. Equally, some patients may not be at risk of a full stomach or can be deferred for sufficient time to reduce the risks of aspiration, and intubation can be carried out with more confidence using a non-depolarizing relaxant. Obviously full consultation with the surgeons is required in making a decision.

There are of course other factors which raise intraocular pressure and these must be taken into account. Ketamine raises intraocular pressure and should not be used. Crying, struggling or vomiting can raise intraocular pressure by as much as 40 mmHg and therefore there should be no attempt at passing a nasogastric tube to empty the stomach. This may also influence induction and gaseous induction may be appropriate. This has been performed satisfactorily on numerous occasions and is an acceptable alternative in experienced hands.

Laryngoscopy and intubation also produce a significant rise in intraocular pressure and this aspect requires further attention. Lignocaine 1.5 mg/kg intravenously attenuates the rise in intraocular pressure following intubation (Lerman and Kiskis, 1985) and may be helpful, and alfentanil 20 μg/kg attenuates the hypertensive response (Morton and Hamilton, 1986). This latter action should modify the intraocular pressure rise and the other short-acting narcotics can be expected to have a similar effect.

In those difficult situations where the eye is at risk and regurgitation is a concern, the following technique has been shown to provide good early intubating conditions without raising intraocular pressure and should be considered (Mirakhur et al, 1987). A secure intravenous line is established and fentanyl 2 µg/kg is given, followed by vecuronium 1.5 mg/kg. At the first sign of muscle weakness, thiopentone 5 mg/kg is given and cricoid pressure applied. Intubation can be performed 80–90 s after the vecuronium, which is approximately 60 s after loss of consciousness. A nerve stimulator is useful in indicating when full relaxation has occurred.

Maintenance of anaesthesia is a matter of personal preference since most general anaesthetic agents produce a modest decrease in intraocular pressure, ketamine being an exception. The stomach should be emptied as much as possible before the end of anaesthesia and to prevent coughing on the tracheal tube it is the author's practice, once relaxation has been reversed and the patient is breathing satisfactorily, to extubate while the patient is still asleep. Because of the risk of regurgitation this should be performed with the patient on his or her side.

BURNS

Children are unfortunately very susceptible to burns and scalds and anaesthetics are frequently involved early, both for resuscitation and where anaesthesia is required for airway protection, fasciotomy or early wound debridement. Because of the large ratio of surface area to weight in children, burns are relatively more important in this age group and mortality is greater than in adults with the same size burn.

In the immediate post-burn period several important problems may be encountered. These include resiratory tract involvement, fluid loss, intravenous access, acute gastric dilatation and temperature regulation. Loss of skin integrity also predisposes to infection and strict aseptic techniques should be adopted from the outset.

Burns of the face and neck are frequently accompanied by upper airway oedema, suggested by hoarseness and a croaky cry. This can be rapidly progressive and early tracheal intubation to protect the airway is of great importance. The lower airway may also be compromised by the inhalation of smoke, steam or toxins such as aldehydes, ketones and acrolein. This results in varying degrees of respiratory epithelial damage and hypoxia, and a high inspired oxygen concentration should always be administered. Systemic poisoning may also occur from the inhalation of cyanide and arsenic (Chi-Shing Chu, 1981). If carbon monoxide poisoning has occurred 100% oxygen will be necessary. Pulmonary oedema may also occur, either from the noxious gases or from injudicious fluid replacement and ventilatory support may be needed.

Where there has been a major hypoxic insult cerebral oedema may be present and hyperventilation for cerebral protection may be required. These inhalational pulmonary complications of course may also occur without skin damage.

One of the most difficult aspects of burns management is fluid replacement. Skin damage leads to an enormous loss of fluid, including plasma and all its protein fractions, from damaged capillaries at the burn site. The release of vasoactive substances such as serotonin and histamine from the injury causes further capillary dilatation and disordered permeability, with a massive shift of fluid from the vascular compartment into the burned tissue. Changes in vascular integrity also occur in other areas of the body, particularly the lungs and soft tissues, with further loss of protein and fluid from the vascular compartment.

Pulmonary oedema thus occurs readily even in the absence of inhalational injury. Because of these protein losses plasma colloid osmotic pressure is low, exacerbating the generalized tissue oedema. This fluid loss is directly proportional to the burn severity and can lead rapidly to hypovolaemic shock, though the systemic blood pressure is initially well maintained due to the release of catecholamines and antidiuretic hormone. Both the volume and nature of the replacement fluid have become controversial issues in the attempt to restore circulating volume without increasing oedema. There are numerous formulae for calculating volume replacement, some based on weight and others on surface area. There are theoretical advantages to those formulae that use surface area, but it is not always practical to assess this as it requires both height and weight. Since the different formulae are all apparently successful it suggests that none is ideal. More contentious is whether colloid or crystalloid should be used as the replacement fluid. Few centres now use colloid during the first 12–24 h postburn as it is thought to leak into the tissues, particularly the lungs, increasing oedema. Colloid that has leaked also tends to remain in the extravascular space long after the capillary leak has stopped, exerting an osmotic effect and prolonging the oedema. The capillary leak generally seals within about 24 h, after which time colloid will remain in the circulation and can be given to restore the colloid osmotic pressure.

The opposing view holds that the tissue oedema is in fact caused by the low colloid osmotic pressure and that colloid is necessary in the first 24 h to correct this and adequately maintain the circulation. Hypertonic saline has also been suggested in order to limit fluid requirements and oedema but this is inappropriate in children because of the high salt load. It would appear sensible to limit the amount of colloid given to about 25–30% of the fluid replacement in the first 24 h and use Ringer's lactate in 5% dextrose for the remainder (Solomon, 1985).

In calculating the fluid replacement required in children it is necessary to estimate the percentage burn. The classical 'rule of nines' has to be modified because of the disproportionately large head. This represents 18% at birth, reducing by about 1% per year until age 9 years, with the lower limbs reduced accordingly (Figure 18.4). Fluid requirements are 3 ml/kg/% burn, with half given in the first 8 h and the rest over the following 16 h. This is in addition to normal daily requirements. It is important to remember that this formula is only a guide and that it should be modified according to the response. Every effort should be made to protect the kidneys which are at risk of acute tubular necrosis from hypovolaemia and the added insults of myo- and haemoglobinuria from tissue damage. A urine flow of 1 ml/kg/h indicates satisfactory volume replacement and renal perfusion.

General anaesthesia is rarely required in the acute burn period unless fasciotomy is necessary, either for a limb or following a circumferential thoracoabdominal burn.

Tracheostomy is rarely necessary unless there are major burns involving the head and neck, and should be avoided if possible as it predisposes to

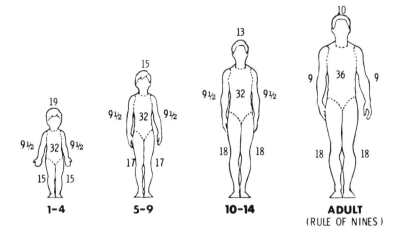

Figure 18.4. The assessment of percentage burn in children. A modified 'rule of nines' from Carvajal, with permission.

life-threatening sepsis. Burns involving large areas may give rise to difficulties in establishing intravenous access, and there may also be difficulties in securing the lines. It is important that reliable access is established, especially for early wound debridement, as blood loss can exceed twice the blood volume.

Monitoring may also be a problem, often demanding much ingenuity, and invasive techniques may be preferable. Cardiac output is reduced following major burns and it appears that there may be circulating myocardial-depressant polypeptides and lipoproteins. Within 4–5 days however cardiac output is supranormal.

One of the biggest problems is temperature regulation and a warming blanket, heated humidifier, and blood warmer should be used. The operating theatre temperature should also be high.

Halothane is best avoided because of its cutaneous vasodilatation and its propensity to cause postoperative shivering. Gastric dilatation is common following major burns, increasing the risk of regurgitation, and gastric contents are very acidic. The incidence of gastric ulceration in children is approximately twice that in adults and antacids are necessary.

One of the unfortunate effects of burns is that treatment is prolonged, necessitating multiple general anaesthetics for debridement, scar revision, skin-grafting and dressing changes. Many of the simple procedures can be accomplished satisfactorily under ketamine anaesthesia, but more major procedures need full general anaesthesia. The most important point to note is that the use of suxamethonium in burned patients is associated with a dangerous rise in serum potassium (Gronert and Theye, 1975). This has been attributed to physicochemical changes in the muscle, so that the entire membrane acts as a neuromuscular junction end-plate. The same process may account for the resistance to non-depolarizing relaxants seen in these patients, who may require up to five times the normal dosage (Martyn et al, 1983; Dwersteg et al, 1986). This phenomenon begins around 5 days after the burn and may last a year (see p 106). The pharmacokinetics of many drugs are altered after burn injury and this subject has recently been comprehensively reviewed by Martyn (1986). Late problems are further discussed in Chapter 12.

REFERENCES

Adams RW, Gronert GA, Sundt TM & Michenfelder JD (1972) Halothane, hypocapnia and cerebrospinal fluid pressure in neurosurgery. *Anesthesiology* **37:** 510–517.

Baumgart S, Engle WD, Fox WW & Polin RA (1981) Radiant warmer power and body size as determinants of insensible water loss in the critically ill neonate. *Pediatric Research* **15:** 1495–1499.

Bencini A & Newton DEF (1984) Rate of onset of good intubating conditions, respiratory depression and hand muscle paralysis after vecuronium. *British Journal of Anaesthesia* **56:** 959–965.

Berquist WE, Rachelefsky GS, Kadden M et al (1981) Gastroesophageal reflux-associated recurrent pneumonia and chronic asthma in children. *Pediatrics* **68:** 29–35.

Blitt CD, Gutman HL, Cohen DD, Weisman H & Dillon JB (1970) Silent regurgitation and aspiration during general anesthesia. *Anesthesia and Analgesia* **49:** 707–712.

Bohn DJ, James I, Filler RM et al (1984) The relationship between $PaCO_2$ and ventilation parameters in predicting survival in congenital diaphragmatic hernia. *Journal of Pediatric Surgery* **19:** 666–671.

Bohn DJ, Tamura M, Perrin D, Barker G & Rabinovitch M (1987) Ventilatory predictors of pulmonary hypoplasia in congenital diaphragmatic hernia, confirmed by morphologic assessment. *Journal of Pediatrics* **111:** 423–431.

Brock-Utne JG, Rubin J, McAravey R et al (1977) The effect of hyoscine and atropine on the lower oesophageal sphincter. *Anaesthesia and Intensive Care* **5:** 223–225.

Buck N, Devlin HB & Lunn JN (1987) *The Report of a Confidential Enquiry into Perioperative Deaths.* London: Nuffield Provincial Hospitals Trust.

Cameron JL, Mitchell WH & Zuidema GD (1973) Aspiration pneumonia. Clinical outcome following documented aspiration. *Archives of Surgery* **106:** 49–52.

Carre IJ (1984) Clinical significance of gastro-oesophageal reflux. *Archives of Disease in Childhood* **59:** 911–912.

Carvajal HF (1987) Burns. In Behrman RE & Vaughan VC (eds) *Nelson's Textbook of Pediatrics,* 13th edn, pp 223–227. Philadelphia: Saunders.

Chi-Shing Chu (1981) New concepts of pulmonary burn injury. *Journal of Trauma* **21:** 958–961.

Colombani PM, Buck JR, Dudgeon DL, Miller D & Haller JA (1985) One-year experience in a regional pediatric trauma center. *Journal of Pediatric Surgery* **20:** 8–13.

Coté CJ, Goudsouzian NG, Liu LMP, Dedrick DF & Szyfelbein SK (1982) Assessment of risk factors related to the acid aspiration syndrome in pediatric patients—gastric pH and residual volume. *Anesthesiology* **56:** 70–72.

Cotton BR & Smith G (1981a) Single and combined effects of atropine and metoclopramide on the lower oesophageal sphincter pressure. *British Journal of Anaesthesia* **53:** 869–874.

Cotton BR & Smith G (1981b) Comparison of the effects of atropine and glycopyrrolate on the lower oesophageal sphincter pressure. *British Journal of Anaesthesia* **53:** 875–879.

Dear GL, Hammerton M, Hatch DJ & Taylor D (1987) Anaesthesia and intra-ocular pressure in young children. A study of three different techniques of anaesthesia. *Anaesthesia* **42:** 259–265.

Dwersteg JF, Pavlin EG & Heimbach DM (1986) Patients with burns are resistant to atracurium. *Anesthesiology* **65:** 517–520.

Eger EI (1981) Isoflurane: a review. *Anesthesiology* **55:** 559–576.

Fallis JC (1987) Multiple injuries in paediatric emergencies, 1979. In Black JA (ed) *Multiple Injuries in Paediatric Emergencies*, 2nd edn, pp 14–31. London: Butterworths.

Fell D, Cotton BR, & Smith G (1983) I.m. atropine and regurgitation. *British Journal of Anaesthesia* **55:** 256–257.

Feneck RO & Cook JH (1983) Failure of diazepam to prevent the suxamethonium-induced rise in intra-ocular pressure. *Anaesthesia* **38:** 120–127.

Feurle GE (1975) Effect of rising intragastric pH induced by several antacids on serum gastrin concentration in duodenal ulcer patients and in a control group. *Gastroenterology* **68:** 1–7.

Gibbs CP, Schwartz DJ, Wynne JW, Hood CI & Kuck EJ (1979) Antacid pulmonary aspiration in the dog. *Anesthesiology* **51:** 380–385.

Gramstad L, Lilleaasen P & Minsaas BB (1983) Comparative study of atracurium, vecuronium (Org NC45) and pancuronium. *British Journal of Anaesthesia* **55 (suppl):** 95S–86S.

Graves SA (1982) Pediatric Blood and Fluid Therapy. In *Abstracts of the American Society of Anesthesiologists*, p 224. Las Vegas: American Society of Anesthesiologists.

Grisoni ER, Gauderer MWL, Ferron J & Izant FJ (1984) Nonoperative management of liver injuries following blunt abdominal trauma in children. *Journal of Pediatric Surgery* **19:** 515–518.

Gronert GA & Theye RA (1975) Pathophysiology of hyperkalemia induced by succinylcholine. *Anesthesiology* **43:** 89–99.

Hardesty RL, Griffith BP, Debski RF, Jeffries MR & Borovetz HS (1981) Extracorporeal membrane oxygenation. Successful treatment of persistent fetal circulation following repair of congenital diaphragmatic hernia. *Journal of Thoracic and Cardiovascular Surgery* **81:** 556–563.

Harrison GG (1978) Death attributable to anaesthesia. A 10 year survey (1967–1976). *British Journal of Anaesthesia* **50:** 1041–1046.

Henderson JM, Spence DG, Clarke WN, Bonn GG & Noel LP (1987) Sodium citrate in paediatric outpatients. *Canadian Journal of Anaesthesia* **34:** 560–562.

Herbst JJ (1981) Gastroesophageal reflux. *Journal of Pediatrics* **98:** 859–870.

Hester JB & Heath ML (1977) Pulmonary acid aspiration syndrome. Should prophylaxis be routine? *British Journal of Anaesthesia* **49:** 595–599.

Holdsworth JD, Furness RMB & Roulston RG (1974) A comparison of apomorphine and stomach tubes for emptying the stomach before general anaesthesia in obstetrics. *British Journal of Anaesthesia* **46:** 526–529.

Horton JM (1976) The anaesthetist's contribution to the care of head injuries. *British Journal of Anaesthesia* **48:** 767–771.

Hovi-Viander M (1980) Death associated with anaesthesia in Finland. *British Journal of Anaesthesia* **52:** 483–489.

Hunt PCW, Cotton BR & Smith G (1984a) Barrier pressure and muscle relaxants. Comparison of the effects of pancuronium and vecuronium on the lower oesophageal sphincter. *Anaesthesia* **39:** 412–415.

Hunt PCW, Cotton BR & Smith G (1984b) Comparison of the effects of pancuronium and atracurium on the lower oesophageal sphincter. *Anesthesia and Analgesia* **63:** 65–68.

Iritani I (1984) Experimental study on embryogenesis of congenital diaphragmatic hernia. *Anatomy and Embryology* **169:** 133–139.

James CF, Modell JH, Gibbs CP, Kuck EJ & Ruiz BC (1984) Pulmonary aspiration—effects of volume and pH in the rat. *Anesthesia and Analgesia* **63:** 665–668.

Lerman J & Kiskis AA (1985) Lidocaine attenuates the intraocular pressure response to rapid intubation in children. *Canadian Anaesthetists' Society Journal* **32:** 339–345.

Lind JF, Warrian WG & Wanklin WJ (1966) Responses of the gastroesophageal junctional zone to increases in abdominal pressure. *Canadian Journal of Surgery* **9**: 32–38.

Lunn JN, Hunter AR & Scott DB (1983) Anaesthesia-related surgical mortality. *Anaesthesia* **38**: 1090–1096.

Mallaiah S, Eltringham RJ & Magauran DM (1986) Atracurium and vecuronium in emergency eye surgery. *Anaesthesia* **41**: 84–85.

Marsh RHK, Spencer R & Nimmo WS (1984) Gastric emptying and drug absorption during surgery. *British Journal of Anaesthesia* **56**: 161–164.

Martyn JAJ (1985) Cimetidine and/or antacid for the control of gastric acidity in pediatric burn patients. *Critical Care Medicine* **13**: 1–3.

Martyn J (1986) Clinical pharmacology and drug therapy in the burned patient. *Anesthesiology* **65**: 67–75.

Martyn JAJ, Liu LMP, Szyfelbein SK, Ambalavanar ES & Goudsouzian NG (1983) Neuromuscular effects of pancuronium in burned children. *Anesthesiology* **59**: 561–564.

Mayer T, Walker ML, Johnson DG & Matlak ME (1981) Causes of morbidity and mortality in severe pediatric trauma. *Journal of the American Medical Association* **245**: 719–721.

Mendelson CL (1946) The aspiration of stomach contents into the lungs during obstetric anesthesia. *American Journal of Obstetrics and Gynecology* **52**: 191–205.

Michenfelder JD, Sundt TM, Fode N & Sharbrough FW (1987) Isoflurane when compared to enflurane and halothane decreases the frequency of cerebral ischaemia during carotid endarterectomy. *Anesthesiology* **67**: 336–340.

Mirakhur RK, Shepherd WFI, Lavery GG & Elliot P (1987) The effects of vecuronium on intra-ocular pressure. *Anaesthesia* **42**: 944–949.

Morton NS & Hamilton MB (1986) Alfentanil in an anaesthetic technique for penetrating eye injuries. *Anaesthesia* **41**: 1148–1151.

Nimmo WS, Wilson J & Prescott LF (1975) Narcotic analgesics and delayed gastric emptying in labour. *Lancet* **i**: 890-893.

Olsson GL & Hallen B (1982) Pharmacological evacuation of the stomach with metoclopramide. *Acta Anaesthesiologica Scandinavica* **26**: 417–420.

Olsson GL, Hallen B & Hambraeus-Jonzon K (1986) Aspiration during anaesthesia: a computer aided study of 185 358 anaesthetics. *Acta Anaesthesiologica Scandinavica* **30**: 84–92.

Puri P & Gorman WA (1987) Natural history of congenital diaphragmatic hernia: implications for management. *Pediatric Surgery International* **2**: 327–330.

Roberts RB & Shirley MA (1974) Reducing the risk of acid aspiration during cesarian section. *Anesthesia and Analgesia* **53**: 859–868.

Robinson S & Gregory GA (1977) Urine specific gravity as a predictor of hypovolaemia and a hypotensive response to halothane anesthesia in the newborn. *Abstracts of the American Society of Anesthesiologists* p 37. Park Ridge, Ill.: American Society of Anesthesiologists.

Rose J, Valtonen S & Jennett B (1977) Avoidable factors contributing to death after head injury. *British Medical Journal* **2**: 615–618.

Sakai H, Tamura M, Hosokawa Y, Bryan AC, Barker GA & Bohn DJ (1987) Effect of surgical repair on respiratory mechanics in congenital diaphragmatic hernia. *Journal of Pediatrics* **111**: 432–438.

Salem MR, Wong AY & Fizzotti GF (1972) Efficacy of cricoid pressure in preventing aspiration of gastric contents in paediatric patients. *British Journal of Anaesthesia* **44**: 401–404.

Salem MR, Wong AY, Mani M, Bennett EJ & Toyama T (1976) Premedicant drugs and gastric juice pH and volume in pediatric patients. *Anesthesiology* **44**: 216–219.

Sellick BA (1961) Cricoid pressure to control regurgitation of stomach contents during induction of anaesthesia. *Lancet* **ii**: 404–406.

Smith G, Dalling R & Williams TIR (1978) Gastro-oesophageal pressure gradient changes produced by induction of anaesthesia and suxamethonium. *British Journal of Anaesthesia* **50:** 1137–1143.

Solomon JR (1985) Pediatric burns. In Wachtel TL (ed) *Symposium on Burns,* pp 159–173. Philadelphia: Saunders.

Spitz L (1987) Complications in the surgery of oesophageal atresia. *Pediatric Surgery International* **2:** 1–2.

Stirt JA, Grosslight KR, Bedford RF & Vollmer D (1987) 'Defasciculation' with metocurine prevents succinylcholine-induced increases in intracranial pressure. *Anesthesiology* 67: 50–53.

Sumner E & Frank JD (1981) The effect of tolazoline on the treatment of congenital diaphragmatic hernia. *Archives of Disease in Childhood* **56:** 350–353.

Teabeaut JR (1952) Aspiration of gastric contents. An experimental study. *American Journal of Pathology* **28:** 51–67.

Unni VKN, Johnston RA, Young HSA & McBride RJ (1984) Prevention of intracranial hypertension during laryngoscopy and endotracheal intubation. Use of a second dose of thiopentone. *British Journal of Anaesthesia* **56:** 1219–1223.

Vacanti JP, Crone RK, Murphy JD et al (1984) The pulmonary hemodynamic response to perioperative anesthesia in the treatment of high risk infants with congenital diaphragmatic hernia. *Journal of Pediatric Surgery* **19:** 672–679.

Waterston DJ, Bonham Carter RE, Aberdeen E (1962) Oesophageal atresia: tracheo oesophageal fistula. A study of survival in 218 infants. *Lancet* **i:** 819–822.

Wesson DE, Filler RM, Ein SH, Shandling B, Simpson JS & Stephens CA (1981) Ruptured spleen—when to operate? *Journal of Pediatric Surgery* **16:** 324–326.

Wu PYK & Hodgman JE (1974) Insensible water loss in preterm infants: changes with postnatal development and non-ionising radiant energy. *Pediatrics* **54:** 704–712.

Yildiz F, Tryba M, Kuehn K & Hausdoerfer J (1984) Reduction of gastric acid secretion. The efficacy of pre-anaesthetic oral cimetidine in children. *Anaesthesia* **39:** 314–318.

Day-stay surgery in paediatrics

INTRODUCTION

There is little doubt that the first ether and nitrous oxide anaesthetics were administered to those whom we would now regard as day-stay patients. They underwent dental or minor surgical procedures, recovered quickly from light but effective levels of anaesthesia and left their doctors' surgeries soon afterwards. Many of these patients were children.

Day-stay surgery remained important well into the 20th century, so that in 1909, Nicoll reported on 9000 outpatient surgical procedures performed on children in Glasgow. However, concerns arose. Hipsley, in 1952, remembered: 'Children who had had their tonsils removed were sent home soon after the operation; and it is not surprising that an occasional fatality occurred due to postoperative haemorrhage.' Nor is it surprising that, with increasing availability of hygienic and comfortable hospital services and greater expectations on the part of the community, the practice fell into decline.

It is only in the last 20 years that the advantages of day-stay or short-stay admission for paediatric surgery have again been recognized widely. These include cost savings both for the individual patient and the community (Kitz et al, 1987) and a reduction in hospital-acquired infections. Otherson and Clatworthy (1968) reported a 50–70% reduction in cross-infection amongst infants undergoing outpatient herniotomy as compared to an inpatient group having the same operation.

Children aged between 6 months and 4 years are especially benefited by minimizing the duration of separation from their parents and the familiar surroundings of their homes. This results in decreased anxiety and, subsequently, less behavioural disturbance (Steward, 1973).

If the planned procedure, the patient or family circumstances render day-stay admission inadvisable, then limiting the length of hospital stay to the postoperative night helps to maintain these benefits.

Facilities

The appreciation of the advantages of day-care has led to the development of special facilities in established hospitals and free-standing day-surgery centres. Hospital-based units may make use of admission procedures, ward areas and even operating theatres different from those used by other patients. Of these, the most important is a special day-stay ward to which children are admitted and in which the staff are accustomed to the specific needs of this group of patients. Provision must be made for parents to be with their children as much as possible, even during induction of anaesthesia and recovery. In free-standing units, the staffing, equipment and monitoring used in wards, operating theatres and recovery area must be of the same standard as that specified for normal hospitals.

An essential requirement for any day-stay unit is that accommodation must be available should any patient require overnight admission. Consequently, independent units must have standing arrangements for the transfer of patients to regular hospitals, when necessary. The ease with which admission can be arranged from hospital-based units may allow more flexible policies on the types and duration of planned surgery and also may allow a formal programme of overnight admission. In this case, accommodation for parents to stay overnight with their children is desirable. Day-stay facilities in the centre of large cities with great traffic density may not be viable as appointments early in the day may be difficult to keep.

PATIENT SELECTION

The procedure

To maintain the advantages offered by day-stay programmes, the patients must be selected carefully. Initially, this will be on the basis of the planned surgery. The following general criteria, adapted from Lawrie (1964), should be met:

1. There should be minimal risk of bleeding or other surgical or anaesthetic complications occurring postoperatively.
2. No special nursing care should be needed, apart from the mother's loving attention.
3. No special drugs should need to be given postoperatively, apart from simple analgesics.
4. No restraints should be needed postoperatively, except those imposed by the child's own inclination.

Many of the operations of childhood fall within these guidelines, so that most paediatric hospitals perform a large proportion of their surgery on a day-stay basis. This figure is usually of the order of 20–40%, although Steward (1986) reported that 60% of the surgical patients at British Columbia's Children's Hospital were managed in this way. Typical procedures are listed in Table 19.1. None involves entry into a major body cavity.

Whether tonsillectomy and adenoidectomy should be performed on a day-stay basis is controversial. This is mandatory in several states of the USA and Johnson (1983) mentions the strict guidelines under which this

Table 19.1. Paediatric procedures suitable for day-stay

General surgery	*Orthopaedic*
Herniotomy	Change of plaster
Excision of hydrocoele	Manipulations
Orchidopexy	Removal of wires
Frenulectomy	
Skin lesions	*Dental*
Muscle biopsy	Conservations
	Extractions
Urology	
Cystoscopy	*Oncology*
Circumcision	Bone marrow aspiration
Glansplasty	Lumbar puncture
Meatotomy	Testicular biopsy
ENT	*Investigations*
Myringotomy and insertion tubes	Computerized tomography, magnetic
Reduction nasal fracture	resonance imaging scans
Examinations under anaesthesia	Tomography
Laryngoscopy and bronchoscopy	Gastroscopy
? Adenoidectomy	Colonoscopy
? Tonsillectomy	
Ophthalmology	
Probing tear duct	
Examinations under anaesthesia	
Chalazion excision	
Strabismus correction	

surgery is carried out in Ottawa, Canada. However, many other units are unwilling to accept the risk of major postoperative haemorrhage, which requires the return to theatre of almost 1% of patients in the first 24 h (Capper and Randall, 1984). Adenoidectomy alone is demonstrably safer and is undertaken as a day-stay procedure in some hospitals, including the author's own. If any concern arises over the condition of such patients after the operation, they must be admitted overnight. This requirement may preclude such potentially hazardous pharyngeal procedures being performed in free-standing day-surgery centres.

Special consideration also needs to be given if bilateral operations are planned. For instance, the parents of a large proportion of older children having bilateral orchidopexies in the author's hospital reported that simple analgesics, such as paracetamol, provided inadequate pain relief on the night of surgery. Consequently, these patients are scheduled for overnight admission.

The patient

Many units limit day-stay surgery to those children classified as American Society of Anaesthetists (ASA) class I or II. However, ASA class III patients, such as those being treated for a malignancy or with controlled congenital heart disease, may benefit greatly, because of the reduction in cross-infection and emotional upset. Most authorities consider that diabetics or children with other severe metabolic disturbances are unsuitable.

The common infections of childhood result in the postponement of anaesthesia and surgery for a number of children. We have found that viral upper respiratory tract infections (URTI) result in the cancellation of planned day-stay operations in about 5% of our patients. As there is a significant increase in postoperative respiratory complications amongst children who have had an URTI in the preceding 2 weeks, such patients should not be re-scheduled for about 4 weeks (Tait et al, 1983). Despite active immunization programmes, measles and pertussis still appear in many communities. Children who have had these infections retain an especially irritable airway for some time and elective surgery should not be contemplated for at least 6 weeks. Anaesthesia and surgery are probably inadvisable within 4 weeks of polio immunization.

Age is another important factor in patient selection. Healthy, full-term infants need not be excluded from day-stay programmes. On the other hand, prematurely born babies, even those who do not have a history of apnoeic episodes, should have non-essential surgery deferred until they are beyond 46 weeks' conceptual age. If operation cannot be delayed, they should be admitted and monitored for at least 18 h postoperatively (Gregory and Steward, 1983). Overnight admission and monitoring following surgery is advisable until these babies are at least 60 weeks' postconceptual age (Kurth et al, 1987). Prematurely born infants also have a high incidence of respiratory complications (Steward, 1982), probably related to persisting pulmonary pathology; they are often anaemic and are especially susceptible to hypothermia and hypoglycaemia.

Although no causal or temporal relationship has been demonstrated between anaesthesia and sudden infant death syndrome (SIDS), the possibility of an association causes great anxiety to parents who have already lost a child. Partly to allay these fears, we insist that the siblings of SIDS victims, who have an increased risk of sudden death, are admitted and monitored overnight after surgery.

The family

The medical care of any child must take into account his or her whole family situation. This is particularly relevant to day-stay surgery. Some parents are very anxious about taking their child home so soon after an operation, but may be reassured by explanation of the simple care the child will need once home, and the advantages of this form of management. However, there remain those who, because of family commitments, business demands, language difficulties or other disabilities, are unwilling or unable to co-operate. Families who live more than an hour's drive from the unit are usually excluded from day-stay programmes, although this requirement may be modified depending on the surgery and anaesthetic planned and possible complications.

The surgeon has the initial responsibility of deciding on the suitability of the individual patient for day-stay treatment on the basis of these factors. Steward (1980) recommended the use of a medical history questionnaire, completed by the parents, to assist in this process. As with adults, no routine tests apart possibly from haemoglobin are indicated for children undergoing elective day-care procedures, unless their need is suggested by the history or physical examination (Kaplan et al, 1985). Surgical assessment does not preclude the necessity for a preoperative examination by the anaesthetist, either in the day-stay ward on admission or at a special preoperative clinic held a day or two before surgery. Similar preparation is necessary for those patients admitted just before surgery, although scheduled for overnight admission.

PREPARATION FOR SURGERY

Psychological preparation

As one of the major benefits to be gained by day-stay surgery in children is the minimization of psychological trauma, special attention needs to be given to preparing families in this area. In 1978, Robert Smith commented that attempts to gain a child's confidence are useless unless that of the parents has already been won. The process of reassuring and minimizing the anxiety of both must begin in the surgeon's consulting room, with a full explanation in understandable terms of the necessary operation, why it is needed and the advantages and requirements of day-stay procedures.

Although older children should be included in this discussion, the parents are best left to explain what is to happen to toddlers, again in terms that they can understand. It is important to stress to parents that some preparation is necessary for their children, even for the very young.

Psychological preparation for hospitalization can be assisted by appropriate books, audiovisual presentations or photographic albums illustrating hospital procedures. Preoperative classes and hospital tours are of undoubted value in preparing children and their families for admission; unfortunately, the parents who usually take advantage of such programmes are often those whose levels of education and understanding suggest that formal processes may be unnecessary (Rosen et al, 1985).

Printed information and advice, prepared for the particular day-stay unit, must be given to the parents when arrangements are made for the admission. In areas with large immigrant populations, such material should be presented in the range of community languages. This information should include:

1. admission date and time;
2. admission procedures;
3. fluid restriction and fasting requirements;
4. contact telephone numbers for advice, especially if the child develops an intercurrent illness;

5. a reminder that the person caring for the child on the way home should not also attempt to drive.

Preoperative home visits or telephone calls by nurses attached to the unit have been demonstrated to be of value in ensuring that parents understand these instructions, as well as giving early warning of cancellation due to intercurrent illnesses (Postuma et al, 1987).

It is useful to seek parents' opinions regularly on the adequacy of this assistance. Since anaesthetists are involved with patients and their parents during the most stressful part of the day-stay experience, they are in a special position to judge the effectiveness of any preparatory programmes and must play a role in their development and review.

Fasting requirements

Although many studies have provided conflicting results as to whether preoperative fasting induces hypoglycaemia and ketosis in small children, prolonged thirsting certainly may result in dehydration and emotional upset (Meakin et al, 1987). While solids are not usually allowed within the 6 h preceding anaesthesia, children are often allowed clear, sugar-containing liquids until 4 h before, in order to minimize these adverse effects. As healthy, pre-school age children do not become hypoglycaemic after overnight fasting prior to morning surgery (Redfern et al, 1986), it seems unreasonable to wake them in the very early hours; instead, it is often recommended that their parents should rouse them for a drink about 11 p.m. on the preoperative night.

The practice of demand-feeding small babies up to 3 or 4 h preoperatively may heighten the risk of pulmonary aspiration by increasing residual gastric volume above that seen with clear fluids (van der Walt and Carter, 1986). Breast milk may be safer than cows' milk or some formulae, as less curd is formed and gastric emptying times are faster; we allow breastfed babies to follow their usual feeding routine until the 4 h limit; those on more frequent or special regimens may not be suitable for day-case surgery.

As mentioned earlier, parents must be given clear verbal and written instructions on the timing of fasting and the reasons for it. The degree of compliance with these orders is usually so great that equally specific recommendations, that the patient should be given fluids until a particular time, must be included.

Admission

Admission to the day-stay unit must be timed to allow the anaesthetist to meet and examine the child, if this has not been done previously, as well as for the administration of any pharmacological premedication. The fasting state must be checked and appropriate documentation completed. During any waiting periods, children should be allowed to play, preferably in special play areas.

ANAESTHESIA

The anaesthetic technique chosen for a day-stay procedure must provide for:

1. safety;
2. adequate operating conditions;
3. minimal morbidity;
4. rapid recovery;
5. maximum patient acceptance.

This last factor often precludes the use of unsupplemented local anaesthetic techniques in paediatric practice.

Premedication

As part of the process of anaesthesia, any premedication must be chosen to conform with the principles listed above. Drugs may be given preoperatively with the object of:

1. providing sedation and facilitating induction;
2. supplementing the general anaesthetic technique;
3. providing continuing analgesia in the postoperative period;
4. blocking undesirable autonomic reflexes;
5. decreasing airway secretions.

The need to meet the first three of these objectives has been questioned. Several studies have failed to produce evidence that sedative premedication increases the proportion of children who are calm at induction (Beeby and Morgan-Hughes, 1980). Consequently, many authors suggest that such drugs are unnecessary and should not be given, as they may result in prolonged recovery and delay discharge (Steward, 1980).

In contrast, others report that the unallayed anxiety of non-premedicated children frequently prevents smooth gaseous induction because of crying and increased airway secretions (Brzustowicz et al, 1984). This is especially a problem in children less than 5 years old; Rita et al (1985) have demonstrated that induction of patients in this age group is more satisfactory after premedication with midazolam than after morphine or a placebo, while recovery room stay was shorter. This may have been due to decreased anaesthetic requirements; a variety of premedications has been shown to decrease the dose of thiopentone required to induce anaesthesia (Duncan et al, 1984). Oral diazepam has also been recommended as an effective preoperative sedative for anxious children (Steward, 1986). Temazepam or midazolam may be preferable for this purpose for day-stay patients, because of their shorter duration of action.

Drugs which offer both sedative and antiemetic actions, such as trimeprazine and similar antihistamines, also offer advantages. Not only do they decrease the incidence of vomiting (Padfield et al, 1986), but they increase the pH of gastric contents, thus minimizing the risk of acid aspiration (Meakin et al, 1987). This may be an important consideration in procedures such as correction of strabismus or orchidopexy, associated with a high rate of postoperative emesis. The report of Padfield and his colleagues also demonstrated that those children who had received a sedative premedicant displayed fewer behavioural problems during the next 2 weeks at home than their peers who had been given a placebo. As this investigation related to children who had been admitted to hospital overnight, this finding should not necessarily be applied to day-stay patients.

The popularity of opiates for premedication of paediatric day-stay patients has declined because of concern over prolonged sedation and the increased incidence and duration of vomiting associated with their use (Booker and Chapman, 1979; Wilton and Burn, 1986). The realization that 30% of children describe injections as their most disliked experience while in hospital (Doughty, 1959) has also had its effect. However, pain itself causes anorexia, nausea and vomiting in the postoperative period (Anderson and Krohg, 1976). If pain cannot be alleviated or prevented by simple analgesics or local anaesthetic techniques, then narcotics are appropriate. Whether these are given pre-, intra- or postoperatively, the incidence of side-effects is similar, so that many would argue that preoperative sedation with narcotic analgesics is appropriate for painful procedures.

Bellville (1961) reported that pethidine in doses of 1 mg/kg or less decreased the incidence of vomiting after operations. Clark and Hurtig (1981) reported that the same dose did not delay discharge of adults after day-stay procedures. Thus, pethidine may be a more appropriate premedicant than other narcotics, such as morphine or papaveretum. New formulations, such as oral transmucosal fentanyl citrate, prepared as sweets which children can suck, may have a role. However, further assessment of these is necessary, especially in relation to a possible increase in residual gastric volume (Leiman et al, 1987).

Children have brisk vagal reflexes, with bradycardia a possible response to a variety of surgical stimuli. This is typically seen in the oculocardiac reflex, but occurs even with instrumentation of the airway. The administration of succinylcholine also often causes a significant reduction in heart rate. It has been demonstrated that the reduction of cardiac output which accompanies the administration of halothane in children is reversed by atropine (Barash et al, 1978). Consequently, despite the controversy over the benefits and needs for sedative premedication, it is generally agreed that children benefit from preoperative administration of an anticholinergic. In addition, this will decrease airway secretions, already mentioned as a possible cause of difficulties during gaseous induction.

Atropine is the most commonly favoured of the anticholinergic drugs for paediatric patients. It may be given orally in increased dose, when its absorption is effective although slow, as well as rectally, intramuscularly or intravenously at induction if no premedication has been given. Hyoscine is less favoured, because of its central effects and poor absorption, while glycopyrrolate may provide less protection against vagal reflexes.

From the contrasting views presented, it is apparent that the premedication requirement of each child is different. While calm, well prepared children often need no premedication, anxious ones, especially those in the younger age group, may benefit from preoperative sedation. If postoperative pain is anticipated, then narcotic administration may be justified, even if this requires an intramuscular injection. Similarly, if nausea and vomiting are seen commonly after a procedure, then antiemetic premedication is useful. In general, drugs given orally are preferred by children and those caring for them, both parents and nurses. Finally, the need for and type of premedication will be influenced by the particular day-surgery unit's structure and functioning, such as the availability of a quiet preoperative area close to the operating theatre, as well as by the circumstances surrounding the induction of anaesthesia.

Induction and maintenance

Despite the temptation to regard day-surgery as minor, day-case or overnight-stay patients require the same standard of anaesthetic care as do those undergoing more complex operations. The availability of trained assistants for the anaesthetist, as well as resuscitation and other equipment, must conform at least to the minimum standards accepted by professional or governmental bodies. Monitoring needs will vary depending on the patient's condition and the duration and complexity of the surgery. If lack of access or vision restricts direct clinical monitoring, pulse oximetry is advisable. Certainly minimal monitoring standards, such as those suggested by Cass et al (1988), must be attained in day-surgery areas.

Unless fasted for an inordinately long period, few day-stay children need intravenous fluids during surgery, as they usually resume drinking soon after they awake. However, during procedures associated with a high incidence of vomiting or a reluctance to swallow because of postoperative discomfort, appropriate volumes of glucose-containing fluids should be given.

Parental presence

One of the major benefits of day-stay treatment for children is to lessen the emotional upset occasioned by separation from parents. It has been suggested that having a parent present at induction maintains this advantage and allows sedative premedication to be omitted. Hannallah and Rosales (1983) showed that fewer children were upset at the start of their anaesthetics if accompanied by a parent, but failed to show any difference in their recovery or subsequent behaviour at home. Others argue that the anaesthetist's prime responsibility is to the physical well-being of the patient and that a parent's presence may distract from this, while offering no long-term benefit (Vivori, 1981).

Obviously, the resolution of this argument must be left to the individual anaesthetist caring for a particular child and the decision will partly depend on whether access for parents to the anaesthetic area is feasible. Special consideration must be given in the cases of blind or deaf children, or those with other communication difficulties, while those in the 1–3-year age group, who most vigorously resent separation from their parents and are most upset at induction, may also benefit from the practice (Rosen et al, 1985).

Intravenous agents

Intravenous agents offer the advantage of rapid and pleasant onset of anaesthesia. The skilled insertion of a small disposable needle provokes little complaint from most children, especially if it is kept concealed and the patient, having been warned to expect a 'scratch', is distracted by a parent or an experienced assistant. The use of EMLA cream will further reduce the pain of intravenous injection.

Thiopentone remains the most commonly used drug for this purpose. The usual dose is 4–5 mg/kg, which may need to be almost doubled in the unpremedicated child (Duncan et al, 1984). Beyond the first 15 min after anaesthesia, there is no difference in the recovery of patients given a single dose of thiopentone and those who have had a gaseous induction (Steward, 1975).

Methohexitone, in a dose of 1.5–2 mg/kg, offers a slightly more rapid recovery than thiopentone. Again, this advantage is not maintained beyond 15 min, and is gained at the cost of venous pain. Hiccuping, coughing and involuntary movements are frequent and interfere with the smooth uptake of inhalational agents.

Similarly, *propofol* allows rapid recovery but causes venous pain, even if injected in the large veins of the antecubital fossa. This pain and a high incidence of excitatory effects resulted in unsatisfactory induction in 33% of a group of children given 2.5 mg/kg after narcotic premedication (Purcell-Jones et al, 1987). These authors warned that propofol should not be injected into the smaller veins on the backs of children's hands.

The use of *etomidate* has also been reported in children. Although it allows rapid recovery and causes little respiratory or cardiovascular depression, severe venous pain, coughing and movements during injection have limited its role. Unlike methohexitone and propofol, the addition of lignocaine 1 mg/ml to the injected solution does not decrease the pain accompanying the injection (Kay, 1976).

Ketamine may be used as an intravenous or intramuscular induction agent. Despite its powerful analgesic effect, the possibility of unpleasant dreams and delayed recovery suggests that alternative drugs should be preferred in day-patients.

Rectal induction

The rectal administration of barbiturates provides an alternative method of induction. This is especially useful in children less than 3 years old, in whom venous access appears difficult and who are unlikely to be persuaded to accept gaseous induction. Methohexitone, in a dose of 25 mg/kg, is commonly used and induces sleep in 5–10 min. While recovery is prolonged beyond that seen with intravenous thiopentone, it is rapid enough to be suitable for day-stay patients (Goresky and Steward, 1979) and can be reduced significantly by removing excess unabsorbed drug by suction once anaesthesia is induced (Kestin et al, 1987). Rectal induction may be commenced outside but adjacent to the operating theatre area, allowing a parent to remain with the child until he or she is asleep. If this practice is followed, the anaesthetist must also remain with the patient continuously and full resuscitation equipment must be available immediately.

Gaseous agents

In many institutions the most common induction method is the administration of inhalational anaesthetic agents. These drugs are usually continued throughout the procedure.

Inhalational induction may be frightening, especially for children less than 3 years old, who are too young to understand explanation and accept reassurance. Sedative premedication and parental presence may be helpful, but the anaesthetist's technique is of major importance in achieving a calm induction. The facemask, preferably of clear plastic, should not be applied suddenly to the child's face; instead the gases can be directed towards the patient's nose and mouth through the delivery tubing held in the anaesthetist's cupped hand. Simple conversations and suitable stories or poems can act as a distraction. Allowing children to remain sitting upright or being nursed is sometimes helpful. Liquid food flavourings, painted on to the mask, may be of benefit as another diversion.

Nitrous oxide is used during induction as an initial sedative before the introduction of more potent volatile agents. In the technique of relative analgesia, nitrous oxide provides sufficient sedation and analgesia to allow procedures such as the changing of dressings; for surgical anaesthesia it requires supplementation. It does not seem to result in an increase in the incidence of postoperative vomiting (Muir et al, 1987); day-stay procedures are too brief for methionine synthetase suppression to be a difficulty. Thus, this agent forms the basis of most inhalational anaesthesia in such cases.

Halothane remains the standard against which the use of other volatile agents in paediatrics must be compared. It provides a smooth induction with little breath-holding or coughing, and stable maintenance. Although halothane depresses myocardial contractility, the decrease in cardiac output can be offset by the administration of atropine (Barash et al, 1978). Neither this nor the transient dysrhythmias which may be seen during induction (Kingston, 1986), have been a problem in the healthy children admitted for day-stay or short-stay procedures.

Theoretically, *enflurane* should offer more rapid induction and emergence. In fact, induction is longer because of the frequent occurrence of laryngospasm and coughing as its concentration is increased. Many paediatric anaesthetists find that enflurane does not provide smooth maintenance conditions either, and that the high inspired concentrations necessary produces more cardiovascular and respiratory depression than does halothane (O'Neill et al, 1982).

Isoflurane, when used for induction, results in more laryngospasm and excitement than either of the two preceding agents (Fisher et al, 1985). These difficulties may be minimized as the anaesthetist's experience with the drug increases (Wren et al, 1985) or by using isoflurane for maintenance after another form of induction. Recovery, both in hospital and in return to normal activities once home, is faster than with halothane or enflurane (Steward, 1986), so that isoflurane as a maintenance agent may offer particular benefits to day-stay patients.

Concern over the risk of halothane-related hepatic disease in children has resulted in a recent reappraisal of this drug. However, comparison of the rarity of the complication with the obvious advantages of halothane, particularly at induction, has led to the recommendation of its continued use, even in children who have had the drug before (Walton, 1986; Battersby et al, 1987). The relative cost of these three volatile agents also confers an advantage on halothane.

In some units, *cyclopropane* has retained a role in the rapid induction of anaesthesia. It is unsuitable for maintenance because of the high incidence of vomiting associated with its use. The risk of explosions has further restricted the use of this drug.

Methoxyflurane is clearly unsuitable as an induction agent because of its high blood/gas solubility; the risk of nephrotoxicity makes its prolonged use in high concentrations unacceptable, despite the lower peak fluoride levels seen in children. Nevertheless, it has potent analgesic effects, even in low concentrations; these may continue into the postoperative period because of its slow elimination. During spontaneous breathing techniques for laryngoscopy and bronchoscopy, the addition of 0.2–0.5% to oxygen and halothane prevents the sudden changes in depth of anaesthesia which may otherwise occur with air dilution. This agent is not now universally available.

Intubation

Spontaneous breathing techniques, using a facemask, are suitable for maintenance of anaesthesia for most paediatric day-stay surgery. When indicated, intubation should not be avoided, as the incidence of postintubation stridor is minimal after gentle laryngoscopy and the use of correctly sized, non-reactive, uncuffed tubes. If no leak can be demonstrated around a tracheal tube when a positive pressure of 20–30 cm H_2O is applied, the tube is too large and must be replaced. Although stridor usually develops rapidly, the protocols of many day-stay units insist that children should be observed for 4 h after extubation: the same time is usually required after diagnostic laryngoscopy and bronchoscopy.

Muscle relaxants

The use of muscle relaxants both facilitates intubation and reduces the amount of volatile agent needed to allow adequate operating conditions.

Succinylcholine may cause a bradycardia in children, even after a single dose; its use must be preceded by the administration of atropine, either as a premedication or intravenously after induction. Although muscle pains are uncommon in young children (Bush and Roth, 1961), their incidence may be increased in older day-stay patients who are likely to be active postoperatively. Pretreatment with a small dose of a non-depolarizing agent, such as d-tubocurarine 50 µg/kg reduces this complication.

Of the non-depolarizing relaxants, *atracurium* and *vecuronium* are especially suitable for use in day-stay patients, because of their relatively brief duration of action and lack of residual effects. If neuromuscular function is monitored, pharmacological reversal may be unnecessary in many patients, thus avoiding the adverse effects of the anticholinesterase drugs. New ultra-short-acting non-depolarizing agents seem likely to play an important role in day-case anaesthesia.

In summary, the choice of agents and techniques for induction and maintenance of anaesthesia must aim at meeting the need for minimal morbidity, rapid recovery and patient comfort and acceptance.

THE POSTOPERATIVE PERIOD

Recovery

Following surgery, patients should be returned to an appropriately staffed and equipped recovery area. The use of pulse oximetry has demonstrated that oxygen should be given to all children postoperatively, at least until they reject the face mask. By this time, the need for supplemental oxygen has declined, as haemoglobin saturation in patients breathing air improves once they are awake (Motoyama and Glazener, 1986).

Observations of temperature, circulation, respiration and state of consciousness should be recorded. A scoring system developed for the particular unit may be helpful in assessing recovery and determining fitness for discharge. In some day-stay units patients are allowed to go home directly from the recovery area; the criteria for their discharge must be more demanding than for either day-stay or overnight-stay patients returning to a ward.

Parents should be allowed to be with their children during recovery, assisting in their care and comforting. When they are adequately awake, the children should be encouraged to take small quantities of clear fluids.

Complications

The possibility of severe pain, protracted vomiting, haemorrhage or other complications following anaesthesia and surgery is one of the main determinants of whether a child should be selected for day-stay care or for overnight admission.

Pain

Pain is the most common complication of surgery and itself increases the incidence of other adverse effects, including nausea and vomiting. It is sometimes difficult to assess the severity of pain in children, especially the very young, and it must be distinguished from distress caused by separation from parents, thirst, hunger or other discomforts. The value of parents being present to alleviate this distress has already been mentioned.

The treatment of pain introduces further complications. As discussed earlier, narcotic analgesics may increase the incidence of nausea and vomiting, cause respiratory depression and prolonged sedation and thus delay discharge. Accepting these effects, single doses of narcotics given in the perioperative period are useful in the control of pain in some children undergoing day-surgery. Small doses of pethidine, codeine and fentanyl are commonly used for this purpose. Procedures which necessitate the repeated administration of narcotic analgesics for pain control are unsuitable and should not be done on a day-stay basis.

If pain-free when they awake from their anaesthetic, most patients undergoing superficial procedures obtain adequate analgesia from *paracetamol*, 10 mg/kg orally. This may be given safely to small infants, provided they are not jaundiced and have no hepatic disease. *Aspirin* is avoided, both because of its effects on platelet function and its possible relationship to the development of Reye's syndrome.

The non-steroidal anti-inflammatory agents may also have a role in postoperative analgesia, although their use has yet to be adequately assessed in children. In adults, their potency appears to be between that of paracetamol and the narcotics; diclofenac suppositories (100 mg or 2 mg/kg in suspension) have been shown to provide effective analgesia for tonsillectomy in adults (Dommery and Rasmussen, 1984) and children (dose 1–2 mg/kg t.d.s.; Bone and Fell, 1988). Ibuprofen, which is available as a suspension, may be the appropriate drug for paediatric use (5 mg/kg 6-hourly).

Regional nerve blocks, performed under anaesthesia but before surgery is begun, can provide effective pain relief. By allowing a reduction in the depth of anaesthesia and the need for potent analgesics, they speed recovery and decrease morbidity for day-stay patients (Langer et al, 1987). As local anaesthetic techniques are dealt with elsewhere in this volume, discussion here is limited to this role.

Ilioinguinal and iliohypogastric nerve blocks are useful for herniotomy and orchidopexy. The blocks may be performed by the surgeon intraoperatively, allowing accurate placement of the anaesthetic agent and decreasing the risk of haematoma. Infiltration around the skin incision for a variety of superficial procedures is also best left to the surgeon.

Caudal blocks are widely used in paediatric practice and provide effective analgesia in 80–90% of children undergoing circumcision, inguinal or perineal operations. They are simple to perform, have a low incidence of complications if 0.25% bupivacaine is used and may be used for day-stay patients (Broadman et al, 1987a). Before being allowed to go home, children who have had caudals must have no postural hypotension or dizziness and must have passed urine. Although these conditions may be met earlier, many units insist on a 4-h observation period to ensure full recovery.

For patients having circumcisions, several additional techniques have been employed. Dorsal penile nerve block is effective, but has been viewed with some concern because of reported complications associated with its use. These include intravascular injection of local anaesthetic agents, haematoma formation and ischaemia of the glans (Sara and Lowrey, 1985). Ring block of the shaft of the penis should be safer; it provides effective analgesia in 80% of patients (Broadman et al, 1987b). Lignocaine jelly, applied to the circumcision wound, while of no benefit during the procedure, relieves pain in the immediate postoperative period. Parents may be given a tube of the jelly to apply at home and this can be used to provide relief of pain and tenderness for up to 48 h (Tree-trakarn et al, 1987). Provided anaesthetists are open to the possibility, many other local anaesthetic techniques are of occasional use in day-surgery, achieving the same benefits as those specifically mentioned.

If an operation results in prolonged severe pain then it is not appropriate for it to be done on a day-stay basis. The more complex drugs and techniques mentioned above should only be necessary for the relief of pain in the immediate postoperative period and must allow reasonably prompt discharge. If this cannot be anticipated, then patients must be admitted overnight or for longer periods.

Vomiting (see also p. 247)

Apart from pain, nausea and vomiting are the most common undesired sequelae to anaesthesia and surgery in children. Their incidence varies according to the nature of the operation, but more than 50% vomit after strabismus surgery, tonsillectomy and orchidopexy. Those younger than 3 years are less affected than older children (Rowley and Brown, 1982). Persistent vomiting is the chief reason for unplanned admission of paediatric day-stay patients (Patel et al, 1986).

Measures which reduce this complication include the avoidance of narcotics, substituting other forms of analgesia whenever possible, and the use of antiemetics. Droperidol 75 µg/kg significantly decreases the incidence and frequency of vomiting after strabismus surgery (Abramowitz et al, 1983). Although these children were not fit for discharge for 6 h because of sedation, an untreated group was equally delayed by severe nausea and vomiting. A recent study at this hospital has demonstrated that trimeprazine 2 mg/kg is similarly effective (Baines, unpublished data).

Children must tolerate drinking clear fluids before they can be discharged from a day-care unit. For those who vomit more than twice, we have found that metoclopramide 150 µg/kg is helpful, even though discharge is again postponed.

Approximately 20% of day-stay patients vomit at home; many of these have not done so prior to discharge. This may be related to motion sickness. Parents should be warned of this possibility and advised to restrict their children to a light diet until the next day.

Other complications

Many patients complain of sore throats postoperatively. This is related especially to intubation, but also occurs after the use of oropharyngeal airways (Steward, 1975; Booker and Chapman, 1979). Postintubation stridor is potentially a major problem and has resulted in full admission from some units (Patel et al, 1986), although not our own. Children with croupy coughs but no signs of airway obstruction may be allowed home if no deterioration has been noted after several hours' observation.

Headaches and muscular aches are also frequent complaints. These respond to simple analgesics, although the latter can often be prevented by avoiding the use of succinylcholine without pretreatment. When lifting or positioning unconscious patients, care must be taken to avoid undue strain on muscles and ligaments, as well as to prevent pressure damage to skin or nerves.

Other less specific problems include regressive behaviour and sleep disturbances. These may be treated expectantly and are probably related to the psychological stress of hospitalization and surgery; as such, their incidence, duration and significance may well be decreased by day-stay or overnight-stay admission.

Inevitably, some children cannot be discharged at the expected time. The most common reasons for this are protracted vomiting, haemorrhage, extension of surgery beyond that originally planned, fever, drowsiness, stridor, severe pain and parental anxiety which has only become apparent postoperatively. These patients usually make up 1–2% of those admitted for day-stay procedures, although the proportion has been reported as ranging from 0.26% (Johnson, 1983) to 8% (Jones and Smith, 1980). This variation is probably explained by different policies of patient selection, with some units entering children into day-stay programmes with the knowledge that overnight admission is readily available.

Planned overnight admission provides a different approach, when it is anticipated that prolonged observation or the continuing use of potent analgesics may be necessary, or when social factors render day-care inadvisable. This allows better use of resources and provokes less anxiety for both patients and parents than does unexpected retention in hospital.

Whether children are discharged from the day-stay unit or next morning from a surgical ward, their parents need to be given adequate information about the simple care of the surgical wound, analgesia, diet and return of patients to normal activity. These instructions will vary according to the nature of the procedure but must always include a telephone number to report complications and seek advice. Even when this information has been given before admission, reinforcement at the time of discharge is essential.

REFERENCES

Abramowitz MD, Oh TH, Epstein BS, Ruttiman UE & Friendly DS (1983) The antiemetic effect of droperidol following outpatient strabismus surgery in children. *Anesthesiology* 59: 579–583.

Andersen R & Krohg K (1976) Pain as a major cause of postoperative nausea. *Canadian Anaesthetists' Society Journal* 23: 366–369.

Barash PGF, Glanz S, Katz JD, Taunt K & Talner NS (1978) Ventricular function in children during halothane anesthesia. *Anesthesiology* 49: 79–85.

Battersby EF, Glover WJ, Bingham R et al (1987) Halothane hepatitis in children. *British Medical Journal* 295: 117.

Beeby DG & Morgan-Hughes JO (1980) Behaviour of unsedated children in the anaesthetic room. *British Journal of Anaesthesia* **52**: 279–281.

Bellville JW (1961) Postanesthetic nausea and vomiting. *Anesthesiology* **22**: 773–780.

Bone ME & Fell D (1988) A comparison of rectal diclofenac with intramuscular papaveretum or placebo for pain relief following tonsillectomy. *Anaesthesia* **43**: 277–280.

Booker PD & Chapman DH (1979) Premedication in children undergoing day-care surgery. *British Journal of Anaesthesia* **51**: 1083–1087.

Broadman LM, Hannallah RS, Norden JM & McGill WA (1987a) 'Kiddie caudals': experience with 1154 consecutive cases without complications. *Anesthesia and Analgesia* **66**: S18.

Broadman LM, Hannallah RS, Belman AB et al (1987b) Post-circumcision analgesia—a prospective evaluation of subcutaneous ring block of the penis. *Anesthesiology* **67**: 399–402.

Brzustowicz RM, Nelson DA, Betts EK, Rosenberry KR & Swedlow DB (1984) Efficacy of oral premedication for pediatric outpatient surgery. *Anesthesiology* **60**: 475–477.

Bush GH & Roth F (1961) Muscle pains after suxamethonium chloride in children. *British Journal of Anaesthesia* **33**: 151–155.

Capper JWR & Randall C (1984) Postoperative haemorrhage in tonsillectomy and adenoidectomy in children. *Journal of Laryngology and Otology* **98**: 363–365.

Cass NM, Crosby WM & Holland RB (1988) Minimal monitoring standards. *Anaesthesia and Intensive Care* **16**: (in press).

Clark AJM & Hurtig JB (1981) Premedication with meperidine and atropine does not prolong recovery to street fitness after outpatient surgery. *Canadian Anaesthetists' Society Journal* **28**: 390–393.

Dommery H & Rasmussen OR (1984) Diclofenac (Voltaren): pain relieving effects after tonsillectomy. *Acta Otolaryngologica (Stockholm)* **98**: 185–192.

Doughty AG (1959) The evaluation of premedication in children. *Proceedings of the Royal Society of Medicine* **52**: 823–834.

Duncan BBA, Zaimi F, Newman GB, Jenkins JG & Aveling W (1984) Effect of premedication on the induction dose of thiopentone in children. *Anaesthesia* **39**: 426–428.

Fisher DM, Robinson S, Brett CM, Perin G & Gregory GA (1985) Comparison of enflurane, halothane and isoflurane for diagnostic and therapeutic procedures in children with malignancies. *Anesthesiology* **63**: 647–650.

Goresky GV & Steward DJ (1979) Rectal methohexitone for induction of anaesthesia in children. *Canadian Anaesthetists' Society Journal* **26**: 213–215.

Gregory GA & Steward DJ (1983) Life threatening perioperative apnoea in the 'ex premie'. Editoral. *Anesthesiology* **59**: 495–498.

Hannallah RS & Rosales JK (1983) Experience with parents' presence during anaesthesia induction in children. *Canadian Anaesthetists' Society Journal* **30**: 286–289.

Hipsley PL (1952) *The Early History of the Royal Alexandra Hospital for Children, Sydney. 1880 to 1905.* Sydney: Angus and Robertson.

Johnson GG (1983) Day care surgery for infants and children. *Canadian Anaesthetists' Society Journal* **30**: 553–557.

Jones SEF & Smith BAC (1980) Anesthesia for pediatric day-surgery. *Journal of Pediatric Surgery* **15**: 31–33.

Kaplan EB, Sheiner LB, Boeckmann AJ et al (1985) The usefulness of preoperative laboratory screening. *Journal of the American Medical Association* **253**: 3576–3581.

Kay B (1976) A clinical assessment of the use of etomidate in children. *British Journal of Anaesthesia* **48**: 207–211.

Kestin IG, McIlvaine WB, Lockhart CH, Kestin KJ & Jones M (1987) Pediatric rectal methohexitone induction with and without rectal suctioning after sleep. *Anesthesiology* **67**: A493.

Kingston HGC (1986) Halothane and isoflurane anesthesia in pediatric outpatients. *Anesthesia and Analgesia* **65**: 181–184.

Kitz DS, Lecky JH, Slusarz-Ladden C & Conahan TJ (1987) Inpatient vs. day surgery: differences in resource use, patient volume and anesthesia reimbursement. *Anesthesia and Analgesia* **66**: S97.

Kurth CD, Spitzer AR, Broennie AM & Downes JJ (1987) Postoperative apnea in preterm infants. *Anesthesiology* **66**: 483–488.

Langer JC, Shandling B & Rosenberg M (1987) Intraoperative bupivacaine during outpatient hernia repair in children: a randomized double blind trial. *Journal of Pediatric Surgery* **22**: 267–270.

Lawrie R (1964) Operating on children as day cases. *Lancet* **ii**: 1289–1291.

Leiman BC, Walford A, Rowal N et al (1987) The effects of oral transmucosal fentanyl citrate premedication on gastric volume and acidity in children. *Anesthesiology* **67**: A489.

Meakin G, Dingwall AE & Addison GM (1987) Effects of fasting and oral premedication on the pH and volume of gastric aspirate in children. *British Journal of Anaesthesia* **59**: 678–682.

Motoyama EK & Glazener CH (1986) Hypoxemia after general anesthesia in children. *Anesthesia and Analgesia* **65**: 267–272.

Muir JJ, Warner MA, Offord KP et al (1987) Role of nitrous oxide and other factors in postoperative nausea and vomiting: a randomized and blinded prospective study. *Anesthesiology* **66**: 513–518.

Nicoll JH (1909) The surgery of infancy. *British Medical Journal* **ii**: 753–754.

O'Neill MP, Sharkey AJ, Fee JPH & Black GW (1982) A comparative study of enflurane and halothane in children. *Anaesthesia* **37**: 634–639.

Otherson AB & Clatworthy HW (1968) Outpatient herniorrhaphy for children. *American Journal of Disease in Children* **116**: 78–80.

Padfield NL, Twohig MMcD & Fraser ACL (1986) Temazepam and trimeprazine compared with placebo as premedication in children. *British Journal of Anaesthesia* **58**: 487–493.

Patel RI, Hannallah RS, Murphy LS & Epstein BS (1986) Pediatric outpatient anesthesia—a review of post-anesthetic complications in 8995 cases. *Anesthesiology* **65**: A435.

Postuma R, Ferguson CC, Stanwick RS & Horne JM (1987) Pediatric day-care surgery: a 30 year hospital experience. *Journal of Pediatric Surgery* **22**: 304–307.

Purcell-Jones G, Yates A, Baker JR & James IJ (1987) Comparison of the induction characteristics of thiopentone and propofol in children. *British Journal of Anaesthesia* **59**: 1431–1436.

Redfern N, Addison GM & Meakin G (1986) Blood glucose in anaesthetized children. *Anaesthesia* **41**: 272–275.

Rita L, Seleny FL, Mazurek A et al (1985) Intramuscular midazolam for pediatric preanesthetic sedation: a double-blind controlled study with morphine. *Anesthesiology* **63**: 528–531.

Rosen DA, Rosen KR & Hannallah RS (1985) Preoperative characteristics which influence the child's response to induction of anesthesia. *Anesthesiology* **63**: A462.

Rowley MP & Brown TCK (1982) Postoperative vomiting in children. *Anaesthesia and Intensive Care* **10**: 309–313.

Sara CA & Lowrey CJ (1985) A complication of circumcision and dorsal nerve block of the penis. *Anaesthesia and Intensive Care* **13**: 79–82.

Smith RM (1978) Pediatric anesthesia in perspective. *Anesthesiology* **57**: 634–646.

Steward DJ (1973) Experiences with an outpatient anesthesia service for children. *Anesthesia and Analgesia* **52**: 877–880.

Steward DJ (1975) Outpatient pediatric anesthesia. *Anesthesiology* **43**: 268–276.

Steward DJ (1980) Anaesthesia for paediatric out-patients. *Canadian Anaesthetists' Society Journal* **27**: 412–416.

Steward DJ (1982) Preterm infants are more prone to complications following minor surgery than are term infants. *Anesthesiology* **56:** 304–306.

Steward DJ (1986) Daycare anaesthesia in paediatrics. In *Proceedings of the First European Congress of Paediatric Anaesthesia*. Rotterdam.

Tait AR, Ketcham TR, Klein MJ & Knight PR (1983) Perioperative respiratory complications in patients with upper respiratory tract infections. *Anesthesiology* **59:** A433.

Tree-trakarn T, Pirayavaraporn S & Lertakyamanee J (1987) Topical analgesia for relief of post-circumcision pain. *Anesthesiology* **67:** 395–399.

van der Valt JH & Carter JA (1986) The effects of different preoperative feeding regimes on plasma glucose and gastric volume and pH in infants. *Anaesthesia and Intensive Care* **14:** 352–359.

Vivori E (1981) Induction and maintenance of anaesthesia. In Rees GJ and Gray TC (eds) *Paediatric Anaesthesia—Trends in Current Practice*, pp 101–104. London: Butterworths.

Walton B (1986) Halothane hepatitis in children. *Anaesthesia* **41:** 575–578.

Wilton NCT & Burn JMB (1986) Delayed vomiting after papaveretum in paediatric outpatient surgery. *Canadian Anaesthetists' Society Journal* **33:** 741–744.

Wren WS, McShane AJ, McCarthy JG et al (1985) Isoflurane in paediatric anaesthesia. *Anaesthesia* **40:** 315–323.

Upper airway obstruction in paediatrics

The causes of airway obstruction in children are many and varied, ranging from the acute to the chronic, and are usually classified as congenital or acquired (Table 20.1). Common to all is the potential to develop hypoxaemia to a life-threatening degree. Twenty-five children below the age of 4 died of acquired infections of the upper respiratory tract in Canada in 1985 (Statistics Canada, 1985). These deaths were all theoretically preventable. In both the emergency and non-emergency situations, the anaesthetist may be consulted regarding the differential diagnosis of the patient in addition to providing safe anaesthesia for diagnostic or surgical intervention in these children. The anaesthetist should also be able to recognize and identify potential airway obstructive lesions which might present as incidental findings during direct laryngoscopy for intubation of a patient undergoing unrelated surgery.

Recognition, diagnosis and treatment of upper airway obstruction in the paediatric patient involves the knowledge of the normal anatomical and physiological parameters of the upper airway in the various paediatric age groups and the impact of the many and varied pathological entities upon them. Although these have been mentioned elsewhere (p. 236) they are re-emphasized below in relation to upper airway problems.

ANATOMICAL FACTORS

1. The tongue is large in relation to the mandible in the newborn period and approaches the more normal ratio only in late infancy. Any pathological entity which exaggerates this difference in size, e.g. micrognathia, or which impedes the nasopharyngeal airway, e.g. choanal atresia, will produce upper airway obstruction in these age groups.
2. The mucous membrane of the anterior or lingual surface of the epiglottis is relatively less adherent than that of the posterior or laryngeal surface. Oedema of this looser mucous membrane can rapidly progress and produce upper airway obstruction.
3. The narrowest diameter of the larynx in the paediatric age group up to about the age of 10 years is at the level of the cricoid ring, below the vocal cords. The mucous membrane lining of the larynx is also fixed at this level. Accumulation of oedema in this area will have greater potential to produce airway obstruction.

Table 20.1. Common causes of upper airway obstruction in the paediatric patient

Congenital	Acquired
Choanal atresia	*Infections*
	Croup
	Epiglottitis
	Abscess
	Adenotonsillar
	Diphtheria
	Ludwig's angina
Craniofacial malformations	*Trauma*
Pierre Robin syndrome	Foreign bodies
Treacher Collins syndrome	Thermal and chemical burns
	External trauma
	Postintubation
	Postoperative
Macroglossia	*Neurogenic*
Down's syndrome	Altered consciousness
Beckwith's syndrome	Muscular dystrophies
	Peripheral nerve lesions
Laryngeal	*Neoplastic*
Laryngomalacia	Tumours
Subglottic stenosis	Cysts
Webs	Nodes
Cleft (laryngo-oesophageal)	
Cord palsies	
Tracheal	*Immunological*
Tracheomalacia	Angio-oedema
Congenital stenosis	Juvenile rheumatoid arthritis
Vascular rings	
Congenital tumours and cysts	
Haemangioma	
Lymphangioma	
Cystic hygroma	

The diameter of the airway is 3.5–4 mm at the level of the cricoid ring in the infant age group, and 1 mm of oedema at this level will lead to a decrease in cross-sectional area of 75%. Since the resistance to flow is inversely proportional to the radius of the lumen to the fourth power, there will be a 16-fold increase in resistance to air flow.

4. The cartilaginous supporting structures of the tracheobronchial tree and chest wall in the younger paediatric patients lack the rigidity of the older child or adult due to their more watery matrix. Extraluminal compression may markedly decrease or distort the intraluminal integrity. The lack of rigidity of the chest wall places these younger children at a mechanical respiratory disadvantage should airway obstruction occur.

PHYSIOLOGICAL FACTORS

1. Oxygen consumption in the infant age group is 6–8 ml/kg/min compared with approximately 4 ml/kg/min in the adult. The normal newborn or small infant meets this increased requirement by an increased respiratory rate to 30–40 breaths/min, producing a minute ventilation of 180–240 ml/kg/min, twice that of the average adult. The tidal volumes of the infant and adult are similar (6 ml/kg).
2. The closing volume of the lung in an infant is 12 ml/kg compared to 7 ml/kg for the adult. This is compounded by the high ratio of alveolar ventilation to functional residual capacity in this age group (Keon, 1985).
3. Premature and term infants have fewer type 1 muscle fibres present in their diaphragms and intercostal muscles compared to older children. These are the muscle fibres capable of repetitive contraction (Keens et al, 1978).
4. The normal haemoglobin in the infant age group is 11–12 g%, compared to 14–15 g% in the adult. The oxygen-carrying capacity of the infant is therefore reduced when compared to the adult or older child, thus the consequence of respiratory obstruction is the rapid onset of hypoxia.

SIGNS OF UPPER AIRWAY OBSTRUCTION

Stridor and indrawing of the supraclavicular, intercostal and subdiaphragmatic areas are pathognomonic signs of upper airway obstruction. Inspiratory stridor indicates obstruction at or above the larynx. Hoarseness confirms vocal cord involvement. Biphasic (inspiratory/expiratory) stridor is present when the obstruction is at or below the larynx. Expiratory stridor alone indicates obstruction below the larynx, usually intrathoracic. The volume, pitch, and tonality of the stridor will vary according to the type and size of the obstructive lesion and the age of the child.

Indrawing—the result of increased respiratory effort to overcome the obstruction—occurs when there is an imbalance between the intrapleural forces generated and the rigidity of the chest wall. Both indrawing and stridor occur when the cross-sectional diameter of the airway is reduced by 70%. Indrawing is most pronounced in infants, in whom the chest wall is extremely compliant.

The degree of stridor and indrawing is compounded by the development of an increased negative intrathoracic pressure below the level of the obstruction which, when combined with the infant's compliant cartilaginous supporting structures, leads to a further decrease in the diameter of the trachea (the Bernoulli effect).

As the infant matures, the chest wall and the supporting structures of the trachea become more rigid, and the indrawing and stridor, although always present in a major obstruction, may not be as severe in degree.

Fatigue cannot be measured quantitatively in the clinical setting but the efficiency of the respiratory effort can be assessed by the use of a scoring system such as that developed by Downes and Raphaely (1975; Table 20.2). By serial observations of the clinical signs as set out in this table, the patient may be 'scored'. The same observer will then be able to note the patient's progress or lack of it.

Table 20.2. Clinical croup score

	Score		
	0	1	2
Inspiratory breath sounds	Normal	Harsh with rhonchi	Delayed
Stridor	None	Inspiratory	Inspiratory and expiratory
Cough	None	Hoarse cry	Bark
Retractions and flaring	None	Flaring and supersternal retractions	As under 1, plus subcostal, intercostal retractions
Cyanosis	None	In air	In 40% O_2

From Downes and Raphaely (1975).

Serial blood gas measurements are not, in our opinion, of clinical use in the paediatric patient with upper airway obstruction other than to emphasize that these patients may be hypoxic in room air. It is not uncommon for them to be hypocarbic in the early stages of airway obstruction, and hypercarbia, when it occurs, is a late sign; the clinical status of the patient will have shown obvious deterioration by then.

The recent availability of accurate oximetry by non-invasive means has been a major advance. It ensures the beat-to-beat monitoring of the oxygenation of these children and thus guides oxygen therapy.

OBSTRUCTIVE SLEEP APNOEA

Chronic upper airway obstruction may be associated with obstructive sleep apnoea in which the child becomes totally obstructed intermittently during sleep (Wilms et al, 1982). This chronic obstructive state is usually associated with hypoxia and may potentially lead to pulmonary hypertension and right-sided heart failure (Macartney et al, 1969).

In the clinical assessment of such children, in addition to ascertaining the frequency and duration of the apnoeic spells, assessment of their cardiovascular status and oximetry to quantitate the adequacy of oxygenation is necessary.

RADIOLOGICAL EVALUATION

The radiological appearance of obstructive lesions of the upper airway is often invaluable in determining their site and extent (Swischuk, 1979). However, radiological airway examination should only be undertaken when there is significant doubt as to the diagnosis and/or the child is not clinically compromised. If such a radiological examination is undertaken, it should be done in an appropriate environment where skilled personnel capable of assessing and intervening on an obstructed airway are present.

LABORATORY EVALUATION

Arterial or arterialized capillary gas analysis is seldom necessary in the acutely obstructed child. In the chronically obstructed paediatric patient, it will reveal the degree of chronic hypoxia or hypercarbia present, together with any metabolic compensation. It is uncommon to see significant polycythaemia in these patients. Similarly the serum electrolytes are usually within normal limits.

Obtaining blood from such a child may produce agitation and aggravate an already compromised airway. If deemed necessary, it should be performed by skilled personnel, in a secure environment where the appropriate airway maintenance equipment is available.

GENERAL PRINCIPLES OF MANAGEMENT OF THE PAEDIATRIC PATIENT WITH AIRWAY OBSTRUCTION

The many and varied causes of upper airway obstruction in the paediatric patient, both acute and chronic, mandate certain general principles.

Oxygenation

Most patients with upper airway obstruction, acute or chronic, will exhibit varying degrees of hypoxaemia in room air. This may be evident clinically through the presence of cyanosis, by non-invasive pulse oximetry, or in rare circumstances by blood gas analysis.

The routine administration of oxygen to these children until a definitive diagnosis and specific treatment is initiated is mandatory. The initial method of administration will depend upon the age of the child but in the acute situation, it is usually via a clear non-occlusive facemask with a flow of 6–8 l/min.

Agitation, restlessness or anxiety, should be assumed to be due to hypoxaemia in an obstructed child until this has been ruled out.

Sedation

Attempts to relieve anxiety and the work of breathing by sedating a paediatric patient with airway obstruction are specifically contraindicated.

The clinical assessment of such a child may be misleading on initial examination. Sedation in any form should be withheld until the clinical status has been well established, the diagnosis made, and treatment initiated. Even then, sedation should be used with great discretion, if at all.

The anxiety of such a child is more appropriately met by the calming presence of the parents and attendants. For similar reasons, blood sampling and the establishment of intravenous access should be undertaken only by personnel skilled in their performance. It is prudent in most circumstances of acute airway obstruction to omit such procedures until the child is in an appropriate environment, such as the intensive care unit or the operating room.

Transportation

Not infrequently, a child with acute upper airway obstruction will present at a peripheral hospital where airway assessment or intervention may cause problems. As a minimum requirement, such a child, if being transferred, should be accompanied by personnel including a physician who is capable of the continued assessment of such a child and equipped and adept in airway management.

The prior establishment of an airway before transportation of an acutely obstructed hypoxic child is preferred. The ability to secure an airway will depend on the availability of specific expertise of an anaesthetist or surgeon at the referring hospital.

Transport teams for critically ill newborns are well established entities sent out by the tertiary paediatric centres. Equivalent transport teams for children with airway obstruction would be of equal value, but are not commonly available.

Anaesthesia

Preoperative evaluation

The history of onset, duration and nature of the symptoms should be elicited, in addition to the past medical history, previous anaesthetic experiences, medications and allergies. On clinical examination, respiratory rate, the presence or absence of cyanosis, the type and degree of stridor, and flaring of the nares or indrawing should all be specifically looked for. Auscultation of the chest will reveal any abnormalities in air entry and the presence or absence of additional chest sounds.

As previously indicated, preoperative laboratory investigation and X-ray examination should only be sought in those children whose clinical condition indicates that they do not have a life-threatening situation.

Premedication

An antisialagogue should be given 45 min prior to the induction of anaesthesia to those patients with chronic upper airway obstruction presenting for anaesthesia, to reduce oral and tracheobronchial secretions.

In acute upper airway obstruction atropine 0.02 mg/kg is given intravenously at the induction of anaesthesia to minimize reflex vagal effects on the heart and to reduce secretion. Preoperative hydrogen ion blockers have been recommended to reduce gastric acidity in those children with known gastro-oesophageal reflux or a full stomach (Goudsouzian et al, 1981).

Monitors and equipment should include a pulse oximeter in addition to the standard monitoring of the paediatric patient (precordial stethoscope, blood pressure, electrocardiograph and temperature). A selection of tracheal tubes with lubricated stylets should be available several times smaller than that suggested by the patient's age and size. A similar selection of tracheal tubes are placed in ice to stiffen them. Appropriate-sized rigid and flexible bronchoscopes should also be immediately at hand, together with a tracheostomy set and apparatus for transtracheal ventilation. Means to perform a cricothyrotomy by catheter or incision should be available. An ear, nose and throat surgeon should be present.

Induction of anaesthesia

In an infant less than approximately 46 weeks' postconceptual age, or an obtunded older infant or child, direct laryngoscopy and tracheal intubation preceded by optimal oxygenation without any general anaesthesia is performed. Success in this approach depends not only on the skill of the person performing the direct laryngoscopy, but the availability of an assistant specifically instructed in holding the head straight in the sniffing position. The use of topical Xylocaine 3 mg/kg prior to the direct laryngoscopy may be of help. In a more robust infant or older child who is not obtunded, it will be necessary to give a general anaesthetic. This should be done in a stepwise and deliberate manner.

Anaesthesia is induced with 100% oxygen and halothane. The initial position of the infant or child should be that in which he or she is most at ease—sitting, recumbent or supine. The halothane should be slowly increased in concentration as tolerated to a maximum of 4%. As anaesthesia deepens, respiratory obstruction is minimized by maintaining a tight reservoir bag, and then the ability to assist ventilation is assessed. If an intravenous route has not been established, it should be at this time and atropine 0.02 mg/kg i.v. given.

If assisted ventilation is possible then the halothane concentration is decreased to 2–3% and the induction continued with gentle positive pressure, not exceeding 10 cm H_2O. The depth of anaesthesia at which direct laryngoscopy can be attempted without stimulation may be difficult to determine. A decrease in the systolic blood pressure of 20 mmHg, central small pupils and lax abdominal musculature are all general indications. Ten to 20 min is the usual acceptable period of elapsed time from the start of induction before direct laryngoscopy should be attempted. Topical Xylocaine to a maximum of 3 mg/kg or intravenous Xylocaine 1.5 mg/kg is an effective adjunct in depressing the airway reflexes, cough and potential laryngospasm when direct laryngoscopy is attempted, but given at too tight a plane of anaesthesia, will itself cause laryngospasm.

At any time during induction, if it is not possible to assist the ventilation or if the degree of obstruction is increasing, then direct laryngoscopy and tracheal intubation should be performed at that time. Again appropriate assistance at all stages of the induction is mandatory.

The use of intravenous induction agents and muscle relaxants in the paediatric patient with airway obstruction is beset with danger. Even in experienced hands the abolition of spontaneous ventilation and the subsequent decision to ventilate and rapidly intubate the patient may be a difficult one.

After orotracheal intubation has been performed, the decision to replace it with a nasotracheal tube or perform a tracheostomy will depend upon the specific diagnosis and circumstance.

At all times prior to the induction of anaesthesia in these children equipment for the immediate establishment of an airway should be available, e.g. a needle catheter, bronchoscopes of appropriate size and a surgeon capable of performing a rapid tracheostomy on such a patient. Tracheostomy and cricothyrotomy, an acceptable alternative in the acutely obstructed adult patient or older child, are both difficult to perform in those paediatric patients in whom the larynx is small, difficult to palpate, and in whom the risk of misplacement is high.

If following the initial laryngoscopy tracheal intubation is not successful due to the pathology present, or the lack of visualization of the laryngeal aditus, then inhalation anaesthesia should be resumed to prevent lightening of the patient and potential laryngospasm. When assisted ventilation has been re-established and the depth of the patient is adequate, then a change in the position of the head or alternative appropriate instrumentation, e.g. fibreoptic laryngoscopy rigid and flexible, should be made.

If general anaesthesia is conducted in a step-by-step manner, the appropriate equipment is available, and good assistance is to hand, it is rare that tracheal intubation in these patients is not possible.

CAUSES OF UPPER AIRWAY OBSTRUCTION

Congenital

Craniofacial abnormalities

Bilateral choanal atresia.   This produces severe indrawing and signs of airway obstruction even during quiet respiration in the newborn period, since the newborn is an obligate nose-breather. The failure to pass a suction catheter through either nostril to the pharynx confirms the diagnosis. Initially inserting and fixing in place an oral airway or a nipple in which the aperture has been enlarged is a simple and effective means of supplying an airway. Intubation is rarely required to maintain the airway. Subsequently the obstructing bony or fibrous septum is removed surgically.

Craniofacial malformations.   The Pierre Robin sequence and Treacher Collins syndrome have in common micrognathia and relative macroglossia with the tongue placed more posteriorly than normal (Figure 20.1). Initial treatment of the obstructed airway is to attempt to nurse the newborn infant prone with the head in the sniffing position. A nipple modified as for choanal atresia or a nasopharyngeal airway fixed in place may also be of help (see p. 408). If these simple measures are not sufficient, then intubation should be attempted, and in skilful hands is usually successful. Surgical intervention to fix the tongue forward or perform tracheostomy is rarely needed. The long-term goal is to support the airway until the mandible has grown sufficiently to allow forward movement of the tongue.

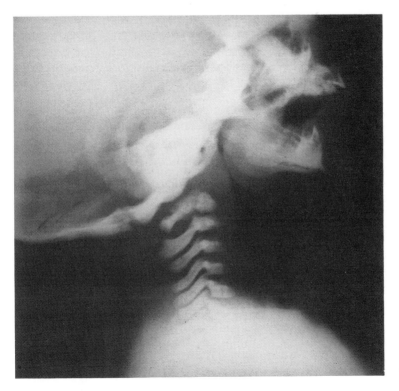

Figure 20.1. Pierre Robin syndrome. Posterior position of base of tongue, micrognathia, and marked narrowing of oropharyngeal airway are easily identifiable.

Macroglossia

Syndromes such as Down's, Beckwith's, congenital hypothyroidism, and glycogen storage disease may result in macroglossia of a sufficient degree to produce airway obstruction. These are rare. Even more uncommonly, lingual tumours may be present in the newborn period of a size sufficient to cause airway obstruction. Maintenance of the airway by mechanical means until the infant has reached sufficient size and age to support his or her own airway, or for the abnormality to be corrected surgically, is the usual approach.

Laryngeal abnormalities

Laryngotracheomalacia.   This is the commonest cause (70%) of congenital stridor and is usually a benign condition (Hollinger and Brown, 1967). It is generally felt to be due to the indrawing of the lax, redundant aryepiglottic folds during inspiration. The onset of the typical high-pitched inspiratory stridor is usually at birth or in the early months of infancy. Feeding problems and respiratory infections are often associated with this condition, which commonly resolves by the second year of life. Mechanical support of the airway is rarely necessary but direct laryngoscopy to exclude less benign causes of stridor in this age group is indicated.

Congenital subglottic stenosis.   This accounts for 6–19% of all congenital laryngeal abnormalities (Maze and Bloch, 1979). Commonly it is a diffuse, firm circumferential ring at the level of the cricoid cartilage. As in any initially asymptomatic congenital airway lesion, a superimposed upper respiratory tract infection and associated oedema may severely compromise the airway in the infant. The symptomatology of subglottic stenosis is biphasic stridor, severe indrawing and the inability to handle secretions. Recurrent episodes of such symptomatology in association with upper respiratory tract infections in an infant should trigger a high index of suspicion that congenital subglottic stenosis is present. It is recommended that direct laryngoscopy and bronchoscopy should be performed to confirm or rule out the diagnosis. If the stenosis is of a mild degree, no active treatment is indicated as the diameter of the lumen of the trachea increases as the child becomes older. With severe stenosis, long-term tracheostomy is indicated with monthly dilatations under general anaesthesia until the diameter of the trachea is of sufficient size.

Surgical correction of the abnormality has been attempted with success in recent years (Evans, 1979). Intubation of these infants requires the availability of stiffened (iced or styletted) tracheal tubes of diameters from one size below that predicated by the age and size of the infant, down to the smallest practical diameter and length. A rigid bronchoscope of appropriate size and facilities to perform a tracheostomy if necessary should be immediately available.

Congenital laryngeal webs.   These occur most commonly at the level of the vocal cords. They usually occupy one-half to two-thirds of the diameter of the anterior parts of the larynx. The web may vary from being a thin, transparent and membranous structure to being fibrous and thick. These infants commonly present in the newborn period with inspiratory stridor, indrawing, and the cry may be abnormal. Diagnosis is made by direct laryngoscopy. Surgical correction varies from the simple splitting of the membranous type to tracheostomy and repeated dilatations for the fibrous type. If the web involves all or most of the length of the vocal cords, a true emergency exists at birth, and rapid forced intubation, cricothyroid split, or emergency tracheostomy are the limited possibilities to establish an airway.

Laryngotracheo-oesophageal cleft. This condition is rare and is diagnosed by direct laryngoscopy and oesophagoscopy. The indrawing is associated with feeding, and aspiration is frequent. Stridor is not always present. The cry is usually abnormally weak. Protection of the airway by nasotracheal intubation prior to the surgical correction is indicated. Breakdown of the surgical repair is not infrequent, requiring continuing vigilance into the postoperative period.

Congenital vocal cord palsies. These may be central in origin and the cord paralysis is then bilateral. When the aetiology is peripheral, the cord paralysis is usually on the left side due to the longer course of the left recurrent laryngeal nerve. In most cases, the left cord palsy is secondary to a congenital cardiovascular anomaly. Birth trauma accounts for some of the congenital bilateral cord palsies, but the aetiology is often obscure and the lesion generally resolves as the infant matures.

Increased intracranial pressure with caudal displacement of the brainstem and subsequent traction and compression of the vagus and cervical nerve roots will lead to vocal cord palsies (Bluestone et al, 1972).

If the injury to the recurrent laryngeal nerves is complete, the cords will take up a neutral abducted position and the airway is usually adequate. There may be no stridor but the cry will be hoarse or faint. With partial injury to the recurrent laryngeal nerves, abduction is lost, and the vocal cords may then be fixed in adduction, with the obstruction being more severe and inspiratory stridor prominent. The diagnosis is confirmed by direct laryngoscopy in the phonating infant. The risk of severe obstruction during the procedure is present. Treatment is directed at the underlying causative factors where they are known. Occasionally, tracheostomy or nasotracheal intubation is indicated when the obstruction is severe or to prevent recurrent aspiration.

Tracheal abnormalities

Tracheomalacia. This is a rare congenital abnormality, sometimes associated with tracheo-oesophageal fistula and vascular ring, producing biphasic stridor with a weak cry and varying degrees of indrawing. Due to the lack of cartilaginous support, the trachea may buckle or be compressed by extrinsic structures, and is a rare cause of sudden infant death. The indrawing is exaggerated by the increased negative intratracheal pressure relative to the atmospheric pressure produced by the obstruction. Diagnosis is made by bronchoscopy and the treatment is by aortopexy where possible (Cohen, 1981).

Congenital tracheal stenosis. This is also a rare anomaly presenting with biphasic stridor, weak cry and indrawing. Diagnosis is made by bronchoscopy with supporting information from soft tissue X-ray of the neck and chest to help elucidate the extent of the stenosis. If airway obstruction is severe, it may be relieved initially by nasotracheal intubation. The placement and the sizing of the tracheal tube are critical factors. Specific surgical correction by dilatation, resection, or by widening of the trachea through the insertion of a stent or a mesh may be successful (Debrand et al, 1979).

Vascular rings.   Vascular rings compressing the trachea may produce congenital stridor. The commonest cause is a double aortic arch. The stridor is biphasic and commonly associated with a barking cough and respiratory indrawing. Feeding difficulties will occur if the oesophagus is also compressed. Difficulties in handling secretions and recurrent pulmonary infection may also occur. Diagnosis is made by barium swallow and possibly bronchoscopy. Arteriography may be performed to give more specific information. If severe respiratory obstruction is present, nasotracheal intubation is indicated preoperatively. Following surgical correction, the nasotracheal tube should be left in situ for at least 24–48 h to splint the trachea at the site of the compression, as the trachea lacks rigidity at this site and has the potential to collapse as in tracheomalacia. The use of nasal continuous positive air pressure following extubation after this initial period of postoperative intubation is of benefit to overcome this potential problem.

Congenital tumours and cysts

Congenital subglottic haemangioma.   This is a vascular abnormality commonly associated with cutaneous haemangiomas. It produces biphasic stridor, a hoarse cry and signs of respiratory obstruction in the first months of life. Soft-tissue lateral X-ray of the neck may show a lesion in the trachea, and the diagnosis is confirmed by bronchoscopy under general anaesthesia. If the degree of respiratory obstruction is severe, a softened nasotracheal tube should be carefully positioned beyond the haemangioma under general anaesthesia. Laser surgery is nowadays the treatment of choice. Tracheostomy is indicated until the haemangioma has regressed, usually after 1 year of age. Other treatment modalities such as corticosteroids (Cohen, 1969) or radiation have been suggested for the treatment of this condition.

Cystic hygroma and laryngeal lymphangiomas.   These may produce signs of upper respiratory tract obstruction either due to extrinsic pressure on the larynx or trachea, or by intrusion into the lumen of the airway. The clinical degree of obstruction and stridor will indicate the need to establish an airway by the use of a nasotracheal tube preoperatively.

Surgical excision of these lesions is usually difficult and incomplete and postoperative recurrence or infection are not uncommon problems.

Congenital cysts.   These are rare and may arise in the hypopharynx, larynx or trachea, the commonest being a laryngocoele. Congenital thyroglossal duct cysts may occasionally produce upper airway obstruction due to extrinsic compression of the trachea. Needle aspiration, deroofing or excision are the treatment modalities. Again, preoperative nasotracheal intubation should be performed if the upper airway obstruction is severe in nature.

Acquired

Infection

In 80% of all paediatric patients with acquired stridor, infection is the cause (Arthurton, 1970). In all, 90% of these infectious cases will be due to laryngotracheobronchitis (croup) whilst approximately 5% are due to epiglottitis.

Laryngotracheobronchitis. This commonly occurs in infants of 6 months to 2 years of age. This disease is usually viral (parainfluenza) in aetiology, occurring in the winter months. The onset is gradual, preceded by the signs of upper respiratory tract infection. In most instances, the infant does not require hospitalization, responding to the humidification of the environment, oral hydration and symptomatic treatment of fever. The inspiratory and expiratory stridor, barking cough and signs of upper airway obstruction will usually resolve over a period of hours. Observation in a holding area, should the child present to the emergency room of a hospital, prior to discharge is recommended. Approximately 10% of the children seen in an emergency department of a children's hospital do require admission to hospital (Mitchell and Thomas, 1980). Routine use of a mist tent with oxygen and intravenous hydration usually suffices; the infant normally responds over a 24–48-h period. The use of steroids is controversial, and not routine in most centres. Similarly, antibiotic therapy is not used unless secondary bacterial infection is identified.

Failure to respond to this conservative therapy, no improvement over a 24-h period, or a deterioration in respiratory status indicates that the child should be cared for in a more intensive environment. Consultation between the anaesthetist and ENT surgeon is usual at this stage.

It has been established that these latter children are hypoxic, with the degree of hypoxia correlating best with respiratory rate (Newth et al, 1972). In the authors' intensive care unit the use of a croup score as suggested by Downes and Raphaely (1974; Table 20.2), on an hourly basis initially and then at increasing intervals as the child improves, is standard. Oxygenation is routinely assessed by the use of a pulse oximeter and arterial blood gases are not usually performed. A chest X-ray to help assess the degree of pulmonary involvement is useful. The use of a mist tent with oxygen to give an inspired concentration of approximately 30% along with the correction of any errors of hydration and the administration of racemic adrenaline is our standard conservative treatment. Attention should be paid to any degree of gastric distension in these children, due to the increased negative intra-abdominal pressures produced by the increased inspiratory effort, and is treated by inserting a nasogastric tube.

The successful use of racemic adrenaline in the treatment of croup was first reported in 1971 by Adair et al. Initially, controversy over the benefits of its routine use followed, but in many centres, including our own, its use is now standard; 0.5 ml of a 2.25% solution of racemic adrenaline is diluted with 4 ml saline and given by nebulization using 100% oxygen and administered with a loose-fitting clear facemask. The ECG is routinely monitored and the administration stopped if the increase in heart rate exceeds 200 beats/min or arrhythmias occur. The croup score is assessed pre- and post-treatment. If no improvement occurs, or after initial improvement the clinical condition again deteriorates, then the administration may be repeated within 1 h. If there are any signs of increasing fatigue or a lack of response to the administration of racemic adrenaline, then active intervention is indicated to secure the airway. This occurs in approximately 2–6% of those children admitted to hospital with laryngotracheobronchitis (Mitchell and Thomas, 1980), and is likely to be necessary if the croup score is 7 or more.

Nasotracheal intubation or tracheostomy can be used to establish an airway, but nasotracheal intubation has become the commonest and most accepted approach. The long-term complication rate of nasotracheal intubation in these children is 1.6% (Schuller and Birk, 1974), but is less than the mortality rate (3%) with tracheostomy in this infant age group.

Intubation is best performed under anaesthesia in the operating room using the stepwise approach with 100% oxygen and halothane as previously described. Tracheal tubes stiffened by icing or threaded with a lubricated stylet should be available and the airway initially secured by the oral route using a tube of the smallest practical diameter and length. This is changed to a nasotracheal tube of a similar diameter after the child has been well oxygenated, suctioned etc. The average duration of intubation for a child with laryngotracheobronchitis is 3–6 days; extubation is indicated when there is a leak present around the tube at 20–30 cm H_2O pressure.

If, following extubation, the signs of subglottic oedema recur and the administration of racemic adrenaline does not improve the clinical status, then re-intubation possibly followed by a tracheostomy is indicated.

Acute epiglottitis.   This is a fulminant bacterial infection usually due to *Haemophilus influenzae*, involving supraglottic structures (the epiglottis, the aryepiglottic folds) leading to acute airway obstruction in 5–15 h. Rapkin (1973) reported a 25% incidence of acute airway obstruction in patients treated conservatively with antibiotics and close observation but without airway intervention. It is commonest in the 2–5-year age group, but may occur at any age. Characteristically, these children look toxic and have a high-grade fever. They will not lie down but sit with the mouth open, the tongue forward, drooling, with the head in the sniffing position. Indrawing and stridor may be minimal. A striking feature in these children is that they tend not to phonate and if they do, then only in a whisper, even though they are obviously afraid (Figure 20.2).

A child presenting with these symptoms and the characteristic posture is in danger of sudden respiratory obstruction and demands immediate and concurrent consultation with the anaesthetist and ENT surgeon. The child should be moved immediately to an intensive care environment accompanied by anaesthesia and/or ENT personnel and together with full airway maintenance equipment.

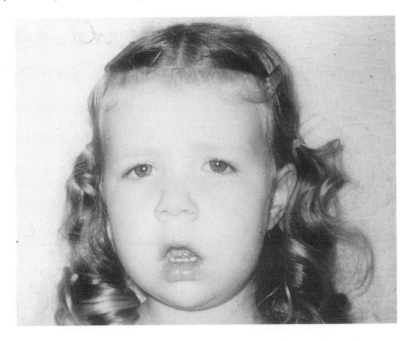

Figure 20.2. Acute epiglottitis. A 3-year-old infant sitting with mouth open, and anxious facies.

The suspicion of epiglottitis should lead to the same procedures, e.g. consultation and transfer to an intensive care environment. Only in that environment should relevant examinations and investigations such as soft-tissue X-ray of the neck be performed to help elucidate the diagnosis (Figure 20.3).

If the diagnosis of epiglottitis remains a *remote* possibility, then one should perform a direct laryngoscopy either in an intensive care environment or in the operating room. This procedure can be performed quickly and simply and will dispel any remaining suspicion of acute epiglottitis which may linger after clinical and X-ray examination have made it a remote possibility. Most commonly, this type of patient will be found to have acute pharyngitis or tonsillitis.

When the diagnosis is clinically apparent or clearly demonstrated by X-ray or direct laryngoscopy, then the child is transferred to the operating room accompanied by anaesthesia/ENT personnel equipped with the appropriate airway maintenance equipment.

In the operating room, it is our practice as well as others' (Hanallah and Rosales, 1978) to anaesthetize the child in the sitting position with the step-by-step approach maintaining spontaneous ventilation at all times. If an i.v. route has not been established before the child arrives at the operating room, then one is preferably started prior to the induction of anaesthesia and intravenous atropine 0.02 mg/kg is given.

As the child becomes obtunded, he or she is slowly placed into the supine position. Commonly, there is minimal difficulty at this time to maintain an airway and anaesthesia may be slowly deepened with the use of 100% oxy-

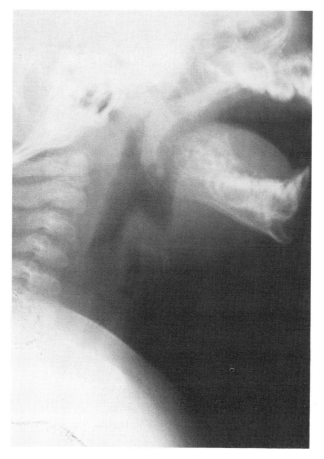

Figure 20.3. Acute epiglottitis. Soft-tissue lateral X-ray of neck showing markedly oedematous epiglottis and aryepiglottic folds.

gen and up to 4% halothane with assisted ventilation and the judicious use (less than 10 cm H_2O) of positive pressure.

Less commonly, on lying supine there is increased airway obstruction; however, support of the airway by the careful, forward manipulation of the jaw, positioning of the head and the use of positive pressure will overcome this. Rarely, on laying the child supine, complete obstruction may occur in spite of airway maintenance manoeuvres. Direct laryngoscopy should be performed immediately in this situation and the airway secured by the oral route.

The appearance of the epiglottic and glottic structure at direct laryngoscopy may vary from a grossly swollen, reddened, cherry-like epiglottis with a slit-like aperture, to an epiglottis which is minimally erythematous and oedematous but with marked oedema of the aryepiglottic folds. It is because of the marked and unpredictable variation in the degree of swelling, potential difficulty in inflating the lungs, and the inability to locate the glottic aperture rapidly in some cases, that the avoidance of barbiturates and relaxants is recommended.

Even in the most experienced hands, intubation of these patients may be an extremely difficult precedure, and the only clue to the position of the larynx may be movement of sputum, caused by spontaneous breathing. The means to obtain an airway by a rigid bronchoscope, emergency tracheostomy, or placement of a catheter via the cricothyroid membrane should always be at hand in the operating theatre prior to the induction of anaesthesia. The immediate availability of a surgeon capable of carrying out a rapid tracheostomy in such an infant or child is also necessary as part of the team approach.

Following the initial oral intubation, a blood culture is obtained if this has not been previously performed. The orotracheal tube is then replaced by a nasotracheal tube of the smallest practical diameter and length. This is securely fixed in place. Intravenous sedation (diazepam/morphine in our hospital) is commenced, a nasogastric tube is inserted and left in situ to minimize gastric distension. The arms are placed on boards to prevent flexion and the patient is then returned to an intensive care environment.

Continuous positive air pressure 2–4 mm H_2O with 30% oxygen is used routinely for all these intubated patients as a high incidence of radiological evidence of pulmonary atelectasis has been shown to exist without its use. The intravenous sedation is continued. Suction and routine care of the nasotracheal tube is performed at 2-hourly intervals, or more frequently if indicated, as is chest physiotherapy.

Antibiotic therapy is initially with cefuroxime 25 mg/kg 6-hourly i.v. until the result of the blood culture is obtained. If sensitivity to ampicillin is shown, then the cefuroxime is discontinued and ampicillin is given for 7 days. If insensitivity to ampicillin is shown then the cefuroxime is continued for a similar length of time. Prior to the availability of cefuroxime, combinant therapy with ampicillin–chloramphenicol was the treatment of choice.

After 24–36 h, if the child is afebrile, swallowing and there is an increased air leak around the tube, in our centre direct laryngoscopy is performed to assess the degree of oedema, if any, of the epiglottis. For this examination, the child is given a sleep dose of sodium pentothal or methohexital preceded by atropine. If the oedema and erythema have resolved or are significantly decreased, then extubation is performed. In some other centres, extubation is preferred when the symptomatology has subsided without prior laryngoscopy (Vernon and Sarnaik, 1986). The child is then placed in a mist tent with 30% oxygen and given nothing by mouth for at least 6 h prior to starting clear fluids, with eventual discharge to a regular nursing unit after a further 6 h. Observation for recurrence of airway obstruction is maintained during this 12-h period. Occasionally stridor may occur following extubation. If there is no response to two doses of racemic adrenaline, then the child should be re-intubated, usually for a further 24–48 h.

The presence of an inflammatory process of both the supraglottic and infraglottic areas may occur simultaneously. Whilst uncommon, when it does occur, management and treatment are as for epiglottitis with the expectation that the duration of intubation will be longer—up to 4 or 5 days.

Pulmonary oedema in association with acute severe upper airway obstruction such as may occur with acute epiglottitis or laryngospasm has been reported (Kantor and Watchko, 1984). The markedly increased negative intrapleural pressure produced in association with the obstruction, and increased pulmonary blood flow have both been implicated in the aetiology. Treatment using continuous positive air pressure or intermittent positive pressure ventilation, and occasionally diuretics, produces rapid resolution.

Peritonsillar abscess.   This, and more commonly, a retropharyngeal abscess may produce obstruction of the upper airway. The infection is usually due to β-haemolytic streptococcus and the child, in addition to having the signs of upper airway obstruction, will also be toxic. Diagnosis is made by the careful direct examination of the pharynx and confirmed by lateral soft-tissue X-rays of the neck, which for both of these lesions will show markedly thickened prevertebral tissue with narrowing of the oropharynx (Figure 20.4).

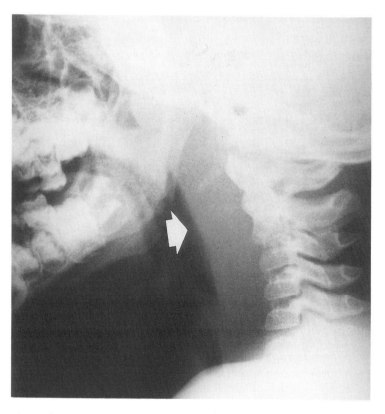

Figure 20.4. Retropharyngeal abscess. The markedly thickened prevertebral tissue is indicated by the arrow.

Incision and drainage of an abscess of the upper airway in a child is difficult to accomplish without a general anaesthetic. General anaesthesia induced with 100% oxygen and halothane and deepened stepwise until careful laryngoscopy can be performed is the technique of choice. Atraumatic intubation to secure and protect the airway from aspiration of infected material during the procedure is mandatory. Theoretically, it is advantageous to perform the induction with the child head-down in the left lateral position to limit the potential for aspiration of infected material should laryngoscopy or intubation be traumatic. The practicalities of inducing the child head-down in the supine position may in less skilled hands outweigh this advantage.

Tonsillar and adenoid hypertrophy.

Acute infection of the tonsils may occasionally produce an obstructive picture similar to acute epiglottitis in acuteness of onset and symptomatology. The differentiation is made on soft-tissue X-ray examination of the neck and on direct examination of the pharynx and larynx. Induction of anaesthesia for children with this degree of airway obstruction must take into account the probability of preoperative hypoxia and is again best accomplished with 100% oxygen and halothane. A relaxant used to facilitate intubation should only be considered when the ability to assist ventilation has been established.

In the chronic obstructive state due to hypertrophy of adenoidal tissue (Figure 20.5), the airway may continue to be obstructed postoperatively following the removal of the tonsils for 1–2 weeks. As these children are obligate mouth-breathers, the method of induction of anaesthesia should take this into account. Extubation should only be performed when the child is fully awake, and postoperative sedation given judiciously as there is the potential for continued obstruction of the airway. Similarly, when a nasopharyngeal pack has been used in the treatment of postadenoidectomy bleeding, sedation should be limited, if used at all, and observation of the child for airway obstruction is mandatory whilst such a pack is in situ.

Diphtheria.

Although rare, diphtheria must be considered in the differential diagnosis of stridor in a child who has not received the appropriate immunization. The symptomatology of upper airway obstruction is gradual in onset and the obstructing grey, shaggy membrane characteristic of this infection may be visible on the pharyngeal wall or tonsillar bed on direct examination of the pharynx. Nasotracheal intubation is indicated if clinically the obstruction is severe.

Ludwig's angina.

This is caused by the marked 'woody' swelling of the floor of the mouth, usually due to staphylococcal or β-haemolytic streptococcal infection of the sublingual space. Rarely seen in this antibiotic era, the child assumes an opisthotonic posture, with the tongue protruding and elevated. The oedema of the floor of the mouth and the immobility of the tongue make direct laryngoscopy and intubation a very difficult, if not impossible manoeuvre. Blind nasotracheal intubation or fibreoptic intubation, if the child is severely obstructed, should be performed before a tracheostomy is carried out. If severely obstructed, and tracheal intubation is not possible by any means, then a tracheostomy should be performed under local anaesthesia.

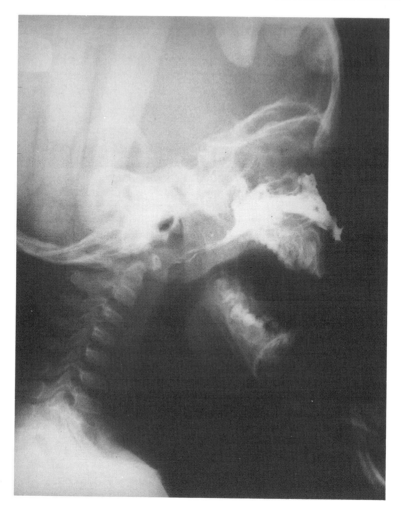

Figure 20.5. Adenoid hypertrophy. The obstruction to flow into the nasopharynx of barium placed in the nares is easily identifiable.

Trauma

Foreign body.   This is a leading cause of death from airway obstruction due to the intrinsic occlusion of the lumen or by extrinsic pressure especially in the infant age group. Children with debilitating disease and who have concomitant pathology, usually of a congenital, neurological, or cardio-vascular nature, are especially at risk of aspiration, usually with feeding.

   However, aspiration of food and foreign objects occurs not infrequently in infants and children who are otherwise healthy. An acute episode of cough-ing with or without cyanosis may occur at the time of aspiration. Periods of coughing may ensue accompanied by stridor or wheezing depending on the location, size and nature of the foreign body. History of the acute episode may often be lacking and the diagnosis is made retrospectively following clinical examination and X-ray studies. A comparison of the inspiratory and expiratory X-ray studies of the chest showing poor deflation on the affected side is often diagnostic if the foreign body is in the main stem bronchus, producing a ball-valve effect or if the foreign body is radiolucent. The anaesthetic management for removal of a foreign body is discussed on p. 419.

The posterior wall of the trachea being musculomembranous, a foreign body in the upper oesophagus may produce signs of upper airway obstruction due to the extrinsic pressure on the trachea. The upper oesophagus should therefore be examined in those children with a history and a clinical picture of aspiration of a foreign body when the foreign body cannot be located in the tracheobronchial tree.

Following bronchoscopy, the child should be observed for the potential development of subglottic oedema due to the instrumentation. The use of a mist tent postoperatively and adequate hydration are necessary and oedema, should it develop, is treated by the administration of racemic adrenaline given by nebulization and dexamethasone 0.25 mg/kg i.v.

Thermal and chemical burns.   Around the face burns must be assumed to be associated with erythema and oedema of the upper airway and the potential for the development of upper airway obstruction. Such a child should be observed in an intensive care environment for a 24–48-h period for signs of upper airway obstruction. If these develop, racemic adrenaline may be of help in alleviating the condition, but if the obstruction increases, then nasotracheal intubation should be performed. When the burn is such that intubation is impractical, then a tracheostomy is necessary.

Inhalation of chemical gases, the products of combustion, and smoke may produce oedema and sloughing of the mucosa of the larynx and trachea extending into the tracheobronchial tree. Nasotracheal intubation should be performed to facilitate the toilet to the tracheobronchial tree if signs of airway obstruction develop in such a child.

Ingestion of toxic chemicals is a common occurrence in children. Chemical burns of the glottis may occur, producing an upper airway obstruction. Direct laryngoscopy under general anaesthesia will demonstrate the extent of the lesion. Steroids, to limit the extent of the reaction, and the use of racemic adrenaline by nebulization may alleviate mild symptomatology. Intubation or tracheostomy, depending on the extent and the severity of the lesion is indicated if the airway obstruction is severe.

External trauma.   Although very rare, external trauma may produce anatomical disruption of the larynx to the extent that upper airway obstruction results. There may be extrinsic pressure on the trachea due to haematoma formation or swelling. Direct bronchoscopy confirms the clinical diagnosis and nasotracheal intubation or tracheostomy is indicated according to the pathology found.

Postintubation.   Subglottic oedema may occasionally occur following routine tracheal intubation, usually due to the use of an inappropriate size of tracheal tube. Stridor and signs of upper airway obstruction develop early in the postoperative period and usually respond to the administration of humidified oxygen and dexamethasone. If they persist, then racemic adrenaline given by nebulization usually results in a rapid resolution (see p. 244).

Postoperative.   Excision of lesions of the neck such as thyroglossal duct cysts in infants and children may be followed in the postoperative period by signs of upper airway obstruction. This may be due to the movement of the tracheal mucosa over the tracheal tube by surgical manipulation intraoperatively, leading to mucosal swelling postoperatively. This will respond well to humidification and/or racemic adrenaline if necessary.

Haematoma or postoperative swelling may produce extrinsic pressure, narrowing the tracheal lumen. Routine drainage of neck wounds postoperatively for a 24-h period usually prevents such haematoma formation.

Neurogenic

Altered consciousness.   Airway obstruction of varying degrees may accompany a depressed conscious state. Lack of attention to the airway may accentuate and exacerbate the already depressed conscious state. Simple airway management manoeuvres will often suffice to correct the obstruction. If the degree of airway obstruction is severe or the child markedly obtunded, then intubation to secure and protect the airway and to ensure oxygenation is indicated.

Acquired peripheral neurological lesions.   The muscular spasms associated with tetanus may affect the laryngeal musculature, producing airway obstruction. Sedation with for example diazepam may suffice to relieve the obstruction but commonly sedation combined with paralysis and nasotracheal intubation is indicated. Rarely, diseases of viral aetiology such as poliomyelitis or ascending myelitis may affect pharyngeal and laryngeal musculature, leading to the signs of upper airway obstruction.

Neoplastic

Intrinsic tumours.   Intrinsic tumours of the airway are uncommon in children, but may occur at any level of the larynx or trachea. They produce stridor and indrawing, the extent of which depends on the size and location of the mass. The commonest in the paediatric age group is juvenile laryngeal papillomatosis. This is often a benign condition but may spread rapidly and unpredictably, leading to a relatively rapid onset of upper airway obstruction. Direct laryngoscopy and excision by laser surgery are the treatments of choice (see p. 422). Occasionally, tracheostomy is indicated to secure the airway, but it is avoided if at all possible as it is associated with the spread of the papilloma. Many of these children require repeated anaesthetics, halothane remaining the drug of choice, despite the remote risk of hepatotoxicity.

Extrinsic pressure from benign or neoplastic nodes, tumours or cysts of the neck or mediastinum may be associated with obstruction. Often the extrinsic pressure produces a softening of the trachea, necessitating careful observation of the child in an intensive care environment following the surgical excision of the mass. Occasionally it is prudent to leave a nasotracheal tube in situ postoperatively until the postoperative swelling has subsided.

Immunological

Angio-oedema.   Triggered by a variety of allergens, angio-oedema may specifically produce oedema of the larynx. Rapid in onset, the administration of subcutaneous adrenaline, intravenous steroids or antihistamines is usually effective in reducing this oedematous swelling. Oral intubation, cricothyrotomy, or tracheostomy may be life-saving if the obstruction is severe.

Juvenile rheumatoid arthritis.   This is a rare disease in children but signs of upper airway obstruction may occur if the disease process affects the small joints of the larynx. The symptomatology of cricoarytenoid arthritis is a feeling of fullness in the throat similar to the sensation of a foreign body. This may be accompanied by hoarseness or stridor. Specific diagnosis is made by direct laryngoscopy when the mucosa overlying the joints may be seen to be erythematous and oedematous. The glottic opening may also be narrowed.

REFERENCES

Adair JC, Ring WH & Jordan WS (1971) Ten year experience with IPPB in the treatment of acute laryngotracheobronchitis. *Anesthesia and Analgesia (Cleveland)* **50:** 649–653.

Arthurton MW (1970) Stridor in a paediatric department. *Proceedings of the Royal Society of Medicine* **63:** 712–714.

Bluestone CD, Delerne AN & Samuelson GH (1972) Airway obstruction due to vocal cord paralysis in infants with hydrocephalus and meningomyelocoele. *Annals of Otolaryngology* **81:** 778.

Cohen D (1981) Tracheopexy, aortotracheal suspension for severe tracheomalacia. *Australian Paediatric Journal* **17:** 117–126.

Cohen SR (1969) Unusual lesions of the larynx, trachea and bronchial tree. *Annals of Otolaryngology* **78:** 476–489.

Debrand M, Tseudo K & Browning S (1979) Anesthesia for extensive resection of congenital tracheal stenosis in an infant. *Anesthesia and Analgesia* **58:** 431.

Downes JJ & Raphaely RC (1975) Pediatric intensive care. *Anesthesiology* **43:** 238–250.

Evans JNG (1979) Laryngotracheoplasty. *Otolaryngology Clinics of North America* **10:** 119–123.

Goudsouzian N, Cote CJ & Liu LMP (1981) The dose–response effects of oral cimetidine on gastric pH and volume in children. *Anesthesiology* **55:** 533.

Hanallah K & Rosales JK (1978) Acute epiglottitis: current management and review. *Canadian Anaesthetists' Society Journal* **25:** 84–91.

Hollinger PH & Brown WT (1967) Congenital webs, cysts, laryngocoeles and other anomalies of the larynx. *Annals of Otology, Rhinology, Laryngology* **76:** 744.

Kantor RK & Watchko JF (1984) Pulmonary oedema associated with upper airway obstruction. *American Journal of Diseases of Childhood* **138**: 356–358.

Keens TG, Bryan AC, Levison H et al (1978) Developmental pattern of muscle fiber types in human ventilatory muscles. *Journal of Applied Physiology* **44**: 909–913.

Keon TP (1985) Anesthesia for airway surgery. In Godinez RI (ed) *Special Problems in Pediatric Anesthesia*, pp 87–116. Boston: Little, Brown.

Macartney FJ, Panday J & Scott O (1969) Cor pulmonale as a result of chronic nasopharyngeal obstruction due to hypertrophied tonsils and adenoids. *Archives of Diseases of Childhood* **44**: 585–592.

Maze A & Bloch E (1979) Stridor in pediatric patients. *Anesthesiology* **50**: 132–145.

Mitchell DP & Thomas RL (1980) Secondary airway support in the management of croup. *Journal of Otolaryngology* **9**: 419–422.

Newth CJL, Levison H & Bryan AC (1972) The respiratory status of children with croup. *Journal of Pediatrics* **81**: 1068–1073.

Rapkin RH (1973) Tracheostomy in epiglottitis. *Paediatrics* **42**: 426–429.

Schuller DE & Birk HG (1974) The safety of intubation in croup and epiglottitis. An eight year follow up. *Laryngoscope* **85**: 33–46.

Statistics Canada (1985) *Causes of Death*.

Swischuk LE (1979) *Emergency Radiology of the Acutely Ill or Injured Child*. Baltimore: Williams & Wilkins.

Vernon DD & Sarnaik AP (1986) Acute epiglottitis in children. A conservative approach to diagnosis and management. *Critical Care Medicine* **14**: 23–25.

Wilms D, Popovitch J, Fujita S et al (1982) Anatomic abnormalities in obstructive sleep apnoea. *Annals of Otology, Rhinology and Laryngology* **91**: 595–596.

Unusual conditions in paediatric anaesthesia

INTRODUCTION

This chapter will present an approach to the evaluation of children with congenital anomalies or syndromes, including those anomalies with obvious implications for anaesthesia management or monitoring, and some syndromes with subtle or hidden potential problems. After a general presentation of preoperative evaluation, specific congenital syndromes, their anaesthetic-related problems and alternatives for management will be discussed. A more complete list of syndromes grouped by area of potential anaesthetic impact appears in Table 21.1, which expands and reorganizes the indexes of Jones and Pelton (1976) and of Steward (1985). Finally a discussion of malignant hyperthermia, its presentation, diagnosis and treatment will complete the chapter.

PREOPERATIVE EVALUATION

Thorough preoperative evaluation is essential to assure optimum perioperative monitoring and care, and to identify the patient needing subspecialty consultation prior to surgery.

Past anaesthetic records can provide a wealth of information concerning airway, respiratory, cardiovascular, and metabolic function. Unsuspected problems may have been identified and treated, and potential problems may have been resolved during past anaesthetics.

The general health of the child may be assessed by reviewing height and weight, including percentiles from growth grids. Many syndromes cause alterations in overall growth (Table 21.2).

The upper airway evaluation seeks to identify conditions that will modify anaesthesia planning. If abnormalities are found, parents may be informed of potential problems and therapeutic plans. A history of snoring which wakens the child reveals significant airway obstruction. The child with micrognathia who may present difficulties with intubation can be identified if the child's face, especially in profile, is examined (Figure 21.1). Stehling (1984) reported in adults that if the distance from the lower border of the mandible to the thyroid notch, measured with the neck extended, is less than 6 cm, visualization of the larynx by direct laryngoscopy will be impossible. A distance of 6.5 cm, if associated with prominent upper teeth or limited cervical or temporomandibular motion will also lead to difficult direct laryngoscopy. The equivalent distance in paediatric patients has not been reported.

Table 21.1. Congenital syndromes affecting anaesthesia—listed by body system

a. Airway (difficulty intubation or mask fit: J = micrognathia; C = cervical spine instability or limited motion; M = soft tissue mass or macroglossia; L = small larynx; S = increased secretions)

Aaskog–Scott—C	Hunter's—S, M
Achondroplasia—C	Hurler's—S, M
Anderson's—midface hypoplasia	I-cell disease—C, J
Angioneurotic oedema—L (swelling)	Juvenile rheumatoid arthritis—C
Aglossia–adactylia—J	Klippel–Feil—C
Apert's—J	Kniest's—C
Arthrogryposis multiplex—C, J	Larsen's—C
Beckwith–Wiedemann—M	Meckel's—J
Behçet's—ulcers of pharynx	Median cleft face—J, cleft
Carpenter's—J	Moebius—J
CHARGE association—J; choanal atresia	Morquio—C
	Multiple mucosal neuroma—M
Cherubism—M	Myositis ossificans—C
Christ–Siemens–Touraine—J	Noack's—J
Chotzen—J	Noonan's—C
Cretinism—M	Orofacial–digital—cleft
Cri du chat—M	Patau (trisomy 13)—J, cleft
Crouzon—J	Pendred—M
Cystic hygroma—M	Pierre Robin—J, cleft
Diastrophic dwarfism—C, J	Pompe's disease—M
Down's (trisomy 21)—C, M	Rieger—abnormal teeth
Dyggue–Melchior–Clausen's—C	Russell–Silver dwarf—J
Edward's (trisomy 18)—J	Scleroderma–small mouth
Epidermolysis bullosa—see text, L	Smith–Lemli–Opitz—J
Farber's disease—L	Spondylometaphyseal dysplasia—C
Freeman–Sheldon—small mouth	Spondyloepiphyseal dysplasia—C
Goldenhar (hemifacial microsomia)—J	Sprengel's—C
	Treacher Collins—J, small mouth
Goltz–Gorlin—abnormal teeth, C	Turner's—C, J
Hallermann–Strief—J, small mouth	Urbach–Wiethe disease—L
Hallervorden–Spatz—torticollis, trismus	von Recklinghausen's disease—M
	Weaver—J
Hand–Schüller–Christian—L	

b. Ventilation problems (L = intrinsic lung disease; W = muscle weakness; C = chest wall deformity)

Amyotonia congenita—W, see text	Jeune's—C
Central core myopathy—W	Kartagener's—L
Chronic granulomatous disease—L	Kugelberg–Welander muscular atrophy—W
Cretinism—W	
Cutis laxa—L	Letterer–Siwe disease—L
Cystic fibrosis—L	Marfan's—L, C
Duchenne muscular dystrophy—W	Maroteaux–Lamy—C
Ehlers–Danlos—L (pneumothorax)	McArdle's disease—W
Familial periodic paralysis—W	Morquio s.—C
Gaucher's disease—L (aspiration)	Myasthenia congenita—W
Guillain–Barré—W	Myasthenia gravis—W
Hand–Schüller–Christian—L	Myositis ossificans—C (stiff)
I-cell disease—L, C (stiff)	Myotonic dystrophy—see text

Table 21.1.b. (*cont.*)

Niemann–Pick disease—L	Rubinstein—L
Osteogenesis imperfecta—C	Scleroderma—L
Polycystic kidneys—L (cysts in 33%)	Smith–Lemli–Opitz—L
Pompe's disease—W	VATER—L
Prader–Willi—W (in infancy)	Werndig–Hoffman disease—W
Prune belly—W	Wilson–Mikity—L
Riley–Day—L	

c. Cardiovascular C = congenital heart disease; M = cardiomyopathy; A= autonomic or arrhythmias; I = ischaemic; T = thrombotic)

Albright's osteodystrophy—A	Laurence–Moon–Biedl—C
Apert's—C	Leopard—C
Asplenia (Ivemark)—C	Marfan's—C
CHARGE association—C	Maroteaux–Lamy—M
Conradi's—C	Meckel's—C
Cretinism—M	Myotonic dystrophy—M
DiGeorge's—C	McArdle disease—M
Down's (trisomy 21)—C	Noonan—C
Duchenne muscular dystrophy—M	Patau (trisomy 13)—C
Edward's (trisomy 18)—C	Polysplenia—C
Ehlers–Danlos—T	Pompe's disease—M
Ellis–Van Creveld—C	Progeria—I
Fabry's disease—I	Riley–Day—A
Farber's disease—M	Rubinstein—C
Freidrich's ataxia—M	Sebaceous naevi—C
Gullain–Barré—A	Shy–Drager—A
Goldenhar—C	Sipple—A
Groenblad–Strandberg—T	Stevens–Johnson—M
Holt–Oram—C	William's—C
Homocystinuria—T	Tangier's disease—I
Hunter's—M	TAR—C
Hurler's—M	VATER—C
I-cell disease—C (valvular)	Werner—I
Jervell–Nielson—A	Wolff–Parkinson–White—A

d. Endocrine (S = steroid coverage perioperatively; P = phaeochromocytoma; T = thyroid)

Adrenogenital—S	Epidermolysis bullosa—S (often)
Behçet's—S (often)	Hand–Schuller–Christian—S
Blackfan–Diamond—S	Kasabach–Merritt s.—S
Chediak–Higashi—S	Multiple mucosal neuroma (multiple
Collagen vascular diseases—S (often)	endocrine adenomatosis type
Dermatomyositis	IIb)—P
Juvenile rheumatoid arthritis	Myositis ossificans—S (often)
Scleroderma	Pendred—T
Lupus	Sipple—T, P
Periarteritis nodosa	von Hippel–Lindau—P
Cretinism—T	von Recklinghausen disease—P

Table 21.1. (*cont.*)

e. Metabolic (G = glucose; E = electrolyte; C = calcium problems)

Adrenogenital—E	Laurence–Moon–Biedl—E (diabetes
Albers–Schönberg—C	insipidus)
Albright's osteodystrophy—C	Leprechaunism—G
Albright–Butler—E	Lesch–Nyhan—uric acid
Alström—G	Lipodystrophy—G
Andersen's disease—G	Lowe—C
Bartter's—E	Maple syrup urine disease—E, G
Beckwith—G	McArdle's disease—G
Cretinism—G, E	Paramyotonia congenita—E
DiGeorge's—C	Phenylketonuria—G
Down's—G	Prematurity—G, E, C
Familial periodic paralysis—E	Prader–Willi—G
Fanconi—E	von Gierke's disease—G
Hand–Schüller–Christian—E (diabetes	Wermer syndrome (multiple endo-
insipidus, rarely)	crine adenomatosis I)—G, C
Homocystinuria—G	Werner—G, C
	William's syndrome—C

f. Skin problems (careful positioning, intravenous access may be difficult)

Behçet's—ulcers in mouth	Groenblad–Strandberg
Christ–Siemens–Touraine	Osler–Weber–Rendu
Cutis laxa	Ritter's disease
Ehler–Danlos	Scleroderma
Epidermolysis bullosa—mucosal and	Stevens–Johnson
skin ulcers	

g. Orthopaedic (limited joint mobility or fragile bones)

Albers–Schönberg disease	Osteogenesis imperfecta
Marfan's	Scheie disease
Ollier's	

h. Haematological (anaemia, platelet decrease or dysfunction, or clotting disturbance)

Albers–Schönbeg	Letterer–Siwe disease
Blackfan–Diamond	Lipodystrophy
Chediak–Higashi	Maroteaux–Lamy
Christmas disease	Moschkowitz disease
Collagen vascular diseases	Niemann–Pick disease
Favism	Sickle cell disease—avoid pneumatic
Gaucher's disease	tourniquets
Hand–Schüller–Christian	Tangier disease
Hermansky	TAR
Homocystinuria	von Willebrand's disease
Kasabach–Merritt	Wiskott–Aldrich
Klippel–Trenaunay	Wolman's disease

Table 21.1. (*cont.*)

i. Renal (renal dysfunction affects use of drugs such as muscle relaxants)

Alport	Lesch–Nyhan
Alström	Lowe
Bowen's (cerebrohepatorenal)	Meckel's
Chotzen's	Orofacial–digital
Conradi's	Prune belly syndrome
Edward's (trisomy 18)	Tuberous sclerosis
Fabry's disease	VATER
Fanconi	von Hippel–Lindau
Farber's disease	Wermer
Laurence–Moon–Biedl	Wilson's disease

Table 21.1. (*cont.*)

j. Pharmacology (S = avoid succinylcholine; M = careful use of muscle relaxants or barbiturates; H = avoid halothane; B = avoid barbiturates)

Amyotonia congenita—M	Lipodystrophy—H
Arthrogryposis multiplex—M	McArdle's disease—S
Bowen's—M	Myotonia congenita—M, S
Central core myopathy—M	Myotonic dystrophy—S, H, M
Duchenne's muscular dystrophy—M	Paramyotonia congenita—S, H, M
Familial periodic paralysis—M	Phenylketonuria—M
Guillain–Barré—S	Porphyria—B
Hallervorden–Spatz disease—S	Wilson's disease—M

Table 21.2. Syndromes associated with altered growth parameters

Small stature	
Chromosomal abnormality, including	Non-chromosomal abnormality, including
Trisomy 21	Bloom syndrome
Trisomy 18	CHARGE association
Trisomy 13	Cornelia De Lange syndrome
Trisomy 8	Fetal alcohol syndrome
Cri du chat	I-cell disease
4 p$^-$	Noonan syndrome
13 q$^-$	Russell–Silver syndrome
18 q$^-$	Seckel syndrome
Cat-eye syndrome	Smith–Lemli–Opitz
Turner syndrome	Williams syndrome

Tall stature/obesity	
XXY, Klinefelter syndrome	Beckwith–Wiedemann
XYY syndrome	Sotos syndrome
	Weaver syndrome
	Prader–Willi (after infancy)

A complete history and physical examination of the respiratory system will identify patients with poor pulmonary reserve. A history of infant respiratory distress syndrome requiring mechanical ventilation, cystic fibrosis, recurrent pneumonia, asthma or muscular dystrophy will identify patients at risk for intraoperative or postoperative respiratory problems. Pulmonary function testing in older children with advanced pulmonary disease or weakness may guide perioperative care and family counselling.

A search for congenital heart disease, use of cardiac medications (digoxin, diuretics, propranolol), exercise tolerance of the child, or a history consistent with arrhythmias (syncopal episodes or paroxysmal tachycardia) guide the cardiovascular assessment. The signs and symptoms of congestive heart failure in infants are non-specific and can be subtle. Tachypnoea, nasal flaring, or grunting respirations are often present; the infant may feed slowly, tire during feeding, or sweat profusely. The older child may tire more quickly than playmates. Physical examination may reveal a cardiac murmur, tachycardia at rest or irregular rhythms, hepatomegaly, cyanosis,

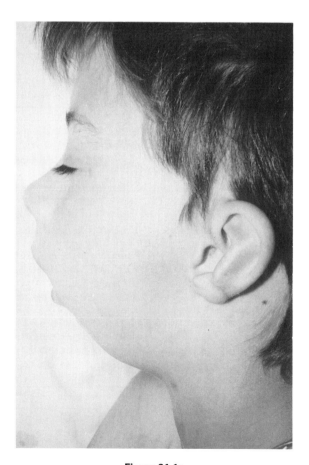

Figure 21.1a

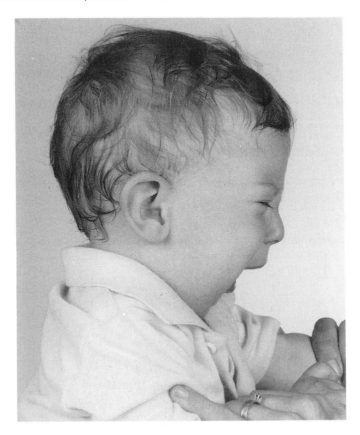

Figure 21.1b

Figure 21.1a, b. Profiles showing micrognathia.

or clubbing of the fingers. Cardiology evaluation should be reviewed or obtained to aid perioperative care. Cardiac evaluation should be considered when major anomalies are present in other systems, such as gastrointestinal (e.g. omphalocoele, duodenal atresia) or extremity malformations (Holt–Oram syndrome, VATER syndrome; see Table 21.3).

In congenital syndromes known to affect blood chemistries (Table 21.1), metabolic studies should include evaluation of glucose levels, acid–base status, electrolytes, or calcium concentrations. General neurological development is assessed in children with congenital anomalies since it affects anaesthetic plans. Focal findings such as spastic diplegia or hemiparesis may affect placement of intravenous or arterial catheters or choice of anaesthesia (general compared with regional techniques). The infant with hydrocephalus requires a smooth induction and intubation to avoid potential problems with increases in intracranial pressure.

Musculoskeletal abnormalities may also affect anaesthesia choices. In the myotonia syndromes succinylcholine is avoided; Duchenne's muscular dystrophy may be associated with malignant hyperthermia and suggests the

Table 21.3. Congenital syndromes frequently associated with congenital heart defects

Syndrome	Findings	Congenital heart lesion	Incidence
Apert	Craniosynostosis, midfacial hypoplasia, syndactyly of extremities	VSD, TOF	
Blackfan–Diamond	Anaemia in infancy	VSD	
Carpenter	Synostosis of coronal, sagittal, or lambdoid sutures		
	Brachydactyly and partial syndactyly of hands and feet, polydactyly of feet	PDA, VSD	
CHARGE association	Coloboma choanal atresia, retarded growth, retarded mental development, microphallus, cryptorchidism, micrognathia/cleft palate, ear anomalies/deafness	Vascular ring or interrupted aortic arch, AV canal, TOF, truncus arteriosus, DORV c̄ AV canal, VSD, PDA	60–70%
Cri du chat	Slow growth, mental deficiency, microcephaly, hypertelorism, strabismus, simian crease	VSD, ASD	25%
Crouzon	Craniostenosis, shallow orbits	Coarctation of aorta	
DiGeorge	Hypoparathyroidism, hypocalcaemia, deficient T-call-mediated immunity	Truncus arteriosus, double aortic arch (vascular ring), right aortic arch, TOF	
Ehlers–Danlos	Hyperextensible, joints, blue sclerae, easy bruising, parchment scars, scoliosis, hernias, pes planus	Mitral insufficiency	50%
Ellis-van Creveld	Short distal extremities, polydactyly, hypoplastic nails, dysplastic teeth, small thorax	ASD	50%
Fetal alcohol	Microphthalmos, microcephaly, mental retardation, growth failure	VSD, PDA	
Goldenhar	See text	TOF, VSD	

Syndrome	Features	Cardiac defect	%
Holt–Oram	Radial club hand or hypoplasia, proximal thumb placement	ASD, VSD	
Homocystinuria	Lens dislocation (downward), slender, pectus, osteoporosis, malar flush	Thrombotic events	
Hurler	See text	Aortic insufficiency, mitral insufficiency	
Ivemark (asplenia)	Absent spleen, infection risk increased, situs inversus of abdominal viscera	Dextrocardia, complex cyanotic heart disease (e.g. TGA; single ventricle)	
Marfan	Long thin limbs and fingers, joint laxity with scoliosis, pectus excavatum, tall stature, upward lens dislocation	Aortic aneurysm, aortic regurgitation, mitral valve prolapse	
Multiple lentigines (Leopard)	Hypertelorism, dark lentigenes especially on face or trunk, prominent ears sensorineural deafness	PS	95%
Noonan	See text	PS, ASD	
Rubella	Cataract, deafness, retardation, cryptorchidism	PDA, PS (peripheral), VSD	
TAR (Thrombocytopenia, absent radius)	Decreased platelets and megakaryocytes, bilateral radial hypoplasia/aplasia	TOF	
Trisomy 13	Small-for-age, severe retardation, deafness, microcephaly, retinal dysplasia, cleft lip/palate (80%), polydactyly, parieto-occipital scalp, skin defects	VSD, dextroversion	90%
Trisomy 18	Growth deficiency, retardation, low-set ears, micrognathia, short sternum, clenched hand	VSD, PDA, PS	99%
Trisomy 21	See text	AV canal, ASD, VSD	50%

Table 21.3. (cont.)

Syndrome	Findings	Congenital heart lesion	Incidence
Tuberous sclerosis	Adenoma sebaceum, ash-leaf spots, café-au-lait spots, hamartoma of brain, seizures, mental deficiency	Rhabdomyomas	
Turner	Pterygium colli, infantile lymphoedema, short stature, webbed neck, low hairline	Coartation, AS	35%
VATER	Vertebral anomalies, anal atresia, T-O fistula, radial dysplasia	VSD	20–30%
Williams	Prominent lips, hoarse voice, mental deficiency, talkative, hypercalcaemia in infancy (20%), blue eyes with stellate pattern	AS, PS	

VSD = ventricular septal defect; TOF = tetralogy of Fallot; PDA = patent ductus arteriosus; AV = arteriovenous; ASD = atrial septal defect; TGA = transposition of great arteries; PS = pulmonary stenosis; AS = aortic stenosis; DORV c̄ AV canal = double outlet right ventricle with atrio-ventricular canal; T-O = tracheo-oesophageal.

use of a non-triggering anaesthetic technique, one which avoids succinylcholine or potent inhalational agents. Children with unusual facies or defects in multiple systems can be identified and seen by genetic or dysmorphology consultants to aid preoperative diagnosis and management.

SYNDROMES AFFECTING AIRWAY MANAGEMENT (see Chapter 12)

The infant or child with a compromised airway can be identified at the preoperative examination by the presence of an obstructing mass (e.g. cystic hygroma or a large tongue), micrognathia, limited mouth or neck mobility, or by symptoms such as stridor. In these children, preoperative sedation should usually be avoided, since its effect on airway patency is unpredictable. Drying of oral secretions and blockade of vagal stimulation during laryngoscopy are indications for an anticholinergic agent. Atropine (0.01–0.02 mg/kg) intravenously assures complete absorption and eliminates an unnecessary intramuscular injection for the child. A variety of facemasks, laryngoscope blades, endotracheal tubes, and stylets should be assembled along with functioning suction equipment. The Vital Signs (Totowa, New Jersey) anaesthesia mask, with its soft air-filled cushion, facilitates mask fit when distortions of facial anatomy are present. Use of the oxyscope in infants allows delivery of oxygen to the pharynx during laryngoscopy, giving an additional 30–60 s for visualization during direct laryngoscopy. A modified oxyscope may be obtained for older children by taping a feeding tube or suction catheter to the back of the laryngoscope blade. A 3.0 tracheal tube adapter is inserted into the end of the catheter, and connected to the anaesthesia circuit, allowing oxygen to be delivered to the pharynx, as in infants.

In severe cases the surgeon and the equipment needed to perform an emergency cricothyrotomy or tracheostomy should be present before laryngoscopy is undertaken. Awake laryngoscopy is our usual procedure in infants under 6 weeks of age, and may be used in the co-operative older child or adolescent, though this is not universal practice. Lack of understanding and the risk of damage to oral or pharyngeal tissues usually mandate another approach in the young child or the retarded child.

An inhalation induction with spontaneous ventilation may be used in the unco-operative child presenting for elective surgery. It is often modified in children with associated congenital heart disease who may develop hypotension or an increase in right-to-left shunting under deep inhalation anaesthesia with the associated systemic vasodilatation. When inhalation induction is elected, halothane is the agent used, and the induction is begun with the child positioned comfortably (often sitting or lying laterally). An airtight mask fit allows assisted ventilation during induction if increasing airway obstruction occurs when the child is positioned supine. Demonstration of the ability to ventilate with a mask must precede the use of any muscle relaxants. Airway obstruction during early induction may be decreased by the use of a nasopharyngeal airway.

If laryngoscopy under deep inhalational anaesthesia allows visualization of the vocal cords, intubation under direct vision may be accomplished. If the vocal cords are not visible but the epiglottis is, the use of a stylet to direct the tracheal tube just below the epiglottis may allow intubation if the tube can be gently advanced into the trachea. The importance of an assistant holding the child's head in the midline, 'sniffing' position cannot be overemphasized. If the larynx cannot be visualized directly, alternate methods of intubation are employed.

Blind nasotracheal intubation may be attempted following topical anaesthesia to the nares, with 4% cocaine spray, and to the pharynx and larynx with 4 or 10% lignocaine to a maximum dose of 3 mg/kg. Intravenous sedation with thiopentone (2 mg/kg), diazepam (0.1–0.2 mg/kg), midazolam (0.05–0.1 mg/kg) and/or fentanyl (1–2 μg/kg) is carefully titrated to maintain spontaneous ventilation while allowing maximal patient comfort (Lynn et al, 1988). With the child sitting tilted head-up at 60° and with the chin lifted, in the 'sniffing' position, the nasal tube is advanced while listening for maximal breath sounds. Entry into the oesophagus causes loss of breath sounds. If direct laryngoscopy and blind nasal intubation are not successful, fibreoptic laryngoscopy can be employed. A tracheal tube greater than a 4.5 mm internal diameter and an operator experienced in the use of fibreoptic laryngoscope are prerequisites (Stehling, 1984). Alfery et al (1979) reported the use of the fibreoptic laryngoscope via one nostril for visualization, while a tracheal tube was manipulated into the trachea via the other nostril. When fibreoptic laryngoscopy is considered, it is best used early before attempts at intubation obscure the pharynx with secretions or blood. Recently even smaller fibreoptic catheters (as small as 1.3–3.6 mm) have become available, although current models cannot be deflected (Visicath, Microvasive, Milford, Massachusetts).

If inhalational induction with a mask is possible, it may be followed by laryngeal nerve block with 2 mg/kg of lignocaine to each side of the neck, with passage of a guide wire retrograde through the cricothyroid membrane into the oral or nasopharynx. A tracheal tube may then be advanced into the trachea while the guide wire is held taut. Once the tracheal tube enters the proximal trachea, the guide wire is pulled through the tracheal tube while the tube is advanced into a more secure position in the trachea (Lopez, 1968). This procedure has been fairly, but not uniformly, successful in children over 6 years in Seattle. It is not a procedure recommended for use in infants. If mask ventilation can be established, tracheostomy can be done in this manner.

Finally, tracheostomy with local anaesthesia is possible with a cooperative patient. Some of the congenital syndromes that may present problems in airway management will now be described.

Pierre Robin syndrome, or the Robin anomalad includes micrognathia, glossoptosis, and a U-shaped cleft palate (Figure 21.2). In utero, mandibular hypoplasia displaces the tongue posteriorly, interfering with closure of the soft palate. These children may present in infancy for glossopexy or tracheostomy if the tongue and small mandible cause severe airway obstruction with cyanosis and apnoea. This condition is seen in otherwise normal children, and growth of the mandible in the first year of life is possible, resulting in a normal jaw in later childhood. However, the Robin anomalad may be seen as part of other syndromes, including Stickler, DeLange, Hallerman–Strief or femoral hypoplasia syndromes.

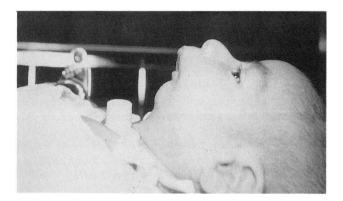

Figure 21.2. Infant with Pierre Robin syndrome. Severe airway obstruction necessitated tracheostomy.

Goldenhar syndrome (hemifacial microsomia) occurs as a defect in development of the first and second branchial arches (Figure 21.3). These children show asymmetric hypoplasia of malar, maxillary and mandibular areas, which may include soft tissues and the tongue. Goldenhar's is the diagnosis if epibulbar dermoids, congenital heart disease, or cervical vertebral defects accompany the facial defects. If involvement is primarily facial, then hemifacial microsomia is the diagnosis given, but these probably represent gradations of the same defect in morphogenesis (Smith, 1976). The mouth often has a cleft-like extension on the affected side, making mask fit during anaesthesia a problem. A deformed to absent external pinna or a preauricular skin tag is often associated with deafness. Cardiac defects, especially ventricular septal defect (VSD) or tetralogy of Fallot (TOF) are associated conditions in the Goldenhar syndrome. These children present for reconstructive surgery of their mandibles or external ear. Induction of general anaesthesia may present difficulties in maintaining a patent airway and in laryngoscopy and intubation.

Treacher Collins syndrome is an autosomal dominant mandibulofacial dysostosis with down-slanting palpebral fissures, eyelid colobomata, malar and mandibular hypoplasia and malformation of the external pinna and ear canal. Conductive deafness is seen in 40% of these children. Laryngeal hypoplasia may be part of the syndrome constellation. Mental development is normal. Mandibular osteotomies and cosmetic surgery to eyes or ears are scheduled during childhood in severely affected children. Difficulty with intubation is seen with severely hypoplastic, retrognathic mandibles.

Moebius syndrome is a rare defect resulting from agenesis or hypoplasia of cranial nerve nuclei, in particular cranial nerves VI and VII. The facial nerve palsies can be associated with poor mandibular growth and secondary micrognathia; XII nerve involvement may limit tongue movement. A small number (approximately 10%) of affected children have other brain anomalies. Difficulties in intubation in these children relate mainly to the degree of micrognathia.

The *Klippel–Feil anomalad* shows fusion of cervical vertebrae causing a short neck with limited mobility. This may interfere with positioning for intubation, making visualization of the larynx difficult. Frequently associated findings in these children are neurological defects, deafness, congenital heart disease (VSD) and scoliosis.

Arthogryposis multiplex congenita results from a number of in-utero neuropathic or myopathic problems which lead to limited fetal joint mobility and cause congenital joint contractures. The immobile joints are most obvious in the extremities, but of most concern to anaesthetists when limited temporomandibular and cervical spine movement make intubation difficult. These patients are discussed in detail by Hall (1983); two-thirds of these children have a good prognosis for mental development but one-third will have severe central nervous abnormalities and most of the latter group die in infancy. Similar limitations in joint mobility in jaw and neck may be seen in children with *juvenile rheumatoid arthritis*.

The *mucopolysaccharidoses* are lysosomal storage disorders characterized by the progressive diffuse accumulation of mucopolysaccharides in

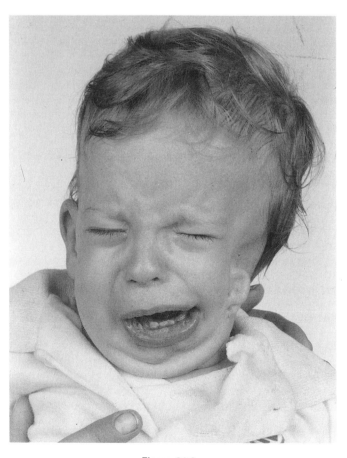

Figure 21.3a

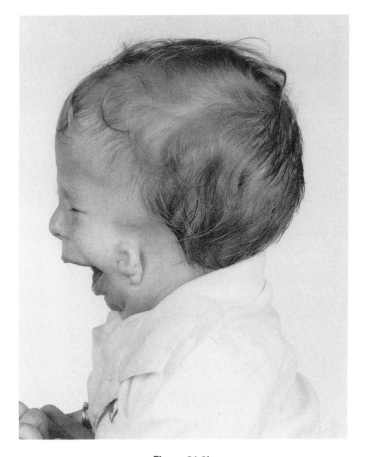

Figure 21.3b

Figure 21.3a, b. A 16-month-old child with severe hemifacial microsomia. His profile from the unaffected side is shown in Figure 21.1b.

lysosomes in bone, muscle, visceral organs and in the soft tissues of the mouth and pharynx. Classification of these disorders is based on clinical, biochemical and/or genetic differences. *Hurler's syndrome*, mucopolysaccharidosis type I, shows the most severe involvement with coarse facies, macroglossia, infiltration of pharyngeal and laryngeal soft tissues, short neck, kyphosis, corneal opacities, claw hand and limited cardiac function as distinctive features (Figure 21.4). Profuse secretions from upper and lower airways are usual, and severe mental retardation is obvious by 3 years of age. *Hunter's syndrome*, mucopolysaccharidosis type II, differs only in the more gradual onset of symptoms, lack of corneal opacities and presentation only in males. The combination of mental deficiency with a limited ability to co-operate, profuse airway secretions, and increasing soft-tissue infiltration with the mucopolysaccharides makes airway management and intubation a major anaesthetic problem, particularly in the child past infancy.

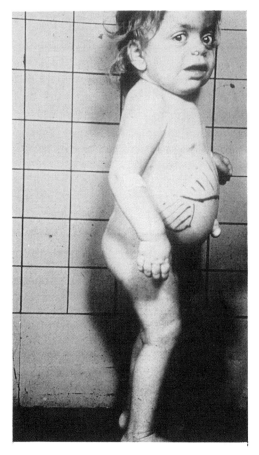

Figure 21.4. Hurler's syndrome (mucopolysaccharidosis type I). Note thickened facial features, short neck and nasal secretions. (Courtesy Dr V. A. McKusick.)

Baines and Keneally (1983) reported their experience with these children. Some 50% of their patients had difficulties with airway management during anaesthesia. Profuse secretions occluding a tracheostomy, coughing spasms, difficulty maintaining a patent airway during mask anaesthesia and a failed intubation were problems they described. Inhalation inductions were used in the majority, with small amounts of intravenous agents to aid induction in unco-operative children. Maintaining spontaneous ventilation until airway control is secured and preoperative atropine were recommended.

Morquio syndrome, mucopolysaccharidosis type IV, presents less problems with soft-tissue infiltration of the upper airway and mental development is usually normal (Figure 21.5). Chest wall deformities result in limited ventilatory reserve. These children have odontoid hypoplasia, putting them at risk of anterior dislocation of the C1 vertebra with resultant cord compression. This can occur during head positioning for tracheal intubation, so

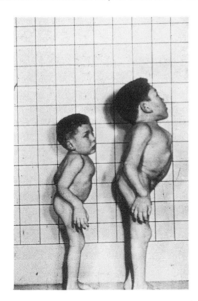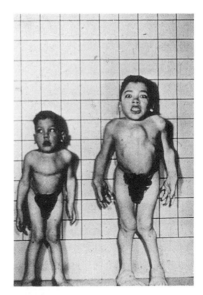

Figure 21.5. Brothers with Morquio's syndrome. From McKusick (1972).

extreme flexion should be avoided by having an assistant hold the head in the neutral position during laryngoscopy. Several other congenital syndromes associated with odontoid hypoplasia have been included in Table 21.1a.

Cleft lip and/or palate may be seen as part of many syndromes, including the CHARGE association, fetal hydantoin syndrome, orofacial–digital syndrome, and trisomy 18, but it is an isolated defect in 90–95% of affected children. Airway management and intubation are usually straightforward, but may be difficult if the cleft displaces intraoral tissues so that palatal tissues mechanically interfere with placing the tracheal tube at the glottis. Visualization of the larynx is usually not a problem. Following palate closure, the tongue may cause airway obstruction, so these children should be extubated when they are fully awake. Practical management of these patients is covered more fully on p. 293.

Haemangiomas and lymphangiomas (cystic hygromas) are congenital benign tumours, but can cause significant airway problems, particularly if intraoral extension limits airway access or their large size causes tracheal compression extrinsically (Figure 21.6). Haemangiomas, if present elsewhere, can be a clue to their presence in the trachea and, like laryngeal webs or cysts, they may present with stridor and symptoms of airway obstruction.

Beckwith–Wiedemann syndrome includes omphalocoele, macroglossia, large size and neonatal hypoglycaemia (Figure 21.7). Because omphalocoeles are also seen in 10–50% of infants with trisomy 13 or 18, chromosomal studies are indicated in all infants with omphalocoeles (Smith, 1976). Congenital heart disease is seen in 20% of infants with omphalocoeles, and genitourinary defects including extrophy of the bladder have been reported frequently (Stehling and Zauder 1980). Because of the Beckwith–

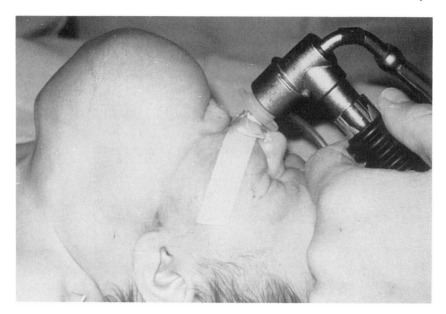

Figure 21.6. Infant with large cystic hygroma.

Wiedemann association of omphalocoele and neonatal hypoglycaemia, anaesthesia in these infants should include frequent blood sugar determinations. Extubation is attempted only when the infant has demonstrated adequate spontaneous ventilation following repair, since limitation of diaphragmatic excursion often necessitates a period of postoperative mechanical ventilation.

SYNDROMES AT RISK OF RAPID INTRAOPERATIVE BLOOD LOSS

Craniostenosis, premature fusion of one or more of the skull sutures, is seen in several syndromes including *Crouzon, Saethre–Chotzen, Pfeiffer, Carpenter* and *Apert* syndromes. All but Crouzon syndrome are associated with syndactyly; most patients with these disorders are of normal intellect. These children present at several months of age for craniectomy or for more extensive revision of the skull and orbital area. The anaesthetic management of these syndromes is discussed on p. 392.

There are many other congenital anomalies which carry an equal risk of blood loss, including separation of conjoined twins (Furman et al, 1971; Towey et al, 1979), correction of kyphoscoliosis in a child with Morquio's syndrome or resection of a sacrococcygeal teratoma.

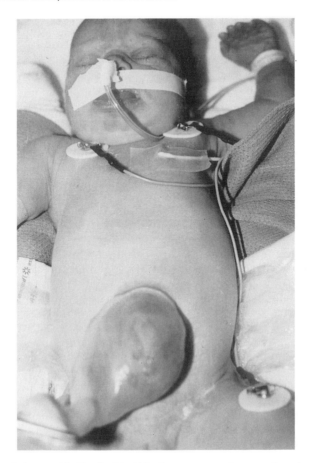

Figure 21.7. Infant with Beckwith–Wiedemann syndrome showing omphalo-coele, macroglossia and large size (birthweight 4.1 kg). Hypoglycaemia responded to intravenous 10% dextrose solution.

SYNDROMES WITH RESPIRATORY PROBLEMS

Ventilation difficulties may be present before surgery, may develop intraoperatively or in the postoperative period. They may be caused by intrinsic lung disease, chest wall deformities, or muscular weakness (Table 21.1).

Myotonic dystrophy, an autosomal dominant disorder, is characterized by myotonia (the inability to relax muscles), cataracts, frontal baldness, testicular atrophy in males and the expressionless 'myopathic' facies. Presentation in late adolescence is most common with progressive muscle weakness and swallowing difficulties, but subtle symptoms have been reported in childhood. Cardiac conduction abnormalities are present in over 50% of patients. *Myotonia congenita*, another autosomal dominant disorder, shows hypertrophied muscle and more severe myotonia but no weakness or cardiac involvement. *Paramyotonia* presents as myotonia and weakness induced by exposure to cold; potassium levels should be evaluated in these patients since myotonia may be seen in patients with *Familial periodic paralysis*.

Anaesthetic management in the myotonia syndromes is influenced by several special considerations. Since cold or shivering increase myotonia, a warm environment is essential and some authors avoid halothane to minimize postoperative shivering (Kaufman et al, 1983). The depolarizing muscle relaxants are absolutely contraindicated, since generalized myotonia has been seen following succinylcholine, making ventilation difficult to impossible for several minutes (Ellis, 1974). Non-depolarizing muscle relaxants may be used safely with a transcutaneous nerve stimulator to titrate dosage, but are ineffective if local manipulation causes myotonia. Direct injection of local anaesthetic into the affected muscle has been suggested to treat local myotonia (Gregory, 1983). Demonstration of adequate spontaneous ventilation prior to extubation should include an inspiratory effort greater than -30 cm H_2O and a tidal volume greater than 5 ml/kg. The use of muscle relaxants in these children is discussed further on p. 105.

Inadequate ventilation may be seen in congenital syndromes associated with weakness or inadequate cough, such as Werdnig–Hoffmann, myasthenia gravis, nemaline myopathy, central core disease, or the muscular dystrophies, Duchenne's being the most common and most severe. Careful titration of muscle relaxants, if any are used, and assisted or controlled ventilation intraoperatively guide intraoperative care. Assessment of chest wall and diaphragmatic function should include inspiratory effort (normal > -30 cm H_2O) and vital capacity (≥ 15 ml/kg) prior to extubation. Children with central core disease, nemaline myopathy and Duchenne's muscular dystrophy are at risk for malignant hyperthermia (see final section for anaesthetic management).

Cystic fibrosis, an autosomal recessive disorder, involves abnormal sweat and mucus production with diffuse effects, but it is the pulmonary involvement which impinges most directly on anaesthetic management. The ventilatory problems include inspissated secretions, ventilation–perfusion mismatching with resultant hypoxaemia and infection of large and small airways with multiple organisms, often including *Pseudomonas*. Advanced pulmonary disease results in cor pulmonale. The use of chest percussion, postural drainage and antibiotics preoperatively to optimize pulmonary function has been generally recommended (Gregory, 1983). Atropine will cause drying of secretions. Ketamine is best avoided because of its stimulation of airway reflexes. General anaesthesia with tracheal intubation allows intraoperative suctioning of secretions as needed, and controlled or assisted ventilation is used to minimize atelectasis. Inhalation anaesthesia with halothane is well tolerated, but induction may be prolonged due to ventilation–perfusion mismatching. Intra-arterial monitoring for serial blood gases is indicated in the presence of severe lung disease or cor pulmonale. Adequacy of ventilation must be demonstrated prior to extubation, as detailed above, with inspiratory effort and tidal volume and, in the severely affected child, by blood gas measurement during spontaneous ventilation. Postoperative chest physiotherapy and close observation remain necessary, since deterioration in lung function has been reported following general anaesthesia (Richardson et al, 1984).

Prune belly syndrome results from a congenital deficiency of the abdominal musculature, associated with genitourinary anomalies (Figure 21.8; Henderson et al, 1987). The long-term prognosis in these children is determined by the degree of compromise of their renal function. The abdominal musculature deficiency raises the potential problem of inadequate cough before, during, or following anaesthesia. For anaesthetic management see p.282.

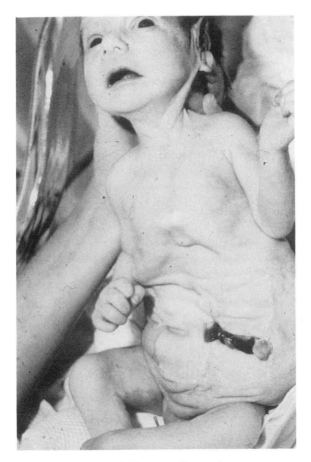

Figure 21.8. Prune belly syndrome.

SYNDROMES ASSOCIATED WITH CARDIOVASCULAR PROBLEMS

An extensive discussion of congenital heart disease and its implications for anaesthesia is beyond the scope of this chapter. Recent literature presents discussion in depth (Gregory, 1983; Hickey and Hansen, 1984; Lake, 1987). Table 21.3 lists syndromes frequently associated with congenital heart disease. The anaesthetic management of cardiovascular problems is discussed in Chapter 13.

Trisomy 21 (Down's syndrome) is a chromosomal disorder involving all body systems. The characteristic flat facies, protruding tongue, inner canthal folds, up-slanting palpebral fissures, hypotonia and hyperflexible joints, mental retardation, and short broad hand with simian creases are easily recognized. Some 40–50% of these children have congenital heart disease, most commonly endocardial cushion defects or VSD. The hyperflexible joints necessitate careful intubation, since cervical dislocation with spinal cord damage has been reported (Kobel et al, 1982).

Turners's syndrome should be suspected in any female with short stature. Ovarian dysgenesis with failure of sexual maturation at puberty and infertility, as well as short neck with posterior webbing or pterygium are additional findings. Thirty per cent of these children have cardiac defects, usually coarctation of the aorta. Chromosome studies demonstrate the XO karyotype.

Noonan syndrome represents the phenotype of Turner's syndrome with normal chromosomal studies. Short stature, webbed neck, and cryptorchidism in males are findings similar to Turner's; mental retardation and pectus excavatum are more common in Noonan's and the congenital heart disease seen is commonly pulmonary stenosis rather than coarctation.

William's syndrome is a sporadic disorder which includes prominent lips, wide mouth, elfin facies, mild growth retardation and mental deficiency, hypercalcaemia in infancy (20%), and valvular or supravalvular aortic stenosis. These children have a distinctive hoarse voice and talkative manner.

Arrhythmias are the major feature in *Romano–Ward syndrome* (prolonged QT), *Jervell–Lange–Nielsen* (prolonged QT and deafness) and *Wolff–Parkinson–White syndrome* (aberrant arteriovenous conduction, with a short PR interval and delta waves on ECG). Placement of a transvenous pacemaker for perioperative care is the safest course for the prolonged QT syndromes, but left stellate ganglion block has also been used with success (Callaghan et al, 1977). In patients with Wolff–Parkinson–White syndrome, avoidance of tachycardia and excitation is recommended. If supraventricular tachycardia appears, the use of propanolol 0.01 mg/kg increments intravenously, or verapamil 0.1 mg/kg slowly intravenously, has been successful in converting the rhythm to normal sinus rhythm. However, in recalcitrant cases, synchronized DC cardioversion should be available for intraoperative use.

Tuberous sclerosis, a disease characterized by hamartomatous lesions that may involve multiple systems, is dominantly inherited with many cases representing fresh mutations. The skin changes appear in early to mid childhood, have been called adenoma sebaceum (a misnomer) and prominently affect nasolabial folds. Affected children have ash-leaf spots (hypopigmented areas) and café-au-lait spots in infancy. Seizures and mental deficiency are seen in most affected children. Cardiac involvement with rhabdomyomas may present with arrhythmias or signs of obstruction to blood flow. Anaesthetic management should avoid possible arrhythmogenic agents, e.g. halothane, and should maintain normal vascular volume to minimize vertricular outflow obstruction.

Children with congenital heart disease should be examined for other anomalies. If abnormalities of vertebrae, anus (imperforate), or arms (radial dysplasia) are found, careful evaluation for the presence of tracheo-oesophageal fistula is mandatory; this symptom complex represents the

VATER association: *v*ertebral anomalies, imperforate *a*nus, *t*racheo-oesophageal fistula, *r*adial or renal anomalies (Quan and Smith, 1973). Congenital heart disease, both cyanotic and acyanotic, is seen in 20–30% of these children.

Familial dysautonomia (Riley–Day syndrome)

Disturbances of autonomic function with this condition have profound anaesthetic implications (Stenqvist and Sigurdsson, 1982). There may be a defect in the formation of noradrenaline from levodopa which is manifest clinically by cardiovascular and temperature instability, hypotonia, no tear production and insensitivity to pain. Recurrent pulmonary aspiration after gastro-oesophageal reflux is common so that lung function deteriorates with the age of the child and is usually the eventual cause of death. Nissen's fundoplication and feeding jejunostomy are frequently required (Cox and Sumner, 1983).

The absence of compensatory cardiovascular reflexes may make anaesthesia hazardous. Respiratory-depressant analgesics should be used with great care and in reduced doses. Premedication with a benzodiazepine is satisfactory, but atropine should be avoided where possible. There is no contraindication to the use of muscle relaxants, but inhalational agents must also be used with care. Hypovolaemia is poorly tolerated. Hypotension may be controlled by fluid administration and hypertension by increasing the dose of inhalational agent. Postoperative respiratory support may be necessary.

SYNDROMES THAT REQUIRE SPECIAL CARE IN PATIENT MOVEMENT OR POSITIONING

Difficulties with positioning occur in the infant with meningomyelocoele or in thoracopagus conjoined twins. Intubation is usually possible with these infants in a lateral position.

Epidermolysis bullosa is a genetically inherited group of skin disorders which result in vesicles and bullae, occurring either spontaneously or with minimal trauma or friction. Both dominant and recessively inherited forms of the disorder have been described. The most severely involved are the recessive forms, where bullae heal with scarring that can result in significant contractures and syndactyly. Involvement of oral mucosa in these patients can result in microstomia and involvement of mucosa in the larynx and pharynx has been reported (Stehling, 1982). James and Wark (1982) reported no tracheal or laryngeal problems after anaesthesia with tracheal intubation in 131 patients with epidermolysis bullosa dystrophica. Special care is essential to prevent trauma to skin or mucosa. Tape is avoided; soft cotton padding under the blood pressure cuff, needle electrodes for electrocardiogram monitoring, and securing the tracheal tube with umbilical tape help to protect skin. Lubricating the facemask, laryngoscope, and face with hydrocortisone ointment and using a tracheal tube 0.5–1 mm internal diameter smaller than predicted have been recommended (Gregory, 1983).

Ketamine and halothane have both been used successfully. When tracheal tubes have been used the pharynx and vocal cords should be visualized prior to extubation to look for bullae formation.

Children with ectodermal dysplasia (Christ–Siemens–Touraine syndrome) have no sebaceous or sweat glands, absent hair and absent teeth (partial or complete). Full expression of this sex-linked recessive disorder is seen in males, and the facial features include depressed nasal bridge, deformed external ears, thick lips and underdeveloped maxilla and mandible. Airway management may be a problem in these children. Thermoregulation is defective because of the lack of sweat glands; therefore cooling measures should be available (cooling mattress, cool i.v. solutions) and temperature should be closely monitored. Anticholinergic medication is avoided to minimize its effect on temperature.

Patients with *osteogenesis imperfecta* or with *osteopetrosis* are at risk of fractures and joint dislocations with minimal trauma. Care in moving and positioning these patients extends to intubation, since their teeth are more fragile than normal.

MALIGNANT HYPERTHERMIA

Malignant hyperthermia is a rare, potentially lethal disorder most commonly triggered by anaesthetic agents. Some of the children mentioned above are at risk of this reaction during anaesthesia (Table 21.4).

Table 21.4. Congenital syndromes associated with malignant hyperthermia

Central core disease
Duchenne's muscular dystrophy
King–Denborough syndrome
Nemaline myopathy
Osteogenesis imperfecta

Malignant hyperthermia is an inherited disorder of skeletal muscle characterized by intermittent hypermetabolic crises, it may be triggered by the potent inhalational anaesthetics (halothane, enflurane, isoflurane), succinylcholine, ketamine or large doses of amide local anaesthetics. Stress has also been suggested to be a trigger, and this is seen in susceptible swine, the animal model. Its incidence is reported as 1:15 000 in children and 1:50 000 in adults.

A clinical diagnosis of malignant hyperthemia is made when the signs and symptoms listed in Table 21.5 appear during anaesthesia. The earliest signs are given in italic and are always present; the others appear in fulminant cases or when diagnosis is delayed. All reflect the hypermetabolism seen; hence tachycardia and tachypnoea with immediate rise in end-tidal CO_2 are the earliest and most sensitive signs. Temperature increases may be rapid or more insidious. If succinylcholine has been used, masseter spasm may be the first sign of malignant hyperthermia reaction. Children with any of the myotonic syndromes (myotonia congenita, myotonic dystrophy, paramyotonia) may develop masseter spasm following succinylcholine, but whether this represents a malignant hyperthermia reaction or myotonia is unclear. Current controversy exists about how to classify and treat patients who develop masseter muscle spasm following succinylcholine, which may occur in up to 1% of paediatric patients. Schwartz (1984) reported positive muscle biopsy results in 100% of such patients; others report 50–65% incidence (Flewellen and Nelson, 1982; Ellis and Halsall, 1984; Rosenberg and Fletcher, 1986). When metabolic demands exceed supply, venous desaturation, lactic acidosis and hyperkalaemia develop. A high index of suspicion will stimulate blood gas and potassium determinations in the event of unexpected tachycardia, tachypnoea, temperature rise (>0.5°C) or masseter spasm.

Table 21.5. Signs and symptoms of malignant hyperthermia

Symptoms	Signs
Tachycardia	*Venous oxygen desaturation*
Tachypnoea	*Venous hypercarbia*
Arrhythmias	*Metabolic acidosis*
Cyanosis	*Respiratory acidosis*
Mottling of skin	Hyperkalaemia
Fever	Myoglobinaemia/myoglobinuria
Rigidity	Elevated creatine phosphokinase
Sweating	Disseminated intravascular
Labile blood pressure	coagulation
Masseter spams (after succinylcholine)	

No single laboratory screen is available; serial (at least 3) serum creatine phosphokinase (CPK) determinations will show elevated baseline levels in 70% of susceptible patients. Following a malignant hyperthermia reaction CPK levels rise, with peak values in 8–12 h. Muscle biopsy testing is the best diagnostic test currently available—susceptible muscle shows contracture to halothane and to low concentrations of caffeine. Unfortunately, the contracture testing is technically difficult, performed only in selected centres, is invasive (requiring fresh muscle) and is not usually undertaken in prepubertal subjects. In both Europe and the USA uniform criteria for performing and interpreting the results are being established.

Malignant hyperthermia is an inherited disorder and genetic evaluation is usually consistent with an autosomal dominant pattern. The pathophysiology of the disorder is incompletely understood. Research has been facilitated by the presence of an animal model (several breeds of pig) which undergoes a similar hypermetabolic crisis in response to stress. Current understanding is that the hypermetabolism is related to a defect in calcium metabolism in susceptible skeletal muscle. This leads to high levels of intracellular calcium and stimulates actin–myosin coupling, causing sustained contraction. The contraction generates heat and metabolic by-products, eventually leading to muscle degeneration with release of myoglobin, potassium and CPK.

Patients at risk for malignant hyperthermia include:

1. those with a past history of a malignant hyperthermia event or with a positive muscle biopsy;
2. first-degree relatives of patients with malignant hyperthermia, if CPK is elevated;
3. patients with muscular dystrophy, osteogenesis imperfecta or central core myopathy (see Table 21.4).

These patients are given anaesthesia with non-triggering agents. Nitrous oxide, thiopentone, droperidol, morphine, fentanyl, pethidine (demerol), fentanyl derivatives such as sufentanil or alfentanil and non-depolarizing muscle relaxants such as pancuronium, vecuronium or atracurium have been used safely in such patients. Careful monitoring of electrocardiogram for heart rate and rhythm, blood pressure, end-tidal CO_2 and temperature are mandatory with blood sampling for blood gas and electrolytes if any signs of malignant hyperthermia occur.

Pretreatment with dantrolene may be given but is avoided if muscle biopsy is to be obtained during surgery.

Treatment of a malignant hyperthermia event must include:

1. elimination of the triggering agents, i.e. stop halothane, enflurane or isoflurane, change anaesthesia circuit (tubing, CO_2 absorber) and machine if possible, converting to nitrous oxide–narcotic–relaxant technique and stop surgery as soon as possible;
2. drawing blood gas, potassium, and initial CPK level to corroborate diagnosis;
3. hyperventilation with 100% O_2 and $NaHCO_3$ i.v. are used to treat respiratory and metabolic acidosis;
4. cooling meaures for fever (cooling mattress, cold saline for bladder, gastric or even peritoneal lavage, cool i.v. solutions);
5. aborting the muscle hypermetabolism with dantrolene which is continued until the patient has been asymptomatic and afebrile for 24 h;
6. maintaining good urine output with fluid therapy, and mannitol or frusemide if necessary;
7. repeating CPK level at 8 and 24 h after the event (levels over 20 000 units are diagnostic; over 10 000 are highly suggestive).

Close cardiovascular and temperature monitoring (usually in an intensive care unit) are necessary for 24–48 h following an event.

Dantrolene has become the mainstay in treatment of a malignant hyperthermia crisis. It is a hydantoin derivative which blocks intracellular calcium release and is used to abort malignant hyperthermia crises, given prophylactically to prevent their occurrence. Since absorption after oral doses can be variable, intravenous use is favoured. Swine studies have demonstrated effective malignant hyperthermia prophylaxis with dantrolene; blood levels which are protective in swine can be achieved in humans for 6 h following administration of 2.4 mg/kg of dantrolene intravenously. In treating a crisis, increments of 1 mg/kg up to 10 mg/kg may be necessary to reverse the hypermetabolism. Lerman et al (1988) recently reported dantrolene kinetics in children and found more rapid clearance than in adults. Blood levels in children remain protective (>3.0 μg/ml) for 5 h following an intravenous bolus of 2.4 mg/kg. Thus supplemental doses may be needed more frequently in children than in adults.

REFERENCES

Alfery DD, Ward CF, Harwood IR et al (1979) Airway management for a neonate with congenital fusion of the jaws. *Anesthesiology* **51**: 340.

Baines D & Keneally J (1983) Anaesthetic implications of the mucopolysaccharidoses: a 15-year experience in a children's hospital. *Anaesthesia and Intensive Care* **11**: 198–202.

Callaghan ML, Nichols AB & Sweet RB (1977) Anaesthetic management of prolonged Q–T syndrome. *Anesthesiology* **47**: 67–69.

Cox RG & Sumner E (1983) Familial dysantonomia. *Anaesthesia* **38**: 293.

Ellis FR (1974) Neuromuscular disease and anaesthesia. *British Journal of Anaesthesia* **46**: 603–612.

Ellis FR & Halsall PJ (1984) Suxamethonium spasm—a differential diagnositic conundrum. *British Journal of Anesthesia* **56**: 381.

Flewellen EH & Nelson TE (1982) Masseter spasm induced by succinylcholine in children; contracture testing for malignant hyperthermia. *Canadian Anaesthetists' Society Journal* **129**: 432–449.

Furman EB, Roman DG, Hairabet J et al (1971) Management of anesthesia for surgical separation of newborn conjoined twins. *Anesthesiology* **34**: 95–101.

Gregory GA (1983) *Pediatric Anesthesia*, vols 1 and 2. Philadelphia: Churchill Livingstone.

Hall JG (1983) Arthrogryposes In Emery AEH & Rimoin DL (eds) *Principles and Practice of Medical Genetics*, pp 781–811. Philadelphia: Churchill Livingstone.

Henderson AM, Vallis CJ & Sumner E (1987) Anaesthesia in the prune belly syndrome *Anaesthesia* **42**: 54–60.

Hickey PR & Hansen DD (1984) Fentanyl and sufentanil–oxygen–pancuronium anesthesia for cardiac surgery in infants. *Anesthesia and Analgesia* **63**: 117–124.

James I & Wark H (1982) Airway management during anesthesia in patients with epidermolysis bullosa dystrophica. *Anesthesiology* **56**: 323–326.

Jones AEP & Pelton DA (1976) An index of syndromes and their anesthetic implications. *Canadian Anaesthetists' Society Journal* **23**: 207–226.

Kaufman J, Friedman JM & Sadowsky D (1983) Myotonic dystrophy: surgical and anesthetic considerations during orthognathic surgery. *Journal of Oral and Maxillofacial Surgery* **41**: 667–671.

Kobel M, Creighton RE & Steward DJ (1982) Anaesthesia considerations in Down's syndrome; experience with 100 patients and a review of the literature. *Canadian Anaesthetists' Society Journal* **29**: 593–599.

Lake CL (ed) (1987) *Pediatric Cardiac Anesthesia*. East Norwalk, Connecticut: Appleton Lange.

Lerman J, Derdemezi J, Strong HA & McLeod ME (1988) Pharmacokinetics of intravenous dantrolene in malignant hyperthermia susceptible pediatric patients. *Anesthesia and Analgesia* **67**: S133.

Lopez NR (1968) Mechanical problems with the airway. *Clinical Anesthesia* **3**: 16.

Lynn AM, Morray JP & Furman EB (1988) Short-acting barbiturate sedation: effect on arterial pH and $PaCO_2$ in children. *Candian Journal of Anaesthesia* **35**: 76–79.

Quan L & Smith DW (1973) The VATER association. Vertebral defects, anal atresia, T-E fistula with esophageal atresia, radial and renal dysplasia: A spectrum of associated defects. *Journal of Pediatrics* **82**: 104–107.

Richardson VF, Robertson CF, Mowat AP et al (1984) Deterioration in lung function after general anaesthesia in patients with cystic fibrosis. *Acta Paediatrica Scandinavica* **73:** 75–79.

Rosenberg H & Fletcher JE (1986) Masseter muscle rigidity and malignant hyperthermia susceptibility. *Anesthesia and Analgesia* **65:** 161–164.

Schwartz L, Rockoff MA & Koka BV (1984) Masseter spasm with anesthesia: incidence and implications. *Anesthesiology* **61:** 772–775.

Smith DW (1976) *Recognizable Patterns of Human Malformation*, 2nd edn. Philadelphia: W.B. Saunders.

Stehling LC (1982) *Common Problems in Pediatric Anesthesia*. Chicago: Yearbook Medical.

Stehling LC (1984) The difficult intubation and fiberoptic techniques. In *ASA Annual Refresher Course Lectures*, p 230. American Society of Anesthesiologists.

Stehling LC & Zauder HL (1980) *Anesthetic Implications of Congenital Anomalies in Children*. New York: Appleton-Century-Crofts.

Stenqvist O & Sigurdsson J (1982) The anaesthetic management of a patient with familial dysautononomia. *Anaesthesia* **37:** 929–932.

Steward DJ (1985) *Manual of Pediatric Anesthesia*, 2nd edn. New York: Churchill Livingstone.

Towey RM, Kisia AKL, Jacobacci S et al (1979) Anaesthesia for the separation of conjoined twins. *Anaesthesia* **34:** 187–192.

Paediatric anaesthesia in developing countries

INTRODUCTION

Technology and techniques, in whatever field, should always be appropriate to all the circumstances of their application and exercise. This fact has particular relevance for Third World anaesthesia. The term 'Third World' is often replaced by the descriptive term 'developing world'. Conditions and degrees of development, vis-à-vis first (Western) or second (Eastern Block) world development, vary considerably from country to country, and within countries, so that, as least in parts of a country, the environment in which hospital medicine is practised may be in many respects little different from that in parts of Europe or the USA.

However, to any observer other than the most casual, it may well be obvious that the existence and apparent success of a Western style of medical practice in a developing country depends upon the continuing influence of Western design and structure and/or the actual presence of expatriate staff. Elsewhere, it may be all too obvious that a Western structure has collapsed or is in the process of doing so, with nothing or not enough on hand to replace it. For historical reasons, European ideas and influences played some part in the development of modern medical services virtually everywhere in the Third World. It might be said, that all the medical facilities established by expatriates in the developing world are inappropriate and always were despite their apparent success for varying periods of time. This would be a judgement made with the benefit of hindsight; it is less easy to decide whether such a judgement could have been made at the time of their conception.

It is the firm conviction of the writer that the practice of medicine can only be optimum or first-rate if it conforms to the principle of appropriateness at every level. What follows in this chapter is the practical consequence of that conviction. As basic premises, it is pointed out:

1. the 'appropriateness' in anaesthesia and other branches of medicine applies to and is determined by two factors: the human elements—patient and attendants—and the technology elements—equipment, drugs, techniques.
2. that techniques taught and practised in the main centres in a country must in general be applicable throughout the country.

RESOURCES

Realism requires that the practice of medicine should take account of available resources and their limitations, otherwise appropriateness in incomplete or non-existent. With respect to the practice of anaesthesia, resources include personnel, equipment and drugs. If some resource is always lacking, then a method of procedure excluding it will be in operation; it is the intermittent, particularly the unexpected, shortage that is hazardous. It is essential that the techniques of anaesthesia taught are always applicable and appropriate throughout the region or country. However it is vital that the organization of the anaesthetic services also provides for the unexpected.

Personnel

Of significance here are not only the level of training and expertise of the anaesthetist and surgeon but also the quality of the support staff, including skilled assistance for the anaesthetist.

The anaesthetist may be a non-physician anaesthetist, i.e. a paramedical person, or a physician anaesthetist; the latter category includes non-specialists and specialists of varying grades.

An inexperienced anaesthetist working with an inexperienced surgeon (e.g. intern, house officer or paramedical officer) is certainly undesirable but this occurs despite intentions and efforts to prevent or minimize its happening. In situations where numbers are few, the non-availability of a particular worker is always a possibility, and must be provided for in the organizational structures for junior and/or paramedical staff. If guidelines for alternative arrangements in such situations are not set down, disasters may rapidly occur.

Drugs and equipment

In the developing world, the supply of drugs and equipment may be unreliable for a variety of reasons and the source of supply may vary. Shipments of donated or subsidized supplies of both drugs and equipment arrive intermittently from a variety of government and non-government sources. It is not unknown for such items to be drugs in concentrations no longer recommended in the country of origin, or even drugs withdrawn from the home market for some reason, or drug batches which have expired or are about to expire. The local purchasing authority, if poorly or inadequately advised, may accept tenders for drugs (and equipment) from countries using an unfamiliar language. In this case, as also with donated or subsidized drugs and equipment, the package labelling or instructions may be in a language unknown to the potential users. Another possibility is the failure of the user to recognize that a particular preparation of a drug is a different concentration from that normally used; for example, there are available both 5% and 1% aqueous solutions of suxamethonium salts. While one may expect that provision will be made for translation and suitable re-labelling, particular attention should be drawn to the concentration. This is by no means always done and the risks, especially regarding drug usage are obvious. Training and instruction, particularly of junior and paramedical staff, must cover these eventualities.

Anaesthetic drugs, which according to the manufacturer's dating are expired have probably suffered no change more serious than a reduction in potency, and this possibly not until the expiry period is significant—for example, a year or more. However, this presumes storage under suitable or prescribed conditions. Aqueous preparations of suxamethonium salts hydrolyse at a rate directly related to the temperature, and unless refrigerated may demonstrate significantly reduced potency.

Diethyl ether, although not expiry-dated, is decomposed by exposure to light, heat and air, to acetaldehyde and peroxides, with a resultant decrease in potency.

Donated and unwisely purchased equipment also brings the possibility of another significant problem—the negation of the principle of standardization of equipment. The importance of this principle is widely recognized, in particular with regard to matching connections and user familiarity, especially for the non-specialist. Related to this is the difficulty and cost of servicing and spares for a variety of models of equipment. Above all, safety is compromised.

Supplies of compressed gas may also be a cause for concern. The supply may be unreliable or non-existent for a variety of reasons: manufacturing plant problems, transport problems, cost etc. and there may be failure or non-availability, for other reasons, of associated equipment. Thus nitrous oxide may often be unavailable and in some areas never available; the supply of oxygen may be unreliable or even non-existent.

At the present stage of oxygen concentrator technology, particularly with reference to the domiciliary models, a source of supplementary oxygen dependent only on electrical power is now available to even very small health care facilities in situations where compressed gases are not available. These units require careful frequent maintenance or the oxygen output falls providing as little as 35% oxygen. If the unit is small it can be used to fill reservoir cylinders during 'off-peak' periods for later use. Oxygen generators using hydrogen peroxide as fuel are also available and have apparently been found satisfactory.

Another significant item is the supply of intravenous fluids. In this regard a very pertinent question has been asked: 'Why import water?' While many, possibly all, national health authorities in the developing world maintain a facility to manufacture i.v. fluids, distance from peripheral hospitals and other health care facilities, with attendant transport difficulties and cost, may make the possibility of local production highly desirable. 'Do-it-yourself' i.v. fluid plants are available as a package or can be put together by an interested technician, anaesthetist or other professional.

Further, it should be remembered that rehydration may be achieved by routes other than intravenous, and in fact may have to be achieved or attempted in the absence of suitable preparations for i.v. use. If there is no vomiting, oral (or nasogastric) rehydration may be possible, using either commercial oral rehydration salts which are available in packets to be dissolved in water or 'home-made' preparations e.g. 1, three-finger pinch of salt and 2, four-finger scoops of sugar in 0.5 l of drinking water (Woldman, 1987). Fluids can be administered by the rectal route, and thus do not have to fulfil the standards for parenteral fluid; again 'home-made' fluids can be used. Subcutaneous and intraperitoneal fluid administration requires fluid of parenteral standards, but not necessarily an i.v. giving set—a syringe may be used.

EQUIPMENT AND TECHNIQUES APPROPRIATE TO PAEDIATRIC ANAESTHESIA IN DEVELOPING COUNTRIES

What follows is not an exhaustive study of techniques, but merely an indication of necessary or recommended modifications or adaptations of recognized paediatric techniques, making them more appropriate to local circumstances.

The use of conduction (or regional) anaesthesia in paediatric patients in the Third World is certainly less than in the First World. The frequent absence of skilled assistance for the anaesthetist renders the production of a (regional) block after induction of general anaesthesia (probably the commonest form of its use in the First World) a hazardous undertaking, and one which the wise 'occasional' paediatric anaesthetist will be reluctant to attempt, and which others should have been discouraged from undertaking during training.

General anaesthesia techniques include the inhalational, the parenteral and perhaps the rectal route. Total intravenous anaesthesia, while requiring a minimum of equipment, presents certain problems in its exercise, e.g. the accurate titration of the drug used, which in the hands of a non-specialist may pose too great a risk of excessive dosage to be tolerated. A pair of anaesthetists (e.g. 'buddy system'; see p. 549) may well develop a successful and safe technique. Intramuscular ketamine may be satisfactory, either as induction or total anaesthesia for short procedures, but in children under 10 kg response can be unpredictable. Rectal anaesthesia technique should be known for the occasions when nothing else is available, but occasional techniques are never wise, especially in the hands of the non-specialist.

Inhalational anaesthesia is the most common and usually the best technique. The supply of compressed gases may be unreliable or even non-existent. Therefore inhalational techniques independent of compressed gases must be available, i.e. a draw-over technique. The agent or agents used should be safe in the user's hands, as well as versatile and cheap.

An agent whose versatility includes the possibility of its safe use with environmental air as the carrier gas in a spontaneously breathing patient should be available. Agents such as halothane which cause respiratory depression can be used safely with air in conjunction with intermittent positive pressure ventilation (IPPV) though the latter may not always be possible. Ether is the only inhalational agent which can be safely used with air as the carrier gas in a spontaneously breathing patient, as, unlike other inhalational agents, it stimulates respiration at surgical levels of anaesthesia.

However, in altitudes above 1500 m (5000 feet), hypoxia is possible and it is advisable to add supplementary oxygen if available.

Of the other volatile agents currently in use, halothane and trichloroethylene may be generally available and enflurane and isoflurane possible. If suitable draw-over vaporizers are available, which can be commercial or home-made. These agents can be used in the spontaneously breathing patient with supplementary oxygen, or in its absence with IPPV. The actual technique used will depend among other things on what is available. The T-piece can be used with draw-over vaporizer apparatus; some method of providing continuous gas flow is required, such as the Oxford inflating bellows.

Notes on draw-over vaporizers

The draw-over vaporizer, functioning in the demand or intermittent flow mode, is economical of the anaesthetic agent and has a considerably lower atmosphere-polluting potential than, for example, a Magill breathing system. In addition it is not dependent on compressed gas for its functioning; it uses room air with oxygen supplementation when possible or necessary. The simplest form of the draw-over vaporizer is a glass jar with two holes in the lid, to one of which is attached a length of tubing—the patient line. Air and supplementary oxygen enter the system via the other hole. The insertion of a T-piece or similar device in the patient line permits an increased degree of control—with the side arm open the concentration of the anaesthetic agent is approximately halved (Figure 22.1).

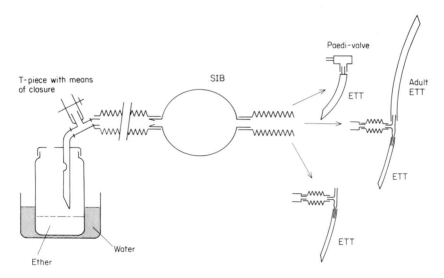

Figure 22.1. Equipment for draw-over anaesthesia. An improvised vaporizer with breathing system. The 'water bath' retards the rate of temperature, and therefore concentration drop with time. SIB = self-inflating bag; ETT = endotracheal tube. (After TB Boulton with kind permission.)

The addition of a self-inflating bag or bellows in the line between the vaporizer and the patient provides the facility to assist or control the ventilation. As vaporization of the agent proceeds, the temperature of the liquid remaining in the jar falls with a consequent progressive decrease in the vapour concentration. The rate of this decrease in temperature and concentration can be reduced by standing the jar in a container of water; the water acts as a heat reservoir, and thus as a temperature stabilizer (Boulton, 1966).

The EMO (Epstein Macintosh Oxford—Penlon) is a draw-over ether vaporizer incorporating a water jacket and a thermostat which automatically compensates for temperature change within the normal working range of temperature. The ether chamber is lined with wicks; by means of the control lever, ether concentrations of approximately 2–20% can be selected (Cole and Parkhouse, 1963). Though the accuracy of the EMO has been challenged (Schaefer and Farman, 1984), the potential error is on the safe side because the concentration is lower than indicated (apart from the high-range induction settings); in any case clinical assessment of the level of anaesthesia should always take precedence over theoretical considerations. A paediatric bellows is available for the Oxford inflating bellows, the ventilating device normally used with the EMO.

Supplementary oxygen and the EMO

Supplementary oxygen may be added to draw-over vaporizers via an open-ended piece of 2.5-cm diameter corrugated tubing 20 cm or more in length, attached at the air inlet. Oxygen enters this tube close to the vaporizer either via a side arm or via a fine gas feed tube passed up from the open end and secured by a stitch or by passing it through a hole cut in the corrugated tubing near its open end.

The corrugated tubing serves as a reservoir for oxygen when there is no movement of gas flowing through the vaporizer, i.e. during expiration and the respiratory pause. This technique of oxygen supplementation is economical of oxygen.

For the relationship between inspired concentration of oxygen (FiO_2) minute volume and flow of supplementary gas, see Farman (1973) or calculate the FiO_2. (Note: the supplementary oxygen should not be added at the Oxford inflating bellows—(tap-on older models)—during anaesthesia.)

Dräger produces a draw-over ether vaporizer, the AFYA, similar in function to the EMO, though temperature compensation is not automatic—adjustment is made according to the temperature of the ether in the chamber. A paediatric breathing system is provided with the AFYA. The PAC range of draw-over vaporizers includes an ether vaporizer, the Ether-Tec; a halothane vaporizer, the Fluotec, and the Pentec for methoxyflurane.

Penlon also produces the Oxford miniature vaporizer (OMV and OMV 50) which can be used in both the draw-over and plenum modes. The OMV comes in two versions—right-to-left flow for draw-over use in conjunction with the EMO etc. and left-to-right for use on the Boyle's and similar machines. The OMV can be used to vaporize halothane, trichlorethylene and chloroform; though the scale must be changed accordingly. The OMV has a capacity of 30 ml; the newer OMV 50 has a capacity of 50 ml. Both models incorporate a water jacket, but are not temperature-compensated. The greater volume of the newer model and, therefore, less frequent re-filling, means that there is a potential for a temperature-related fall in delivered concentrations. However in practice this does not seem to pose significant problems. Penlon's Tri-Service kit, developed for military use, contains two OMV 50 vaporizers.

Another vaporizer still in use, but not now manufactured, is Penlon's Bryce Smith induction unit (BSIU). This is a simple device, without controls, which delivers a measured dose of halothane (or trichlorethylene) for induction. The delivered concentrations vary inversely with the minute volume, so that in small children there is a risk of overdose, but duration of any such overdose is small by virtue of the limited maximum volume of charge (about 3 ml) and this can of course be further reduced by charging the wick with a smaller volume of agent.

A halothane vaporizer should be located downstream of an ether vaporizer, and a trichloroethylene vaporizer downstream of both to avoid the possibility of one agent dissolving in the other to any extent.

DRAW-OVER VAPORIZERS IN CLINICAL USE

Draw-over vaporizers, in general, when used with low flow rates, deliver lower concentrations than the control lever indicates. This fact needs to be taken into account when such vaporizers are used in paediatric practice, and a technique adopted which is suitable to the particular vaporizer.

The AFYA system has been subjected to a laboratory study (Swai et al, 1985) which demonstrated that: 'the system is suitable for spontaneous and controlled ventilation of the lungs in both adults and children'.

The standard EMO however is not suitable for spontaneous ventilation in the high-frequency, low tidal volume pattern; the output of ether vapour is very low. The OMV under the same conditions, with halothane, is unlikely to produce useful anaesthesia, and with trilene the output is far too low to be effective (Schaefer and Farman, 1984).

Using a T-piece

Both the EMO and the OMV can be used with the T-piece and this is extremely successful with either spontaneous or controlled ventilation. As noted above, a continuous gas flow must be provided.

If compressed gas is available and plentiful, then an appropriate flow can be directed into the inlet of the vaporizer. If compressed gas flow is limited, then an entrainer, such as the Farman oxygen entrainer, may be used, so that an air/oxygen mix is produced (see below). In these situations, the draw-over vaporizer is being used in a plenum mode, and inaccuracies will occur regarding concentrations; the delivered concentration will be closest to the indicated concentration with a continuous flow of about 10 l/min (Schaefer and Farman, 1984). However, ultimate reliance should not be placed on the concentration indicator of the vaporizer, but on clinical observations, so no problem should arise. In the absence of compressed gas, a self-inflating bag (SIB) or bellows (normally located between the patient and the draw-over vaporizer) can be used to produce a virtually continuous flow of gas. Though a second person is needed to do this it is quite satisfactory. It is advisable to practise this technique without a patient but with a gas flow meter (e.g. a Wright's respirometer) to determine the most suitable procedure. With the adult Oxford inflating bellows, a rapid filling followed by emptying over about 10 s and continued repetition of the sequence will usually be satisfactory.

It is possible to make an improvized T-piece by attaching an adult tracheal tube to the suction port of the paediatric connector of the Cobb type (Houghton et al; Figure 22.2).

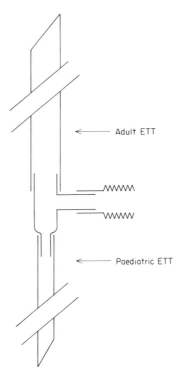

Figure 22.2. Improvised T-piece for spontaneous ventilation. The reservoir tube is an adult endotracheal tube (ETT) attached, for example, to an open suction union. After Houghton et al, with permission.

Another possibility needs no valve and employs the adult draw-over arrangement with IPPV. For induction, the anaesthetic mixture can be blown across the face of the child by operating the bellows with the mask held a little above the face. For maintenance, an open suction union is used on the tracheal tube; the suction port is occluded by a finger during inflation while expiration is via the non-occluded port (Cole and Parkhouse, 1963; Houghton et al; Figure 22.3). This technique requires a second person to attend to any task other than ventilation; the ventilator should of course be monitoring both the ventilation and the heart sounds via a precordial or oesophageal stethoscope.

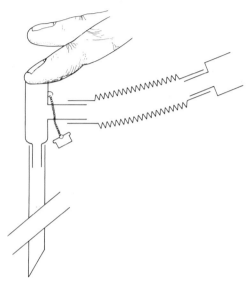

Figure 22.3. An improvised T-piece for controlled ventilation. The suction union is closed with the finger during compression of a self-inflating bag or bellows. After Houghton et al, with permission.

Farman entrainer

This device operates on the Venturi principle; a flow of oxygen, sufficient to register 100 mmHg on a sphygmomanometer connected to a side-tube on the device, entrains air at a ratio of about 5:1 air:oxygen. Thus it can be used when supplies of oxygen are limited. However, indications for its use are wider than just the need for economy in the use of oxygen. High concentrations of oxygen may be detrimental, with both the nature and severity of lesions being time-related, so that in the absence of nitrous oxide an air/oxygen mixture may be highly desirable.

Using a paediatric non-rebreathing valve

If a paedi-valve (e.g. AMBU or similar valve) is available, then an adult draw-over arrangement is adaptable; it is advisable to ventilate (control or assist) all except fit children over 12 kg. Spontaneous ventilation may be permitted in smaller children, using the adult bellows as a reservoir and re-filling it as necessary. However, if the tidal volume is very small, the time to empty the bellows may be sufficiently prolonged for some 'layering' of the heavy ether vapour to occur inside the bellows, with resultant variations in the inspired concentration. The writer has insufficient experience with the technique to elaborate on this point, having restricted this particular form of the technique to the end of surgery phase, when satisfactory spontaneous ventilation has been re-established. When used with a Farman entrainer the increased flow may prevent the expiratory valve from closing during breathing and dilution will take place.

INDUCTION

This may be parenteral, inhalational or rectal. Inhalational induction is usually safer for the non-specialist. It may be slow, and perhaps stormy, with ether. If a BSIU or OMV is available, then induction may be rendered more pleasant for the patient and quicker by using a limited amount of halothane, even if the drug to be used for maintenance is ether. In the absence of a halothane vaporizer, 2–3 ml halothane measured in a glass (not plastic) syringe may be injected into the tubing between the bellows and the patient, ensuring that the liquid cannot reach the patient. In a small baby, induction may be easier using an open mask (Figure 22.4) and dripping a measured amount (2 ml from a glass syringe) of trichloroethylene or halothane on to the gauze. It is advisable to direct a flow of oxygen under the mask via a small catheter.

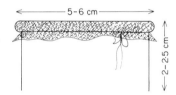

Figure 22.4. An improvised open mask for infants. The end is cut off a small food can of 5–6 cm diameter to give a cylinder of 2–2.5 cm height. The cut end is smoothed and several layers of gauze are tied over one end (sufficient layers so that liquid will not run through, but not so many that breathing is impeded—light should be visible through the full thickness). A piece of plastic foam of 8–9 cm diameter (as found in the top of a pharmacy tablet container), with a hole cut for the mouth and nose, will provide a seal when the mask is placed on the face. A flow of oxygen, e.g. 250–500 ml/min, is ideally directed under the mask via a fine catheter.

Intubation

The widely held view that the non-specialist or occasional anaesthetist should intubate virtually every patient is sound. Competence must be achieved and maintained, otherwise even a moderately difficult intubation may end in disaster. Less frequently offered is the advice to this category of anaesthetist to intubate the spontaneously breathing patient in order to obviate the hazards of prolonged or even failed intubation. To intubate such a patient when he or she is deeply anaesthetized with ether is not difficult, and, if a careful technique is practised, is not a prolonged procedure in a paediatric patient.

Muscle relaxation

In the hands of the inexperienced anaesthetist, especially when working alone, the use of both depolarizing and competitive muscle relaxants is usually contraindicated and is unnecessary especially when ether is used.

Monitoring

Equipment for monitoring will vary from place to place; if the purpose and functioning of what is available are understood by the prospective user, if its use can be safely initiated, and does not distract him or her from contact with the patient, then presumably it should be used. Such equipment may include a pulse monitor, ECG, temperature probe and a device for recording blood pressure. Certainly a sphygmomanometer should be used if possible. However, in many if not most situations other than in central hospitals, the paediatric anaesthetist will have only a precordial or oesophageal stethoscope. The latter is a particularly useful item; accurately placed and secured before the start of surgery, it provides the means for continuous and easy monitoring of both the respiratory and cardiovascular systems. An oeso- phageal stethoscope may be prepared by tying a rubber glove finger over the end of a piece of tubing of suitable diameter and length. If a length of tubing is interposed between the stethoscope earpiece and the patient end, a useful degree of mobility is obtained without interruption of auditory surveillance. The chest piece of a paediatric precordial stethoscope should be small and light and can be made in the hospital workshop. A single earpiece made from plastic foam allows this stethoscope to be used as a continuous monitor.

Hypothermia

Even in tropical climates hypothermia in small children is possible. The usual devices used in the developed world for maintaining body tempera- ture may be lacking and surgery may be slow if carried out by inexperienced surgeons. Available means must be used to minimize heat loss, these will include ensuring that the child is not lying in a pool of skin-cleaning liquid; is not lying on a wet drape; that parts of the body of a neonate or infant not needing to be exposed, particularly the head, are wrapped in for example cotton wool and that theatre air conditioning, if it exists, is adjusted accord- ingly. The temperature of the child should be checked at the end of the surgery, and if found to be low should be returned to normal by active means. If no other form of hot water bottle is available, and this method seems to be indicated, intravenous fluid bottles can be used.

Suction equipment

Because proper functioning of suction equipment is essential, and unreliability is potentially life-threatening, manual apparatus should be available as a back-up whenever and wherever the electric power supply is less than absolutely certain. Compressed gas-driven (e.g. oxygen) suction apparatus is available, but is not feasible for regular use in situations where compressed gases are in short supply. Manual equipment is necessary. Foot-operated suckers are commercially available in both paediatric and adult versions. A useful suction pump can be made by modifying a foot-operated motor vehicle pump to suck instead of pump. It is advisable to use unbreakable bottles with this type of equipment.

PREOPERATIVE ASSESSMENT

Non-surgical pathology present in children being assessed in preparation for surgery will include conditions peculiar to specific areas, in particular parasitic infestation. The anaesthetist should be aware of the local problems. Also frequently encountered will be calorie or protein malnutrition.

Anaemia

Probably the most commonly occurring preoperative problem in Third World paediatric practice is anaemia. The acceptable dividing line between anaemia and a normal haemoglobin displays a regional variation. In the developing world a haemoglobin of 10 g/100 ml may be classified as normal in an adult, or at least acceptable as a preoperative level. In developed regions, because the average haemoglobin is significantly higher, there is a tendency for this higher figure to be seen as the required normal. In developing world paediatric practice haemoglobin of not less than 10 g/100 ml of blood is frequently required, but in fact a level of 8 g/100 ml may be quite satisfactory, and in children with sickle cell disease the recommendation is that a haemoglobin of 8 g/100 ml should be considered optimum.

When deciding what haemoglobin level is acceptable in a particular case possible intraoperative and postoperative blood loss must be taken into account, as well as the availability of supplementary oxygen and blood for transfusion. In many parts of the developing world banked blood is not routinely available, and if a transfusion is needed suitable donors must be found. The high incidence of acquired immune deficiency syndrome (AIDS) in some parts of the world is relevant in this context.

Ancylostomiasis is common in children aged 2–5 years and the resultant anaemia may be compounded by various nutritional deficiencies (iron, folates, vitamin B_{12}, etc.) and associated infections. Premature infants and breastfed infants may exhibit iron deficiency anaemia while older children may have multiple deficiency anaemias. Among the congenital haemolytic anaemias sickle cell disease, thalassaemia major and glucose 6-phosphate dehydrogenase (G6-PD) deficiency are of particular importance in relevant areas. Malaria is a frequent cause of anaemia in children, commonly presenting as acute haemolysis in children aged 4 months to 8 years, and as chronic anaemia in older children. Schistosomiasis causes chronic blood loss from the gut and/or urinary tract.

It is important to find and correct the cause of anaemia preoperatively in all but emergency situations. It is possible that this is of far greater significance to the welfare of the patient than the proposed surgery.

Malnutrition

In addition to its part in the aetiology of anaemia, protein malnutrition probably increases susceptibility to infection, and causes delayed healing even in the absence of infection. It may be advisable to defer surgery, and send the patient away with clear guidelines for nutritional supplementation; the assistance of a primary health care centre may need to be sought. In times and areas of famine or of severe economic hardship, it will be necessary to recognize that sending the patient away for supplementary feeding is futile, and some form of in-hospital preparation should be attempted.

Other aspects of preoperative preparation

Sickle cell disease needs to be recognized preoperatively, so that pre- and intraoperative management is appropriate and designed to minimize the risk of a sickling crisis. The sickle cell syndrome involves the presence of an abnormal haemoglobin (HbS), which in the deoxygenated state (PaO_2 of less than about 5.5 kPa) gels or forms liquid crystals—tactoids—which distort the red cells, which in turn occlude vessels, causing multiorgan infarctions. The abnormal gene occurs predominantly in people of African and West Indian origin. Screening for the presence of sickle cells in people at risk should be carried out preoperatively unless the diagnosis is already established. In the presence of a positive screening test, haemoglobin electrophoresis will determine the severity of the disease; however, this is unlikely to be available in many or most parts of the developing world. If the sickle test is positive and the haemoglobin is less than 10 g/100 ml, sickle cell disease is probable.

The heterozygous state or sickle cell trait does not normally cause perioperative problems. The homozygous state or sickle cell disease presents significant risks during anaesthesia and surgery. Preoperative transfusion of packed red cells over several days or exchange transfusion may be carried out to reduce or suppress erythropoiesis and reduce the level of abnormal haemoglobin to below 40%. However, in the developing world this is often not practicable, and the most one can hope to achieve with blood transfusion preoperatively is to raise the haemoglobin to 8 g/100 ml. (A higher level of haemoglobin may cause a deleterious increase in blood viscosity.) Maintenance of adequate hydration before, during and after the operation is important.

Essentially, both systemic and regional tissue hypoxia and acidosis must be avoided. Some clinicians advise the preoperative use of sodium bicarbonate as prophylaxis against intraoperative acidosis; however, this is not without risks, and a meticulous anaesthetic technique is perhaps the best protection.

G6-PD deficiency should also be documented, although there does not seem to be agreement about the risk of using barbiturates in such patients.

Communication

In some, perhaps most, Third World countries problems of language are encountered in medical practice, especially in central or referral hospitals where there may be patients drawn from a number of tribal areas. Communication with the patient and his or her attendants may have to be through a third person. In this situation there is a risk of the interpreter imposing nuances on or even new meanings to both question and answer, either because of personal unrecognized bias, or deliberately, in order for example to produce the 'right' response. Similarly, when giving explanations and preoperative instructions, for example with regard to fasting, the medical team's intentions may be misunderstood for a variety of reasons. A possible source of confusion is the existence of different methods for designating the time of day.

Always to be borne in mind, but probably particularly in emergency situations, is the possibility of the patient having been given some native or traditional medicine beforehand.

Late presentation

Major problems for both surgeon and anaesthetist arise from the late presentation of all types of pathology; almost certainly this happens with greater frequency in the Third World than in the First World; ignorance, fear, and isolation are some of the reasons. The consequence is often a child in a very poor condition to tolerate anaesthesia and surgery. When neglected or late-presentation surgical pathology involves the mouth or airway, by direct involvement or because of distortion or displacement of tissues by an adjacent tumour, the anaesthetist may face significant problems of initial airway management. In such cases awake intubation may be more suitable and practical in most situations is preliminary tracheostomy under local anaesthesia. In the case of haemorrhagic tumours, attempts at nasal or oral intubation may be disastrous. Proper preparation of the child with adequate and appropriate explanation will, more often than not, result in patient co-operation for tracheostomy, when indicated.

TRAINING

Training for anaesthesia in the developing world encompasses both the preparation of the anaesthetists, medical and paramedical, and the preparation of other medical personnel for working with non-physician anaesthetists.

In addition, preparation of ancillary anaesthetic staff must be ensured. The fact that in parts of the developing world anaesthesia is barely, if at all, recognized as a discipline in its own right, presents difficulties that need to be addressed at all levels in the area of training. Realistic and informed attitudes, especially in national health authority officers and hospital administrators, play a large part in the success of any local training scheme; contrary attitudes do the reverse.

The argument that given the shortage of doctors in the developing world, physician anaesthetists are an unaffordable luxury, is not necessarily valid, and in the opinion of this writer, not valid at all. Surgery is a technical matter much of the time and the nature of the surgical condition in most cases does not alter during the surgery. Paramedics can be trained to do specific surgical procedures. It may be more appropriate for the physician to care for the whole patient and oversee the paramedic performing the surgery. Of course, the physician anaesthetist does much more than merely give anaesthesia for surgery.

Physician anaesthetists

The training of the specialist anaesthetist in the developing world is, in theory at least, no different from training in the First World. It may be that part or all of the training must be in a regional centre, for example in a neighbouring country. The concept of regional centres is important; training gained in such a centre is almost certainly more appropriate, in both the technical and philosophical senses, than that received in the totally different setting of Europe or the USA vis-à-vis Black Africa, for example.

At present, most if not all of the specialist anaesthetists in the developing world are working in the major centres, much of the time supervising the work of non-physician anaesthetists while in peripheral hospitals non-physician anaesthetists work alone. A satisfactory compromise may well be the promotion of the concept of the semi-specialist—the 1-year postgraduate training for the Diploma in Anaesthesia or equivalent could equip the doctor to combine the practice of anaesthesia with, for example, general practice. Such an arrangement apparently works well in parts of the First World, and is satisfactorily established in parts of the Third World. The author believes that this may be a very suitable arrangement.

Young graduates in rural hospitals

A more elementary version of the general practitioner–anaesthetist is the young medical graduate (say, 2 or 3 years after graduation) in an up-country hospital, with 1 or 2 colleagues perhaps of equal inexperience. The internship is an important period of preparation for this very demanding type of medical practice. With this category in mind, the World Health Organization (WHO) is preparing a set of five manuals to guide the young rural hospital doctor. The national health authority should use the internship as a thorough preparation for the next phase in the medical officer's career. In this context, a 2 year internship offers certain advantages. The WHO manuals will, it is hoped, serve as a suitable guide concerning the scope of this stage of formation.

Ideally, the intern will be posted to the department of anaesthesia for a term—at least 10 weeks—in which he or she will undergo an apprenticeship designed to prepare him or her for a rural posting. From the point of view of anaesthesia and surgery, this preparation should assume that only surgery which cannot be referred to a larger hospital will be undertaken. The WHO manuals on surgery and anaesthesia address this concept.

If the young graduate at the end of the internship knows and understands what the anaesthesia manual is attempting to teach him or her, and has some dexterity in the necessary skills, he or she would go to his or her first up-country appointment with a certain justifiable degree of confidence in his or her ability to conduct safe anaesthesia after adequate preoperative preparation.

For the reasons noted above, the surgery will often be emergency surgery that cannot be referred elsewhere, and therefore resuscitation in all its aspects, care of unconscious patients and transport of seriously ill or injured patients will be included in this training.

The expatriate physician anaesthetist

The last category of medical anaesthetist is the expatriate, who having trained in his or her own country, perhaps in the First World, goes to work in a Third World area. There are formal courses for such people and also instruction on a one-to-one basis available in the First World and perhaps elsewhere. Some such preparation is necessary, even for a specialist anaesthetist.

Non-physician anaesthetists

Training ranges from formal government courses with staged examinations to relatively brief but possibly far more effective apprenticeships in non-government hospitals with individual assessment by the trainer. The candidates are selected from a variety of sources, but the most appropriate are health workers with a proven commitment to health care and appropriate clinical experience prior to specialist training. The grade of medical assistant or clinical officer (or paramedical doctor) seems the most suitable; registered general nurses can also be trained.

The design of the training programme should be such that the purpose of the training is never forgotten. Sufficient basic sciences to understand clinical practice should be expected, and great emphasis placed on safety. Techniques taught should be simple and applicable in all situations. Irrelevant material and inappropriate techniques should not find a place in the training programme. Continuous assessment is advisable, so that unsuitable trainees are not retained in the programme. After successful completion of the training course, a period of internship is highly desirable. A programme of continuing education is necessary and some form of continuing assessment should exist.

In at least one African country non-physician anaesthetists employed in the central hospital do not engage in paediatric anaesthesia (and some other subspecialties), and when working in peripheral hospitals are advised to refer such cases to a centre where a medical anaesthetist is available. However, this will not always be possible, and anaesthetists in developing countries should be trained in all aspects of the specialty with certain obvious exceptions, such as open heart surgery. This is usually concentrated in particular centres, and if it occurs at all may constitute a very small part of the national workload.

The most suitable working arrangement for paramedical anaesthetists is one in which they are supervised by a physician anaesthetist. However, in many situations the non-physician anaesthetist will be working nominally under the supervision of the surgeon; in practice, this means that he or she is essentially working independently. There is much to be said for a system in which non-physician anaesthetists are trained to work in pairs; more hands and mutual supervision should improve the standard of care and, therefore, safety. This system has been termed 'buddy care' or the 'buddy system'.

The buddy system

If justification is needed for the establishment of this system, and health authorities may be more interested in economy than efficiency and safety, it is not hard to find. In the most sophisticated theatre environments, anaesthesia is often provided by a team of anaesthetists—two or even more depending upon circumstances: nature of case, training programme, etc. In addition, the 'skilled assistance for the anaesthetist' specified as part of minimal requirements by all bodies responsible for setting up and maintaining standards of safe practice (e.g. Faculty of Anaesthetists, Royal Australasian College of Surgeons, 1978) is often lacking in the developing world. There may be no provision for assistance for the anaesthetist during induction, and at the end of surgery, the anaesthetist may find him- or herself alone with the patient. Vigorous efforts must be made, by those responsible for the anaesthetic services, to remedy these serious shortcomings in theatre procedure. However the problem is less potentially serious when the buddy system is in operation. A well trained pair of anaesthetists can be expected to render good service, and this is surely a desirable feature of paediatric anaesthesia in the developing world.

THE FUTURE FOR PAEDIATRIC ANAESTHESIA IN THE DEVELOPING WORLD

The future arises out of the present, and the future for paediatric anaesthesia in developing countries has roots in both the developing and the developed worlds.

It seems essential that anaesthesia everywhere should be accorded its rightful status as a major independent discipline, and that anaesthetists should ensure that both the medical profession and the lay public are brought to an adequate understanding of the significance of their work. Until this happens in the First World, it is unlikely that efforts to achieve it in the Third World will be entirely successful. Thus, standards of practice which are less than satisfactory will continue.

First World involvement in Third World anaesthesia exists in several forms:

1. assistance in the form of personnel;
2. assistance with, and participation in, regional meetings in the Third World;
3. organization of and assistance with regional workshops and refresher courses;
4. assistance with donated or subsidized drugs and equipment;
5. assistance with donated or subsidized journals, books and other teaching materials.

First World prospective donors of items to the Third World should exercise responsible judgement about the appropriateness of the items in question, whether they are drugs, equipment, books, etc. 'If in doubt, send it out' is not the right approach. Far better is to make enquiries so that a great deal of time and money may be saved.

Individuals wanting to offer themselves and organizations offering personnel should carefully assess all aspects of the relevance of the assistance offered, including qualifications and experience of the person, duration of stay, etc. Proper consultation and exchange of information with those 'in the field' is essential if maximum benefit is to be derived from these generous offers. Organizations and special-purpose groups with accumulated experience of assistance to the developing world would seem to be the most suitable medium through which aid can be channelled. This applies both to the determining of the suitability of material goods and for selecting and preparing personnel. Such organizations include national associations of anaesthesiologists, specialist groups such as World Anaesthesia (UK), universities and faculties etc.

Personnel of all grades, properly prepared and suitably placed, could usefully contribute to and themselves benefit from a time of work in the Third World. Perhaps the most suitable category, for professional and personal reasons, is the newly qualified or senior trainee specialist anaesthetist (e.g. UK senior registrar). In fact, one could go so far as to suggest that it is highly desirable that such people do rotate through Third World posts for periods of 6–12 months or longer. Apart from more philanthropic reasons, the fact that the world is increasingly small and its security increasingly at risk are compelling arguments. The First World anaesthesiologist would gain experience, and it is hoped, proficiency in techniques little used in the First World, but which should be known, since they are techniques which a major disaster may promote to firstline procedures in his or her own region. The local anaesthetists (both physician and non-physician anaesthetists) would benefit from the exchange of ideas and knowledge, and the discipline itself may perhaps grow in status in the eyes of the uninitiated. More senior anaesthesiologists, e.g. consultants, would rarely be available for 6–12 months unless they had retired from full-time practice. However, such people are probably most profitably involved as visiting lecturers to a country or region, or as participants in workshops or refresher courses. In the area of paediatric anaesthesia, regional work-shops and refresher courses have a special relevance, providing a means for continuing reinforcement of skills and update of knowledge.

Consideration should be given to planned regional production and distribution of videotapes on various aspects of paediatric anaesthetic practice. Some excellent tapes already exist, for example those produced by Dr TCK Brown's unit in Melbourne, Australia, but regionally produced teaching tapes would have the advantage of greater relevance and appropriateness. Co-operation between anaesthesiologists from developed and developing world in such a project would be valuable means of furthering the interests and development of the subspecialty.

In developing countries, planning for the future of paediatric anaesthesia means active commitment to, and involvement in, continuing education of all levels of anaesthetists and support staff, and on-going search and research for the means to improve all aspects of practice. Much that is relevant here has already been discussed under the section on Training, above. However, mention should be made of undergraduate (medical) teaching. The teaching of anaesthesia to medical undergraduates, or 'teaching by anaesthetists', as has been suggested as more accurate (Zorab, 1985), is important and ideally should begin early in the clinical years, e.g. year 3 of a 5 year course, ending only towards the end of the final year, with the bulk of the teaching being in the penultimate year. Whether this teaching can produce medical graduates able to perform a safe anaesthetic is doubtful, but will depend on a number of factors, principally the amount of practical tuition and experience that can be afforded each student. However, basic principles must be presented and assimilated, and interest must be stimulated and maintained. Out of this interest should develop the right attitudes to the practice of anaesthesia in postgraduate years and should encourage in some the decision to enter the specialty.

Included in the basic principles taught by the anaesthetist will be primary care of the critically ill and injured. A large proportion of patients presenting to the medical services in the developing world are children, in whom the margin for error is narrower, so that the consequences of error develop more rapidly and more seriously than in adults. The anaesthetist–teacher must emphasize these aspects of medical care in his or her teaching. For example, one of the critical situations an anaesthetist in the Third World may often have to manage is a patient with tetanus who could be a neonate, an older child or adult. The anaesthetist will therefore be prompted to include in his or her clinical teaching both the prevention and the treatment of tetanus.

Perhaps the most important influence that 'teaching by the anaesthetist' may exercise is that of bringing students to discover within themselves and further develop some degree of the resourcefulness and inventiveness that is a characteristic of many anaesthetists, and which can be so valuable in the developing world.

APPENDIX 1: SOME SIGNIFICANT FACTS ABOUT THE CLINICAL USE OF DIETHYL ETHER

Ether has been in continual use as a general anaesthetic agent since 1846. In parts of the developed world its use is forbidden at present because of its inflammability, but in the developing world it remains an extremely useful agent, and many thousands of satisfactory ether anaesthetics have been performed. Ether is a safe and reliable agent; without doubt, it is the safest inhalational agent in the hands of a non-expert. As mentioned earlier in this chapter, it is virtually the only inhalational agent which can be safely used with air as the carrier gas in a spontaneously breathing patient; this is because ether causes respiratory stimulation at clinically suitable levels of anaesthesia.

Ether is a good analgesic even at sub-sleep levels, and at moderate levels of surgical anaesthesia muscle relaxation is adequate, even in most instances for abdominal surgery. Thus ether can be used as a sole anaesthetic agent, a practice in contrast to that of balanced anaesthesia; the latter, in the hands of an experienced anaesthetist certainly has advantages, but when attempted by the inexperienced may be hazardous.

Ether can be used for induction, although it may be quite a prolonged procedure even without the difficulties created by its unacceptable (to some) smell. It has a high blood solubility and this, combined with possible breath-holding and coughing, due to its irritant effect on the respiratory tract, means that induction is slow. An ether vaporizer such as the EMO may be used with the concentration initially at 2%, the mask held above the face and the bellows slowly operated to create an atmosphere of ether vapour; concentration is slowly and steadily increased as tolerated. An 'open mask' (Schimmelbush or equivalent) is simpler and probably easier in a small child. In both situations—the EMO and the 'open mask'—the mask should not be placed fully on the face before the patient is asleep.

Ether burns in air at concentrations between 1.85 and 36.5% and may explode in oxygen at concentrations between 2 and 82%. Therefore it is essential that such concentrations should not be exposed to sparks. Sources of sparks that might cause ignition include faulty switches, static electricity sparking and diathermy. Equipment for active scavenging may not be available. If a non-return valve is being used, a length of wide-bore corrugated tubing can be employed to carry the expired gas to the floor or even outside the theatre. Such passive scavenging is not easy to arrange when using a T-piece. However, it has been convincingly demonstrated (Blackburn, 1982) that provided any source of sparking is beyond 25 cm from the expiratory valve, the situation is safe—the ether is diluted to non-inflammable mixtures.

Regarding <u>static electricity</u>, considerable protection is afforded by <u>increasing the humidity</u> if it is low. This can be done by having a boiling water sterilizer in the theatre, or some other source of steam.

APPENDIX 2: TECHNIQUES FOR USE OF DRAW-OVER VAPORIZERS IN PAEDIATRIC PRACTICE

Choice of technique I

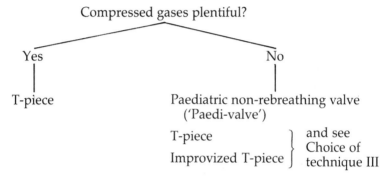

Compressed gases plentiful?

Yes — T-piece

No — Paediatric non-rebreathing valve ('Paedi-valve')

T-piece
Improvized T-piece } and see Choice of technique III

Choice of technique II

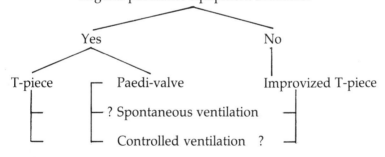

Regular paediatric equipment available?

Yes

No

T-piece   Paedi-valve   Improvized T-piece

? Spontaneous ventilation

Controlled ventilation ?

Choice of technique III

Is means of providing 'continuous' gas flow when supply of compressed gas Limited: 1 or Absent: 2

1. Oxygen air-entrainer
1, 2. Bellows or self-inflating bag

REFERENCES

Blackburn JP (1982) Explosions. In Scurr C & Feldman S (eds) *Scientific Foundations of Anaesthesia*, 3rd edn, pp 566–569. London: Heinemann.

Boulton TB (1966) Anaesthesia in difficult situations. 3 General anaesthesia—technique. *Anaesthesia* **21:** 513–545.

Cole PV & Parkhouse J (1963) Clinical experience with the EMO inhaler. *Postgraduate Medical Journal* **39:** 476–479.

Faculty of Anaesthetists, Royal Australasian College of Surgeons (1978) *Recommended Minimum Facilities for Safe Anaesthetic Practice in Non-teaching Hospitals.* Melbourne: FARACS.

Farman JV (1973) *Anaesthesia and the EMO System,* p 157. English Language Book Society, Hodder & Stoughton.

Houghton IT, Boulton TB & Sanders CD Notes on clinical use of 'Tri-Service' anaesthetic apparatus. Appendix to 7610–99–211–5656 *Manual, Technical, User, for Anaesthesia Apparatus.* Oxford Miniature (RAMC Publication).

Schaefer HG & Farman JV (1984) Anaesthetic vapour concentrations in the EMC system. *Anaesthesia* **39:** 171–180.

Swai EA, Brooks AM & Meckleburgh JS (1985) The AFYA anaesthesia system—a laboratory study. *Anaesthesia* **40:** 1213–1218.

Waldman R (1987) Problems with home oral rehydration salts. *Dialogue on Diarrhoea* **3:** 6–7.

Zorab JSM (1985) Editoral. *World Federation of Societies of Anaesthesiologists Newsletter* **10:** July.

Resuscitation in paediatrics

Paediatrics has for a long time been recognized as an individual specialty requiring those who practise it to have specialized training. Hatch (1984) recognized the need for specialized expertise in paediatric anaesthesia not only in the designated centres but also in the district general hospital. Although the figures are difficult to obtain, Hatch concluded that the majority of paediatric anaesthetics, including just under 50% of neonatal anaesthetics, were carried out in non-specialty units. There has been a postulated increase in the incidence of cardiac arrest following anaesthesia and surgery in children (Salem et al, 1975) which when associated with the concern over the apparent state of advanced cardiac life support as practised by adult anaesthetists (Schwartz et al, 1979, 1982), leads one to consider how much, if any, training has been given in paediatric resuscitation. How many joules of energy are required to be given to defibrillate an 8 kg baby, for example? How many micrograms, or millilitres of 1 in 10 000 solution of adrenaline should be given to a 14 kg child? Such answers should be instantly available, for to be effective resuscitation requires immediate emergency treatment. Delays, as well as mistakes, kill!

Figure 23.1 (Oakley, 1988) is likely to reduce mistakes made with paediatric resuscitations.

RESUSCITATION TECHNIQUES

Resuscitation is divided into two stages. Basic life support is defined as resuscitation without equipment. Advance life support can similarly be defined as resuscitation performed using drugs and equipment. A mixture of both is usually essential to be successful: basic life support is maintained while the equipment and drugs are prepared.

Basic life support

Although the first resuscitation attempt described in literature was a paediatric case, where basic life support was successful alone (2 Kings 4, verse 34), little has been formally written on the subject until recently. In 1974 the American Heart Association published recommendations on standards for

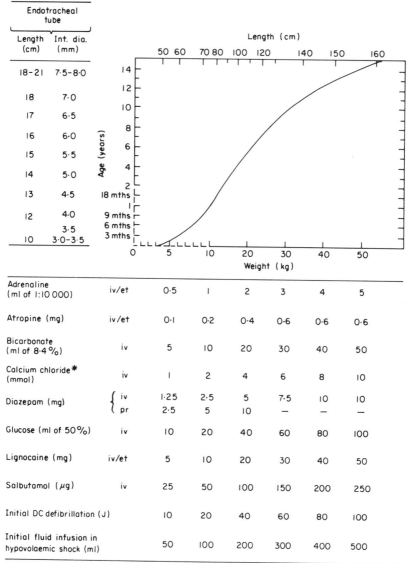

Figure 23.1. Paediatric resuscitation chart. Key: iv = intravenous; et = endotracheal; pr = per rectum. From Oakley (1988) with permission.

cardiopulmonary resuscitation and emergency cardiac care. It contained three short paragraphs on basic life support in infants and children. It was estimated that 12 million Americans were trained with these standards (CPR, 1977). In 1980 the American Heart Association published revised recommendations and included a section on basic life support in infants and children. Unfortunately many of these recommendations were based on the adult model and little was included as a result of practical experience. The most recent revision of these recommendations (American Heart Association, 1986) includes a detailed section (part IV) on paediatric basic life support. In the same year the British Medical Journal published the recommendations of the Resuscitation Council (UK) for the resuscitation of infants and children (Zideman, 1986).

In basic life support for children the airway, breathing, circulation (ABC) sequence holds true. It should be emphasized that in contrast to the adult, the child is more likely to have an airway or breathing problem, followed by a cardiac arrest rather than vice versa.

Airway

It is essential to open and clear the paediatric airway as soon as possible. The head-tilt manoeuvre is the simplest way of achieving this. Over-extension of the neck in infants has been advised against as it may kink or obstruct the relatively soft infant trachea. In practice this is extremely rare. More commonly, because of the relatively large occiput in infants, tilting the head lifts the upper chest off the bed, and it is the weight of the thorax which will distort the trachea. Thus support under the shoulders is a most useful adjunct to airway control in small infants. Kinking of the airway will probably occur if the American Heart Association's recommendation of head-tilt is augmented by neck-lift, with maximum obstruction occurring at the apex of the lift. The chin-lift method is to be recommended as it will displace the relatively large tongue forward, but it must only be achieved by lifting the mandible from behind the angle and not by the soft tissues in the floor of the mouth. To establish a good mandible position, Ludwig and Kettrick (1983) recommended the alignment of the alveolar ridges or teeth (if present). Maintaining the paediatric airway, even in experienced hands, is a matter of trial and error as no two children are the same. It should be remembered that infants are primarily nose-breathers and that this is the child's built-in mechanism for overcoming obstruction caused by its relatively large tongue.

Having opened the airway, the rescuer must then check that it is not obstructed by any obvious cause, for example a foreign body, vomit or even a toy. If a foreign body is present it must be carefully removed as an indifferent technique may lead to trauma, resulting in haemorrhage and oedema of the upper airway, or further impaction of the foreign body. Blind finger sweeps are therefore not recommended. The technique of inverting the child accompanied by back blows may dislodge the object, thus preventing total obstruction. When one foreign body is found, a further one must always be suspected.

Not all airway obstructions are caused by foreign bodies; infectious diseases of the upper airway will cause serious and even fatal obstruction if not recognized quickly and dealt with properly.

Breathing

Initially, by checking for breathing, the rescuer assesses the patency of the child's airway and looks at the chest to see if it is moving with a normal pattern. Any intercostal recession, sternal recession or see-saw movement of the chest and abdomen indicates residual airway obstruction. The nares should be inspected to see if flaring is occurring, similarly indicating residual obstruction. The rescuer should listen and feel for breath sounds at the nose and mouth. Not only will this assess airway patency, but it will give an excellent indication of the cause of any residual airway obstruction (croup, epiglottitis).

If the child is not breathing and the airway is clear, then expired air resuscitation should be initiated. Holding the airway open, the rescuer covers the mouth or nose and mouth of the child with his or her own mouth. By breathing gently into the child and watching the chest move upwards, the rescuer can judge the correct amount of ventilation. Although expired air resuscitation is described as a hyperventilation technique, this can only be achieved in children by varying the ventilatory rate and not the tidal volume. Raising the latter could result in a pneumothorax. Excessive ventilation, either in volume or airway pressure, will result in air entering the stomach rather than the lungs (Melker, 1984). This could cause regurgitation of the stomach contents.

Initially two breaths should be given (the rescue-breathing manoeuvre). Any airway obstruction should then be noted and dealt with as described above. If breathing alone is required, then a breath should be given every 2–4 s (15 to 30 times/min), the slower rate being applicable to older children (Table 23.1).

Table 23.1. Recommendations for basic life support in relation to age

	Baby	Toddler	Child	Adolescent	Adult
Heart rate (beats/min)	120	100	90	80	60
ECC rate (per min)	120	100	90	80	60
Depth (cm)	1–1.5	1.5–2	2–3	3–4	4–5
Respiratory rate (breaths/min)	37	30	20	16	12
EAR rate (per min)	24	20	18	16	12

ECC = external chest compressions; EAR = expired air resuscitation.

Circulation

As stated above, a primary circulatory arrest in a child is rare, but an extreme bradycardia or asystole will rapidly follow hypoxia. Cyanosis is too unreliable as a sign; the child may be cyanosed already as a result of congenital heart disease. Hypoxic infants do not become cyanosed but are usually described as ashen, pale or grey as the circulation begins to fail.

The most reliable sign is the palpation of a peripheral pulse. The site chosen to palpate the pulse may very according to experience and skill, but a choice of the carotid, femoral or brachial should be made. The carotid is the most relevant but probably the most difficult because of the relatively short, fat neck found in infants. Cavallaro and Melker (1983) found that parents were able to assess the brachial pulse more accurately than the apical impulse. An undiagnosed coarctation of the aorta, although rare, may interfere with an assessment made by palpation of the left brachial or the femoral arteries. The right axillary artery is a common site for cardiac catheterization and Blalock shunts may have obliterated an arm artery. It is therefore important that operation scars should be looked for in the axillae and on the chest and abdomen; these may give some clue as to an absent pulse. It is now suggested that two major arteries are palpated before a diagnosis of asystole is made.

If an adequate pulse is present but the child is still apnoeic, ventilation alone should continue. Frequent monitoring of the pulse will indicate any deterioration in the effectiveness of ventilation. Should the pulse be slow, impalpable or extremely weak, then the circulation must be supported by external chest compressions. Rainer and Bullough (1957) reported the successful use of knee-to-chest compression in children, but it was not until Kouwenhoven et al substantiated the effectiveness of closed-chest cardiac compressions in 1960 that this technique began to be accepted.

In infants external chest compressions can be applied to the sternum by the tips of two fingers. Alternatively, the chest can be encircled with the hands, the sternum compressed with the thumbs and additional support gained by interlacing the fingers behind the infant's back (Thaler and Stobie, 1963). In 1986, Phillips and Zideman showed that the anatomical centre of the heart lies under the lower third of the sternum in small children. Orlowski (1986) confirmed these findings in larger children and suggested that compressions should be applied to a position either one finger-breadth above the xiphisternum or the same distance below the internipple line. It is very important to remember that chest compressions must only be applied to the sternum. Thaler and Stobie (1963) showed that no damage occurred to the liver when compressions were limited to the chest. Superficial damage to the hepatic capsule occurred when pressure was applied to the xiphister-num, but rupture of the liver resulted from simultaneous compression of both the chest and abdomen as this prevented the downward, protective movement of the liver during chest compressions.

The combination of external chest compressions and expired air respi-ration is known as basic life support. For infants and small children, it is recommended that one ventilation is given for every five compressions. In older children (aged 8 or older) a ratio of 15 compressions to two ventilations is more appropriate. The depth of compression will also vary with the size of the child. Compressions should be smooth and even, not sharp. The com-pression phase should last for at least 50% of the compression–relaxation cycle. Accuracy of the rate and depth of compressions is not of vital impor-tance; the recommendations given in Table 23.1 are only a guide. The effectiveness of compressions should be regularly assessed by monitoring the character of the pulse; varied rate and depth of compressions produce the best result.

Advanced life support

The 1986 American Heart Association standards and guidelines, together with the recommendations published in the British Medical Journal (Zideman, 1986), include detailed specifications for the practice of advanced life support—resuscitation performed with the use of equipment.

The use of equipment in paediatric resuscitation requires skill and experience and a specific choice or preference of equipment usually accompanies this. The use of adult mannequins to improve and standardize the required adult skills has been well established. Unfortunately, at present, paediatric mannequin models are not as sophisticated as adult models, though new models are being developed.

Airway

The simplest airway adjunct is the Guedel oropharyngeal airway. Sizes vary from 000 to 4; the correct size must be selected to be effective. The selection of too small a size will, on insertion of the airway, only result in forcing the tongue backwards into the pharynx, causing airway obstruction. Attempts to insert too large a size airway will cause trauma to the pharynx with resultant bleeding. Nasopharyngeal airways are also useful; the correct size is that which fits comfortably through the anterior nares. A tracheal tube of suitable size, cut short, can often be substituted as an effective nasopharyngeal airway (a safety pin through the distal end will ensure that the tube does not disappear into the nose). Melker and colleagues (1981) described the development of the paediatric gastric tube airway. Their study showed that the distance from the cricoid cartilage to sternal notch accurately predicted the nares-to-carina and nares-to-gastro-oesophageal junction length in 24 children aged 6 months to 16 years. They reported that a prototype was being tested.

Intubation with tracheal tube is the only foolproof method of guaranteeing the airway. Intubation should only be attempted when the correct equipment is available, including a full range of tracheal tube sizes. The choice of laryngoscope and blade is a matter of personal preference and experience. A straight laryngoscope blade is recommended in infants and children as this will allow direct elevation of the epiglottis with the tip of the blade. Nevertheless in extreme emergencies, and with great care, intubation can be achieved with an adult curved Macintosh laryngoscope blade. Blind nasotracheal intubation is not recommended in the resuscitation situation. Breath sounds, which are not usually present, are used to guide and position the tube correctly and considerable skill and practice are needed to be successful with this technique.

Tracheal tube size and length are best and most rapidly determined by using one of the many formulae (e.g. size = age/4 + 4) or tables currently available (Table 23.2). A complete range of sizes of tracheal tubes should be available. The correct size of tube is that which passes easily through the glottis and subglottic region leaving a slight leak around the tube. Tracheal tubes precut to the appropriate length may save time, but occasionally a smaller size tube may be required than that estimated using a formula or table. Here one may be left with a precut tube too short to be effective. It is therefore essential to have a matching set of uncut, full-length tracheal tubes accessible. Hinckle (1988) describes a reliable method of determining tube size depending on body length and has devised a tape-measure system for use in an emergency.

Table 23.2. Recommended tracheal tube dimensions for children

	Tracheal tube			
Age	Internal diameter (mm)	Oral	Nasal	Suction catheter
Premature	2.5–3.0	11	13.5	6F
Newborn	3.5	12	14	8F
1 year	4.0	13	15	8F
2 years	4.5	14	16	8F
4 years	5.0	15	17	10F
6 years	5.5	17	19	10F
8 years	6.0	19	21	10F
10 years	6.5	20	22	10F
12 years	7.0	21	22	10F
14 years	7.5	22	23	10F
16 years	8.0	23	24	12F

A full set of tracheal tube connectors must also be available. These must be able to fit or be adapted to fit the breathing/ventilation circuit used in the hospital. The 15 mm connector is the current international standard and will fit directly into most resuscitation bags. If the Oxford, Cardiff or Magill systems are used then suitable adaptors must be provided (see Chapter 6); 8.5 mm connectors are now widely available for use in paediatrics and disposable adaptors are fully interchangeable with the 15 mm international standard.

Having successfully achieved intubation of the trachea, the length and position of the tracheal tube should be checked by observing symmetrical chest wall movement and by the auscultation of both chest cavities for equal breath sounds. The tube must then be firmly secured in position to ensure it will not be moved, dislodged or inadvertently removed during further resuscitative manoeuvres. Suction catheters of an appropriate size to fit the selected tracheal tube should also be at hand.

Breathing

Breathing can be supplemented with oxygen by using a head box, facemask, nasal cannulas or an oxygen tent. Selection depends on the availability of the equipment and the tolerance of the child. In the resuscitation situation, oxygen tents are not recommended as they tend to hinder direct observation of the child. Any oxygen given should be heated and humidified to prevent the drying of secretions and temperature loss from the airway.

Resuscitation bags, although apparently easy to use, may lead to a false sense of security in inexperienced hands. First, the correct size of mask must be selected to fit the child's face snugly with minimal gas leakage. The Rendell–Baker design is favoured at present, due to its minimal dead space. These are now available in clear plastic to allow the observation of the airway and the child's colour without removing the mask. Circular masks with inflatable rims, made of a soft plastic, are also useful as they fit a larger range of children's faces. They have also been found to be more successfully used by the inexperienced.

The resuscitation bags are of two types: the self-inflating or the gas-filled Jackson Rees modification of the Ayre's T-piece. The self-inflating bag is manufactured in three sizes—infant, child and adult. Most are supplied with a pressure-limiting valve, thus preventing enthusiastic over-inflation of the lungs. Oxygen can be added to enrich the entrained air, the resultant percentage of oxygen delivered depending on the volume of oxygen supplied and the rate and volume of ventilation. Spontaneous respiration is possible through the self-inflating bag; resistance is about 5 cm H_2O. The gas-filled Jackson Rees modification of the Ayre's T-piece is more adaptable and is usually preferred by the skilled operator. It is limited by the need for a constant gas supply, which, if it fails, renders the circuit useless. Experience is necessary to use this system as it requires the operator to occlude the open tail of the reservoir bag correctly whilst squeezing the bag. Similarly it must be released during expiration. Over-inflation and over-ventilation can very easily be achieved. Portable adult automatic resuscitators have been modified for use in children by increasing the available range of respiratory rates and by delivering smaller tidal volumes. They may be considered useful when transportation of a ventilated child is required but their life is limited by the volume of gas supply. Their use in children has not yet been fully evaluated. They are therefore not recommended for the inexperienced or unsupervised paramedical use.

Circulation

Until now, the circulation has been solely supported by external chest compressions which can achieve up to 50% of normal cardiac output; effectiveness is monitored by palpation of a major pulse. Blood pressure can also be monitored with either a simple hand-inflated machine or by an automated self-timing device. A range of blood pressure cuff sizes should be supplied; the blood pressure measured is a function of the cuff size used and the diameter of the limb. Direct intra-arterial blood pressure monitoring is usually considered an unnecessary luxury at this stage.

Further support for the circulation is dependent on gaining intravenous access. High-risk patients where cardiovascular instability is likely should have appropriate venous access established in anticipation of possible problems. There is no doubt that placing an intravenous cannula is a major problem, not only for the experienced, but more so for the inexperienced.

Peripheral access is not adequate due to the existing poor peripheral circulation during resuscitation. Central venous access is mandatory in this situation and results in higher peak concentrations of drug than those achieved by a peripheral route (Hedges et al, 1984). There are four sites readily accessible for central venous cannulation:

1. The *external jugular vein* is probably the simplest, as in most resuscitation victims it is grossly distended and thus visible on the side of the neck.
2. The *internal jugular vein* is a popular vein in the hands of the experienced and has been reported to have a low complication rate (Cote, 1979). In the arrested patient it may be difficult to distinguish between carotid artery and jugular vein.
3. The *subclavian vein* is a popular site in adults but is difficult, via a percutaneous technique, in children during resuscitation (Groff and Ahmed, 1974). The risk of complications, such as a pneumothorax, is high.
4. The *femoral vein* is a useful short-term venous access point (Ludwig and Kettrick, 1983). Infection and femoral vein thrombosis are the complications of long-term cannulation.

Both the internal jugular vein and femoral vein may have to be found in the absence of an accompanying arterial pulsation as a landmark. Dalsey et al (1984) have shown that drugs are better delivered centrally by injections from above the diaphragm than from below. Whichever site is chosen, either a direct percutaneous technique or a Seldinger (1953) technique should result in the reliable placement of an appropriate-size cannula. If percutaneous venous access fails a cut-down insertion of a cannula, for example in the groin or antecubital fossa, should be considered. A 22 SWG cannula is probably of sufficient size to administer all the drugs required during resuscitation. If massive haemorrhage accompanied by hypovolaemia are the cause of the cardiac arrest a larger-gauge cannula should be considered. It must be emphasized that it is central venous access that is essential and that a wide-bore cannula, whose placement may be more difficult or even impossible, is not usually necessary. Once established the cannula should be well secured and connected to an intravenous infusion of 5% dextrose or 4% dextrose in 18% saline, to be run at a minimal rate to keep the intravenous access open.

The central venous route is the optimal choice for the administration of drugs, but because of the difficulty in achieving this early in the resuscitation procedure two other routes should be considered. Adrenaline, atropine and lignocaine are suitable for administration via the tracheal tube and are subsequently rapidly absorbed from the pulmonary vascular bed. Secondly, direct intracardiac injections may be attempted in extreme emergencies. The effectiveness of these injections is low and the reported complication rate high (Sabin et al, 1983).

DRUGS

Paediatric resuscitation drug therapy is based on a dose per kg body weight system. It has been suggested that a dose per m^2 body surface area is better when dealing with children, but this requires a knowledge not only of the weight but also the height of the child and reference to a nomogram to obtain the surface area. This is totally impractical in the emergency situation. Children admitted routinely to hospital are all weighed, but during an emergency admission a weight may not be immediately available and an estimate has to be made. In these cases a weight/age nomogram may be of assistance.

A weight/height nomogram may also be a useful asset; length is simply obtained by laying a tape-measure along the side of the infant. Having determined the correct weight, and thence the correct dose of drug, it is then necessary to work out its equivalent in ml of solution of the drug present-ation supled. Under stress and in the rush of a paediatric resuscitation attempt, mistakes can easily be made and it is recommended that a chart should be made available to perform the direct conversion from body weight to ml of solution. Alternatively an individual resuscitation drug chart can be prepared for each sick child with all the doses and volumes precalculated.

Oxygen

Mention has already been made of the fact that the majority of paediatric cardiac arrests are primarily respiratory in origin. It therefore cannot be over-emphasized that establishing efficient ventilation is a priority and that ventilation must continue despite all other manoeuvres if resuscitation is to be successful. The addition of oxygen to raise the inspired oxygen concen-tration will rapidly correct any hypoxaemia (Fillmore et al, 1970) and this alone may correct any cardiac arrhythmia to sinus rhythm (Ayres and Grace, 1969). Oxygen should therefore be administered in the highest possible concentration; considerations of oxygen toxicity (e.g. retrolental fibroplasia) should not preclude the use of 100% oxygen in the acute resuscitation situation.

The remainder of the drugs are preferably administered intravenously. Small volumes should be used wherever possible so as not to fluid-overload the child, thus adding further to his or her problems.

Atropine 0.02 mg/kg (minimum 0.1 mg)

Atropine is a parasympathetic blocking drug, used mainly for its action in blocking the cardiac effects of the vagus nerve. Thus it is useful for the treatment of a severe bradycardia accompanied by hypotension (Goldberg, 1974). It should be considered in the management of second- and third-degree heart block and slow idioventricular rhythms (Greenblatt et al, 1976). Atropine may cause both atrial and ventricular tachyarrhythmias (Massumi et al, 1972).

It cannot be over-emphasized that the majority of bradycardias seen in children will respond to adequate ventilation and oxygenation together with atropine and will require no further therapy.

Adrenaline 10 μg/kg (0.1 ml/kg of 1 in 10000 solution)

Adrenaline is an α- and β-adrenergic receptor stimulator. It is the front-line drug in the treatment of anaphylactic shock (0.01 ml/kg of 1:1000 subcutaneously). It increases both the inotropic and chronotropic activity of the heart, thus raising the heart rate and blood pressure. In asystole it may be given either intravenously or by the tracheal route. Adrenaline's action is less effective in the presence of a metabolic acidosis. It may also be used as an infusion in the management of hypotension in a dose of 0.02–0.05 μg/kg/min but peripheral vasoconstriction will result if doses greater than 0.5 μg/kg/min are given.

Sodium bicarbonate 1 mmol/kg (1 ml/kg of 8.4% solution)

Bicarbonate is used to correct the acidosis that accompanies resuscitation. If the ventilation and the circulation are adequate, this correction is not always necessary. It should only be used in a direct therapeutic titration to the results of repeated blood gases (body weight × 0.2 × base deficit = mmol HCO_3^-). An empirical dose of 0.5–1 mmol/kg can be given at the outset or if blood gases are not immediately available. The repeated use of bicarbonate, even in its most concentrated form, may easily lead to fluid overload. Some authors recommend the use of 4.2% bicarbonate in patients younger than 6 months but this makes the fluid-loading problem worse and there is no need to use it. Excessive use will result later in an unwanted metabolic alkalosis (Lawson et al, 1973), hypernatraemia (Worthley, 1976) and a hyperosmolar state (Mattar et al, 1974). An alternative is to use tris-hydroxy methyl amino methane (THAM), which has a low sodium content but has the potential to cause hypoglycaemia and is rarely used nowadays. Administration of sodium bicarbonate should always be accompanied by efficient ventilation. It should never be mixed with any other drugs as it will chemically react with calcium salts and will inactivate adrenaline.

Calcium

Chloride 5–10 mg/kg (0.25 ml/kg of 10% solution)

Gluconate 30 mg/kg (1 ml/kg of 10% solution)

The calcium ion increases myocardial contractility and prolongs systole and may be very effective. In the digitalized child it may cause an unresponsive asystole or augment coronary artery spasm causing myocardial ischaemia (Dembo, 1981). More recently the role of calcium in resuscitation has been questioned again. White et al (1983) have implicated the calcium ion in the final common pathway of cell death. Calcium should not be given to patients with myocardial infarction from right or left outflow obstruction. Calcium administration is therefore not as popular as it used to be.

There are two formulations currently available; the gluconate requires three times the dose (and volume) of the chloride. This is because of the difference in ionic binding properties. Calcium chloride is a highly sclerosing solution, which should never be administered through a peripheral vein. Serum ionized calcium levels, if available, may be useful in deciding if calcium administration will be of use.

Dextrose 1 g/kg (2 ml/kg of 50% solution)

Hypoglycaemia is a well documented cause of sudden collapse, as small infants have low stores of glycogen. This is especially so in the chronically sick child. Immediate diagnosis and treatment by administration of dextrose is necessary to prevent permanent damage occurring.

The mixture of dextrose with insulin (1 g/kg with 0.25 u/kg) is frequently used to improve myocardial function and to encourage the return of potassium into the cells.

Lignocaine 1 mg/kg (0.1 ml/kg of 1% solution)

Lignocaine decreases the automaticity of the heart and is used to treat multifocal ventricular extrasystoles, ventricular tachycardia and bigeminy. As these arrhythmias are infrequent in children, lignocaine is thought of as a useful rather than a frontline drug. The dose can be repeated every 5 min or an infusion may be established of 0.1 mg/kg/min and titrated to the required effect.

Diuretics

Two diuretics are considered useful in paediatric resuscitation:

1. *Mannitol* up to 1 g/kg (5 ml/kg of 20% solution). Volume overload is the main problem with its use and no more than 0.5 g/kg should be given in the first instance.
2. *Frusemide* 1 mg/kg. Serum potassium levels should be measured following administration. Frusemide is ototoxic when administered rapidly.

Dopamine

Dopamine is a precursor of adrenaline that has α- and β-receptor stimulant activity dependent on the dose used. In low dosage (1–5 μg/kg/min) it will improve renal blood flow and increase cardiac output. In high doses (10–20 μg/kg/min) α effects predominate, resulting in systemic vasoconstriction. The dose is rapidly calculated by adding 3 × body weight in mg of dopamine to 50 ml of 5% dextrose and running the infusion in ml/h equivalent to the calculated dose in µg/kg/min required (5 ml/h = 5 µg/kg/min). Increased concentrations are used when fluid restriction is required.

Isoprenaline infusion (0.05–0.1 µg/kg/min)

Isoprenaline is an adrenergic stimulant with purely β effects. It is used, in an infusion, as an intravenous pacemaker. It may also be used as a bronchodilator.

Defibrillation (2 J/kg)

Ventricular fibrillation and ventricular tachycardia, the two main indications for defibrillation, are rare in children. Nevertheless, when they occur, defibrillation must be carried out immediately on diagnosis. The recommendations on the dose of energy to be administered varies considerably but Gutgesell and colleagues (1976) found a 91% response to 2 J/kg using 4.5 or 8 cm paddles (100% at 4 J/kg). Energy overdosage can cause damage to the myocardium (Crampton, 1980) but the paddle size and position seem to have little effect (Kerber et al, 1981). Some defibrillators only charge to preset levels (20, 50, 100, 200 or 400 J), whilst others have a preset maximum dose (100 J) when paediatric paddles are connected.

At present, an initial dose of 2 J/kg using a paddle size and position appropriate to the child's chest size would seem the best option. The dose should be doubled if the initial dose is not effective.

Temperature

Hypothermia will cause an additional strain on the cardiovascular system. It is therefore vitally important, especially in the baby and smaller infant, that efforts should be made to maintain the temperature of the child during the resuscitation attempt. A warming mattress, infrared heater, and an incubator together with warm coverings should therefore be considered an essential part of paediatric resuscitation equipment.

NEW METHODS

Abdominal compression

In 1967, Harris et al found that they could augment carotid blood flow during resuscitation by sustained manual compression of the abdomen. They found it was associated with an increased incidence of laceration of the liver, but Redding (1971), when re-examining the technique, found the same result without any hepatic damage. Chandra et al (1981) assessed the effect of brief periods of abdominal binding in man. By inflating a 30-cm square bladder, bound to the anterior abdominal wall, to between 60 and 110 cm H_2O for 4 min intervals, they were able to raise the mean arterial blood pressure from 53.9 ± 7.1 to 67.2 ± 8.4 mmHg in patients undergoing standard cardiopulmonary resuscitation. No associated abdominal visceral injuries were found at post-mortem.

Sustained abdominal compression does not seem to be a technique applicable to children. It has already been mentioned that Thaler and Stobie (1963) postulated that damage occurred to the hepatic capsule in children if the downward movement of the liver was impaired during chest compressions. Intermittent (10–15/min) abdominal compression is a useful adjunct to other therapy for severe right heart failure.

Rogers and Hillman (1970) found an improved resuscitation rate in hypothermic rats following intermittent abdominal compressions prior to artificial respiration and rewarming.

Ralsten et al (1982), using intermittent abdominal compression in dogs, raised the brachial artery blood pressure from 58/16 to 87/32 mmHg and the cardiac output from 13.8 ± 2.5 to 24.2 ± 5.7 ml/min/kg. This technique of intermittent abdominal compression needs full and proper evaluation in man before it can be recommended.

'New CPR' (cardiopulmonary resuscitation)

In 1976 Criley et al sustained consciousness for 92 s during ventricular fibrillation by making the patient cough repeatedly. They called this 'cough–CPR'. Further investigation showed that the right heart flow occurred during the relaxation phase and was greatly augmented by the pre-cough inspiration (Criley et al, 1981). Cough–CPR was the first demonstration of the passive role of the heart during resuscitation. In 1980 Rudikoff and colleagues demonstrated identical pressures in the right atrium, pulmonary artery, left ventricle and aorta during standard cardiopulmonary resuscitation. They then generated a high intrathoracic pressure and were able to raise the pressure in all the intrathoracic structures and the extrathoracic arteries. The same raised intrathoracic pressure caused the thin-walled intrathoracic veins to collapse. The result was a raised pressure within the carotid artery, with a minimal rise in jugular venous pressure, thus creating an arteriovenous pressure gradient required for antegrade blood flow. The Johns Hopkins group had formulated the 'chest pump' theory as opposed to the previously accepted 'heart pump' theory of Kouwenhoven et al (1960). Pressure-synchronized cineangiography in dogs (Nieman et al, 1981) and two-dimensional echocardiography in man (Rich et al, 1981; Werner et al, 1981) further confirmed that during external chest compressions there was little change in cardiac chamber size in man and that the aortic and mitral valves opened simultaneously.

In 1980 Chandra et al showed in man that by performing chest compressions at a rate of 40/min with a 60% compression duration, together with simultaneous ventilation at airway pressures between 60 and 110 cm H_2O, they were able to increase mean systolic arterial pressure by 13 mmHg and increase carotid blood flow by 252%. The synchronization of ventilations and compressions was obtained by using a preprogrammed computer to link the ventilator and mechanical chest compressor. The results were in comparison with those obtained by a standard resuscitation methodology; the computer switched between techniques every 30 s. This new technique was named 'new CPR' and is now known as synchronized ventilation and compression CPR or SVC–CPR.

Despite these results, 'new CPR' has been greeted with cautious optimism. Other workers have been unable to produce any difference in cardiac output or regional blood flow in groups of animals receiving inter-posed or simultaneous ventilations and compressions (Bircher and Safar, 1981; Redding et al, 1981; Babbs et al, 1982a). Saunders and colleagues (1982) found that five out of six dogs receiving standard cardiopulmonary resusci-tation were resuscitated, whereas none of the six receiving the 'new' methodology were resuscitated. They suggested, as did others (Ditchley et al, 1982), that although carotid blood flow was improved during new CPR, because of the low pressure gradient across the coronary bed, perfusion of the coronary arteries may be impaired.

When applied to children, the technique seems to have little to offer. Synchronization of ventilation and compression is important to the tech-nique, for without peak inspiration coinciding with peak compression the raised blood pressures and cardiac outputs would not occur. The resulting squeeze from outside (chest compression) and from inside (high-pressure ventilation) the chest could cause rupture of intrathoracic structures in a child. Some authors required abdominal binding in their models to achieve their improved results, the implications of which have already been described. Rogers et al (1981) pointed out that any rise in intrathoracic pressure may well be associated with a reciprocal rise in intracranial pressure and a resultant fall in intracranial perfusion. Babbs et al (1982b) suggested that the successful groups practising new CPR used larger animal and adult human models, whereas the unsuccessful groups used smaller dogs. This could reflect the fact that the results of the different methods of resuscitation depend on the relative shape and size of the thoracic cavity.

Thus, although the physiological principles of the 'chest pump' theory seem to have been reasonably established in adults, they have yet to be verified in children. The application of the synchronized compression, ventilation cardiopulmonary resuscitation methodology may not offer any substantial advantage over the more established conventional techniques.

RESULTS

It is generally believed that the results of cardiopulmonary resuscitation in children are good. Ehrlich et al (1974) reported on 239 paediatric cardiac arrests in 6 years. There was a 78% initial response to therapy (a return of cardiac function); 67% survived for 24 h, 53% at 5 days and 47% were discharged from the intensive care unit in a satisfactory condition. Similar figures were reported by the Royal Alexandra Hospital for Children in Sydney (Wark and Overton, 1984); 66% showed an initial response and 42%

survived to leave hospital. The best figures were reported from the Children's Hospital of Philadelphia (Ludwig and Kettrick, 1983); in 130 patients there was an 81% immediate survival and 55% were discharged from hospital.

In contrast, Friesen and co-authors (1982) reported on 66 unexpected cardiac arrests in children. They found that only 9% survived to discharge, of which only half were considered neurologically and physically normal. This was a multicentre study and included cardiac arrests occurring inside and outside the hospital from urban and rural Manitoba. Their main conclusion was that the survivors had a significantly shorter time (2.3 min) to the application of basic life support than the non-survivors (6.5 min). They found no relationship between the duration of the initial resuscitation to the eventual outcome.

It could be surmised that better results from the first three studies were from specific paediatric units with specific protocols for paediatric resuscitation. Even so, Ludwig and Kettrick in Philadelphia reported results from their Emergency Department as 56% immediate survival and 29% survival to discharge. The authors recognized two factors with a deleterious effect on outcome: firstly, late recognition of the arrest (especially in the sudden infant death syndrome) and secondly, minimal prehospital phase treatment.

It is always difficult to compare separate studies, but the above results suggest that specific paediatric training and specific paediatric protocols produce better resuscitation results. They also demonstrate the importance of the immediate recognition and treatment at both basic and advanced life support levels.

Three papers have challenged the ability and knowledge of doctors to perform basic and advanced life support (Lowenstein et al, 1981; Casey, 1984; Skinner et al, 1985). Lowenstein and colleagues (1981) found that only 29% of house officers could adequately compress and ventilate the mannequin and only one-third could intubate in less than 35 s. They further reported that most house officers tested displayed helplessness and anxiety during the simulated resuscitation attempt. Wynne et al (1987) challenged the ability of nurses to perform adult resuscitation with very similar disturbing results. There have been no specific trials of the ability of doctors or nurses to perform paediatric resuscitation. In view of the emotional overlay of the event and for the other reasons already discussed above the results would probably be little better.

Paediatric resuscitation is neither an adult nor a neonatal technique. Formal guidelines have now been drawn up (American Heart Association, 1986; Zideman, 1986) and training of all those involved in the care of infants and children should begin in earnest. Until this is properly established there must be some doubt as to the true efficacy of paediatric resuscitation.

NEONATAL RESUSCITATION

Neonatal resuscitation is unique in that most events can be forecast, managment planned and treatment carried out in well defined and controlled conditions. It is therefore not surprising that it is a well developed and researched subject.

The classic neonatal resuscitation is the treatment of birth asphyxia. Clinically the neonate is apnoeic; this may be the result of respiratory depression caused by asphyxia or may be drug-induced. Birth asphyxia is defined as an apnoeic interval of 2 min. It has a quoted incidence of 13.6% for singleton deliveries (Russel et al, 1975). The physiological changes associated with asphyxia have been reviewed by Dawes (1968; Figure 23.2) and by Robertson and Rosen (1982). It is the understanding of these physiological changes that has not only allowed for the prediction of neonates likely to require resuscitation but has also provided a logical and standardized approach to the methodology.

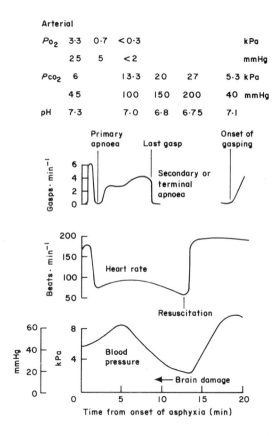

Figure 23.2. Continuous asphyxia after primary apnoea causes gasping breaths which stop with a severe metabolic and respiratory acidosis. Before final cardiac arrest there is terminal or secondary apnoea. If oxygen is supplied during primary apnoea, regular respiration will begin. Brain damage occurs without effective resuscitation once terminal apnoea is established. From Dawes (1968).

The publication of the recommended guidelines for advanced neonatal resuscitation by the American Heart Association (1986) and by the Resuscitation Council in the UK (Milner, 1986) has provided an excellent baseline from which to work. Many publications have reviewed the same topic (Hey, 1977; Hatch and Sumner, 1981; Robertson and Rosen, 1982) and most textbooks on paediatrics and anaesthesia have more than adequate descriptions of the methodology.

Neonatal assessment and prognosis have for a long time been related to a 1-min and 5-min Apgar score, i.e. the scoring of colour, heart rate, respiration, muscle tone and activity (Apgar and James, 1962; Table 23.3). The popularity of the system has remained, despite comments on its lack of prognostic value (Auld et al, 1961). Chamberlain and Banks (1974), when assessing the various modalities of the Apgar score, found that an assessment of heart rate at 1 min and the time to the neonate's first breath or cry were the most useful parameters and suggested the use of these as a simpler scoring system. No matter which system has been selected, resuscitation should not be delayed by the assessment. The airway must be cleared, care being taken not to stimulate the hypopharynx causing a reflex bradycardia (Codero and Hoe, 1971). Meconium aspiration must be prevented and this may require a joint obstetric and paediatric approach to airway clearance (Carson et al, 1976). If the liquor is meconium-stained, the mouth should be suctioned, the trachea intubated and suctioned before the lungs are ventilated.

Table 23.3. Apgar score (Apgar and James, 1962)

	0	1	2
Colour	White	Blue	Pink
Heart rate (beats/min)	0	<100	>100
Activity in response to pharyngeal suction	Nil	Grimace	Cough
Respiration	Absent	Gasping or irregular	Regular or crying lustily
Muscle tone	Limp	Reduced or normal with no active movements	Normal with active movements

Facemask resuscitation is recommended as a primary manoeuvre in the apnoeic neonate with an initial inflation of 30 cm H_2O maintained for 1 s to provide initial aeration of the lung and the formation of a functional residual capacity (Hey, 1977). Vyas et al (1983) showed that oesophageal inflation and gastric distension did not occur until a mean inflation pressure of 5.4 kPa was exceeded; Milner et al (1984) found facemask resuscitation to be relatively inefficient. Despite the limitations of their method—they could only measure expired gas volumes—they showed that during facemask resuscitation tidal volumes of only one-third the value seen after intubation were obtained for the same inflating pressure. It would therefore seem that early intubation is the answer to successful neonatal resuscitation. The fact that facemask resuscitation was successful was, according to the authors, due to stimulation of the Head's reflex (inspiratory efforts being reflexly stimulated by inflation pressure). Facemask resuscitation is important as intubation is considered a skilled procedure and is not always immediately available. Furthermore, in the same paper the authors comment that intubation seemed to delay the onset of spontaneous respiratory efforts (facemask 7.8 s, intubation 21.3 s).

Mention has already been made of initial inflation pressures. The recognized way of inflating the newborn lung has been to use an inflation pressure of 30 cm H_2O maintained for 1 s. In 1981 Vyas and colleagues produced a twofold increase in inflation volume by maintaining the initial inflation pressure for approximately 5 s. This improved inflation volume always led to the formation of a functional residual capacity. Furthermore it was felt that the conventional objections to prolonging the inflation pressure (impedance of venous return, reduced cardiac output, increased risk of pneumothorax) were not valid as the inflation pressures used were less than those measured during the first spontaneous breaths. It was not recommended that these prolonged inflations should be maintained once expansion of the lung had been established.

Ventilation is of primary importance in neonatal resuscitation and most bradycardias will respond to ventilation alone. In a severe or prolonged bradycardia, external chest compressions may be considered. The use of drugs in this type of resuscitation is limited. If they are required the best access is via the umbilical vessels; catheterization of these vessels is considered a skilled task. The method of chest compression and the drugs and dosages used have been described earlier in this chapter. In addition it may be necessary to counteract the effect of any opiate analgesic given to the mother prior to delivery, which may be the cause of respiratory depression in the neonate. Naloxone 40 µg/kg intravenously or 70 µg/kg intramuscularly is the treatment of choice. Hypovolaemia may have to be considered one of the causes of circulatory collapse; this requires an infusion of a plasma expander or blood to maintain the neonatal blood volume. It must be remembered that whilst all these manipulations are being carried out ventilation must continue uninterrupted.

In-utero transfer of 'at risk' neonates to specialized delivery and neonatal units is now considered optimal. In-utero resuscitation has been reported on a 19-week-old fetus who was being treated by intrauterine blood transfusion for severe rhesus isoimmunization. The authors, aided by ultrasound, compressed the fetal heart at 40 compressions/min by compressing the mother's abdomen. At 32 weeks' gestation a 1900 g anaemic baby was delivered by elective caesarean section; subsequent growth and behaviour have been reported as normal (Nicholaides and Rodeck, 1984). This encouraging result would seem to herald the beginning of a new era in neonatal resuscitation.

REFERENCES

American Heart Association (1974) Standards for cardiopulmonary resuscitation (CPR) and emergency cardiac care (ECC). *Journal of the American Medical Association* **227**: 833–868.

American Heart Association (1980) Standards and guidelines for cardiopulmonary resuscitation (CPR) and emergency cardiac care (ECC). *Journal of the American Medical Association* **244**: 453–509.

American Heart Association (1986) Standards and guidelines for cardiopulmonary resuscitation (CPR) and emergency cardiac care (ECC). *Journal of the American Medical Association* **255**: 2905–2992.

Apgar V & James LS (1962) Further observations of the newborn scoring system. *American Journal of Diseases of Children* **104**: 419–428.

Auld PAM, Rudolph AJ, Avery ME et al (1961) Responsiveness and resuscitation in the newborn. The use of the Apgar score. *American Journal of Diseases of Children* **101**: 713–724.

Ayres SM & Grace WJ (1969) Inappropriate ventilation and hypoxaemia as causes of cardiac arrhythmias. The control of arrhythmia without antiarrhythmic drugs. *American Medical Journal* **46**: 495–505.

Babbs CF, Fitzgerald KR, Voorhess WD & Murphy RJ (1982a) High-pressure ventilation during CPR with 95% O_2:5% CO_2. *Critical Care Medicine* **10**: 505–508.

Babbs CF, Tacker WA, Paris RL, Murphy RJ & Davis RW (1982b) CPR with simultaneous compression and ventilation at high airway pressure in 4 animal models. *Critical Care Medicine* **10**: 501–504.

Bircher N & Safar P (1981) Comparison of standard and 'new' closed chest CPR and open chest CPR in dogs. *Critical Care Medicine* **9**: 384–385.

Carson BS, Losey RW, Bowes WJ Jr & Simmons MA (1976) Combined obstetric and paediatric approach to prevent meconium aspiration syndrome. *American Journal of Obstetrics and Gynecology* **126**: 712–715.

Casey WF (1984) Cardiopulmonary resuscitation, a survey of standards amongst junior staff doctors. *Proceedings of the Royal Society of Medicine* **77**: 921–924.

Cavallaro DL & Melker RJ (1983) Comparison of two techniques for detecting cardiac activity in infants. *Critical Care Medicine* **11**: 189–190.

Chamberlain G & Banks J (1974) Assessment of the Apgar score. *Lancet* **ii**: 1225–1228.

Chandra N, Rudikoff MT & Weisfeldt ML (1980) Simultaneous chest compression and ventilation at high airway pressure during cardiopulmonary resuscitation. *Lancet* **i**: 175–178.

Chandra N, Snyder LD & Weisfeldt ML (1981) Abdominal binding during cardiopulmonary resuscitation in man. *Journal of the American Medical Association* **246**: 351–353.

Codero L & Hoe EH (1971) Neonatal bradycardia following nasopharyngeal suction. *Journal of Paediatrics* **78**: 441–447.

Cote CJ, Jobes DR, Schwartz AJ & Ellison N (1979) Two approaches to cannulation of a child's internal jugular vein. *Anesthesiology* **50**: 371–373.

CPR Lifesaving Techniques. (1977) Princeton, NJ: Gallup Poll.

Crampton R (1980) Accepted, controversial and speculative aspects of ventricular defibrillation. *Progress in Cardiovascular Disease* **23**: 167–186.

Criley JH, Blaufuss AH & Kissel GL (1976) Cough-induced cardiac compressions. *Journal of the American Medical Association* **236**: 1246.

Criley JH, Niemann JT, Rosborough JP, Ung S & Suzuki J (1981) The heart is a conduit in CPR. *Critical Care Medicine* **9**: 373–374.

Dalsey WC, Barsan WG, Joyce SM et al (1984) Comparison of superior vena caval and inferior venal caval access using a radioisotope technique during normal perfusion and cardiopulmonary resuscitation. *Annals of Emergency Medicine* **13**: 881–884.

Dawes GS (1968) Birth asphyxia, resuscitation and brain damage. In Dawes GS (ed) *Fetal and Neonatal Physiology*, pp 237–250. Chicago: Year Book Medical Publishers.

Dembo DH (1981) Calcium in advanced life support. *Critical Care Medicine* **9**: 358–359.

Ditchley RV, Winkler JV & Rhodes CA (1982) Relative lack of coronary blood flow during closed chest resuscitation in dogs. *Circulation* **66**: 297–302.

Ehrlich R, Emmett SM & Rodriguez-Torres R (1974) Pediatric cardiac resuscitation team. A 6 year study. *Journal of Pediatrics* **84:** 152–155.

Fillmore SJ, Shapiro M & Killip T (1970) Serial blood gas studies during cardiopulmonary resuscitation. *Annals of Internal Medicine* **72:** 465–469.

Friesen RM, Duncan P, Tweed WA & Bristow G (1982) Appraisal of pediatric cardiopulmonary resuscitation. *Canadian Medical Association Journal* **126:** 1055–1058.

Goldberg AH (1974) Cardiopulmonary Arrest. *New England Journal of Medicine* **290:** 381–385.

Greenblatt DJ, Gross PL & Bolognini V (1976) Pharmacotherapy of cardiopulmonary arrest. *American Journal of Hospital Pharmacology* **33:** 579–583.

Groff DB & Ahmed N (1974) Subclavian vein catheterization in the infant. *Journal of Paediatric Surgery* **9:** 171–174.

Gutgesell HP, Tacker WA, Geddes LA et al (1976) Energy dose ventricular defibrillation of children. *Pediatrics* **58:** 898–891.

Harris L, Kirimili B & Safar P (1967) Augmentation of artificial circulation during cardiopulmonary resuscitation. *Anesthesiology* **28:** 730.

Hatch DJ (1984) Anaesthesia for children. *Anaesthesia* **39:** 405–406.

Hatch DJ & Sumner E (1981) Resuscitation of the newborn. In *Neonatal Anaesthesia*. Current Topics in Anaesthesia no 5, pp 174–186. London: Edward Arnold.

Hedges JR, Barsan WB, Doan LA et al (1984) Central versus peripheral intravenous routes in cardiopulmonary resuscitation. *American Journal of Emergency Medicine* **2:** 385–390.

Hey EN (1977) Resuscitation at birth. *British Journal of Anaesthesia* **49:** 25–33.

Hinckle AJ (1988) A rapid and reliable method of selecting endotracheal tube size in children. *Anesthesia and Analgesia* **67(Suppl S92)**.

Kerber RE, Jensen SR, Grayzel J, Kennedy J & Hoyt R (1981) Effective cardioversion: influence of paddle-electrode location and size on success rates and energy requirements. *New England Journal of Medicine* **305:** 658–662.

Kouwenhoven WB, Jude RJ & Knickerbocker CG (1960) Closed-chest cardiac massage. *Journal of the American Medical Association* **173:** 1064.

Lawson NW, Butler CG & Ray CT (1973) Alkalosis and cardiac arrhythmias. *Anesthesia and Analgesia* **52:** 951–964.

Lowenstein SR, Hansborough JF, Libby LS et al (1981) Cardiopulmonary resuscitation by medical and surgical house officers. *Lancet* **ii:** 679–681.

Ludwig S & Kettrick RG (1983) Pediatric resuscitation for the non-pediatrician. In Jacobsen S (ed.) *Clinics in Emergency Medicine (Resuscitation)*, vol. 2, pp 101–112. Edinburgh: Churchill Livingstone.

Massumi RA, Mason DT & Amsterdam EA (1972) Ventricular fibrillation and tachycardia after intravenous atropine. *New England Journal of Medicine* **287:** 336–338.

Mattar JA, Weil MH & Shubin H (1974) Cardiac arrest in the critically ill. II. Hyperosmolar states following cardiac arrest. *American Journal of Medicine* **56:** 162–168.

Melker R (1984) Asynchronous and other alternative methods of ventilation. *American Emergency Medicine* **13:** 758.

Melker R, Cavallaro D & Krischer J (1981) A pediatric gastric tube airway. *Critical Care Medicine* **9:** 426–427.

Milner AD (1986) ABC of resuscitation: resuscitation at birth. *British Medical Journal* **292:** 1657–1659.

Milner AD, Vyas H & Hopkin IE (1984) Efficiency of facemask resuscitation at birth. *British Medical Journal* **289:** 1563–1565.

Nicholaides KH & Rodeck CH (1984) In utero resuscitation after cardiac arrest in a fetus. *British Medical Journal* **288:** 900–901.

Nieman JT, Rosborough JP, Hausknecht M, Gardner D & Criley JM (1981) Pressure-synchronized cineangiography during experimental cardiopulmonary resuscitation. *Circulation* **64:** 985–991.

Oakley P (1988) Inaccuracy and delay in decision making in paediatric resuscitation, and a proposed chart to reduce error. *British Medical Journal* **297:** 817–819.

Orlowski JP (1986) Optimum position for external cardiac compression in infants and young children. *Annals of Emergency Medicine* **15:** 667–673.

Phillips GWL & Zideman DA (1986) Relation of the infant heart to the sternum: its significance in cardiopulmonary resuscitation. *Lancet* **i:** 1024–1025.

Rainer EH & Bullough J (1957) Respiratory and cardiac arrest during anaesthesia in children. *British Medical Journal* **2:** 1024.

Ralsten SH, Babbs CF & Niebauer MJ (1982) Cardiopulmonary resuscitation with interposed abdominal compression in dogs. *Anesthesia and Analgesia* **61:** 645–651.

Redding JS (1971) Abdominal compression in cardiopulmonary resuscitation. *Anesthesia and Analgesia* **50:** 668–675.

Redding JS, Haynes RR & Thomas JD (1981) 'Old' and 'new' resuscitation manually performed. *Critical Care Medicine* **9:** 165.

Rich S, Wix HL & Shapiro EP (1981) Clinical assessment of heart chamber size and valve motion during cardiopulmonary resuscitation by two-dimensional echocardiography. *American Heart Journal* **102:** 368–373.

Robertson NRC & Rosen M (1982) Safer resuscitation of the newborn. *Clinics in Obstetrics and Gynaecology* **9:** 415–435.

Rogers P & Hillman H (1970) Recovery from hypothermia. *Journal of Applied Physiology* **29:** 58–60.

Rogers MC, Weisfeldt ML & Trayston RJ (1981) Cerebral blood flow during cardiopulmonary resuscitation. *Anesthesia and Analgesia* **60:** 73–75.

Rudikoff MT, Maughan WL, Effron M, Freund P & Weisfeldt ML (1980) Mechanisms of blood flow during cardiopulmonary resuscitation. *Circulation* **61:** 345–352.

Russel G, Lydon Y & Tunstall M (1975) Antenatal prediction of neonatal asphyxia. *Anaesthesia* **30:** 118.

Sabin HI, Khunti K, Coghill SB & McNeill GO (1983) Accuracy of intracardiac injections determined by post-mortem studies. *Lancet* **ii:** 1054–1055.

Salem MR, Bennett EJ, Schweiss JF et al (1975) Cardiac arrest related to anesthesia. *Journal of the American Medical Association* **233:** 238–241.

Saunders AB, Ewy GA, Alferness CA, Taft T & Zimmerman M (1982) Failure of one method of simultaneous chest compression, ventilation and abdominal binding during CPR. *Critical Care Medicine* **10:** 509–513.

Schwartz AJ, Orkin FK & Ellison N (1979) Anesthesiologists' training and knowledge of basic life support. *Anesthesiology* **50:** 191–194.

Schwartz AJ, Ellison N, Ominsky AJ & Orkin FK (1982) Advanced CPR—student, teacher, administrator, researcher. *Anesthesia and Analgesia* **61:** 629–630.

Seldinger SI (1953) Catheter placement over the needle in percutaneous arteriography. *Acta Radiologica* **39:** 368–376.

Skinner DV, Camm AJ & Miles S (1985) Cardiopulmonary resuscitation skills of preregistration house officers. *British Medical Journal* **290:** 1545.

Thaler MM & Stobie GHC (1963) An improved technique of external cardiac compression in infants and young children. *New England Journal of Medicine* **269:** 606–610.

Vyas M, Milner AD, Hopkin IE & Boon AW (1981) Physiological responses to prolonged and slow rise inflation in the resuscitation of the asphyxiated newborn infant. *Journal of Pediatrics* **99:** 635–639.

Vyas H, Milner AD & Hopkin IE (1983) Facemask resuscitation: does it lead to gastric distension? *Archives of Diseases in Children* **58:** 373–375.

Wark H & Overton JH (1984) A paediatric 'cardiac arrest' survey. *British Journal of Anaesthesia* **56:** 1271–1274.

Werner JA, Green HL, Janko CL & Cobb LA (1981) Visualization of cardiac valve motion in man during external chest compression using two-dimensional echocardiography. Implications regarding the mechanism of blood flow. *Circulation* **63:** 1417–1421.

White BC, Winegar CD, Wilson RF et al (1983) Possible role of calcium blockers in cerebral resuscitation. A review of the literature and synthesis for future studies. *Critical Care Medicine* **11:** 202–207.

Worthley LIG (1976) Sodium bicarbonate in cardiac arrest. *Lancet* **ii:** 903–904.

Wynne G, Marteau TM, Johnston M et al (1987) Inability of trained nurses to perform basic life support. *British Medical Journal* **294:** 1198.

Zideman DA (1986) ABC of resuscitation: resuscitation of infants and children. *British Medical Journal* **292:** 1584–1588.

Appendix 1

Drugs in common use in paediatric anaesthetic practice

All drugs given on the basis of body weight (kg)

SEDATIVES (e.g. night-time preoperatively)—all given *orally*

1. **Chloral hydrate**
   Dose   up to 30 mg/kg; not more than 1 g in a single dose (chloral mixture BPC 100 mg/ml)

2. **Diazepam** (Valium; e.g. as pre-premedication 4 h preoperatively)
   Dose   0.4 mg/kg

3. **Nitrazepam** (Mogadon)
   Dose   15–30 kg: 2.5 mg
           over 30 kg: 5 mg
   Preparation   5 mg tablets

4. **Promethazine** (Phenergan)
   Dose   0.5–1.0 mg/kg to a maximum of 50 mg (elixir BPC 5 mg/5 ml)

5. **Temazepam** (Normison)
   Dose   5–10 mg

6. **Trichloral syrup**
   Dose   about 30 mg/kg
   Preparation   100 mg/ml

7. **Trimeprazine tartrate** (Vallergan)
   Dose   3 mg/kg (Vallergan Forte 6 mg/ml)

PREMEDICATION

Routine premedication (except cardiac, ENT or neurosurgery)

1. *Infants up to 6 months of age*: Atropine only. Some infants just below this age who are having major surgery or repeated anaesthetics may require sedation.

2. *Small children (6–15 kg)*: Atropine plus some sedation depending on the surgical operation. e.g. Pethidine injection compound.
3. *Older children (over 15 kg)*: Papaveretum and hyoscine.

1. **Atropine** 0.02 mg/kg
   The Hospital for Sick Children, Great Ormond Street, London
   Doses   up to 2.5 kg: 0.15 mg
             2.5–8 kg: 0.2 mg
             8–15 kg: 0.3 mg   } i.m. 45 min preoperatively
           15–20 kg: 0.4 mg
           over 20 kg: 0.5 mg
   (Caution with pre-existing pyrexia and tachycardia)
   Oral administration e.g. with trimeprazine—double dose.

2. **Diazepam** (Valium)
   Dose   0.4 mg/kg orally 90 min preoperatively
   Preparation
   syrup: 2 mg/5ml
   tablets: 2, 5 and 10 mg
   rectal sachets (5 or 10 mg): 2.5–10 mg

3. **Papaveretum and hyoscine** (Omnopon and Scopolamine)
   Dose   Papaveretum: 0.4 mg/kg   } i.m. 90 min preoperatively
            Hyoscine: 0.008 mg/kg
   Maximum dose of papaveretum   15 mg

4. **Pethidine compound injection** (Inj. Peth. Co.)
   Dose   0.06–0.08 ml/kg i.m. 1 h preoperatively
   (This has a pethidine content of 1.5–2 mg/kg)
   Preparation
   Pethidine   25 mg
   Promethazine   6.25 mg } in 1 ml
   Chlorpromazine 6.25 mg
   Maximum dose   1.5 ml

5. **Trimeprazine tartrate** (Vallergan)
   Dose   2–4 mg/kg orally 2 h preoperatively

Special circumstances

1. *Cardiac investigations*

   These are performed under *basal sedation* supplemented if required by i.v. diazepam (0.1–0.2 mg/kg).
   No atropine
   a. Trichloral syrup: 30 mg/kg orally nocte then trimeprazine 3 mg/kg orally 3 h pre-catheter.
   b. Premedication: (all given i.m. *30 min pre-catheter*)
       (i) Newborns–1 month of age: may have pethidine injection compound up to 0.05 ml/kg
          No trimeprazine

   (ii) 1 month of age–15 kg: pethidine injection compound 0.1 ml/kg preceded by trimeprazine in infants over 5 kg body weight. Maximum dose 1.5 ml. Smaller babies in poor condition should have a reduced dose.

   (iii) Over 15 kg: papaveretum and hyoscine preceded by chloral/vallergan:

   Papaveretum   0.4–0.5 mg/kg
   Hyoscine   0.008–0.01 mg/kg
   (maximum dose papaveretum 15 mg).

   (iv) Tetralogy of Fallot: morphine 0.25 mg/kg i.m. 30 min pre-catheter.

Children over 2.5 years of age who are just under 15 kg body weight are usually better sedated if given papaveretum and hyoscine rather than pethidine injection compound. Most children require the full dose of sedation. The timing is important because of the patient preparation time and the duration of the investigation.

2. *Cardiac surgery*

a. Closed heart operations as routine—may have injection pethidine compound 0.05 ml/kg i.m. 1 h preoperatively if over 4 kg.

b. Bypass surgery:
   (i)   Under 4 weeks of age atropine only.
   (ii) Between 4 weeks and 6 kg, pethidine injection compound 0.05 ml/kg + atropine.
   (iii) 6–15 kg, pethidine injection compound 0.07 ml/kg + atropine.
   (iv) Over 15 kg, papaveretum and hyoscine.

Sedation the night before surgery should be given to patients having papaveretum and hyoscine, e.g. trimeprazine 3 mg/kg orally.

3. *Cleft palate*

Atropine only. Never prescribe heavy preoperative sedation for any child with micrognathia or other anatomical deformity of the respiratory tract because of possible airway obstruction.

4. *ENT*

a. Adenotonsillectomy:
   (i)   Under 7 years of age—oral trimeprazine 3–4 mg/kg with atropine 0.05 mg/kg orally 2 h properatively.
   (ii) Over 7 years of age—papaveretum and hyoscine in dose 0.3 mg/kg.
   (iii) Postoperative sedation—codeine phosphate only, 1 mg/kg i.m. before leaving theatre.

b. Endoscopy: atropine i.m. only. Some older children and those with tracheostomy may have sedation, e.g. diazepam or pethidine injection compound.

5. *Neurosurgical investigations*

Cerebral arteriography ⎫
Lumbar air encephalography ⎬ Atropine only
Myelography ⎭
Non-neurological investigations—normal premedication
a. Computerized tomography (CT) scan:
    Either performed under general anaesthetic or under sedation with-
    out general anaesthetic.
       G.A.—Neuro—Atropine only.
             Body —Normal premedication.

Sedation for CT scan

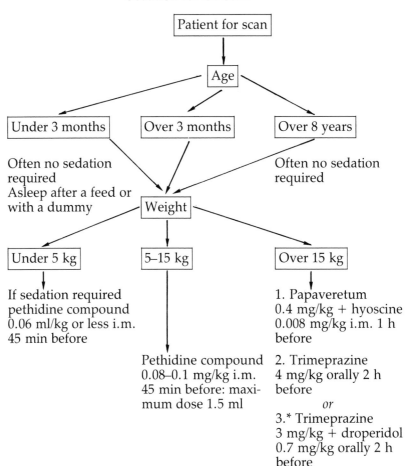

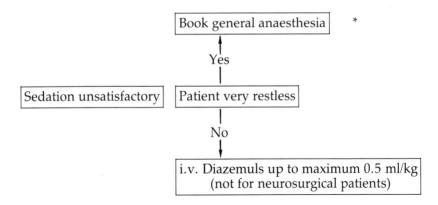

NB:
1. Patients with raised ICP or potentially raised ICP should be sedated with great care or not at all.
2. Patients with airways obstruction (actual or potential) should not be sedated, e.g. some craniofacial abnormalities.
3. Ex-premature babies should not receive opiates until over 2 months' corrected gestational age and should receive other sedation with great caution because of the risk of apnoea.
4. No mentally retarded or hyperactive child should have a general anaesthetic scan as the first option.
5. If in doubt it is better to book a general anaesthetic scan than risk respiratory problems in the scan room.
This regimen results in successful scans in over 90% of children.

*Preferred regime in subnormal patients with neurological diseases.

NB: Sedatives are contraindicated in the presence of raised intracranial pressure (ICP).
  Metrizamide, sometimes used in myelography, is incompatible with phenothiazines.
  Phenobarbitone 2 mg/kg i.m. is given following intrathecal metrizamide before returning to the ward.
  b. Magnetic resonance imaging (MRI)
  Atropine only for general anaesthesia.
  Sedation as for CT scan.

6. *Neurosurgery*

  a. Cranial operations—atropine only + dexamethasone 0.25 mg/kg i.v. on induction where indicated.
  b. Non-cranial cases—may receive sedation according to age and weight but care should be taken to avoid respiratory depression in patients with muscular weakness.

STEROID COVER FOR SURGERY

The Anaesthetic Department should be responsible for prescribing steroid cover for the operation and subsequent 24 h, but further management of the dosage should be the responsibility of the clinician in charge of the patient.

1. On steroids at present

I.m. hydrocortisone with premedication and 6-hourly postoperatively until oral steroids can be recommenced: 25 mg below 10 kg; 50 mg 10–30 kg; 100 mg over 30 kg.

The dose should be reduced to the maintenance level after 1–4 days depending on the nature of the surgery and the condition of the patient.

2. Off steroids within·preceding 2 months

I.m. hydrocortisone with premedication and 6-hourly postoperatively for 24–48 h depending on the nature of the surgery and the condition of the patient. The appropriate dose of oral steroid may be substituted when practicable.

3. Off steroids longer than 2 months

No cover—but hydrocortisone should be available.

ANAESTHETIC AGENTS

All are given intravenously

INDUCTION

1. Ketamine
induction: i.v. 2 mg/kg; i.m. 10 mg/kg
(increments i.v. 1 mg/kg)
(may also be given rectally or orally 10 mg/kg)

	Dose	Preparation
2. **Methohexitone**	1.5–2 mg/kg	10 mg/ml
3. **Propofol**	2–3 mg/kg	10 mg/ml
4. **Thiopentone**	4–6 mg/kg	25 mg/ml

RELAXANTS

1. **Atracurium** 0.5 mg/kg 10 mg/ml
   (increments 0.25 mg/kg)
   infusion: 8 µg/kg/min

2. **Pancuronium**
   a. Infants and
      children 0.1 mg/kg 0.4 mg/ml
   b. Neonate 0.06 mg/kg 0.2 mg/ml

3. **Suxamethonium**
   Intubation 1–2 mg/kg 50 mg/ml
   Intermittent use in
   neonates
      Initial dose 1 mg/kg 2.5 mg/ml
      Supplements 0.5 mg/kg)
      Total dose 5–20 mg (up to 5 mg/kg)

4. **Tubocurarine**
   a. Infants and
      children 0.4 mg/kg 1–1.5 mg/ml
   b. Neonates 0.2 mg/kg 0.25 mg/ml

5. **Vecuronium** 0.1 mg/kg 0.4 mg/ml
   Infusion 1.5–2 µg/kg/min

ANALGESICS (intraoperative)

(Use with care after opiate premedication)

Dose

1. **Alfentanil** 30–50 µg/kg

2. **Fentanyl**
   With assisted ventilation
   After opiate sedation 3–5 µg/kg
   Atropine only premed up to 10 µg/kg
   Cardiac surgery up to 25 µg/kg

3. **Morphine** 0.2 mg/kg
   (Open heart surgery up to 1 mg/kg total dose)

4. **Pethidine** 1 mg/kg

REVERSAL

1. **Atropine** 0.02 mg/kg

2. **Glycopyrrolate** 4–8 µg/kg
   (maximum dose—200 µg)

3. **Neostigmine** 0.05 mg/kg

OTHERS

1. **Chlorpromazine**   1 mg increments up to
                                         0.5 mg/kg

2. **Dantrolene**
   Pretreatment   2.5 mg/kg i.v.
   Malignant hyperthermia   1–10 mg/kg i.v.

3. **Dexamethasone**
   Prophylactic use in prevention of laryngeal oedema following traumatic
   intubation or instrumentation of the airway.

   Not to be used routinely.

   Dose   Initial 0.25 mg/kg i.v., then 0.1 mg/kg 6-hourly for three doses i.v.
   or i.m.

                                         Dose
4. **Droperidol**   0.3 mg/kg

5. **Frusemide**   Up to 1 mg/kg repeatable
                                         Infusion 50 mg in 50 ml *0.9% saline* 1 mg/kg/hr

6. **Heparin**   bypass   3 mg/kg
   (1 mg ≡ 100 u.)   shunts   1 mg/kg
                                         infusion 1.5–4 mg/kg/h

7. **Hydralazine**   0.2 mg/kg then 1.5–3 mg/kg/day

8. **Indomethacin**   0.2 mg/kg × 3

9. **Labetalol**   Increments up to 1 mg/kg
                                         Infusion 1–3 mg/kg/h

10. **Mannitol**   Up to 1 g/kg

11. **Methoxamine**   dilution to 0.5 mg/ml
                                         increments of 0.25 mg to achieve desired result

12. **Methylprednisolone** 30 mg/kg

13. **Naloxone**   10 µg/kg repeatable after 20 min

14. **Nitroglycerine**   5 µg/kg/min (3 mg/kg in 50 ml 5% dextrose;
                                         1 ml/hr = 1 µg/kg/min)

15. **Nitroprusside**   3 mg/kg in 100 ml 5% dextrose
                                         1 ml/hr = 0.5 µg/kg/min
                                         Do not exceed 1–1.5 mg/kg total dose per 24 h
                                         Dose: 0.5–8 µg/kg/min

16. **Phentolamine** dilution to 1 mg/ml
increments to achieve desired effect

17. **Practolol** dilution to 1 mg/ml—maximum dose of
0.5 mg/kg

18. **Propranolol** dilution to 0.1 mg/ml—maximum dose of
0.05 mg/kg

19. **Prostacyclin** 4–20 ng/kg/min

20. **Protamine** 6 mg/kg *slowly*

21. **Ranitidine** 0.5–1 mg/kg *slowly* (diluted to 5 ml) 6-hourly

22. **Theophylline** 8 mg/kg then 1–3 mg/kg/day

23. **Tolazoline** 1–2 mg/kg over 3 min, then infuse same dose/h

24. **Trimetaphan** dilution 250 mg in 100 ml 5% dextrose

NEBULIZED AGENTS

1. **Racemic adrenaline**—2.25%   0.5 ml in 2 ml saline

2. **Atrovent**—0.025%   0.5 ml in 2 ml saline

LOCAL ANAESTHETIC AGENTS

Lignocaine to tracheobronchial tree
10% solution. Maximum dose 3 mg/kg
(metered dose = 10 mg)

CAUDAL ANALGESIA

1. Sacral roots
e.g. circumcision ⎤
    hypospadias ⎦ up to 0.5 ml/kg 0.25% bupivacaine (plain)

2. Lumbar roots
e.g. inguinal hernia—up to 1.0 ml/kg 0.25% bupivacaine (plain)

3. Up to T10 e.g. orchidopexy—up to 1.25 ml/kg of 0.25% bupivacaine
diluted with saline to give 0.175%

Higher doses not recommended.
Maximum dose in any 4 h period should not exceed 2 mg/kg.

SPINAL ANALGESIA

Heavy bupivacaine—0.13 ml/kg

CARDIAC DRUGS

Dilutions only given. The effect of administration must be monitored. The strength may be increased if fluid restriction is necessary. Start at rate of 5–10 ml/h.

1. **Adrenaline**　　0.01–0.5 µg/kg/min
   30 µg/kg in 50 ml
   1 ml/h = 0.01 µg/kg/min

2. **Aminophylline**　0.8 mg/kg/hr

3. **Amiodarone**　　5 mg/kg slow i.v.

4. **Cardioplegia**　　1 amp. in 1 l Ringer's solution (ice-cold)
   30 ml/kg; half-doses after 30 min

5. **Dextrose/insulin**　Dextrose 1 g/kg + insulin 0.25 u/kg

6. **Digoxin**　　　50 µg/kg orally total digitalizing dose

7. **Dobutamine**　　5–10 µg/kg/min

8. **Dopamine**　　6 mg/kg in 100 ml 5% dextrose 1 ml/h = 1 µg/kg/min
   At a dose not exceeding 10 µg/kg/min little alpha-adrenergic action

9. **Isoprenaline**　up to 1 mg in 100 ml 5% dextrose—usually 0.25–0.5 mg in 100 ml 5% dextrose

10. **Nifedipine**　0.5 mg/kg/day in divided dose

11. **Nitroglycerine**　3 mg/kg in 50 ml 5% dextrose—start at 1 ml/h

12. **Nitroprusside**　0.5–8 µg/kg/min

13. **Noradrenaline**　0.01–0.5 µg/kg/min—30 µg/kg in 50 ml
    1 ml/kg = 0.01 µg/kg/min

14. **Phenoxybenzamine** 0.5–1 mg/kg i.v. 8-hourly

15. **Prostaglandin E$_2$**　90 µg in 50 ml 5% dextrose—1 ml/kg/h

16. **Salbutamol**　2.5–5 mg in 100 ml 5% dextrose
    3–5 ml/h as initial dose

17. **Verapamil**　0.1 mg/kg slow i.v.

POSTOPERATIVE AGENTS

Analgesics

1. **Codeine phosphate** 1–1.5 mg/kg i.m. 4–6-hourly p.r.n. Must never be given i.v.—severe falls in cardiac output seen

2. **Codeine phosphate/ Phenobarbitone** — 1 mg/kg of each i.m. 4–6-hourly p.r.n. For neurosurgical patients

3. **Diclofenac** — 2 mg/kg suspension (100 mg suppository)

4. **Distalgesic** (Soluble)
   Dose   Child 6–9 years   1 tablet } 6–8-hourly orally
           Over 10 years   2 tablets
   Preparation   Paracetamol 325 mg } in one tablet
                 Dextropropoxyphene 32.5 mg

5. **Fentanyl** — Infusion 4–8 µg/kg/h
   100 µg/kg in 50 ml 50% dextroxe
   2 ml/h = 4 µg/kg/h

6. **Ibuprofen** — 5 mg/kg suspension

7. **Morphine** — 0.1–0.2 mg/kg i.m. 4–6-hourly p.r.n. or infusion of 2 ml/h i.v. of 0.5 mg/kg in 50 ml 5% dextrose

8. **Papaveretum** — 0.2–0.3 mg/kg i.m. 4–6-hourly p.r.n.

9. **Paracetamol elixir paediatric bpc**—Oral (4-hourly p.r.n.)
   Dose   15 mg/kg 6-hourly
           maximum 60 mg/kg/day
   Preparation   120 mg in 5 ml

10. **Pethidine** — 1 mg/kg i.m. 4–6-hourly p.r.n.

Sedatives

Midazolam — Bolus 20 µg/kg h i.v.   10 mg in 2 ml
Infusion   2–5 µg/kg/min   dilute in dextrose

Baclofen — 5–15 mg 6-hourly orally

Neonates

Codeine phosphate   1 mg/kg i.m. 1 dose only
Rarely–morphine infusion 5–10 µg/kg/h

Antimetics (not required routinely)

1. **Metoclopramide**
   Dose   Child   5 years   2.5 mg ⎤
                10 years   5 mg   ⎦ 2–3 times daily i.m. or oral
         (maximum total daily dose 0.5 mg/kg)
   Oral preparation   syrup 5 mg in 5 ml

2. **Prochlorperazine** (over 10 kg only)
   Dose   0.18–0.25 mg/kg i.m. 8-hourly
         (maximum 12.5 mg)
       Ampoule 12.5 mg/ml
       Tablets 2.5 mg, 5 mg
       Syrup 5 mg in 5 ml
       Suppository 5 mg

DRUGS USED IN CARDIOPULMONARY RESUSCITATION

Administration

1. **Adrenaline** (1/10 000)
   Dose   0.1 ml/kg   Centrally i.v. or intracardiac

2. **Atropine** (0.5 mg/ml)
   Dose   0.02 mg/kg   i.v.

3. **Calcium chloride** (10%)
   Dose   bolus of 0.25 ml/kg   Centrally i.v. slowly or intracardiac

4. **Dexamethasone**
   Dose   0.25 mg/kg   i.v. 6-hourly

5. **Diazepam** (5 mg/ml)
   Dose   0.2 mg/kg   i.v.

6. **Dopamine** (40 mg/ml)
   Dose   5–10 µg/kg/min   i.v. infusion 5–10 ml/h of 6 mg/kg in
                               100 ml 5% dextrose

7. **Hydrocortisone** (50 mg/ml)
   Dose   10 mg/kg   i.v.

8. **Isoprenaline**
   a. (20 µg in 2 ml)
      Dose   bolus of 0.5 ml   i.v.
      (approx. 0.1 ml/kg)
   b. (1 mg/ml for dilution)
      Dose   1 µg/kg/min   i.v. infusion of 0.4 mg in 100 ml 5%
                               dextrose = 4 µg/ml

$$Administration$$

9. **Lignocaine** (1%)
   Dose   1 mg/kg   i.v.

10. **Methylprednisolone**
    Dose   30 mg/kg   i.v.

11. **Naloxone**
    (Neonatal 0.02 mg/ml)
    (Adult 0.4 mg/ml)
    Dose   0.01 mg/kg   i.v.

12. **Sodium bicarbonate** (8.4%)

    Dose   To correct base excess ×   i.v.
    (kg weight/5)
    mmol HCO_3^- ($\equiv$ ml 8.4%)
    Initial dose 1 ml/kg

Antibiotics   Intravenous dosage

1. **Amikacin**   10 mg/kg then 7.5 mg/kg 12-hourly

2. **Ampicillin**   0– 1 year 62.5 mg ⎫
                         1– 2 years 125 mg ⎬ 6-hourly
                         2–10 years 250 mg ⎭

3. **Cefuroxime**   25 mg/kg 6-hourly

4. **Chloramphenicol**   50 mg/kg/day divided doses 8-hourly

5. **Erythromycin**   25 mg/kg/day divided doses 8-hourly

6. **Flucloxacillin**   0– 1 year 62.5 mg ⎫
                         1– 2 years 125 mg ⎬ 6-hourly
                         2–10 years 250 mg ⎭

7. **Gentamicin**   2 mg/kg 8-hourly

8. **Metronidazole**   7.5 mg/kg 8-hourly

9. **Penicillin**   30 mg/kg/day divided doses

10. **Vancomycin**   20 mg/kg i.v. over 1 h 8-hourly

Dental prophylaxis

Amoxycillin   50 mg/kg orally 4 h pre-treatment or i.v. after
                         induction

With penicillin allergy:
Vancomycin 20 mg/kg i.v. over 1 h
          + gentamicin 2 mg/kg

Appendix 2

Normal physiological values in the neonate and adult

	Neonate	Adult
Haematocrit (packed cell volume)	50–60%	45%
Haemoglobin	18–25 g/dl	15 g/dl
Blood volume	70–125 ml/kg	70 ml/kg
Extracellular fluid (% body weight)	35%	20%
Water turnover per 24 h (% body weight)	15%	9%
Serum K^+	5–8 mmol/l	3–5 mmol/l
Na^+	136–143 mmol/l	135–148 mmol/l
Cl^-	96–107 mmol/l	98–106 mmol/l
HCO_3^-	20 mmol/l	24 mmol/l
Blood urea nitrogen	1.3–3.3 mmol/l	6.6–8.6 mmol/l
pH	7.35	7.40
$PaCO_2$	4.7 kPa (35 mmHg)	4.7–6.0 kPa (35–45 mmHg)
PaO_2	8.7–10.7 kPa (65–80 mmHg)	10.7–12.7 kPa (80–95 mmHg)
Base excess	−5	0
Total bilirubin	10 μmol/l	2–14 μmol/l
Total Ca^{2+}	1.48 –2.68 mmol/l	2.13–2.6 mmol/l
Mg^{2+}	0.7–1.1 mmol/l	0.6–1.0 mmol/l
Phosphate	1.15–2.8 mmol/l	1.0–1.4 mmol/l
Glucose	2.7–3.3 mmol/l	2.4–5.3 mmol/l
Total proteins	46–74 g/l	60–80 g/l
Albumin	36–54 g/l	35–47 g/l
Serum osmolality	270–285 mOsmol/l	270–285 mOsmol/l
Urine osmolality	50–600 mOsmol/l	50–1400 mOsmol/l
Na^+	50 mmol/l	30 mmol/l
Specific gravity	1005–1020	1005–1035

Index